WHAT TO EXPECT®
WHEN YOU'RE EXPECTING

FOURTH EDITION

by Heidi Murkoff
and Sharon Mazel

Foreword by Charles J. Lockwood, MD

*The Anita O'Keefe Young Professor of Women's Health
and Chair, Department of Obstetrics, Gynecology and
Reproductive Sciences, Yale University School of Medicine*

WORKMAN PUBLISHING • NEW YORK

To Emma and Wyatt, my greatest expectations
To Erik, my everything
To Arlene, with so much love, always and forever
To all the moms, dads, and babies everywhere

Copyright © 1984, 1988, 1991, 1996, 2002, 2008 by What to Expect LLC

What to Expect is a registered trademark of What to Expect LLC

What to Expect® When You're Expecting and the What to Expect® series were conceived by Heidi Murkoff, Arlene Eisenberg, and Sandee Hathaway.

Library of Congress Cataloging-in-Publication Data is available.
ISBN-13: 978-0-7611-4857-9 (paperback)
ISBN-13: 978-0-7611-5079-4 (hardcover)

Book design: Lisa Hollander
Cover design: John Seeger Gilman
Cover illustrations: Tim O'Brien
Cover quilt: Lynette Parmentier, Quilt Creations
Cover photography: Davies + Starr
Interior illustrations: Karen Kuchar
Medical illustrations: Tom Newsom

Workman books are available at special discounts when purchased in bulk for premiums and sales promotions as well as for fund-raising or educational use. Special editions or book excerpts can also be created to specification. For details, contact the Special Sales Director at the address below.

Workman Publishing Company, Inc.
225 Varick Street
New York, NY 10014-4381
www.workman.com

Printed in the United States of America
First printing March 2008
10 9 8 7 6 5 4 3 2 1

MORE THAN I CAN SAY, TO ARLENE EISENBERG, MY FIRST PARTNER
IN WHAT TO EXPECT AND MY MOST IMPORTANT ONE.
YOUR LEGACY OF CARING, COMPASSION, AND INTEGRITY LIVES ON FOREVER;
YOU'LL ALWAYS BE LOVED AND ALWAYS BE REMEMBERED.

Thanks A Lot (More)

IF I'VE LEARNED TWO THINGS OVER the last 23 years, it's that kids don't raise themselves—and books don't write themselves (no matter how long you look at a blank screen).

Fortunately, I haven't had to take either job on by myself. For the kid raising (officially finished, though, let's face it—does it really ever end?), I've had the best partner-in-parenting out there, my husband, Erik—who also happens to be my partner in What to Expect. For the book writing, I've had dozens of colleagues and friends pitch in—contributing support, insight, and ideas in the creation (and re-creation . . . and re-creation . . . and re-creation) of four editions of *What to Expect® When You're Expecting*.

Some of those helpers have come and gone—but others have stood by since day one, and edition one. Thanks a lot to:

Sandee Hathaway, for all your valuable contributions to What to Expect. You're a great sister and an even greater friend.

Suzanne Rafer, editor and friend, who has faithfully guided What to Expect from conception through delivery four times over—dotting every "i," crossing every "t," deleting every misguided pun (and pair of parens). What's in a name? When it comes to What to Expect, a lot—and we have Suzanne to thank for the memorable moniker that helped launch not only 29 million copies, but hundreds of headlines, cartoons, and parodies.

Peter Workman, a publisher of uncommon integrity and uncompromising commitment—who believed in our book when bookstores didn't, who let What to Expect's grass roots take their slow and steady time sprouting, who never gave up on the little series that could, and did.

Everyone else at Workman who's helped with our latest delivery: David Matt, for believing in evolution (of Cover Mom), taking artistic chances, and overseeing our very challenging—and very successful—Extreme Makeover. John Gilman, for your extreme patience in this extreme makeover—and for making illustration magic happen. Lisa Hollander, for always being my favorite designing woman, as well as to Weiheng Tang. Tim O'Brien for bringing to life Cover Mom, The Next Generation—and for finally getting her off her rocker. Lynette Parmentier for re-creating as an actual quilt our iconic illustrated quilt. Karen Kuchar for inking our hot mamas (almost makes me want to run out and get pregnant again!) and Tom Newsom for our fabulous fetuses. Irene Demchyshyn for going with the flow and keeping the flow going. And my other phenomenal friends at Workman, including Suz2 (Suzie Bolotin), Helen Rosner, Beth Doty, Walter Weintz, Jenny Mandel, Kim Small, and Amy Corley.

My other partner, Sharon Mazel. You're my mini-me, my other (better) half, my BFF—and I love you. To the beautiful Daniella, Arianne, Kira, and Sophia, for sharing your amazing mom with me (and for getting sick and breaking bones only when absolutely necessary). And to the doctor in the house, Jay, for his great biology lessons and his good nature—but mostly, for letting me be the other woman in Sharon's life.

Dr. Charles Lockwood, our remarkable medical advisor, for your concise and precise advice, your meticulous attention to detail (medical and otherwise), and your obvious compassion for moms and babies. It's truly incredible how much you know, how much you do (I get exhausted just reading your CV), and how much you care.

Steven Petrow (MG), Mike Keriakos, Ben Wolin, Jim Curtis (CSOB), Sarah Hutter, and all my wonderful friends and partners at Waterfront Media, for making our vision of whattoexpect.com and My What to Expect a reality. Thanks, also, to the amazing community of moms—not only for making our site the special place that it is, but for sharing your bellies, babies, and toddlers with me every day.

The two other guys in my life (a girl could get spoiled): Marc Chamlin, for your keen legal eagle eye, your business smarts, your unflagging friendship and support; and Alan Nevins, for your masterful management, phenomenal finessing, endless patience, persistence, and hand-holding.

Jennifer Geddes and Fran Kritz, for helping us get our facts straight (check . . .

check . . . check!). Dr. Jessica Wu, for your impeccable pregnancy skin care counsel, and Dr. Howie Mandel, for being such a good sport about the What to Expect questions I'm always sneaking in at my annuals. And always, to always-inspiring Lisa Bernstein, Executive Director of the What to Expect Foundation, for making miracles happen (plump, full-term miracles), and to Zoe, Oh-That-Teddy, and Dan Dubno.

To Erik, my partner in everything I do, always and forever, for all the reasons listed above, and more than I can list. There's no one I'd rather mix business and pleasure with, and I love you forever. And speaking of love, to my pride and joy (I'm not saying who's who), Emma (the baby who started it all) and Wyatt (the baby who followed). I love you guys—you've made me one lucky mama.

The adorable Howard Eisenberg, father and friend (not necessarily in that order); Victor Shargai (and John Aniello) for your love and support; and to the world's best (and newly trimmest) in-laws, Abby and Norman Murkoff. And to Rachel, Ethan, and Liz, Sandee's fantastic three, and to Tim, her Numero Uno.

To ACOG, for being advocates for women and babies, and to all of the doctors, midwives, nurses, and nurse practitioners who work every day to make pregnancy safer and happier for expectant families. Most of all, to all the expectant, new, and old moms (and dads) who've helped make each edition of What to Expect better than the last. I've said it before, and I'll say it again, parents are my most invaluable resource—so keep those cards, letters, and e-mails coming!

Thanks again, and again, everybody . . . and may all your greatest expectations come true!

Contents

Part 1: First Things First

Why Millions of Moms, Dads, and Doctors Love *What to Expect*® *When You're Expecting*

"I love these books! They're full of useful information."
—SUZY A. THOMPSON, MD

♦ ♦ ♦

"I started reading *What to Expect When You're Expecting* the
moment I found out I was pregnant. [It] provided me with a road
map to a stress-free pregnancy."
—CAROLINE GOLDSTEIN, MOTHER

♦ ♦ ♦

"Excellent to allay patients' fears and provide information. . . .
I recommend it highly."
—DONNICA L. MOORE, MD

♦ ♦ ♦

"This book revolutionized prenatal care in America."
—JAMES FAHERTY, MD

♦ ♦ ♦

"I read them faithfully for my two pregnancies and as a pediatrician
find them to be right on."
—SUSAN WALTER MANGIAMELI, MD

♦ ♦ ♦

"This is the only book I recommend to my patients!"
—ELIZABETH DOYLE, MD

♦ ♦ ♦

"This is the 'must have' book for any expectant mother,
whether it's your first baby or your fifth!"
—SOFIA GARCIA, MOTHER

♦ ♦ ♦

"As a maternity designer and as a mother myself, I know
that there is no other book that means so much to so many
pregnant women everywhere."
—LIZ LANGE
MOTHER, FOUNDER AND CEO, LIZ LANGE MATERNITY

Part 2: Nine Months & Counting:
From Conception to Delivery

Chapter 9: The Fourth Month

Chapter 12: The Seventh Month

Chapter 13: The Eighth Month

Chapter 14: The Ninth Month

Part 3: Twins, Triplets & More:
When You're Expecting Multiples

Part 4: After the Baby Is Born

Part 5: For Dads

Part 6: Staying Healthy When You're Expecting

Part 7: The Complicated Pregnancy

Foreword to the Fourth Edition

By Charles J. Lockwood, MD

The Anita O'Keefe Young Professor of Women's Health and Chair, Department of Obstetrics, Gynecology and Reproductive Sciences, Yale University School of Medicine

THE OTHER DAY I RECEIVED A wonderful, heartfelt thank-you letter from a patient. Enclosed was a picture of a strapping college hockey player—whom I had delivered 19 years before! I have the best job on earth. I get to share in the most joyful, exciting, and wondrous moment that human beings will ever experience— the birth of their child—only I get to experience it over and over and over. Sure, being an obstetrician has its share of tough moments—some very tiring ones at 3 A.M., and some very frustrating ones, when the pace of a patient's labor appears to be glacial. There is the occasional adrenaline rush, the patient with the challenging symptom, and the inevitable flood of complex emotions, but mostly it's just plain fun.

In a way, my job is a lot like your pregnancy will probably be—every day will bring a little adventure, but most of them will be fun. *What to Expect When You're Expecting* is like having a personal obstetrician to guide you through that adventure. I have been recommending this book for years and thoroughly enjoyed reading the fourth edition— because the best just got better. All new, it's packed with information and useful advice, the kind you would hear from

your favorite doctor or midwife—one who is wise but funny, thorough but practical, experienced but enthusiastic, organized but empathetic.

The book starts you off before conception with solid recommendations on what to—and what not to—do before you are expecting. It then gently guides you through conception to your first visit to a provider. It explains what changes you'll need to make in your lifestyle, job, and diet. One of the book's best features is a month-by-month—in fact a week-by-week—guide to how your baby is developing and what she or he is doing in your uterus. This is accompanied by a description of how *you* are developing—and not just your belly but everywhere, from your hair to your toes—and what you should be feeling. It tells you what your provider will do at each visit, and reviews what tests will be ordered and why. Toward the end, it prepares you for the big day, however you might be delivering—vaginally or by cesarean. You'll learn about birthing plans, how to recognize real labor from false labor, and which laboring positions work. Your questions about back labor, fetal monitoring, episiotomy, pain relief, and anesthesia will be answered, even if you didn't know to ask. Then *What to*

Expect guides you through all aspects of the incredible process of birth.

The book also covers the postpartum period, providing tips for differentiating the "blues" from depression. In an important chapter, it covers complications that you can read about if they occur, or skip over if they don't. It covers pregnancy in women with common medical conditions, such as asthma, high blood pressure, and diabetes—and how to maximize your chances of a normal pregnancy. It also covers what to do if you experience a pregnancy loss, and does it with a wonderful mix of compassion and practicality. Partners are not forgotten: The book provides a very practical guide to being a great coach. And parents-to-be of multiples are included, too. An entire chapter is devoted to their undoubtedly doubled questions and concerns.

As a maternal-fetal medicine specialist, I am impressed by just how much is covered in this book. As an editor, I am impressed by the clear, cogent, and concise writing. As a husband and father, I am impressed that the authors know just what moms-to-be and their partners need to know. The best judges of this book, however, have been the hundreds of patients who have raved about it to me, my staff, and other patients in the waiting room.

If you are reading these words, it's likely you are either newly pregnant or about to become so. Congratulations! My advice to you is lie back, get comfortable, and read on—you are about to embark on the adventure of a lifetime.

Why This Book Was Born Again, Again

TWENTY-FOUR YEARS AGO, I DELIV-ered a daughter and conceived a book within a few hours of each other (it was a busy day). Nurturing both those babies, Emma Bing and *What to Expect When You're Expecting* (as well as the next baby, my son, Wyatt—and the other *What to Expect* offspring) as they've grown and evolved over the years has been at once exhilarating and exhausting, fulfilling and frustrating, heartwarming and nerve-racking. And like any parent, I wouldn't trade a day of it. (Though there was that week when Emma was thirteen . . . okay, make that a year. Maybe two.)

And now I'm thrilled to announce yet another delivery. A brand-new book that I couldn't be prouder to start showing off and sharing: The fourth edition of *What to Expect When You're Expecting*. A cover-to-cover, front-to-back revision that's been completely rewritten from start to finish—a new book for a new generation of expectant parents (you!), featuring a fresh look, a fresh perspective, and a friendlier-than-ever voice.

What's new in the new *What to Expect*? So much that I'm excited about. Week-by-week updates on your little one's transformation from microscopic bundle of cells to cuddly newborn—the

incredible development of your baby-to-be that will make all that heartburn, all those trips to the bathroom, all that gas, all those pains, and all the sleep depriva-tion more than worth it. And (speaking of heartburn and gas), more symptoms and more solutions than ever before—and more of your questions answered (even the ones you didn't know you had yet). There's an expanded section on working during pregnancy (as if being pregnant weren't hard enough work!). And going from the practical to the pampered, a brand-new section on expectant beauty: how to love—or at least cope with—the expectant skin you're in, even when it's blotchy, pimply, rashy, itchy, too oily, and too dry; which skin, hair, nail, and cosmetic regimens you can stick with and which you'll have to ditch until delivery. Lots on your pregnant lifestyle (from sex to travel to exercise to fash-ion), your pregnancy profile (how your obstetrical, medical, and gynecological backstory may—or may not—affect your pregnancy), your relationships, your emotions. A more realistic than ever chapter on expectant eating that responds to every eating style—from at-the-desk to on-the-run, from vegan to low-carb, caffeine-addicted to junk-food dependent. An expanded section on preconception, a new chapter for all you many moms of multiples. Lots more for that very important (but too often neglected) partner in parenting, the dad-to-be. And, of course, the very latest on all things pregnancy (news you can use, on everything from prenatal diagnosis to labor and delivery and beyond).

And because a cover-to-cover revision wouldn't be complete without a new cover, there's one of those, too. Introducing our new cover mom—off her rocker (okay . . . out of that rocking chair, finally), she's embracing her belly and celebrating one of life's most magical experiences (and the fact that pregnant women now get to wear cute clothes). She's thoroughly enjoying her expectant self—and I, for one, couldn't be happier for her. Almost makes me want to run out and get pregnant again (I said almost).

As always, just as important as what's different in this fourth edition is what's the same. When *What to Expect When You're Expecting* was first con-ceived, it was with a single mission in mind: to help parents-to-be worry less and enjoy their pregnancies more. That mission has grown, but it hasn't changed. Like the first three editions, this fourth one was written to answer your questions, reassure you, relate to you, empathize with you, and help you get a better night's sleep (at least as good a night's sleep as you can get when you're busy running to the bathroom or fighting off leg cramps and backaches).

I hope you enjoy my new baby as much as I enjoyed creating it—and that it helps you as you go about creating that new baby of yours. Wishing you the healthiest of pregnancies and a lifetime of happy parenting. May all your greatest expectations come true!

Heidi

About The What to Expect Foundation

Every parent should know what to expect. That's why we created The What to Expect Foundation, a non-profit organization that provides vital prenatal health and literacy support to moms in need—so they, too, can expect healthier pregnancies, safer deliveries, and healthy, happy babies. For more information and to find out ways you can help, please visit our website at whattoexpect.org.

PART 1

First Things First

CHAPTER 1

Before You Conceive

SO YOU'VE MADE THE DECISION TO start a family (or to grow that family you've already started). That's a great—and exciting—first step. But before sperm meets egg to create the baby of your dreams, take this preconception opportunity to prepare for the healthiest pregnancy—and baby—possible. The next steps outlined in this chapter will help you (and dad-to-be) get into tip-top baby-making shape, give you a leg up on conception, and get you to the pregnancy starting gate with all systems go.

If you don't get pregnant right away, relax and keep trying (and don't forget to keep having fun while you're trying!). If you're already pregnant—and didn't have a chance to follow these steps before you conceived—not to worry. Conception often sneaks up on a couple, cutting out that preconception period altogether and making those preconception pointers pointless. If your pregnancy test has already given you the good news, simply start this book at Chapter 2, and make the very best of every day of pregnancy you have ahead of you.

Preconception Prep for Moms

Ready to board that cute little passenger on the mother ship? Here are some preconception steps you can take to make sure that ship is in shape.

Get a preconception checkup. You don't have to choose a prenatal practitioner yet (though this is a great time to do so; see facing page), but it would be a good idea to see your regular gynecologist or internist for a thorough physi-

cal. An exam will pick up any medical problems that need to be corrected beforehand or that will need to be monitored during pregnancy. Plus, your doctor will be able to steer you away from medications that are pregnancy (or preconception) no-no's, make sure your immunizations are up to date, and talk to you about your weight, your diet, your drinking and other lifestyle habits, and similar preconception issues.

Start looking for a prenatal practitioner. It's easier to start looking for an obstetrician or midwife now, when the pregnancy meter's not already running, than when that first prenatal checkup is hanging over your head. If you're going to stick with your regular ob-gyn, then you've got a head start. Otherwise, ask around, scout around, and take your time in picking the practitioner who's right for you (see page 21 for tips on choosing one). Then schedule an interview and a prepregnancy exam.

Smile for the dentist. A visit to the dentist before you get pregnant is almost as important as a visit to the doctor. That's because your future pregnancy can affect your mouth—and your mouth can possibly affect your future pregnancy. Pregnancy hormones can actually aggravate gum and tooth problems, making a mess of a mouth that's not well taken care of to begin with. What's more, research shows that gum disease may be associated with some pregnancy complications. So before you get busy making a baby, get busy getting your mouth into shape. Be sure, too, to have any necessary work, including X-rays, fillings, and dental surgery, completed now so that it won't have to be done during pregnancy.

Check your family tree. Get the scoop on the health history on both sides of the family tree (yours and your spouse's). It's especially important to find out if there's a history of any medical issues and genetic or chromosomal disorders such as Down syndrome, Tay-Sachs disease, sickle cell anemia, thalassemia, hemophilia, cystic fibrosis, muscular dystrophy, or fragile X syndrome.

Take a look at your pregnancy history. If you've had a previous pregnancy with any complications or one that ended with a premature delivery or late preg-

Putting It All Together

Does looking at this list of to-do's make you realize there's a lot to do even before sperm meets egg? Having a hard time knowing where to start? For a list of questions to ask when choosing a prenatal practitioner, a complete personal medical and obstetrical health history, a family health history chart, and plenty of other helpful information to help you get organized for your baby-making journey, see *The What to Expect Pregnancy Journal and Organizer* and whattoexpect.com.

nancy loss, or if you've had multiple miscarriages, talk to your practitioner about any measures that can be taken to head off a repeat.

Seek genetic screening, if necessary. Also ask your practitioner about being tested for any genetic disease common to your ethnic background: cystic fibrosis if either of you is Caucasian; Tay-Sachs disease if either of you is of Jewish-European (Ashkenazi), French Canadian, or Louisiana Cajun descent; sickle cell trait if you are of African descent; one of the thalassemias if you are of Greek, Italian, Southeast Asian, or Filipino origin.

Previous obstetrical difficulties (such as two or more miscarriages, a stillbirth, a long period of infertility, or a child with a birth defect) or being married to a cousin or other blood relative are also reasons to seek genetic counseling.

Get tested. While you're seeing all your doctors and checking out all your histories, ask if you can get a head start on some of the tests and health workups every pregnant woman receives. Most are as easy as getting a blood test to look for:

- Hemoglobin or hematocrit, to test for anemia.

- Rh factor, to see if you are positive or negative. If you are negative, your partner should be tested to see if he is positive. (If you're both negative, there is no need to give Rh another thought.)

- Rubella titer, to check for immunity to rubella.

- Varicella titer, to check for immunity to varicella (chicken pox).

- Tuberculosis (if you live in a high-incidence area).

- Hepatitis B (if you're in a high-risk category, such as health-care worker, and have not been immunized).

- Cytomegalovirus (CMV) antibodies, to determine whether or not you are immune to CMV (see page 503). If you have been diagnosed with CMV, it's generally recommended you wait six months before trying to conceive.

- Toxoplasmosis titer, if you have an outdoor cat, regularly eat raw or rare meat, or garden without gloves. If you turn out to be immune, you don't have to worry about toxoplasmosis now or ever. If you're not, start taking the precautions on page 80 now.

- Thyroid function. Thyroid function can affect pregnancy. So if you have or ever had thyroid problems, or if you have a family history of thyroid disease, or if you have symptoms of a thyroid condition (see pages 174 and 531), this is an important test to have.

- Sexually transmitted diseases (STDs). All pregnant women are routinely tested for all STDs, including syphilis, gonorrhea, chlamydia, herpes, human papilloma virus (HPV), and HIV. Having these tests before conception is even better (or in the case of HPV, getting the vaccine; see next page). Even if you're sure you couldn't have an STD, ask to be tested, just to be on the safe side.

Get treated. If any test turns up a condition that requires treatment, make sure you take care of it before trying to conceive. Also consider attending to minor elective surgery and anything else medical—major or minor—that you've been putting off. Now is the time, too, to be treated for any gynecological conditions that might interfere with fertility or pregnancy, including:

- Uterine polyps, fibroids, cysts, or benign tumors.

- Endometriosis (when the cells that ordinarily line the uterus spread elsewhere in the body).

- Pelvic inflammatory disease.

- Recurrent urinary tract infections or other infections, such as bacterial vaginosis.

- An STD.

Update your immunizations. If you haven't had a tetanus-diphtheria booster in the past 10 years, have one now. If you know you've never had rubella or been immunized against it, or if testing showed you are not immune to the disease, get vaccinated now with the measles, mumps, and rubella (MMR) vaccine, and then wait one month before attempting to conceive (but don't worry if you accidentally conceive earlier). If testing shows you've never had chicken pox or are at high risk for hepatitis B, immunization for these diseases is also recommended now, before conception.

If you're under 26, also consider getting vaccinated against HPV, but you'd need to get the full series of three before trying to conceive, so plan accordingly.

Get chronic illnesses under control. If you have diabetes, asthma, a heart condition, epilepsy, or any other chronic illness, be sure you have your doctor's okay to become pregnant, your condition is under control before you conceive, and you start taking optimum care of yourself now (if you aren't already). If you were born with phenylketonuria (PKU), begin a strict phenylalanine-free diet before conceiving and continue it through pregnancy. As unappealing as it is, it's essential to your baby-to-be's well-being.

If you need allergy shots, take care of them now. (If you start allergy desensitization now, you will probably be able to continue once you conceive.) Because depression can interfere with conception—and with a happy, healthy pregnancy—it should also be treated before you begin your big adventure.

Get ready to toss your birth control. Ditch that last package of condoms and throw out your diaphragm (you'll have to be refitted after pregnancy anyway). If you're using birth control pills, the vaginal ring, or the patch, talk your game plan over with your practitioner. Some recommend holding off on baby-making efforts for several months after quitting hormonal birth control, if possible, to allow your reproductive system to go through at least two normal cycles (use condoms while you're waiting). Others say it's okay to start trying as soon as you want. Be aware, though, that it may take a few months or even longer for your cycles to become normal and for you to begin ovulating again.

If you use an IUD, have it removed before you begin trying. Wait three to six months after stopping Depo-Provera shots to try to conceive (many women aren't fertile for an average of 10 months after stopping Depo, so time accordingly).

Improve your diet. You may not be eating for two yet, but it's never too early to start eating well for the baby you're planning to make. Most important is to make sure you're getting your folic acid. Not only does getting enough folic acid appear to boost fertility, but studies show that adequate intake of this vitamin in a woman's diet before she conceives and early in her pregnancy can dramatically reduce the risk of neural tube defects (such as spina bifida) and preterm birth. sFolic acid is found naturally in whole grains and green leafy vegetables, and by law it is also added to most refined grains. But taking a prenatal supplement containing at least 400 mcg of folic acid is also recommended (see page 103).

It's also a good idea to start cutting back on junk food and high-fat foods and begin increasing whole grains, fruits, vegetables, and low-fat dairy products (important for bone strength). You can use the Pregnancy Diet (Chapter 5) as a good basic, balanced food plan, but you'll need only two protein servings, three calcium servings, and no more than six whole-grain servings daily until you conceive—plus you won't have to start adding those extra calories (and if you need to lose some weight preconception, you might need to cut some calories out).

Start modifying your fish consumption according to the guidelines for expectant moms (see page 114). But don't cut out fish, because it's a great source of baby-growing nutrients.

If you have any dietary habits that wouldn't be healthy during pregnancy (such as periodic fasting), suffer or

It Takes Two, Baby

Sure, you're closer than ever physically now that you're trying to make a baby (that's something baby-making efforts just about guarantee)—but what about your love connection? As you strive to form that perfect union (of sperm and egg), are you neglecting the other significant union in your lives (the two of you)?

When expanding your twosome becomes your number one priority, when sex becomes functional instead of recreational, when it's less about getting it on than getting it done (and when foreplay consists of running to the bathroom to check your cervical mucus), relationships can sometimes show the strain. But yours definitely doesn't have to—in fact, you can keep it healthier than ever. To stay emotionally connected while you're trying to conceive:

■ **Get out.** Been-there, done-that moms will tell you that *now's* the time for you and your spouse to get out of town—or at least out of the house. Once baby's on board, your days (and nights) of picking up and taking off will be numbered. (Maternity leave? More like maternity *stay*!) So take that mini vacation you've been saving up for—or that second honeymoon (you can call it a baby-to-be-moon). No time for a vacation? Try something new on the weekends—preferably something that you won't be able to do once conception cramps your lifestyle (horseback riding or white-water rafting, anyone?). Need something more tame as a twosome? Slip off to a museum on a weekend afternoon, catch a late-night movie (or two) at the multiplex, or just linger over dinner at your favorite restaurant (no babysitters necessary).

■ **Rev up the romance.** Pee-on-a-stick ovulation tests and the pressure to perform (now!) can make sex seem too much like hard work. So bring fun back into the bedroom. Turn up the heat—and not just your basal temperature—with a sexy little nightie, a steamy movie, a sex toy or two, a round of strip poker or nude twister, a new position (kama sutra will be considerably trickier once that belly gets in the way), a new location (serve yourself up on the dining table), or a new tactic (hot fudge on each other instead of on ice cream). Adventurous isn't in your comfort zone? Ratchet up the romance with a moonlight stroll, dinner by candlelight, cuddling in front of the fireplace.

■ **Stay on the same page.** Worried that your spouse is more interested in charting the stock market than helping you chart your basal body temperature? Get the feeling that he's blasé about baby making? Go easy on him. Just because he might not be obsessing over ovulation or going ga-ga every time he passes a baby boutique doesn't mean he's not as eager as you are to get the baby show on the road. Maybe he's just being a guy (laid-back, instead of worked up). Maybe he's just keeping his tension about conception to himself (so he doesn't stress you out, too). Maybe he's focusing on the business end of baby making (he's working longer hours because he's concerned about providing a nest egg for the nestling you'll be creating). Either way, remember that taking the plunge into parenthood is a huge step for both of you—but that you're taking it as a team. To stay on the same page (even if you're using different words), communicate as you try to procreate. You'll both feel better knowing you're in this together—even if you're approaching it a little differently.

have suffered from an eating disorder (such as anorexia nervosa or bulimia), or are on a special diet (vegan, macrobiotic, diabetic, or any other), tell your practitioner.

Take a prenatal vitamin. Even if you're eating plenty of foods high in folic acid, it's still recommended that you take a pregnancy supplement containing 400 mcg of the vitamin, preferably beginning two months before you try to conceive. Another good reason to start taking a prenatal supplement preconception: Research indicates that women who take a daily multivitamin containing at least 10 mg of vitamin B_6 before becoming pregnant or during the first weeks of pregnancy experience fewer episodes of vomiting and nausea during pregnancy. The supplement should also contain 15 mg of zinc, which may improve fertility. Stop taking other nutritional supplements before conceiving, however, since excesses of certain nutrients can be hazardous.

Get your weight in check. Being overweight or very underweight not only reduces the chances of conception, but, if you do conceive, weight problems can increase the risk of pregnancy complications. So add or cut calories in the preconception period as needed. If you're trying to lose weight, be sure to do so slowly and sensibly, even if it means putting off conception for another couple of months. Strenuous or nutritionally unbalanced dieting (including low-carbohydrate, high-protein diets) can make conception elusive and can result in a nutritional deficit, which probably isn't the best way to start your pregnancy. If you've been extreme dieting recently, start eating normally and give your body a few months to get back into balance before you try to conceive.

Shape up, but keep cool. A good exercise program can put you on the right track for conception, plus it will tone and strengthen your muscles in preparation for the challenging tasks of carrying and delivering your baby-to-be. It will also help you take off excess weight. Don't overdo that good thing, though, because excessive exercise (especially if it leads to an extremely lean body) can interfere with ovulation—and if you don't ovulate, you can't conceive. And keep your cool during workouts: Prolonged increases in body temperature can interfere with conception. (Avoid hot tubs, saunas, and direct exposure to heating pads and electric blankets for the same reason.)

Check your medicine cabinet. Some—though far from all—medications are considered unsafe for use during pregnancy. If you're taking any medications now (regularly or once in a while, prescription or over-the-counter), ask your practitioner about their safety during preconception and pregnancy. If you need to switch a regular medication that isn't safe to a substitute that is, now's the time to do it.

Herbal or other alternative medications shouldn't necessarily move front and center in your medicine cabinet, either. Herbs are natural, but natural doesn't automatically signal safe. What's more, some popular herbs—such as echinacea, ginkgo biloba, or St. John's wort—can interfere with conception. Do not take any such products or supplements without the approval of a doctor familiar with herbals and alternative medicines and their potential effect on conception and pregnancy.

Cut back on caffeine. There's no need to drop that latte (or switch to decaf) if you're planning on becoming pregnant

Pinpointing Ovulation

Knowing when the Big O (ovulation) occurs is key when doing the Baby Dance (aka trying to conceive). Here are a few ways to help you pin down the big day—and pin each other down for baby-making activities.

Watch the calendar. Ovulation most often occurs halfway through your menstrual cycle. The average cycle lasts 28 days, counting from the first day of one period (day 1) to the first day of the next period. But as with everything pregnancy related, there's a wide range of normal when it comes to menstrual cycles (they can run anywhere from 23 days to 35 days), and your own cycle may vary slightly from month to month. By keeping a menstrual calendar for a few months, you can get an idea of what's normal for you. (And when you become pregnant, this calendar will help give you a better estimate of your baby's due date.) If your periods are irregular, you'll need to be more alert for other signs of ovulation (see below).

Take your temperature. Keeping track of your basal body temperature, or BBT (you'll need a special basal body thermometer to do this), can help you pinpoint ovulation. Your BBT is the baseline reading you get first thing in the morning, after at least three to five hours of sleep and before you get out of bed, talk, or even sit up. Your BBT changes throughout your cycle, reaching its lowest point at ovulation and then rising dramatically (about half a

degree) within a day or so after ovulation occurs. Keep in mind that charting your BBT will not enable you to predict the day you ovulate, but rather it gives you evidence of ovulation two to three days after it has occurred. Over a few months, it will help you to see a pattern to your cycles, enabling you to predict when ovulation will occur in future cycles.

Check your underwear. Another sign you can be alert for is the appearance, increase in quantity, and change in consistency of cervical mucus (the stuff that gets your underwear all sticky). After your period ends, don't expect much, if any, cervical mucus. As the cycle proceeds, you'll notice an increase in the amount of mucus with an often white or cloudy appearance—and if you try to stretch it between your fingers, it'll break apart. As you get closer to ovulation, this mucus becomes even more copious, but now it's thinner, clearer, and has a slippery consistency similar to an egg white. If you try to stretch it between your fingers, you'll be able to pull it into a string a few inches long before it breaks (how's that for fun in the bathroom?). This is yet another sign of impending ovulation, as well as a sign that it's time to get out of the bathroom and get busy in the bedroom. Once ovulation occurs, you may either become dry again or develop a thicker discharge. Combined with cervical position (see below) and BBT on a

or even once you become pregnant. Most experts believe that up to two cups of caffeinated coffee (or the equivalent in other caffeinated beverages) a day is fine. If your habit involves more than that, though, it would be smart to

start moderating. Some studies have linked downing too much of the stuff to lowered fertility.

Cut down on alcohol. Start thinking before drinking. Although a daily drink single chart, cervical mucus can be an extremely useful (if slightly messy) tool in pinpointing the day on which you are most likely to ovulate—and it does so in plenty of time for you to do something about it.

Get to know your cervix. As your body senses the hormone shifts that indicate an egg is about to be released from the ovary, it begins to ready itself for incoming hordes of sperm to give the egg its best chance of getting fertilized. One detectable sign of oncoming ovulation is the position of the cervix itself. During the beginning of a cycle, your cervix—that necklike passage between your vagina and uterus that has to stretch during birth to accommodate your baby's head—is low, hard, and closed. But as ovulation approaches, it pulls back up, softens a bit, and opens just a little to let the sperm through on their way to their target. Some women can easily feel these changes, others have a tougher time. If you're game to try, check your cervix daily, using one or two fingers, and keep a chart of your observations.

Stay tuned in. If you're like 20 percent of women, your body will let you know when ovulation is taking place by sending a bulletin in the form of a twinge of pain or a series of cramps in your lower abdominal area (usually localized to one side, the side where you're ovulating). Called mittelschmerz—German for "middle pain"—this monthly reminder of fertility is thought to be the result of the maturation or release of an egg from an ovary.

Pee on a stick. Ovulation predictor kits (OPKs) are able to pinpoint your date of ovulation 12 to 24 hours in advance by measuring levels of luteinizing hormone, or LH, which is the last of the hormones to hit its peak before ovulation actually occurs. All you have to do is pee on a stick and wait for the indicator to tell you whether you're about to ovulate (talk about easy).

Watch your watch. Another option in the ovulation test arsenal is a device you wear on your wrist that detects the numerous salts (chloride, sodium, potassium) in your sweat, which differ during different times of the month. Called the chloride ion surge, this shift happens even before the estrogen and the LH surge, so these chloride ion tests give a woman a four-day window of when she may be ovulating, versus the 12 to 24-hour window that the standard pee-on-a-stick OPKs provide. The key to success in using this latest technology is to make sure to get an accurate baseline of your ion levels (which means you'll need to wear the device on your wrist for at least six continuous hours to get a proper baseline).

Spit a little. Another ovulation predictor is a saliva test, which tests the levels of estrogen in your saliva as ovulation nears. When you're ovulating, a look at your saliva under the test's eyepiece will reveal a microscopic pattern that resembles the leaves of a fern plant or frost on a windowpane. Not all women get a good "fern," but this test, which is reusable, can be cheaper than those pee-on sticks.

will not be harmful in your pregnancy-preparation phase, heavy alcohol consumption can interfere with fertility by disrupting your menstrual cycle. Plus, once you're actively trying to conceive, there's always the possibility that you'll

have succeeded—and drinking during pregnancy isn't recommended.

Quit smoking. Did you know that smoking can not only interfere with fertility but also cause your eggs to age?

Conception Misconceptions

You've heard plenty of old wives'— and new Internet—tales about how best to make a baby. Here are a few that are ready to be taken off the circuit:

Myth: Having sex every day will decrease sperm count, making conception more elusive.

Fact: Though this was once believed to be true, more recent research has shown that having sex every day around the time of ovulation is slightly more likely to end in pregnancy than having sex every other day. More, apparently, is more.

Myth: Wearing boxer shorts will increase fertility.

Fact: Scientists have yet to rule definitively on the boxers versus briefs debate, but most experts seem to think that the underwear a man favors has little effect on the baby race. Though there is something to be said for keeping the testicles cool and giving them a little breathing room (see page 13).

Myth: Missionary position intercourse is the best way for sperm to reach their target.

Fact: The cervical mucus that turns thin and stretchy around the time of ovulation is the perfect medium for sperm, helping those boys swim up the vaginal tract, through the cervix, past the uterus, and up the fallopian tubes to the awaiting egg. Unless sperm have a motility problem, they'll reach their target no matter what position you're in while you're doing it. It doesn't hurt, however, to lie down for a while after intercourse so the sperm don't run out of the vagina before they even get a running start.

Myth: Lubricant will help the sperm hitch a ride to Egg Central.

Fact: Actually, the opposite is true. Lubricants can change the pH balance in the vagina, creating an inhospitable environment for the sperm. So lay off the Astroglide until after your conception mission is accomplished.

Myth: Daytime sex helps you conceive faster.

Fact: Sperm levels do seem to be higher in the morning, but no clinical evidence supports that making hay while the sun shines will increase your chances of conception. (But don't let that stop you if you'd like to grab a quickie before you grab your lunch-break sandwich!)

That's right—a 30-year-old smoker's eggs act more like 40-year-old eggs, making conception more difficult and miscarriage more likely. Kicking the habit now is not only the best gift you can give your baby-to-be (before and after birth), but it can make it more likely that you'll conceive that baby-to-be. For some practical tips to help you quit, check out pages 74–75.

Just say no to illegal drugs. Marijuana, cocaine, crack, heroin, and other illicit drugs can be dangerous to your pregnancy. To varying degrees they can prevent your conceiving, and then, if you do succeed, they may be potentially harmful to the fetus and also may increase the risks of miscarriage, prematurity, and stillbirths. If you use drugs, casually or regularly, stop all use immediately. If you can't stop, seek help before trying to conceive.

Avoid unnecessary exposure to radiation. If X-rays are necessary for medical reasons, be sure your reproductive organs are protected (unless they are being targeted) and the lowest radiation doses possible are used. Once you start trying to conceive, inform any technicians taking X-rays that you could be pregnant, and ask them to take all necessary precautions.

Avoid environmental hazards. Some chemicals—though far from all and usually only in very large doses—are potentially harmful to your eggs before conception and, later, to a developing embryo or fetus. Though the risk in most cases is slight or even just hypothetical, play it safe by avoiding potentially hazardous exposure on the job. Take special care in certain fields (medicine and dentistry, art, photography, transportation, farming and landscaping, construction, hairdressing and cosmetology, dry cleaning, and some factory work). Contact the Occupational Safety and Health Administration (OSHA) for the latest information on job safety and pregnancy; also see page 194. In some cases, it may be wise to ask for a transfer to another position, change jobs, or take special precautions, if possible, before trying to conceive.

Because elevated lead levels when you conceive could pose problems for your baby, get tested if you have been exposed to lead in the workplace or elsewhere, such as in your water supply or your home (see page 81). Avoid, too, excessive exposure to other household toxins.

Get fiscally fit. Having a baby can be pricey. So, together with your spouse, reevaluate your budget and begin creating a sound financial plan. As part of your plan, find out if your health insurance pays for the cost of prenatal care, birth, and well-baby care. If coverage will not start until a certain date, consider delaying your pregnancy until then. Or if you plan to switch policies, do so before you become pregnant, since some policies consider pregnancy a preexisting condition. And if you don't have a will yet, now is the time to draw one up.

Work out those work issues. Find out everything you can about your work rights when pregnant (see page 187). If you're planning a job switch, you might want to consider finding that perfect family-friendly job now so you won't have to interview with a belly.

Start keeping track. Become familiar with your monthly cycle and learn the signs of ovulation so you can time intercourse right (see box, page 8). Keeping track of when you have sex will also help you pinpoint conception later on, which will make calculating an estimated date of delivery easier.

Give it time. Keep in mind that it takes an average of six months for a normal, healthy 25-year-old woman to conceive, and longer for women who are older. It may also take longer if your partner is older. So don't stress if baby magic doesn't happen right away. Just keep on having fun trying, and give yourselves at least six months before consulting your practitioner and, if needed, a fertility specialist. If you're over 35, you may want to check in with your practitioner after three months of trying.

Relax. This is perhaps the most important step of all. Of course, you're excited about getting pregnant—and, more than likely, at least a little stressed about it, too. But getting tense and uptight about conception could prevent you from conceiving. Learn to do relaxation exercises, to meditate, and to cut down as much as possible on stress in your daily life.

Preconception Prep for Dads

As a dad-to-be, you won't be pro-viding immediate room and board for your future offspring—but you will be making a vital contribution to the baby-making process (mom can't do it without you). These preconception steps can help you make conception as healthy as possible.

See your doctor. Though you won't be the one carrying the baby—at least not until after delivery—you'll still need a checkup of your own before you begin baby making. After all, making a healthy baby takes the participation of two healthy bodies. A thorough physical can detect any medical conditions (such as undescended testicles or testicular cysts or tumors) that might interfere with conception or a healthy pregnancy for your partner, as well as ensure that any chronic conditions, such as depression, that might interfere with fertility are under control. While you're at the doctor's office, ask about the sexual side effects of any prescription, over-the-counter, or herbal drugs you are tak-ing. Some can cause erectile dysfunction and lower sperm counts—two things you definitely don't want going on when you're in baby-making mode.

Get a genetic screening, if needed. If your spouse is going in for genetic test-ing, consider tagging along, especially if you have a family history of a genetic problem or other indication.

Improve your diet. The better your nutri-tion, the healthier your sperm and the more likely you'll conceive. Your diet should be a balanced, healthy one that includes plenty of fresh fruits and veg-etables, whole grains, and lean protein. To be sure you get adequate amounts of the most important nutrients (espe-cially vitamin C, vitamin E, vitamin D, zinc, and calcium, all of which appear to affect fertility or the health of sperm), take a vitamin-mineral supplement while you are attempting to conceive. The sup-plement should contain folic acid; a low intake of this nutrient in fathers-to-be has been linked to decreased fertility as well as to birth defects.

Look at your lifestyle. All the answers are not yet in, but research is beginning to show that the use of drugs—includ-ing excessive amounts of alcohol—by the male partner prior to conception could prevent pregnancy or lead to a poor pregnancy outcome. The mech-anisms aren't clear, but drug use and daily heavy drinking can apparently damage sperm as well as reduce their number and can alter testicular func-tion and reduce testosterone levels (not a good scenario when you're trying to conceive). Heavy drinking (equivalent to two drinks a day or five on any one day) during the month before concep-tion could also affect your baby's birth-weight. Keep in mind, too, that if you cut down on or cut out alcohol, it will be much easier for your partner to do likewise. If you are unable to quit drugs or reduce your alcohol intake, seek help now.

Get your weight on track. Men with a very high BMI (or body mass index, a measure of body fat based on height and weight) are more likely to be infer-tile than normal-weight men. Even a 20-pound increase in your weight may increase the chance of infertility by 10 percent, according to researchers. So get your weight in check before trying to conceive.

Stop smoking. No ifs, ands, or butts: Smoking reduces the number of sperm and makes conceiving more difficult. In addition, quitting now will improve the health of everyone in your family, since secondhand smoke is nearly as dangerous to them as firsthand smoke is to you. In fact, it can increase your baby-to-be's risk of dying of SIDS (sudden infant death syndrome).

Don't get zapped. High lead levels, as well as some organic solvents (such as those found in paints, glues, varnishes, and metal degreasers), pesticides, or other chemicals can interfere with a male's fertility, so avoid these or limit your exposure as much as possible in preparation for conception.

Keep 'em cool. Sperm production is impaired when the testicles become overheated. In fact, they prefer to be a couple of degrees cooler than the rest of you, which is why they hang away from your body. So avoid hot tubs and hot baths, saunas, electric blankets, and snug clothing, such as tight jeans. Also avoid synthetic pants and underwear, which can overheat you in hot weather. And keep your laptop off your lap, since the heat from the device can raise your scrotal temperature and reduce your sperm count. Until you conceive, treat it like a desktop.

Keep 'em safe. If you play any rough sports (including football, soccer, basketball, hockey, baseball, or horseback riding), wear protective gear to prevent injury to the genitals, which can damage fertility. Even too much bicycling has the potential to cause problems. According to some experts, the constant pressure on the genitals by a bicycle seat may interfere with conception by damaging arteries and nerves. If you experience genital numbness and/or tingling, and changing seats or lifting yourself off the seat periodically as you ride doesn't help, it would be a good idea to cut down on bicycling during the conception-attempting period. Numb genitals don't perform as well as they should. If the numbness (and/or tingling) doesn't go away, see your doctor.

Relax. Sure, you've got a lot on your mind as you contemplate bringing a baby into your lives—and yes, now you have a preconception to-do list to get busy on before you actually get busy on making baby. But don't forget to take the time to relax, too. Stress doesn't just affect your libido and performance, it also affects your testosterone levels and your sperm production. The less you worry, the more easily you'll conceive. So relax and enjoy trying!

CHAPTER 2

Are You Pregnant?

MAYBE YOUR PERIOD'S JUST A day overdue. Or maybe it's going on three weeks late. Or maybe your period isn't even slated to arrive yet, but you've got a gut feeling (literally, in your gut) that something's cooking—like a brand-new bun in your oven! Maybe the only heads-up your body's given you so far is that missed period. Or maybe you've already developed every conceivable symptom of conception. Maybe you've been giving baby making everything you've got for six months or longer. Or maybe that hot night two weeks ago was your very first contraceptive-free encounter. Or maybe you haven't been actively trying at all. No matter what the circumstances are that have brought you to this book, you're bound to be wondering: Am I pregnant? Well, read on to find out.

What You May Be Wondering About

Early Pregnancy Signs

"A friend of mine said she knew she was pregnant even before she took a pregnancy test. Is there any way to figure out whether or not I'm pregnant that early on?"

The only way to be positively positive that you're pregnant—at least this early on—is to produce that positive pregnancy test. But that doesn't mean your body is staying mum on whether you're about to become a mom. In fact, it may be offering up plenty of conception clues. Though many women never feel any early pregnancy symptoms at all (or don't feel them until weeks into pregnancy), others get lots of hints that there's a baby in the making. Experiencing any of these symptoms or noticing any of these signs may be just the excuse you need to run to the store for a home pregnancy test:

Tender breasts and nipples. You know that tender, achy feeling you get in your breasts before your period arrives? That's nothing compared to the breast tenderness you might be feeling post-conception. Tender, full, swollen, tingly, sensitive, and even painful-to-the-touch breasts are some of the first signs many (but not all) women notice after sperm meets egg. Such tenderness can begin as early as a few days after conception (though it often doesn't kick in until weeks later), and as your pregnancy progresses, it could get even more pronounced. Make that a lot more pronounced.

Darkening areolas. Not only might your breasts be tender, but your areolas (the circles around your nipples) may be changing colors. It's perfectly normal for the areola to darken in hue during pregnancy and even to increase in diameter somewhat in the weeks after conception. You can thank the pregnancy hormones already surging through your body for these and other skin color changes (much more about those hormones in the coming months).

Goose bumps? Well, not really, but early in pregnancy you may notice an increase and enlargement in the tiny bumps on the areola (called Montgomery's tubercles)—bumps you may have never noticed before. They'll resemble goose bumps but are actually glands that produce oils to lubricate your nipples and areolas—lubrication that'll certainly be welcome when your baby starts sucking on your nipples if you're nursing. Another sign your body is planning ahead.

Spotting. Some (but certainly not all) women experience spotting when the embryo implants in the uterus. Such so-called implantation bleeding will likely arrive earlier than your expected monthly flow (usually around five to ten days after conception) and will probably appear light to medium pink in color (rarely red, like a period).

Urinary frequency. Has the toilet become your seat of choice lately? Appearing on the pregnancy scene fairly early (usually about two to three weeks after conception) may be the need to pee with frightening frequency. Curious why? See page 135 for all the reasons.

Fatigue. Extreme fatigue. Make that exhaustion. Complete lack of energy. Super sluggishness. Whatever you call it, it's a drag—literally. And as your body starts cranking up that baby-making machine, it'll only get more draining. See page 127 for reasons why.

Nausea. Here's another reason why you might want to consider moving into the bathroom, at least until the first trimester is finished. Nausea and vomiting—aka morning sickness (if only it were limited to the morning)—can strike a newly pregnant woman fairly soon after conception, though it's more likely to begin around week 6. For a host of reasons why, see page 130.

Smell sensitivity. Since a heightened sense of smell is one of the first changes some newly pregnant women report, pregnancy might be in the air if your sniffer's suddenly more sensitive—and easily offended.

Bloating. Feeling like a walking flotation device? That bloated feeling can creep up (and out) on you very early in a pregnancy—though it may be difficult to differentiate between a preperiod bloat and a pregnancy bloat. It's too soon to attribute any swelling to your baby's growth, but you can chalk it up to those hormones again.

Rising temperature. Basal body temperature, that is. If you've been tracking your first morning temperature with a special basal body thermometer, you might notice that your basal body temperature rises around one degree when you conceive and continues to stay elevated throughout your pregnancy. Though not a foolproof sign (there are other reasons why you may notice a rise in temperature), it could give you advance notice of big—though still very little—news.

Missed period. It might be stating the obvious, but if you've missed a period (especially if your periods generally run like clockwork), you may already be suspecting pregnancy—even before a pregnancy test confirms it.

Diagnosing Pregnancy

"How can I find out for sure whether I'm pregnant or not?"

Aside from that most remarkable of diagnostic tools, a woman's intuition (some women "feel" they're pregnant within moments of conception), modern medical science is still your best bet when it comes to diagnosing a pregnancy accurately. Luckily, these days there are many ways to find out for sure that you've got a baby on board:

The home pregnancy test. It's as easy as one-two-pee, and you can do it all in the privacy and comfort of your own bathroom. Home pregnancy tests (HPTs) are not only quick and accurate, but you can even start using some brands before you've missed your period (though accuracy will get better as you get closer to P-day).

All HPTs measure urinary levels of human chorionic gonadotropin (hCG), a (developing) placenta-produced hormone of pregnancy. HCG finds its way into your bloodstream and urine almost immediately after an embryo begins implanting in the uterus, between 6 and 12 days after fertilization. As soon as hCG can be detected in your urine, you can (theoretically) get a positive reading. But there is a limit to how soon these HPTs can work—they're sensitive, but not always that sensitive. One week after conception there's hCG in your urine, but it's not enough for the HPT to pick up—which means that if you test seven days before your expected period, you're likely to get a false negative even if you're pregnant.

Just can't wait to pee on that stick? Some tests promise 60 percent accuracy four days before your expected period. Not a betting woman? Wait until the day your period is expected, and you'll have about a 90 percent chance of netting the correct result. Test a week later, and the accuracy rate jumps to 97 percent. Whenever you decide to take the testing plunge, the good news is that false positives are much less common than false negatives—which means that if your test is positive, you can be, too. The other good news: Because HPTs provide a very accurate diagnosis very early in pregnancy—earlier than you would probably consider consulting a physician or midwife—they can give you the opportunity to start taking optimum care of yourself within days of conception. Still, medical follow-up to the test is essential. If the result is positive, have it confirmed by a blood test and a complete prenatal checkup.

The blood test. The more sophisticated blood pregnancy test can detect pregnancy with virtually 100 percent accuracy as early as one week after conception (barring lab error), using just a few drops of blood. It can also help date the pregnancy by measuring the exact amount of hCG in the blood, since hCG values change as pregnancy progresses (see page 140 for more on hCG levels).

Many practitioners order both a urine and a blood test to be doubly certain of the diagnosis.

The medical exam. Though a medical exam can be performed to confirm the diagnosis of a pregnancy, with today's accurate HPTs and blood tests, the medical exam—which looks for physical signs of pregnancy such as enlargement of the uterus, color changes in the vagina and cervix, and a change in the texture of the cervix—is almost beside the point. Still, getting that first exam and beginning regular prenatal care isn't (see page 19).

A Faint Line

"When I took a home pregnancy test, it showed a really faint line. Am I pregnant?"

The only way a pregnancy test can give you a positive result is if your body has a detectable level of hCG running through it (or in this case, through your urine). And the only way that your body can have hCG running through it is if you're pregnant. Which means that if your test is showing a line, no matter how faint it is—you're pregnant.

Just why you're getting a faint line instead of that loud-and-clear line you were hoping for has a lot to do with the type of test you've used (some are much more sensitive than others) and how far along you are in your pregnancy (levels of hCG rise each day, so if you test early, there's only a little hCG to tap into).

To figure out just how sensitive your pregnancy test is, check out the packaging. Look for the milli-international units per liter (mIU/L) measurement, which will tell you the sensitivity of the test. The lower the number, the better (20 mIU/L will tell you you're pregnant sooner than a test with a 50 mIU/L sensitivity). Not surprisingly, the more

Testing for the Irregular

So your cycles don't exactly run on schedule? That'll make scheduling your testing date a lot trickier. After all, how can you test on the day that your period's expected if you're never sure when that day will come? Your best testing strategy if your periods are irregular is to wait the number of days equal to the longest cycle you've had in the last six months—and then test. If the result is negative and you still haven't gotten your period, repeat the test after a week (or after a few days if you just can't wait).

expensive tests usually have greater sensitivity.

Keep in mind, too, that the further along in your pregnancy you are, the higher your levels of hCG. If you're testing very early on in your pregnancy (as in a few days before your expected period or even a few days after your expected period), there might not be enough hCG in your system yet to generate a no-doubt-about-it line. Give it a couple of days, test again, and you'll be sure to see a line that'll erase your doubts once and for all.

No Longer Positive

"My first pregnancy test came back positive, but a few days later I took another one and it came back negative. And then I got my period. What's going on?"

It sounds like you may have experienced a chemical pregnancy, a pregnancy that ends practically before it even begins. In a chemical pregnancy, the egg is fertilized and begins to implant in the uterus, but for some reason it never completes implantation. Instead of turning into a viable pregnancy, it ends in a period. Though experts estimate that up to 70 percent of all conceptions are chemical, the vast majority of women who experience one don't even realize they've conceived (certainly in the days before home pregnancy tests, women didn't have a clue they were pregnant until much later). Often, a very early positive pregnancy test and then a late period (a few days to a week late) are the only signs of a chemical pregnancy, so if there's a downside to early home pregnancy testing, you've definitely experienced it.

Medically, a chemical pregnancy is more like a cycle in which a pregnancy never occurred than a true miscarriage. Emotionally, for women like you who tested early and got a positive result, it can be a very different story. Though it's not technically a pregnancy loss, the loss of the promise of a pregnancy can also be upsetting for both you and your spouse. Reading the information on coping with a pregnancy loss on page 576 can help you with your emotions.

If You're Not Pregnant...

If your pregnancy test is negative this time, but you'd very much like to become pregnant soon, start making the most of the preconception period by taking the steps outlined in Chapter 1. Good preconception preparation will help ensure the best possible pregnancy outcome when you do conceive.

And keep in mind the fact that conception did occur once for you means that it'll more than likely occur again soon, and with the happier end result of a healthy pregnancy.

A Negative Result

"I feel as if I'm pregnant, but the three tests I took came back negative. What should I do?"

If you're experiencing the symptoms of early pregnancy and feel, test or no test—or even three tests—that you're pregnant, act as though you are (by taking prenatal vitamins, avoiding alcoholic beverages, quitting smoking, eating well, and so on) until you find out definitely otherwise. Pregnancy tests aren't infallible, especially when they're taken very early. You may well know your own body better than a pee-on-a-stick test does. To find out if your hunch is more accurate than the tests, wait a week and then try again—your pregnancy might just be too early to call. Or ask your practitioner for a blood test, which is more sensitive to hCG than a urine test is.

It is possible, of course, to experience all of the signs and symptoms of early pregnancy and not be pregnant. After all, none of them alone—or even in combination—is absolute proof positive of pregnancy. If the tests continue to be negative but you still haven't gotten your period, be sure to check with your practitioner to rule out other biological causes of your symptoms. If those are ruled out as well, it's possible that your symptoms may have emotional roots. Sometimes, the mind can have a surprisingly powerful influence on the body, even generating pregnancy symptoms when there's no pregnancy, just a strong yearning for one (or fear of one).

Testing Smart

The home pregnancy test is probably the simplest test you'll ever take (you won't have to study for it—but you should read the package directions and follow them to get the most accurate results). The following tips may seem obvious, but in the excitement of the moment (Will I be? Won't I be?), you might forget a couple of things:

■ Depending on the brand, you'll either hold the test stick in your stream of urine for a few seconds or collect your urine in a cup and then dip the stick into it. Most tests prefer you use midstream urine because there's less chance of contamination that way: Urinate for a second or two, stop, hold it, and then put either the stick or the cup in position to catch the rest of the stream.

■ If you'll need to wait for the results, place the sample on a flat surface away from heat and in a place where it won't be disturbed. Read the test after the recommended waiting period; not waiting long enough—or waiting too long—can affect the result.

■ It isn't necessary to use your first-morning urine, but if you're testing early (i.e., before your period is due), you're more likely to get an accurate result if you haven't peed in the past four hours (because your urine will contain more concentrated levels of hCG).

■ Watch for the control indicator (ranging from a horizontal or vertical line to a filled-in circle, or a flashing control symbol in the digital tests) to let you know that the test is working.

■ Look carefully—and before you leap to any conclusions. Any line you see (pink or blue, positive sign, or digital readout), no matter how faint it is (or no matter how faint you feel), means there's hCG in your system— and a baby likely in your future. Congratulations—you're pregnant! If the result isn't positive, and your period still hasn't arrived, consider waiting a few days and testing again. It may have just been too soon to call.

Making the First Appointment

"The home pregnancy test I just took came back positive. When should I schedule the first visit with my doctor?"

Good prenatal care is one of the most important ingredients in making a healthy baby. So don't delay. As soon as you suspect you might be pregnant or have a positive home pregnancy test result, call your practitioner to schedule an appointment. Just how soon you'll be able to come in for that appointment may depend on office traffic and policy. Some practitioners will be able to fit you in right away, while some very busy offices may not be able to accommodate you for several weeks or even longer. At certain practitioners' offices, it's actually routine procedure to wait until a woman is six to eight weeks pregnant for that first official prenatal visit, though some offer a "pre-OB" visit to confirm a pregnancy as soon as you suspect you're expecting (or have the positive HPT results to prove it).

But even if your official prenatal care has to be postponed until midway through the first trimester, that doesn't mean you should put off taking care of yourself and your baby. Regardless of when you get in to see your practitioner, start acting pregnant as soon as you see that positive readout on the HPT. You're probably familiar with many of the basics (take your prenatal vitamins, cut out alcohol and smoking, eat well, and so on), but don't hesitate to call your practitioner's office if you have specific questions about how best to get with the pregnancy program. You may even be able to pick up a pregnancy packet ahead of time (many offices provide one, with advice on everything from diet do's and don'ts to prenatal vitamin recommendations to a list of medications you can safely take) to help fill in some of the blanks.

In a low-risk pregnancy, having the first prenatal visit early on isn't considered medically necessary, though the wait can be hard to take. If the waiting's making you unreasonably anxious, or if you feel you may be a high-risk case (because of a history of miscarriages or ectopic pregnancies, for instance), check with the office to see if you can come in earlier. (For more on what to expect from your first prenatal visit, see page 124.)

Your Due Date

"My practitioner has told me my due date, but how accurate is it?"

Life would be a lot simpler if you could be certain that your due date is actually the day you will deliver, but life isn't that simple very often. According to most studies, only 1 in 20 babies is actually born on his or her due date. Because a normal full-term pregnancy can last anywhere from 38 to 42 weeks, most are born within two weeks either way of that date—which

keeps most parents guessing right up to delivery day.

That's why the medical term for "due date" is EDD, or *estimated* date of delivery. The date your practitioner gives you is only an educated estimate. It is usually calculated this way: Subtract three months from the first day of your last menstrual period (LMP), then add seven days—that's your due date. For example, say your last period began on April 11. Count backward three months, which gets you to January, and then add seven days. Your due date would be January 18.

This dating system works well for women who have a fairly regular menstrual cycle. But if your cycle is irregular, the system may not work for you at all. Say you typically get your period every six to seven weeks and you haven't had one in three months. On testing, you find out you're pregnant. When did you conceive? Because a reliable EDD is important, you and your practitioner will have to try to come up with one. Even if you can't pinpoint conception or aren't sure when you last ovulated, there are clues that can help.

The very first clue is the size of your uterus, which will be noted when your initial internal pregnancy examination is performed. It should conform to your suspected stage of pregnancy. The second clue will be an early ultrasound that can more accurately date the pregnancy. (Note that not all women get an early ultrasound. Some practitioners perform them routinely, but others will only recommend one if your periods are irregular, if you have a history of miscarriages or pregnancy complications, or if the estimated due date can't be determined based on your LMP and physical exam). Later on, there are other milestones that will confirm your date: the first time the fetal heartbeat is heard (at about 9 to 12 weeks with a Doppler), when the first flutter of life is felt (at about 16 to 22 weeks), and the height of the fundus (the top of the uterus) at each visit (for example, it will reach the navel at about week 20). These clues will be helpful but still not definitive. Only your baby knows for sure when his or her birth date will be . . . and baby's not telling.

Choosing and Working with Your Practitioner

We all know it takes two to conceive a baby, but it takes a minimum of three—mother, father, and at least one health-care professional—to make that transition from fertilized egg to delivered infant a safe and successful one. Assuming you and your spouse have already taken care of conception, the next challenge you both face is selecting that third member of your pregnancy team and making sure it's a selection you can live with—and labor with. (Of course, you can make this selection even before you conceive.)

Obstetrician? Family Practitioner? Midwife?

Where to begin your search for the perfect practitioner to help guide you through your pregnancy and beyond? First, you'll have to give some thought to what kind of medical credentials would best meet your needs.

The obstetrician. Are you looking for a practitioner who is trained to handle every conceivable medical aspect of pregnancy, labor, delivery, and the postpartum period—from the most obvious question to the most obscure complication? Then you'll want to look to an obstetrician-gynecologist. Ob-gyns not only provide complete obstetrical care, they can also take care of all your nonpregnancy female health needs (Pap smears, contraception, breast exams, and so on). Some also offer general medical care and thus can act as your primary physician as well.

If yours is a high-risk pregnancy, you will very likely need and want to seek out an ob-gyn. You may even want to find a specialist's specialist, an obstetrician who specializes in high-risk pregnancies and is certified in maternal-fetal medicine. Even if your pregnancy looks pretty routine, you may still want to select an obstetrician for your care—more than 90 percent of women do. If you've been seeing an ob-gyn you like, respect, and feel comfortable with for your gynecological care, there may be no reason to switch now that you're pregnant. If you haven't been seeing an ob-gyn, or you're not sure the one you've been seeing is the practitioner you want to spend your pregnancy with, it's time to start shopping around.

The family physician. Like the general practitioner of years ago, today's family physician (FP) provides one-stop medical service. Unlike the obstetrician, who has had postmedical school training in women's reproductive and general health only, the FP has had training in primary care, maternal care, and pediatric care after receiving an MD.

Birthing Choices

From start (when to conceive) to finish (how to deliver), pregnancy these days is full of personal choices. When it comes to birthing that baby, the array of options is dizzying, even in a hospital setting. Leave the hospital and there's yet more to select from.

Though your delivery preferences shouldn't be your only criteria in picking a practitioner, they should certainly be on the table. The following are among those birthing options that you can consider these days. Ask your potential candidates about their feelings on any of these—or any others—that appeal to you (keeping in mind that no firm birthing decisions can be made until further into your pregnancy, and many can't be finalized until the delivery itself):

Birthing rooms. The availability of birthing rooms in most hospitals makes it possible for you to stay in the same bed from labor through recovery (instead of laboring in one room and then being wheeled into a delivery room when you're ready to push), sometimes even for your entire hospital stay, and for your baby to remain at your side from birth on. Best of all, birthing rooms are cozy and comfy.

Some birthing rooms are used just for labor, delivery, and recovery (LDRs). If you're in an LDR, you (and your baby, if he or she is rooming in) will be moved from the birthing room to a postpartum room after an hour or so of largely uninterrupted family togetherness. If you're lucky enough to be in a hospital that offers LDRP (labor, delivery, recovery, postpartum) rooms, you won't have to do any moving at all. You and baby—and in some cases, dad and even siblings—will be able to stay put from check-in to check-out.

Most birthing rooms boast an "at-home-in-the-hospital" look, with soft lighting, rocking chairs, pretty wallpaper, soothing pictures on the wall, curtains on the windows, and beds that look more as if they came out of a showroom than a hospital supply catalog. Though the rooms are thoroughly equipped for low-risk births and even unexpected emergencies, medical equipment is usually stowed out of sight behind the doors of armoires and other bedroom-type cabinetry. The back of the birthing bed can be raised to support the mom in a squatting or semi-squatting position (a squatting bar can often be attached if desired), and the foot of the bed snaps off to make way for the birthing attendants. After delivery, a change of linens, a few flipped switches, and presto, you're back in bed. Many hospitals and birthing centers also offer showers and/or whirlpool tubs in or adjacent to the birthing rooms, both of which can offer hydrotherapy relief during labor. Tubs for water birth are also available in some birthing centers and hospitals. (See page 24 for more on water birth.) Many birthing rooms have sofas for your support team and/or other guests to hang out on—and sometimes even a pullout for your coach to spend the night on.

Birthing rooms at some hospitals are available only for women who are at low risk for childbirth complications; if you don't fit that profile, you may have no choice but to go to a traditional labor and delivery room, where more technology is readily at hand. And a C-section (cesarean delivery) is always performed in an all-business operating room (no homey look there). Fortunately, though, with the increasing availability of birthing rooms for most women, odds are great that you'll be able to experience unrushed, family-friendly, noninterventionist labor and delivery within a traditional hospital setting.

Birthing centers. Birthing centers, usually freestanding facilities (although they may be attached to—or even located in—a hospital), offer a homey, low-tech, and personalized place for childbirth. You'll be able to get all your prenatal care at a freestanding center—from practitioner visits to childbirth education and breastfeeding classes (in-hospital centers are usually only for childbirth itself). In general, most birthing centers offer the most comfortable childbirth amenities—from nicely decorated private rooms with soft lighting to showers and whirlpool tubs. A kitchen may also be available for family members to use. Birthing centers are usually staffed by midwives, but many have on-call obstetricians; others are located just minutes from a hospital in case any emergencies arise. And though birthing centers generally do not use interventions such as fetal monitoring, they do have medical equipment on hand, including IVs, oxygen for the mother and the infant, and infant resuscitators so emergency care can be initiated (if required) while you're waiting for a transfer to the nearby hospital. Still, only women with low-risk pregnancies are good candidates for delivery in birthing centers. Something else to consider: Unmedicated childbirth is the focus in a birthing center, and though mild narcotic medications are available, epidurals aren't. If you end up wanting an epidural, you'll have to be taken to the hospital.

Leboyer (or gentle) births. When the French obstetrician Frederick Leboyer first offered up his theory of childbirth without violence, the medical community was skeptical. Today, many of the procedures he proposed, aimed at making a newborn's arrival in the world more tranquil, are routine. Babies are often delivered in birthing rooms with-

out the bright lights once deemed necessary, on the theory that gentle lighting can make the transition from the dark uterus to the bright outside world more gradual and less jolting. Upending and slapping the newborn is no longer routine anywhere; less aggressive procedures are preferred for establishing breathing when it doesn't start on its own. In some hospitals, the umbilical cord isn't cut immediately; instead, this last physical bond between mother and baby remains intact while they get to know each other for the first time (and until it stops pulsing). And though the warm bath Leboyer recommended for soothing the new arrival and smoothing the transition from a watery home to a dry one isn't common, being put immediately into mommy's arms is.

In spite of the growing acceptance of many Leboyer theories, a full-on Leboyer birth—with soft music, soft lights, and a warm bath for baby—isn't widely available. If you're interested in one, though, ask about it when you're interviewing practitioners.

Home birth. For some women, the idea of being hospitalized when they aren't sick just isn't the ticket. If that sounds like you—or if you just believe that life should begin at home—you might want to consider a home birth. The upside is obvious: Your newborn arrives amid family and friends in a warm and loving atmosphere, and you're able to labor and deliver in the comfort and privacy of your own home, without hospital protocols and personnel getting in the way. The downside is that if something unexpectedly goes wrong, the facilities for an emergency cesarean or resuscitation of the newborn will not be close at hand.

According to the American College of Nurse-Midwives, if you are considering a home birth, you should meet these guidelines:

(continued on next page)

(continued from previous page)

- Be in a low-risk category—no hypertension, diabetes, or other chronic medical problems, and no history of a previous difficult labor and/or delivery.

- Be attended by a physician or a CNM. If you're using a CNM, a consulting physician should be available, preferably one who has seen you during pregnancy and who has worked with the nurse-midwife before.

- Have transportation available and live within 30 miles of a hospital, if the roads are good and traffic's not an issue, or 10 miles if these standards aren't met.

Water birth. The concept of delivering underwater to simulate the environment of the womb is not widely used in the medical community, but it is more accepted among midwives. In a water birth, the baby is eased from the warm, wet womb into another warm, wet environment, offering familiar comfort after the stresses of delivery. The baby is pulled out of the water and placed in the mother's arms immediately after birth.

And since breathing doesn't begin until the baby is exposed to the air, there is virtually no risk of drowning. Water births can be done at home, in birthing centers, and in some hospitals. Many spouses join the mother in the tub or portable pool, often holding her from behind to provide support.

Most women with low-risk pregnancies can choose a water birth, as long as they can find a willing practitioner and hospital (birthing centers may be more likely to offer the option). If you're in a high-risk category, however, it's probably not a wise option, and it's unlikely you'll find even a midwife who will allow you to try a water birth.

Even if you don't find the idea of a water birth inviting—or don't have the option of one open to you—you might welcome the opportunity to labor in a whirlpool tub or regular bath. Most women find that the water not only provides relaxation, pain relief, and freedom from gravity's pull, but it even facilitates the progression of labor. Some hospitals and most birthing centers offer tubs in the birthing rooms. For more information on water births, go to gentlebirthchoices.org or waterbirth.org.

If you decide on an FP, he or she can serve as your internist, obstetrician-gynecologist, and, when the time comes, pediatrician. Ideally, an FP will become familiar with the dynamics of your family and will be interested in all aspects of your health, not just your obstetric ones. If complications occur, an FP may send you to an obstetrician but remain involved in your care for comforting continuity.

The certified nurse-midwife. If you're looking for a practitioner whose emphasis is on you the person rather than you

the patient, who will take extra time to talk to you not only about your physical condition but also your emotional well-being, who will be more likely to offer you nutritional advice and breastfeeding support, and who will be oriented toward the "natural" in childbirth, then a certified nurse-midwife (CNM) may be right for you (though, of course, many physicians fit that profile, too). A CNM is a medical professional, a registered nurse who has completed graduate-level programs in midwifery and is certified by the American College of Nurse-Midwives. A CNM is thoroughly trained to care for women with low-risk pregnancies and to deliver uncomplicated births. In some cases, a CNM may provide continuing routine gynecological care and, sometimes, newborn care. Most midwives work in hospital settings, others deliver at birthing centers and/or do home births. Though CNMs have the right in most states to offer epidurals and other forms of pain relief, as well as to prescribe labor-inducing medications, a birth attended by a CNM is less likely to include such interventions. On average, midwives have much lower cesarean delivery rates than physicians, as well as higher rates of VBAC (vaginal birth after cesarean) success—but that may be due in part to the fact that they only care for women with low-risk pregnancies, which are less likely to take a turn for the complicated or result in surgical births. Studies show that for low-risk pregnancies, deliveries by CNMs are as safe as those by physicians. Something else to keep in mind: The cost of prenatal care with a CNM is usually less than that of an ob-gyn.

If you choose a certified nurse-midwife (about 8 percent of expectant mothers do), be sure to select one who is both certified and licensed (all 50 states license nurse-midwives). Most CNMs use a physician as a backup in case of complications; many practice with one or with a group that includes several. For more information about CNMs, look online at midwife.org.

Direct-entry midwives. These midwives are trained without first becoming nurses, though they may hold degrees in other health care areas. Direct-entry midwives are more likely than CNMs to do home births, though some also deliver babies in birthing centers. Those who are evaluated and certified through the North American Registry of Midwives (NARM) are called certified professional midwives (CPMs); other direct-entry

midwives are not certified. Licensing for direct-entry midwives is also currently offered in certain states; in some of those states, the services of a CPM are reimbursable through Medicaid and private health plans. In other states, direct-entry midwives cannot practice legally. For more information, call the Midwives Alliance of North America at (888) 923-6262 or check their website at mana.org.

Types of Practice

You've settled on an obstetrician, a family practitioner, or a nurse-midwife. Next you've got to decide which kind of medical practice you would be most comfortable with. Here are the most common kinds of practices and their possible advantages and disadvantages:

Solo medical practice. In such a practice, a doctor works alone, using another doctor to cover when he or she is away or otherwise unavailable. An obstetrician or a family practitioner might be in solo practice; a nurse-midwife, in almost all states, must work in a collaborative practice with a physician. The major advantage of a solo practice is that you see the same practitioner at each visit. This way, you get to know and, ideally, feel more comfortable with this person before delivery. The major disadvantage is that if your practitioner is not available, a backup you don't know may deliver your baby (although arranging to meet the covering physician or midwife in advance helps remedy this potential drawback). A solo practice may also be a problem if, midway in the pregnancy, you find you're not really crazy about the practitioner. If that happens and you decide to switch practitioners, you'll have to start from scratch again searching for one who suits your needs.

Partnership or group medical practice. In this type of practice, two or more doctors in the same specialty care jointly for patients, often seeing them on a rotating basis (though you usually get to stick with your favorite through most of your pregnancy and only start rotating toward the end of your pregnancy, when you're going to the office weekly). Again, you can find both obstetricians and family doctors in this type of practice. The advantage of a group practice is that by seeing a different doctor each time, you'll get to know them all—which means that when those labor pains are coming strong and fast, there's sure to be a familiar face in the room with you. The disadvantage is that you may not like all of the doctors in the practice equally, and you usually won't be able to choose the one who attends your child's birth. Also, hearing different points of view from the various partners may be an advantage or a disadvantage, depending on whether you find it reassuring or unsettling.

Combination practice. A group practice that includes one or more obstetricians and one or more nurse-midwives is considered a combination practice. The advantages and disadvantages are similar to those of any group practice. There is the added advantage of having at some of your visits the extra time and attention a midwife may offer and at others the extra medical know-how of a physician's extensive training and expertise. You may have the option of a midwife-coached delivery, plus assurance that if a problem develops, a physician you know is in the wings.

Maternity center– or birthing center–based practice. In these practices, certified nurse-midwives provide the bulk of the care, and physicians are on call as needed. Some maternity centers are based in hospitals with special birthing rooms, and others are separate facilities. All maternity centers provide care for low-risk patients only.

The advantage of this type of practice is obviously great for those women who prefer certified midwives as their primary practitioners. A potential disadvantage is that if a complication arises during pregnancy, you may have to switch to a physician and start developing a relationship all over again. Or, if a complication arises during labor or delivery, you may need to be delivered by the doctor on call, who may be a complete stranger. And finally, if you are delivering at a freestanding maternity center and complications arise, you may have to be transported to the nearest hospital for emergency care. A big advantage is likely to be the bottom line: CNMs and birthing centers usually charge less than physicians and hospitals.

Independent certified nurse-midwife practice. In the states in which they are permitted to practice independently, CNMs offer women with low-risk pregnancies the advantage of personalized pregnancy care and a low-tech natural delivery (sometimes at home, but more often in birthing centers or hospitals). An independent CNM should have a physician available for consultation as needed and on call in case of emergency—during pregnancy, childbirth, and postpartum. Care by an independent CNM is covered by most health plans, though only some insurers cover midwife-attended home births or births in a facility other than a hospital.

Finding a Candidate

When you have a good idea of the kind of practitioner you want and the type of practice you prefer, where can you find some likely candidates? The following are all good sources:

Division of Labor

Though not yet common practice nationwide, there's a trend that might be coming to a hospital (and an ob practice) near you. Some obstetricians, tired of running from long office hours to long overnights in the hospital delivering babies—and concerned that fatigue can affect the quality of care they provide—are looking for a better way. Enter the ob hospitalists, also known as laborists—obs who work exclusively in the hospital, only attending labors and delivering babies. These laborists don't have an office and don't follow patients through pregnancy.

If your practitioner tells you there's going to be a laborist at your birth, don't worry. But do take some steps to make sure you're comfortable with the arrangement. First, ask your practitioner if he or she and the hospital laborists have worked closely together in the past (and make sure their philosophies and protocols are similar).

You might also want to call the hospital to ask if you can meet the staff docs before labor, so that you're not being attended by a complete stranger during childbirth. Make sure, too, that you arrive at the hospital with extra copies of your birth plan (if you have one) to hand out, so whoever is attending you is familiar with your wishes even if he or she isn't familiar with you.

If you're uncomfortable with the whole arrangement, think about switching practices sooner rather than later. Remember, though, that if you're with a multiple-doc practice already, there's a good chance your "regular" ob won't be on call the day you go into labor anyway. Keep in mind, too, that because hospitalists focus solely on deliveries, they're extra-prepared to give the best possible care during labor. And extra-rested, also, because they work on shifts instead of around the clock.

- Your gynecologist or family practitioner (if he or she doesn't do deliveries) or your internist, assuming you're happy with his or her style of practice. (Doctors tend to recommend others with philosophies similar to their own.)

- Friends or coworkers who have had babies recently and whose personalities and childbearing philosophies are similar to yours.

- An obstetrical nurse who practices locally.

- The local medical society, which can give you a list of names of physicians who deliver babies, along with information on their medical training,

specialties, special interests, type of practice, and board certification.

- The American Medical Association (ama-assn.org) can help you search for a doctor in your area.

- The American College of Obstetricians and Gynecologists Physician Directory has the names of obstetrician-gynecologists and maternal-fetal specialists. Go to acog.org, or call 202-638-5577.

- The American College of Nurse-Midwives if you're looking for a CNM. Go to acnm.org or mybirthteam.com, or call 240-485-1800.

- The local La Leche League, especially if you're strongly interested in breastfeeding.

- A nearby hospital with facilities that are important to you—for example, birthing rooms with whirlpool tubs, rooming-in for both baby and dad, or a neonatal intensive care unit— or a local maternity or birthing center. Ask them for the names of attending physicians.

- If all else fails, check Yellow Book online or the phone book, under "Physicians." Look for the headings "Obstetrics and Gynecology," "Maternal-Fetal Medicine," or "Family Practice."

If your health insurance company hands you a list of practitioners, try to check them out with friends, acquaintances, or another physician to find the one in the bunch that seems right for you. If that's not possible, visit and meet with several of the candidates personally. In most cases, you should be able to find someone who is compatible. If not, finances permitting, you may want to see if you can switch plans.

Making Your Selection

Once you've secured a prospective practitioner's name, call to make an appointment for a consult. Go prepared with questions that will enable you to sense if your philosophies are in sync and if your personalities mesh comfortably. Don't expect that you'll agree on everything—that doesn't happen even in the most productive of partnerships. Be observant, too, and try to read between the lines at the interview (is the doctor or midwife a good listener? A patient explainer? Does he or she seem to take your emotional concerns as seriously as your physical ones?). Now's the time to find out this candidate's positions on issues that you feel strongly about: unmedicated child-birth versus pain relief as needed in childbirth, breastfeeding, induction of labor, use of fetal monitoring or routine IVs, cesarean deliveries, or anything else that's important to you. Knowledge is power—and knowing how your practitioner practices will help ensure there won't be unpleasant surprises later.

Almost as important as what the interview reveals about your potential practitioner is what you reveal about yourself. Speak up and let your true patient persona shine through. You'll be able to judge from the practitioner's response whether he or she will be comfortable with—and responsive to—you, the patient.

You will also want to know something about the hospital or birthing center the practitioner is affiliated with. Does it provide features that are important to you—for example, plenty of LDR or LDRP rooms, breastfeeding support, a tub to labor in, the latest fetal monitoring equipment, a neonatal intensive care unit? Is there flexibility about procedures that concern you (say, routine IVs)? Are siblings allowed in the birthing rooms? Is extended family allowed during a surgical delivery?

Before you make a final decision, think about whether your potential

Pregnant and Uncovered

If you're expecting and uninsured, you're probably more concerned with figuring out how you're going to be able to afford prenatal care than you are with who's going to provide it. For tips that can help you get the care you and your baby need, see page 56.

practitioner inspires trust. Pregnancy is one of the most important journeys you'll ever make; you'll want a copilot in whom you have complete faith.

Making the Most of the Patient-Practitioner Partnership

Choosing the right practitioner is only the first step. The next step is nurturing a good working partnership. Here's how:

- Tell the whole truth, and nothing but the truth. Give your practitioner an accurate and complete general, gynecological, and obstetrical medical history. Fess up about an eating disorder you've battled or eating habits that are otherwise unhealthy. Speak up about any drugs—prescription or over-the-counter (including herbal), legal or illegal, medicinal or recreational, including alcohol and tobacco—that you are currently taking or have taken recently, as well as about any past or present illnesses or surgeries. Remember, what you tell your doctor is confidential; no one else will know.

- When a question or concern that doesn't require an immediate call comes up between visits, write it down and take it to your next appointment. (It may help to keep your PDA handy or to keep pads in convenient places—the refrigerator door, your purse, your desk at work, your bedside table—so that you'll always be within jotting distance of one.) That way you can be sure that you won't forget to ask all your questions and report all your symptoms (you will if you don't write them down; as you'll soon discover, pregnant women are

notoriously forgetful). Along with your list of questions, bring a pen and pad (or your PDA or the *What to Expect Pregnancy Journal and Organizer*) to each office visit so you can record your practitioner's recommendations. If your practitioner doesn't offer up all the information you'll need (side effects of treatments, when to stop taking a medication if one's prescribed, when to check back about a problem situation), ask for it before you leave so there's no confusion once you get home. If possible, quickly review your notes with the practitioner to be sure you've written down just what the doctor (or midwife) ordered.

- When in doubt, call. A symptom has you freaked? A medication or treatment seems to have triggered an adverse reaction? Don't just sit there worrying. Pick up the phone and call your practitioner (or e-mail, if your practitioner prefers to answer non-emergency questions online). Though you won't want to call or e-mail at every pelvic twinge, never hesitate to check in about questions that can't be answered in a book such as this one, and that you feel can't wait until the next visit. Don't be afraid that your concerns will sound silly—if it has you worried, it's not silly. Besides, doctors and midwives expect expectant moms to ask lots of questions, especially if they're first timers. When you do pick up the phone or compose that e-mail, be prepared to be very specific about your symptoms. If you're experiencing pain, be precise about its location, duration, quality (is it sharp, dull, crampy?), and severity. If possible, explain what makes it worse or better—changing positions, for example. If you have a vaginal discharge, describe its color (bright red, dark red, brownish, pinkish, yellowish), when it started, and how heavy it is. Also report accompanying symptoms, such as fever, nausea, vomiting, chills, or diarrhea. (See When to Call Your Practitioner, page 138.)

- Keep up to date. Read those parenting magazines and visit those pregnancy websites, by all means. But also realize that you can't believe everything you read, especially since the media often report medical advances before they are proven safe and effective through controlled studies—or report worrisome pregnancy warnings based on preliminary data that's yet to be backed up. When you read (or hear) about something new in obstetrics, ask your practitioner—usually your best information resource—for his or her take on it.

- When you hear or read something that doesn't correspond to what your practitioner has told you, don't keep it to yourself. Ask for an opinion on what you've heard—not in a challenging way, just so you can get your facts straight.

- If you suspect that your practitioner may be mistaken about something (for example, okaying intercourse when you have a history of incompetent cervix), speak up. You can't assume that he or she, even with your chart in hand, will always remember every aspect of your medical and personal history. As a partner in your own health care, and one who knows your body like the back of your hand (and then some), you share the responsibility of making sure mistakes aren't made.

- Ask for explanations. Find out what the potential side effects of a prescribed medication are, and whether there's a nondrug alternative. Be

So You Won't Forget

Because there'll be times when you'll want to do a little writing with your reading, jot down a symptom so you can share it with your doctor, make a note of this week's weight so you can compare it to next week's, record what needs recording so you'll remember what needs remembering—you'll find plenty of space in the *The What to Expect Pregnancy Journal and Organizer* for all your note taking.

sure you know why a test is ordered, what it will involve, what its risks are, and how and when you'll learn the results.

- Put it in writing. If you find your practitioner doesn't seem to have time to respond to all your questions or concerns, try providing a written list. If it isn't possible for you to get a complete response at the visit, ask if you can get the answers you need through a follow-up phone call or e-mail or a longer visit next time.

- Follow your practitioner's recommendations on appointment schedules, weight gain, bed rest, exercise, medication, vitamins, and so on, unless you have a good reason why you feel you shouldn't or can't (in which case, talk it over with your practitioner before you follow your instincts instead).

- Remember that good self-care is a vital component in good prenatal care. So take the best care of yourself that you can, getting enough rest and exercise, eating well, and steering clear of alcohol, tobacco, and other nonprescribed drugs and medications once you find out you're pregnant, or better still, once you start trying to conceive.

- If you have a gripe about anything—from regularly being kept waiting too long to not getting answers to your questions—speak up, in as nice a way as possible. Letting a problem fester can get in the way of a productive practitioner-patient relationship.

- Insurance companies often serve as mediators between patient and practitioner when there is a conflict or complaint. If you have a problem with your practitioner that good com-munication isn't solving, contact your health organization for help.

If you feel you can't follow your practitioner's instructions or go along with a recommended course of treatment, it might be because you're just not on board with the person you've chosen to care for you and your baby during your pregnancy, labor, and delivery. In such a case—or if, for some other reason, your relationship with your practitioner just isn't working—consider looking for a replacement (assuming that's financially feasible and your medical plan permits it).

CHAPTER 3

Your Pregnancy Profile

HE TEST RESULTS ARE BACK; the news has (sort of) sunk in: You're having a baby! Excitement is growing (along with that uterus of yours), and so is your list of questions. Many, no doubt, have to do with those wild and crazy symptoms you might already be experiencing (more on those later). But many others may have to do with your personal pregnancy profile. What's a pregnancy profile? It's a compilation of your gynecological, general medical, and obstetrical (if you're not a first timer) histories—in other words, your pregnancy backstory. You'll be discussing this backstory (which can actually have a lot of impact on the pregnancy story that's about to unfold) with your practitioner at your first prenatal visit. In the meantime, this chapter can help you take stock of your pregnancy profile and figure out how it may affect—or may not affect—your nine months of baby making.

This Book's for You

As you read *What to Expect When You're Expecting,* you'll notice many references to traditional family relationships—to "wives," "husbands," "spouses." These references are not meant to exclude expectant mothers (and their families) who may be somewhat "untraditional"—for example, those who are single, who have same-sex partners, or who have chosen not to marry their live-in partners. Rather, these terms are a way of avoiding phrases (for instance, "your husband or significant other") that are more inclusive but also a mouthful to read. Please mentally edit out any phrase that doesn't fit and replace it with one that's right for you and your situation.

Keep in mind that much of this chapter may not apply to you—that's because your pregnancy profile (like the baby you're expecting) is unique. Read what fits your profile and skip what doesn't.

Your Gynecological History

Birth Control During Pregnancy

"I got pregnant while using birth control pills. I kept taking them for over a month because I had no idea I was pregnant. Will this affect my baby?"

Ideally, once you stop using oral contraceptives, you'd have at least one normally occurring menstrual cycle before you tried to become pregnant. But conception doesn't always wait for ideal conditions, and occasionally a woman becomes pregnant while taking the Pill. In spite of warnings you've probably read on the package insert, there's no reason for concern. There's just no good evidence of an increased risk to a baby when mom has conceived while on oral contraceptives. Need more reassurance? Talk the situation over with your practitioner—you're sure to find it.

"I conceived while using a condom with spermicides and kept using spermicides before I knew I was pregnant. Should I be worried about birth defects?"

No need to worry if you got pregnant while using a condom or diaphragm with spermicides, a spermicide-coated condom, or just plain spermicides. The reassuring news is that no known link exists between spermicides and birth defects. In fact, the most recent and most convincing studies have found no increase in the incidence of problems even with the repeated use of spermicides in early pregnancy. So relax and enjoy your pregnancy, even if it did come a little unexpectedly.

"I've been using an IUD as birth control and just discovered that I'm pregnant. Will I be able to have a healthy pregnancy?"

Getting pregnant while using birth control is always a little unsettling (wasn't that why you were using birth control in the first place?), but it definitely happens. The odds of its happening with an IUD are pretty low—about 1 in 1,000, depending on the type of device used, how long it's been in place, and whether or not it has been properly inserted.

Having beaten the odds and managed conception with an IUD in place leaves you with two options, which you should talk over with your practitioner as soon as possible: leaving the IUD in place or having it taken out. Which of these options is best in your situation will depend on whether or not your practitioner can—on examination—see the removal cord protruding from your cervix. If the cord isn't visible, the pregnancy has a very good chance of proceeding uneventfully with the IUD in place. It will simply be pushed up against the wall of the uterus by the expanding amniotic sac surrounding the baby and, during childbirth, it will usually deliver with the placenta. If, however, the IUD string is visible early in pregnancy, the risk of infection developing is increased. In that case, chances of a safe and successful pregnancy are greater if the IUD is removed as soon as feasible, once conception is confirmed. If it isn't removed, there is a significant chance that the fetus will spontaneously miscarry; the risk drops to only 20 percent when it is removed. If that doesn't sound reassuring, keep in mind that the rate of miscarriage in all known pregnancies is estimated to be about 15 to 20 percent.

If the IUD is left in during the first trimester, be especially alert for bleeding, cramping, or fever because having an IUD in place puts you at higher risk for early pregnancy complications. Notify your practitioner of such symptoms right away.

Fibroids

"I've had fibroids for several years, and they've never caused me any problems. Will they, now that I'm pregnant?"

Chances are your fibroids won't stand between you and an uncomplicated pregnancy. In fact, most often these small nonmalignant growths on the inner walls of the uterus don't affect a pregnancy at all.

Sometimes, a woman with fibroids notices abdominal pressure or pain. If you do, report it to your practitioner, though it usually isn't anything to worry about. Bed rest for four or five days along with the use of safe pain relievers (ask your practitioner to recommend one) usually brings relief.

Very occasionally, fibroids can slightly increase the risk of such complications as abruption (separation) of the placenta, preterm birth, and breech birth, but these minimal risks can be reduced even further with the right precautions. Discuss the fibroids with your physician so you can find out more about the condition in general and the risks, if any, in your particular case. If your practitioner suspects that the fibroids could interfere with a safe vaginal delivery, he or she may opt to deliver by C-section. In most cases, however, even a large fibroid will move out of the baby's way as the uterus expands during pregnancy.

"I had a couple of fibroids removed a few years ago. Will that affect my pregnancy?"

In most cases, surgery for the removal of small uterine fibroid tumors (particularly if the surgery was performed laparoscopically) doesn't affect a subsequent pregnancy. Extensive surgery for large fibroids could, however, weaken the uterus enough so that it wouldn't be able to handle labor. If, after reviewing your surgical records, your practitioner decides this might be true of your uterus, a C-section will be planned. Become familiar with the signs of early labor in case contractions begin before the planned surgery (see page 358), and have a plan in place for getting to the hospital quickly if you do go into labor.

Endometriosis

"After years of suffering with endometriosis, I'm finally pregnant. Will I have problems with my pregnancy?"

Endometriosis is typically associated with two challenges: difficulty in conceiving and pain. Becoming pregnant means that you've overcome the first of those challenges (congratulations!). And the good news gets even better. Being pregnant may actually help with the second challenge.

The symptoms of endometriosis, including pain, do improve during pregnancy. This seems to be due to hormonal changes. When ovulation takes a hiatus, the endometrial implants generally become smaller and less tender. Improvement is greater in some women than in others. Many women are symptom free during the entire pregnancy; others may feel increasing discomfort as the fetus grows and begins packing a stronger punch, particularly if those punches and kicks reach tender areas. Fortunately, however, having endometriosis doesn't seem to raise any risks during pregnancy or childbirth (though if you've had uterine surgery, your practitioner will probably opt to deliver via C-section).

The less happy news is that pregnancy only provides a respite from the symptoms of endometriosis, not a cure. After pregnancy and nursing (and sometimes earlier), the symptoms usually return.

Colposcopy

"A year before I got pregnant, I had a colposcopy and cervical biopsy performed. Is my pregnancy at risk?"

A colposcopy is usually performed only after a routine Pap smear shows some irregular cervical cells. The simple procedure involves the use of a special microscope to better visualize the vagina and cervix. If abnormal cells are noticed on a Pap smear, as they probably were in your case, your physician performs a cervical, or cone, biopsy (in which tissue samples are taken from the suspicious area of the cervix and sent to the lab for further evaluation), cryosurgery (during which the abnormal cells are frozen), or a loop electrocautery excision procedure (LEEP, during which the affected cervical tissue is cut away using a painless

electrical current). The good news is that the vast majority of women who have had such procedures are able to go on to have normal pregnancies. Some women, however, depending on how much tissue was removed during the procedure, may be at increased risk for some pregnancy complications, such as incompetent cervix and preterm delivery. Be sure your prenatal practitioner is aware of your cervical history so that your pregnancy can be more closely monitored.

If abnormal cells are noted during your first prenatal visit, your practitioner may opt to perform a colposcopy, but biopsies or further procedures are usually delayed until after the baby is born.

HPV (Human Papillomavirus)

"Can having genital HPV affect my pregnancy?"

Genital HPV is the most common sexually transmitted virus in the United States, affecting more than 75 percent of sexually active people, yet most of those who become infected with it never know. That's because most of the time, HPV causes no obvious symptoms and usually resolves on its own within six to ten months.

There are some times, however, when HPV does cause symptoms. Some strains cause cervical cell irregularities (detected on a Pap smear); other strains can cause genital warts (in appearance they can vary from a barely visible lesion to a soft, velvety "flat" bump or a cauliflower-like growth; colors range from pale to dark pink) that will show up in and on the vagina, vulva, and rectum. Though usually painless, genital warts may occasionally burn, itch, or even bleed. In most cases, the warts clear on their own within a couple of months.

Other STDs and Pregnancy

Not surprisingly, most STDs can affect pregnancy. Fortunately, most are easily diagnosed and treated safely, even during pregnancy. But because women are often unaware of being infected, the Centers for Disease Control and Prevention (CDC) recommends that all pregnant women be tested early in pregnancy for at least the following STDs: chlamydia, gonorrhea, trichomoniasis, hepatitis B, HIV, and syphilis.

Keep in mind that STDs don't happen just to one group of people or only at a certain economic level. They can occur in women (and men) in every age group, of every race and ethnic background, at every income level, and among those living in small towns as well as in big cities. The major STDs include:

Gonorrhea. Gonorrhea has long been known to cause conjunctivitis, blindness, and serious generalized infection in a fetus delivered through an infected birth canal. For this reason, pregnant women are routinely tested for the disease, usually at their first prenatal visit. Sometimes, particularly in women at high risk for STDs, the test is repeated late in pregnancy. If infection with gonorrhea is found, it is treated immediately with antibiotics. Treatment is followed by another culture, to be sure the woman is infection free. As an added precaution, an antibiotic ointment is squeezed into the eyes of every newborn at birth. (This treatment can be delayed for as long as an hour—but no longer—if you want to have some unblurry eye-to-eye contact with your baby first.)

Syphilis. Because this disease can cause a variety of birth defects as well as stillbirth, testing is also routine at the first prenatal visit. Antibiotic treatment of infected pregnant women before the fourth month, when the infection usually begins to cross the placental barrier, almost always prevents harm to the fetus. The very good news is that mother-to-baby transmission of syphilis is down in recent years.

Chlamydia. There are more cases of chlamydia in this country than gonorrhea or syphilis, with the disease affecting sexually active women under 26 years old most often. Chlamydia is the most common infection passed from mother to fetus, and it is considered a potential risk to the fetus and a possible risk to mothers. Which is why chlamydia screening in pregnancy is a good idea, particularly if you have had multiple sexual partners in the past, increasing your chance of infection. Because about half the women with chlamydial infection experience no symptoms, it often goes undiagnosed if it's not tested for.

How does genital HPV affect a pregnancy? Luckily, it's unlikely to affect it at all. Some women, however, will find that pregnancy will affect their HPV, causing the warts to become more active. If that's the case with you, and if the warts don't seem to be clearing on their own, your practitioner may recommend treatment during pregnancy. The warts can be safely removed by freezing, electrical heat, or laser therapy, although in some cases, this treatment may be delayed until after delivery.

If you do have HPV, your practitioner will also want to check your cervix to make sure there are no cervical cell

Prompt treatment of chlamydia prior to or during pregnancy can prevent chlamydial infections (pneumonia, which fortunately is most often mild, and eye infection, which is occasionally severe) from being transmitted by the mother to the baby during delivery. Though the best time for treatment is prior to conception, administering antibiotics (usually azithromycin) to the pregnant infected mother can also be effective in preventing infant infection. The antibiotic ointment routinely used at birth protects the newborn from chlamydial, as well as gonorrheal, eye infection.

Trichomoniasis. The symptoms of this parasite-caused STD (also referred to as trichomonas infection, or "trich") are a greenish, frothy vaginal discharge with an unpleasant fishy smell and, often, itching. About half of those affected have no symptoms at all. Though the disease does not usually cause serious illness or pregnancy problems (or affect a baby whose mom is infected), the symptoms can be irritating. Generally, women are treated during pregnancy only if they're having symptoms.

HIV infection. It is becoming increasingly routine for pregnant women to be tested for HIV (human immunodeficiency virus), whether or not they have a prior history of high-risk behavior. Many states actually require doctors to offer HIV counseling and testing to pregnant women, and ACOG recommends that all pregnant women, regardless of risk, be tested. Infection in pregnancy by the HIV virus, which causes AIDS, is a threat not just to the expectant mother but to her baby as well. About 25 percent of babies born to untreated mothers will develop the infection (testing will confirm it in the first six months of life). Luckily, there is plenty of hope with the treatments that are now available. But before taking any action, anyone who tests HIV positive may want to consider a second test (tests are highly accurate but can sometimes be positive in someone who does not have the virus). If a second test is positive, then formal counseling about AIDS and the treatment options is absolutely imperative. Treating an HIV-positive mother with AZT (also known as zidovudine—ZDV—or Retrovir) or other antiretroviral drugs can dramatically reduce the risk of her passing the infection on to her child, apparently without any damaging side effects. Delivering by elective C-section (before contractions begin and before membranes rupture) can reduce the risk of transmission further.

If you suspect that you may have been infected with any STD, check with your practitioner to see if you've been tested; if you haven't, ask to be. If a test turns out to be positive, be sure that you—and your partner, if necessary—are treated. Treatment will protect not only your health but that of your baby.

irregularities. If abnormalities are found, any necessary cervical biopsies to remove the abnormal cells will likely be postponed until after your baby is delivered.

Because HPV is highly contagious, practicing safe sex and sticking with one partner is the best way to prevent reoccurrence. Though there is a vaccine available now to prevent HPV in women under 26, it's not recommended for use during pregnancy. If you started the vaccine course (it's given in a three-dose series) and then became pregnant before completing the series, you'll need to hold off on the remaining doses until after your baby is born.

Herpes

"I have genital herpes. Can my baby catch it from me?"

Having genital herpes during pregnancy is cause for caution but definitely not for alarm. In fact, the chances are excellent that your baby will arrive safe, sound, and completely unaffected by herpes, particularly if you and your practitioner take protective steps during pregnancy and delivery. Here's what you need to know.

First of all, infection in a newborn is quite rare. A baby has only a less than 1 percent chance of contracting the condition if the mother has a recurrent infection during pregnancy (that is, she's had herpes before). Second, though a primary infection (one that appears for the first time) early in pregnancy increases the risk of miscarriage and premature delivery, such infection is uncommon. Even for babies at greatest risk—those whose mothers have their first herpes outbreak as delivery nears (which in itself is rare because it's tested for routinely)—there is an up to 50 percent chance that they will escape infection. Finally, the disease, though still serious, seems to be somewhat milder in newborns these days than it was in the past.

So if you picked up your herpes infection before pregnancy, which is most likely, the risk to your baby is very low. And with good medical care it can be lowered still further.

To protect their babies, women who have a history of herpes and have recurrent herpes during pregnancy are usually given antiviral medications. Those who have active lesions at the onset of labor are usually delivered by cesarean. In the unlikely event a baby is infected, he or she will be treated with an antiviral drug.

After delivery, the right precautions can allow you to care for—and breastfeed—your baby without transmitting the virus, even during an active infection.

Signs and Symptoms of Genital Herpes

It is during a primary, or first, episode that genital herpes is most likely to be passed on to the fetus, so call your practitioner if you experience the following symptoms of infection: fever, headache, malaise, and achiness for two or more days, accompanied by genital pain, itching, pain when urinating, vaginal and urethral discharge, and tenderness in the groin, as well as lesions that blister and then crust over. Healing of the lesions generally takes place within two to three weeks, during which time the disease can still be transmitted.

Your Obstetrical History

In Vitro Fertilization (IVF)

"I conceived my baby through in vitro fertilization. How different will my pregnancy be?"

Some well-deserved congratulations on your IVF success! With all you've been through to get to this point, you've earned some smooth sailing—and happily, you're likely to get it. The fact that you conceived in a laboratory rather than in bed shouldn't affect your pregnancy all that much, at least once the first trimester is over. Early on, however, there will be some differences in your pregnancy and your care. Because a positive test doesn't necessarily mean that a pregnancy will be sustained, because trying again can be so emotionally and financially draining, and because it's not known right off how many of the test-tube embryos are going to develop into fetuses, the first six weeks of an IVF pregnancy are usually more nerve-wracking than most. In addition, if you've miscarried in previous tries, intercourse and other physical activities may be restricted. As an added precaution, the hormone progesterone will likely be prescribed to help support your developing pregnancy during the first two months.

But once this period is past, you can expect that your pregnancy will be pretty much like everyone else's—unless it turns out that you're carrying more than one fetus, as over 30 percent of IVF mothers do. If you are, see Chapter 16.

The Second Time Around

"This is my second pregnancy. How will it be different from the first?"

Since no two pregnancies are exactly alike, there's no predicting how different (or how similar) these nine months will be from the last. There are some generalities, however, about second and subsequent pregnancies that hold true at least some of the time (like all generalities, none will hold true all of the time):

- You'll probably "feel" pregnant sooner. Most second timers are more attuned to the early symptoms of pregnancy and more apt to recognize them. The symptoms themselves may vary from last time—you may have more or less morning sickness, indigestion, and other tummy troubles; you may be more tired (especially likely if you were able to nap in your first pregnancy but now barely have the chance to sit down) or less tired (perhaps because you're too busy to notice how tired you really are or because you're so used to being tired); you may have more urinary frequency or less (though it's likely to appear sooner).

Some symptoms that are typically less pronounced in second and subsequent pregnancies include food cravings and aversions, breast enlargement and sensitivity, and worry (since you've already been there, done that, and lived to tell about it, pregnancy is less likely to induce panic).

- You'll "look" pregnant sooner. Thanks to abdominal and uterine muscles that are more lax (there's no gentler way to put that), you're likely to "pop" much sooner than you did the first time. You may notice, too, that you'll carry differently than you did with baby number one. Baby number two (or three or four) is liable to be larger than your firstborn, so you may have more to carry around. Another potential result of those "loosened-up" abdominals: Backache and other pregnancy pains may be exacerbated.

- You'll probably feel movement sooner. Something else to thank those looser muscles for—chances are you'll be able to feel baby kicking much sooner this time around, possibly as early as 16 weeks (maybe sooner, maybe later). You're also more likely to know it when you feel it, having felt it before. Of course, if the last pregnancy left you with lots of extra abdominal padding that you haven't been able to shed, those first kicks might not be so easy to feel.

- You may not feel as excited. That's not to say you aren't thrilled to be expecting again. But you may notice that the excitement level (and that compulsion to tell everyone you pass in the street the good news) isn't quite as high. This is a completely normal reaction (again, you've been here before) and in no way reflects on your love for this baby. Keep in mind, too, that you're preoccupied (physically and emotionally) with the child who's already here.

- You will probably have an easier labor and a faster delivery. Here's the really good part about those laxer muscles. All that loosening up (particularly in the areas involved in childbirth), combined with the prior experience of your body, may help ensure a speedier exit for baby number two. Every phase of labor and delivery is likely to be shorter, with pushing time significantly reduced.

You may wonder how to tell baby number one about the new baby who's on the way. Realistic, empathetic, and age-appropriate preparation for your firstborn to make the life-changing transition from only child to older child should begin during pregnancy. For tips, see *What to Expect the First Year* and *What to Expect the Toddler Years.* Reading picture books such as *What to Expect When Mommy's Having a Baby* and *What to Expect When the New Baby Comes Home* to your child will also help with older sib preparations.

"I had a perfect first baby. Now that I'm pregnant again, I can't shake the fear that I won't be so lucky this time."

Your chances of hitting the baby jackpot once again are excellent—in fact, better still for already having a successful pregnancy under your reexpanding belt. Also, with each pregnancy you get the chance to up the odds even more, by accentuating all those pregnancy positives (good medical care, diet, exercise, and lifestyle choices).

Your Obstetrical History Repeating Itself

"My first pregnancy was very uncomfortable—I must have had every symptom in the book. Will I be that unlucky again?"

In general, your first pregnancy is a pretty good predictor of future pregnancies, all things being equal. So you are a little less likely to breeze comfortably through pregnancy than someone who already has. Still, there's always the hope that your luck will change for the better. All pregnancies, like all babies, are different. If, for example, morning sickness or food cravings had you down in your first pregnancy, they may be barely noticeable in the second (or vice versa). Though luck, genetic predisposition, and the fact that you've experienced certain symptoms before have a lot to do with how comfortable or uncomfortable this pregnancy will be, other factors—including some that are within your control—can alter the prognosis to some extent. The factors include:

General health. Being in good all-around physical condition gives you a better shot at having a comfortable pregnancy.

Weight gain. Gaining weight at a steady rate and keeping the gain within the recommended guidelines (see page 166) can improve your chances of escaping or minimizing such pregnancy miseries as hemorrhoids, varicose veins, stretch marks, backache, fatigue, indigestion, and shortness of breath.

Diet. It can't offer any guarantees, but eating well (see Chapter 5 to find out how) improves every pregnant woman's chances of having a healthier and more comfortable pregnancy. Not only can it up your odds of avoiding or minimizing the miseries of morning sickness and indigestion, it can help you fight excessive fatigue, combat constipation and hemorrhoids, and prevent urinary tract infections and iron-deficiency anemia—even head off headaches. And if your pregnancy turns out to be uncomfortable anyway, by eating well you'll have bestowed on your baby the best chances of being born healthy.

Fitness. Getting enough and the right kind of exercise (see page 215 for guidelines) can help improve your general well-being. Exercise is especially important in second and subsequent pregnancies because abdominal muscles tend to be more lax, making you more susceptible to a variety of aches and pains, most notably backache.

Lifestyle pace. Leading a harried and frenetic life (and who doesn't these days?) can aggravate or sometimes even trigger one of the most uncomfortable of pregnancy symptoms—morning sickness—and exacerbate others, such as fatigue, headache, backache, and indigestion. Getting some help around the house, taking more breaks away from whatever fries your nerves, cutting back at work, letting low-priority tasks go undone for the time being, or practicing relaxation techniques or yoga can help you chill out—and feel better.

Other children. Some pregnant women with other children at home find that keeping up with their offspring keeps them so busy that they barely have time to notice pregnancy discomforts, major or minor. For others, all the running around that comes with running after kids tends to aggravate pregnancy symptoms. For example, morning sickness can increase during times of stress (the getting-to-school or the getting-dinner-on-the-table rush, for instance); fatigue can be heightened because there doesn't seem to be any time to rest; backaches can be an extra pain if you're doing a lot of child toting; even constipation becomes more likely if you never have a chance to use the bathroom when the urge strikes. You are also more likely to come down with colds and other illnesses, courtesy of older germ-spreading kids. (See Chapter 20 for preventing and dealing with such illnesses.)

It's not realistic to always put your pregnant body first when you've got other kids clamoring for care (the days of pampered pregnancy ended with your first delivery). But taking more time to take care of yourself—putting your feet up while you read that story, napping (instead of vacuuming) while your toddler naps, getting into the healthy snack habit even when there's no time for sit-down meals, and taking advantage of help whenever it's available—can help lighten the load your body's carrying, minimizing those pregnancy miseries.

"I had some complications with my first pregnancy. Will this one be just as rough?"

One complicated pregnancy definitely doesn't predict another one. While some pregnancy complications can repeat, many don't repeat routinely. Others may have been triggered by a onetime event, such as an infection or accident, which means they're extremely unlikely to strike twice. Your complications won't recur, either, if they were caused by lifestyle habits that you've now changed (like smoking, drinking, or using drugs), an exposure to an environmental hazard (such as lead) to which you are no longer exposed, or by not getting medical care early in pregnancy (assuming you've sought care early on this time). If the cause was a chronic health problem, such as diabetes or high blood pressure, correcting or controlling the condition prior to conception or very early in pregnancy can greatly reduce the risk of repeat complications. Also keep this in mind: Even if the complications you faced last time have a chance of reoccurrence, earlier detection and treatment (because you and your practitioner will be on the lookout for a repeat) can make a big difference.

Discuss with your practitioner the complications you had last time and what can be done to prevent them from being repeated. No matter what the problems or their causes (even if no cause was ever pinpointed), the tips in the response to the previous question can help make your pregnancy more comfortable, and safer for both you and your baby.

Back-to-Back Pregnancies

"I became pregnant unexpectedly just 10 weeks after I delivered my first child. What effect will this have on my health and on the baby I'm now carrying?"

Expanding your family (and your belly) again a little sooner than expected? Starting another pregnancy before you've fully recovered from the last one can be hard enough without adding stress to the mix. So first of all, relax. Though two closely spaced pregnancies can take their physical toll on a mom-to-be who just became a mom, there are lots of things you can do to help your body better handle the challenge of back-to-back baby making, including:

■ Getting the best prenatal care, starting as soon as you think you're pregnant.

■ Eating as well as you can (see Chapter 5). It's possible your body has not had a chance to rebuild its stores of vitamins and nutrients, and that can put you at a nutritional disadvantage, particularly if you're still nursing. You may need to overcompensate nutritionally to be sure both you and the baby you are carrying don't get short-changed. Pay particular attention to protein and iron (ask your practitioner whether you should take a supplement) and be sure to continue taking your prenatal vitamins. Try not to let lack of time or energy (you'll have little of both, that's for sure) keep you from eating enough. Healthy grazing may help you fit those nutrients into your busy schedule.

■ Gaining enough weight. Your new fetus doesn't care whether or not you've had time to shed the extra pounds his or her sibling put on you. The two of you need the same weight gain this pregnancy, too, unless your practitioner prescribes otherwise. So shelve any weight loss plans for now. A carefully monitored gradual weight gain will be relatively easy to take off afterward, particularly if it was gained on a high-quality diet, and especially once you have a young toddler and an infant to keep up with. Watch your weight gain carefully, and if the numbers don't start climbing as they should, monitor your calorie intake more closely and follow the tips for increasing weight gain on page 180.

■ Fair-share feeding. If you're breastfeeding your older baby, you can continue as long as you feel up to it. If you are completely exhausted, you may want to supplement with formula or consider weaning altogether. Discuss the options with your practitioner. If you decide to continue breastfeeding, be sure to get enough extra calories to feed both your baby and your fetus (ask your practitioner what to aim for). You will also need plenty of rest.

- Resting up. You need more than may be humanly (and new-motherly) possible. Getting it will require not only your own determination but help from your spouse and others as well—who should take over as much of the cooking, housework, and baby care as possible. Set priorities: Let less important chores or work go undone, and force yourself to lie down when your baby is napping. If you're not breastfeeding, let daddy take over nighttime feedings; if you are, at least have him do the baby fetching at 2 A.M.

- Exercising. But just enough to energize you, not enough to exhaust you. If you can't seem to find the time for a regular pregnancy exercise routine, build physical activity into your day with your baby. Take him or her for a brisk walk in the stroller. Or enroll in a pregnancy exercise class or swim at a club or community center that offers baby-sitting services.

- Eliminating or minimizing all other pregnancy risk factors that apply to you, such as smoking and drinking. Your body and your baby-to-be don't need any extra stress.

Having a Big Family

"I'm pregnant for the sixth time. Does this pose any additional risk for my baby or for me?"

On your way to testing out that cheaper-by-the-dozen theory? Happily—for you and for your large brood—women receiving good prenatal care have an excellent chance of having healthy, normal babies in sixth (and later) pregnancies. In fact, beyond a small jump in the incidence of multiple births (twins, triplets, and so on—which could mean that your large brood could potentially grow even larger still), these more-the-merrier pregnancies are almost as likely to be uncomplicated as any first or second.

So enjoy your pregnancy and your large family. But while you're at it:

- Get rest—all the rest you can get. Sure, you could probably do pregnancy in your sleep by now, but that doesn't mean you should try. Every pregnant woman needs her rest, but pregnant women who are also caring for a houseful of other children (plus the house they're filling) need even more.

- Get help—all the help you can get. This will make getting that rest you need possible (or, at least, somewhat possible). Start with your spouse, who should be shouldering what he can in terms of child and house care, but don't stop there. If you haven't already, teach your older children to be more self-sufficient and assign them age-appropriate chores. Any nonessential chores you can't pass off to someone else, skip for now.

- Feed yourself. Moms with many mouths to feed often neglect to feed their own. Not only does meal skipping or junk-food-grabbing shortchange you these days (leaving you with even less energy than you already have), but it shortchanges the baby you have on board. So take the time to eat well. Making healthy snacking a habit can help a lot (and finishing off PB&J scraps and half-eaten chicken fingers doesn't necessarily count).

- Watch your weight. It's not uncommon for women who've had several pregnancies to put on a few extra pounds with each baby. If that's been the case with you, be particularly careful to eat efficiently and keep your gain on target (a target that should be determined by your practitioner). On the flip side, make sure you're not so busy you don't eat enough to gain adequate weight.

Previous Abortions

"I've had two abortions. Will they affect this pregnancy?"

Multiple first-trimester abortions aren't likely to have an effect on future pregnancies. So if your abortions were performed before the 14th week, chances are there's no cause for concern. Multiple second-trimester abortions (performed between 14 and 27 weeks),

---

Do Tell

Whatever gynecological or obstetrical history is in your past, now's not the time to try to put it behind you. Telling your practitioner everything about your history is more important (and relevant) than you might think. Previous pregnancies, miscarriages, abortions, surgeries, or infections may or may not have an impact on what happens in this pregnancy, but any information you have about them—or any aspect of your obstetrical and gynecological history—should be passed on to your practitioner (all will be handled with confidentiality). The more he or she knows about you, the better care you'll get.

---

however, may slightly increase the risk of premature delivery. In either case, be sure your practitioner knows about the abortions. The more familiar he or she is with your complete obstetrical and gynecological history, the better care you will receive.

Preterm Birth

"I had a preterm delivery in my first pregnancy. I've eliminated all my risk factors, but I'm still worried about having a repeat preterm labor."

Congratulations on doing everything you can to make sure your pregnancy is as healthy as possible this time around—and to give your baby the very best chances of staying on board until term. That's a great first step. Together with your practitioner, there are probably even more steps you can take to minimize the chances for a repeat preterm labor.

First, ask your practitioner about the latest research into preventing preterm labor. Researchers have found that the hormone progesterone—given as shots or a gel during weeks 16 through 36—reduces the risk for preterm birth in women with a prior history of one. If you've had a previous preterm birth, ask your practitioner if you're a good candidate for progesterone.

Second, ask your practitioner if one of the two screening tests available for predicting whether you're at risk for preterm birth would be right for you. Usually, these tests are only recommended for high-risk women since positive test results aren't an accurate predictor of early delivery, but negative results can help avoid unnecessary interventions—and needless anxiety. The fetal fibronectin (fFN) screening test detects a protein in the vagina only present if there has been a separation of the amniotic sac from the uterine wall (an early indicator of labor). If you have a negative fFN test, it's unlikely you'll go into preterm labor within the next few weeks after the test (so you can breathe easy). If it's positive, your risk of going into preterm labor is significantly higher, and your practitioner may take steps to prolong your pregnancy and prepare your baby's lungs for an early delivery.

The second screening test is for cervical length. The length of your cervix is measured via ultrasound, and if there are any signs that the cervix is shortening or opening, your practitioner may take some steps to reduce your risk of early delivery, such as putting you on bed rest or perhaps stitching your cervix closed (if you're before 22 weeks).

Knowledge is always power—but in this case, knowledge can also help prevent your second baby from being born too soon. And that's a very good thing.

Incompetent Cervix

"I had a miscarriage in the fifth month of my first pregnancy. The doctor said it was caused by an incompetent cervix. I just had a positive home pregnancy test, and I'm worried that I'll have the same problem again."

The good news (and there *is* good news here) is that it doesn't have to happen again. Now that your incompetent cervix has been diagnosed as the cause of your first pregnancy loss, your obstetrician should be able to take steps to prevent it from causing another loss. With proper treatment and careful watching, the odds of your having a healthy pregnancy and a safe delivery this time around are greatly in your favor. (If you have a different practitioner now, make sure you share your history of incompetent cervix so you can receive the best care possible.)

An incompetent cervix, one that opens prematurely under the pressure of the growing uterus and fetus, is estimated to occur in 1 or 2 of every 100 pregnancies; it is believed responsible for 10 to 20 percent of all second-trimester miscarriages. It can be the result of genetic weakness of the cervix, extreme stretching of or severe lacerations to the cervix during one or more previous deliveries, an extensive "cone" biopsy done for precancerous cervical cells, or cervical surgery or laser therapy. Carrying more than one fetus can also lead to incompetent cervix, but if it does, the problem will not usually recur in subsequent single-fetus pregnancies.

Incompetent cervix is usually diagnosed when a woman miscarries in the second trimester after experiencing progressive painless effacement (shortening and thinning) and dilation of the cervix without apparent uterine contractions or vaginal bleeding.

To help protect this pregnancy, your ob may perform cerclage (a procedure during which the opening of the cervix is stitched closed) when you're in your second trimester (anywhere from 12 to 22 weeks). Although recent research has seriously questioned the effectiveness of cerclage (more study needs to be done), many practitioners still perform it routinely. More often, however, doctors will only do cerclage when an ultrasound or a vaginal exam shows that the cervix is shortening or opening. The simple procedure is performed through the vagina under local anesthesia. Twelve hours after surgery, you'll be able to resume normal activities, though sexual intercourse may be prohibited for the rest of your pregnancy, and you may need frequent medical exams. When the sutures will be removed depends partly on the doctor's preference and partly on the situation. Usually they're removed a few weeks before your estimated due date.

Your Pregnancy Profile and Preterm Birth

Here's the good news: It's far more likely your baby will be arriving late (as in overdue) than early. Just about 12 percent of labors and births are considered premature, or preterm—that is, occurring before the 37th week of pregnancy. And around half of these occur in women who are known to be at high risk for premature delivery, including the ever-multiplying percentage of moms-to-be of multiples.

Is there anything you can do to help prevent preterm birth if your pregnancy profile puts you at higher risk for it? In some cases, there isn't—even when a risk factor is identified (and it won't always be), it can't necessarily be controlled. But in other cases, the risk factor or factors that might lead to an early birth can be controlled or at least minimized. Eliminate any that apply to you, and you may up the chances that your baby will stay put contentedly until term. Here are some known risk factors for premature labor that can be controlled:

Too little or too much weight gain. Gaining too little weight can increase the chances your baby will be born early, but so can packing on too many pounds. Gaining just the right number of pounds for your pregnancy profile can give your baby a healthier uterine environment and, ideally, a better chance of staying there until term.

Inadequate nutrition. Giving your baby the healthiest start in life isn't just about gaining the right number of pounds—it's about gaining them on the right types of foods. A diet that lacks necessary nutrients (especially folate) increases your risk for premature delivery; a diet that's nutrition packed decreases that risk. In fact, some evidence indicates that eating well regularly can lower the risk of early delivery.

Lots of standing or heavy physical labor. Check with your practitioner to see if you should cut back on the time you spend on your feet, especially later on in pregnancy. Long periods of being on your feet—especially when it involves *heavy* physical labor and lifting—has been linked to preterm labor in some studies.

Extreme emotional stress. Some studies have shown a link between extreme emotional stress (not your everyday "I've got too much to do and not enough time to do it" stress) and premature labor. Sometimes the cause of such excessive stress can be eliminated or minimized (by quitting or cutting back at an unhealthily high-pressure job, for example); sometimes it's unavoidable (as when you lose your job or there's been illness or death in the family). Still, many kinds of stress can be reduced with relaxation techniques, good nutrition, a balance of exercise and rest, and by talking the problem out with your spouse or friends, your practitioner, or a therapist.

Alcohol and drug use. Expectant moms who use alcohol and illegal drugs boost their risk of having a premature delivery.

Smoking. Smoking during pregnancy may be linked to an increased risk of premature delivery. Quitting before conception or as early as possible in pregnancy is best, but quitting at any time in pregnancy is definitely better than not quitting at all.

Gum infection. Some studies show that gum disease is associated with preterm delivery. Some researchers suspect that the bacteria that cause inflammation in the gums can actually get into the bloodstream, reach the fetus, and initiate early delivery. Other researchers propose another possibility: The bacteria that cause inflammation in the gums can also trigger the immune system to produce inflammation in the cervix and uterus, triggering early labor. Practicing good oral hygiene and getting regular dental care can prevent the bacterial infection and possibly lower your risk for an early labor. Treatment for existing infections prior to pregnancy—though not necessarily during pregnancy—may also help lower the risk for a variety of complications, including preterm labor.

Incompetent cervix. The risk of premature delivery as a result of an incompetent cervix—in which a weak cervix opens early (and, unfortunately, can be suspected only after a woman has experienced a late miscarriage or premature labor once before)—can possibly be reduced by suturing the cervix closed and/or by closely monitoring the length of the cervix via ultrasound (see page 45 for more information).

History of premature deliveries. Your chances of premature delivery are higher if you've had one in the past. If you've had a prior preterm labor and delivery, your practitioner may prescribe progesterone during the second and third trimesters of this pregnancy to avoid a repeat preterm birth.

The following risk factors aren't controllable, but in some cases they can be somewhat modified. In others, knowing they exist can help you and your practitioner best manage the risks, as well as greatly improve the outcome if an early birth becomes inevitable.

Multiples. Women carrying more than one fetus deliver an average of three weeks early (though it has been suggested that full term for twins is actually 37 weeks, which might mean that three weeks early isn't early at all). Good prenatal care, optimal nutrition, and the elimination of other risk factors, along with more time spent resting and restriction

of activity as needed in the last trimester, may help prevent a too-early birth. See Chapter 16 for more information.

Premature cervical effacement and dilation. In some women, for reasons unknown and apparently unrelated to an incompetent cervix, the cervix begins to thin out and open up early. Recent research suggests that at least some of this early effacement and dilation may be related to a shorter-than-normal cervix. A routine ultrasound of the cervix midpregnancy uncovers which women are at high risk.

Pregnancy complications. Such complications as gestational diabetes, preeclampsia, and excessive amniotic fluid, as well as problems with the placenta, such as placenta previa or placental abruption, can make an early delivery more likely. Managing these conditions as best as possible may prolong pregnancy until term.

Chronic maternal illness. Chronic conditions, such as high blood pressure; heart, liver, or kidney disease; or diabetes may raise the risk for preterm delivery, but good medical management and self-care may reduce it.

General infections. Certain infections (some sexually transmitted diseases; urinary, cervical, vaginal, kidney, and amniotic fluid infections) can put a mother-to-be at high risk for preterm labor. When the infection is one that could prove harmful to the fetus, early labor may be the body's way of attempting to rescue the baby from a dangerous environment. Preventing the infection or promptly treating it may effectively prevent a too-soon birth.

Under age 17. Teen moms-to-be are often at a higher risk for preterm delivery. Good nutrition and prenatal care can reduce risk by helping to compensate for the fact that both mother and baby are still growing.

In some cases, they may not be removed until labor begins, unless there is infection, bleeding, or premature rupture of the membranes.

You'll have to be alert for signs of an impending problem in the second or early third trimester: pressure in the lower abdomen, bloody discharge, unusual urinary frequency, or the sensation of a lump in the vagina. If you experience any of these, call your doctor right away.

Rh Incompatibility

"My doctor said my blood tests show I am Rh negative. What does that mean for my baby?"

Fortunately, it doesn't mean much, at least now that both you and your doctor know about it. With this knowledge, simple steps can be taken that will effectively—and completely—protect your baby from Rh incompatibility.

What exactly is Rh incompatibility, and why does your baby need protection from it? A little biology lesson can help clear that up quickly. Each cell in the body has numerous antigens, or antenna-like structures, on its surface. One such antigen is the Rh factor. Everyone inherits blood cells that either have the Rh factor (which makes the person Rh positive) or lack the factor (which makes them Rh negative). In a pregnancy, if the mother's blood cells do not have the Rh factor (she's Rh negative) while the fetus's blood cells—inherited from dad—do have it (making the fetus Rh positive), the mother's immune system may view the fetus (and its Rh-positive blood cells) as a "foreigner." In a normal immune response, her system will generate armies of antibodies to attack this foreigner. This is known as Rh incompatibility.

All pregnant women are tested for the Rh factor early in pregnancy, usually at the first prenatal visit. If a woman turns out to be Rh positive, as 85 percent are, the issue of compatibility is moot because whether the fetus is Rh positive or Rh negative, there are no foreign antigens on the fetus's blood cells to cause the mother's immune system to mobilize.

When the mother is Rh negative, as you are, the baby's father is tested to determine whether he is Rh positive or negative. If your spouse turns out to be Rh negative, your fetus will be Rh negative, too (since two "negative" parents can't make a "positive" baby), which means that your body will not consider it "foreign." But if your spouse is Rh positive, there's a significant possibility that your fetus will inherit the Rh factor from him, creating an incompatibility between you and the baby.

This incompatibility is usually not a problem in a first pregnancy. Trouble starts to brew if some of the baby's blood enters the mother's circulation during her first pregnancy or delivery (or abortion or miscarriage). The mother's body, in that natural protective immune response, produces antibodies against the Rh factor. The antibodies themselves are harmless—until she becomes pregnant again with another Rh-positive baby. During the subsequent pregnancy, these new antibodies could potentially cross the placenta into the baby's circulation and attack the fetal red blood cells, causing very mild (if maternal antibody levels are low) to very serious (if they are high) anemia in the fetus. Only very rarely do these antibodies form in first pregnancies, in reaction to fetal blood leaking back through the placenta into the mother's circulatory system.

Prevention of the development of antibodies is the key to protecting the fetus when there is Rh incompatibility. Most practitioners use a two-pronged attack. At 28 weeks, an Rh-negative expectant mom is given a vaccine-like injection of Rh-immune globulin, known as RhoGAM, to prevent the development of antibodies. Another dose is administered within 72 hours after delivery if blood tests show her baby is Rh positive. If the baby is Rh negative, no treatment is required. RhoGAM is also administered after a miscarriage, an ectopic pregnancy, an abortion, chorionic villus sampling (CVS), amniocentesis, vaginal bleeding, or trauma during pregnancy. Giving RhoGAM as needed at these times can head off problems in future pregnancies.

If an Rh-negative woman was not given RhoGAM during her previous pregnancy and tests reveal that she has developed Rh antibodies capable of attacking an Rh-positive fetus, amniocentesis can be used to check the blood type of the fetus. If it is Rh negative, mother and baby have compatible blood types and there's no cause for concern or treatment. If it is Rh positive, and thus incompatible with the mother's blood type, the maternal antibody levels are monitored regularly. If the levels

become dangerously high, ultrasound tests are done to assess the condition of the fetus. If at any point the safety of the fetus is threatened because hemolytic or Rh disease has developed, a transfusion of Rh-negative blood to the fetus may be necessary.

The use of RhoGAM has greatly reduced the need for transfusions in Rh-incompatible pregnancies to less than 1 percent, and in the future may make this lifesaving procedure a medical miracle of the past.

A similar incompatibility can arise with other factors in the blood, such as the Kell antigen, though these are less common than Rh incompatibility. If the father has the antigen and the mother does not, there is again potential for problems. A standard screening, part of the first routine blood test, looks for the presence of circulating antibodies in the mother's blood. If these antibodies are found, the father of the baby is tested to see if he is positive, in which case the management is the same as with Rh incompatibility.

Your Medical History

Rubella Antibody Levels

"I was vaccinated against rubella as a child, but my prenatal blood test shows my rubella antibody levels are low. Should I be concerned?"

There's not much cause for concern when it comes to rubella these days, at least in the United States. Not because the illness isn't still harmful to the unborn (it still can be, particularly in the first trimester; see page 506), but

because it's next to impossible to catch it. The CDC considers rubella to be eradicated in the United States, and since most children and adults have been—and will continue to be—vaccinated against rubella, the chances of being exposed to the illness are virtually nil.

Though you won't be immunized during pregnancy, you will be given a new rubella vaccine right after you deliver, before you even leave the hospital. It's safe then, even if you're breastfeeding.

Immunizations in Pregnancy

Since infections of various sorts can cause pregnancy problems, it's a good idea to take care of all necessary immunizations before conceiving. Most immunizations using live viruses are not recommended during pregnancy, including the MMR (measles, mumps, and rubella) and varicella (chicken pox) vaccines. Other vaccines, according to the CDC, shouldn't be given routinely but can be given if they're needed. These include hepatitis A and pneumococcal vaccine. You also can be immunized safely against tetanus, diphtheria, and hepatitis B with vaccines containing dead, or nonactive, viruses. In the must-have department: The CDC recommends that every woman who is pregnant during flu season (generally October through April) receive a flu shot.

For more information about which vaccines are safe during pregnancy and which, if any, you may need (particularly if you'll be traveling to exotic destinations), check with your practitioner.

Obesity

"I'm about 60 pounds overweight. Does this put me and my baby at higher risk during pregnancy?"

Most overweight—and even obese (defined as someone whose weight is 20 percent or more over her ideal weight)—mothers have completely safe pregnancies and completely healthy babies. Still, obesity always poses extra health risks, and that's the case during pregnancy, too. Carrying a lot of extra weight while you're carrying a baby increases the possibility of certain pregnancy complications, including high blood pressure and gestational diabetes. Being overweight poses some practical pregnancy problems, too. It may be tougher to date your pregnancy accurately without an early ultrasound, both because ovulation is often erratic in obese women and because some of the yardsticks practitioners traditionally use to estimate a due date (the height of the fundus, or top of the uterus, the size of the uterus, hearing the heartbeat) may be difficult to read through layers of fat. The padding may also make it impossible for the practitioner to determine a fetus's size and position (as well as make it harder for you to feel those first kicks). Finally, delivery difficulties can result if the fetus is much larger than average, which is often the case with obese mothers (even among those who don't overeat during pregnancy, and particularly with those who are diabetic). And if a cesarean delivery is necessary, the over-ample abdomen can complicate both the surgery and recovery from it.

Then there's the issue of pregnancy comfort, or rather discomfort—and unfortunately, as the pounds multiply, so do those uncomfortable pregnancy symptoms. Extra pounds (whether they're pounds you already had or pounds you added during pregnancy) can spell extra backache, varicose veins, swelling, heartburn, and more.

Daunted? Don't be. There's plenty you and your practitioner can do to minimize the risks to you and your baby and the discomfort for you—it'll just take some extra effort. On the medical care side, you will probably undergo more testing than the typical low-risk pregnant woman: ultrasound early on to date your pregnancy more accurately, and later to determine the baby's size and position; at least one glucose toler-

Pregnancy After Gastric Bypass

Double congratulations—you've lost a whole lot of weight, and you're expecting! But as you pat yourself on the back (or the belly), you may also be wondering how having had gastric bypass or lap band surgery will affect your pregnancy. Happily, not that much. Chances are you were advised not to become pregnant for at least the first 12 to 18 months after your surgery—the time of the most drastic weight loss and potential for malnutrition. But once you've passed that benchmark, your chances of having a healthy pregnancy and healthy pregnancy outcome are actually even better than they would have been if you hadn't had the surgery and lost the weight. Still, as you probably know, you'll have to work extra hard to ensure the healthiest outcome:

■ Put your weight loss surgeon on your prenatal team. He or she will be best able to advise your ob-gyn or midwife on some of the specific needs of a post–gastric bypass patient.

■ You'll need to keep up with your recommended vitamin supplementation while you're expecting (this is not the time to be at a nutritional disadvantage). A prenatal vitamin is a good start, but you may need more iron, calcium, folic acid, vitamin B_{12}, and vitamin A because of certain malabsorption issues. Be sure to speak to both your prenatal practitioner and your surgeon about your particular supplement needs.

■ Watch your weight closely (with your practitioner, of course). You're used to watching it go down, but now it will have to start going up. If you don't gain enough weight during pregnancy, your baby may not be able to grow to its potential. Make sure you know what your target weight gain is (it may be different than for the average expectant mom), and make sure you have an eating plan in place that will help you reach your weight gain goal.

■ Watch what you eat, too. As a gastric bypass patient, the quantity of food you can eat is limited, so you'll need to focus on quality (not a bad concept when you're expecting, anyway). Try not to waste calories, and instead try to choose foods that efficiently pack the most nutrients into the smallest volume.

■ If at any time you experience abdominal pain and excessive bloating, call your doctor right away.

ance test or screening to determine if you are showing any signs of developing gestational diabetes; and, toward the end of your pregnancy, nonstress and other diagnostic tests to monitor your baby's condition.

As for your part, good self-care will make a big difference. Eliminating all pregnancy risks that are within your control—such as drinking and smoking —will be particularly important for you. Keeping your weight gain on target will

be, too—and it's likely that your target will be smaller than the average expectant mom's and monitored by your doctor more closely. ACOG recommends that overweight women gain 15 to 20 pounds and obese women gain no more than 15 pounds, though your practitioner's recommendations may differ.

Even with a scaled-down bottom line to stick to, your daily diet will have to contain adequate calories and be packed with foods that are concentrated sources of vitamins, minerals, and protein (see the Pregnancy Diet in Chapter 5). Focusing on quality over quantity and making every bite matter will help you make those calories count—and will help your baby get the most nutritional bang for the calories you consume. Taking your prenatal vitamin faithfully will provide extra insurance. (But keep over-the-counter appetite suppressants that you might have been taking prepregnancy off the menu; they can be dangerous during pregnancy. The same goes for beverages that claim to suppress your appetite.) Getting regular exercise, within the guidelines recommended by your doctor, will allow you to eat more of the healthy foods you and your baby need—without packing on too many pounds.

For your next pregnancy, if you are planning on one, try to get as close as possible to your ideal weight before you conceive. It will make everything about pregnancy a lot easier—and less complicated.

Underweight

"I've always been skinny. How will my pregnancy be affected by my being underweight?"

Pregnancy's definitely a time for eating well and gaining weight—for both the skinny and the not-so-skinny. But if you've come into pregnancy on the super-skinny side (with a BMI of 18.5 or less; see page 166 for how to calculate yours), you'll have to be filling up your plate even more. That's because there are some potential risks (such as having a small-for-date baby) associated with being pregnant and extremely underweight, particularly if you're also undernourished. But any added risk can be virtually eliminated with a good diet (one that includes not only extra calories but also fresh fruit and vegetables, which

provide the vitamins and minerals thin people are sometimes short on); prenatal vitamins; and adequate weight gain. Depending on where you started out on the scale, your practitioner may advise you to gain a little extra—possibly 28 to 40 pounds, instead of the 25 to 35 pounds recommended for the average-weight woman. If you've been blessed with a speedy metabolism that makes putting on pounds tricky, see page 181 for some tips. As long as your weight gain stays on track, though, your pregnancy shouldn't encounter any other bumps (besides that belly bump).

An Eating Disorder

"I've been fighting bulimia for the last 10 years. I thought I'd be able to stop the bingeing-purging cycle now that I'm pregnant, but I can't seem to. Will it hurt my baby?"

Not if you get the right kind of help right away. The fact that you've been bulimic (or anorexic) for a number of years means your nutritional reserves are probably low, putting your baby and your body at a disadvantage right off the bat. Fortunately, early in pregnancy the need for nourishment is less than it will be later on, so you have the chance to make up for your body's nutritional shortfall before it can hurt your baby.

Very little research has been done in the area of eating disorders and pregnancy, partly because these disorders cause disrupted menstrual cycles, reducing the number of women who suffer with these problems from becoming pregnant in the first place. But the studies that have been done suggest the following:

- If you get your eating disorder under control, you're just as likely to have a healthy baby as anyone else, all other things being equal.

- It's critical that the practitioner who is caring for your pregnancy know about your eating disorder (so speak up, even if your condition is in the past).

- Counseling from a professional who is experienced in treating eating disorders is advisable for anyone who suffers from such a problem, but it is essential when you're pregnant. You may also find support groups helpful (check online, or ask your practitioner or therapist for a recommendation).

- Continuing to take laxatives, diuretics, and other drugs favored by bulimics and anorexics can harm your developing baby. They draw off nutrients and fluids from your body before they can be utilized to nourish your baby (and later to produce milk), and they may lead to fetal abnormality if used regularly. These medications, like all others, should not be used by any pregnant woman unless prescribed by a physician who is aware of the pregnancy.

- Bingeing and purging during pregnancy (in other words, active bulimia) seems to increase the risk of miscarriage, premature birth, and postpartum depression. Putting those unhealthy habits behind you now will allow you to nourish your baby and yourself well. If you're having trouble doing so, make sure you get the help you need.

- Not gaining enough weight during pregnancy can lead to a number of problems, including preterm delivery and a baby who is small for his or her gestational age.

Just being committed to conquering your eating disorder, so that you can start nurturing that beautiful little baby of yours, is a first and most important step. You'll also need to understand the dynamics of weight gain in pregnancy.

Keep in mind:

- The pregnant shape is universally viewed as healthy and beautiful. Its roundness is normal, a sign that you're growing a baby. Celebrate those curves! Embrace your pregnant self!

- You're supposed to gain weight during pregnancy. The right amount of pregnancy weight gain is vital to your baby's growth and well-being as well as to your own health.

- Weight gained at the right rate, on the right foods, will go to the right places (your baby and those essential baby by-products). If you stay within the recommended guidelines (which are higher for those who begin pregnancy significantly underweight), the weight won't be that difficult to shed once the baby arrives. This strategy (a moderate amount of weight gained steadily on nutritious foods) will help ensure a speedier return to your prepregnancy shape postpartum and help ensure a healthier baby.

- When you starve yourself, you starve your baby. Your baby depends on you for a steady shipment of nutrients. If you don't eat, neither does your baby. If the nutrients you take in are purged (by vomiting, taking laxatives, or taking diuretics), your baby won't have enough left to grow on.

- Exercise can help you keep your weight gain reasonable, while guiding those extra pounds to the right places. But any exercise program you choose should be pregnancy appropriate (check it out with your practitioner first), and strenuous exercise (or too much exercise, which can burn too many calories or raise your temperature excessively) should be avoided.

- All of the weight gain of pregnancy won't drop off in the first few days after delivery. With sensible eating, the average woman returns to close to—but does not hit—her prepregnancy weight about six weeks after delivery. Getting all the weight off and getting back into shape (which requires exercise) can take much longer. For this reason, many women with eating disorders find that negative feelings about their body image cause them to slip back into bingeing and purging or starving during the postpartum period. Because these unhealthy habits could interfere with your ability to recover from childbirth, to parent effectively, and to produce milk if you choose to breastfeed, it's important that you continue professional counseling postpartum with someone experienced in the treatment of eating disorders.

The most important thing to keep in mind: Your baby's well-being depends on your well-being during pregnancy. If you're not well nourished, your baby won't be, either. Positive reinforcement can definitely help, so try putting pictures of cute chubby babies on the fridge, in your office and car, anywhere you might need a reminder of the healthy eating you should be doing. Visualize the food you eat making its way to your baby (and your baby happily gobbling up the meals).

If you can't seem to stop bingeing, vomiting, using diuretics or laxatives, or practicing semistarvation during pregnancy, discuss with your physician the possibility of hospitalization until you get your disorder under control.

Having a Baby After 35

"I'm 38 and pregnant with my first baby. I've read so much about the risks of pregnancy after 35 and wonder whether I should worry."

Becoming pregnant after 35 puts you in good—and growing—company. While the pregnancy rate among women in their 20s has dropped slightly in recent decades, it has increased nearly 40 percent among women over 35. And though the number of babies born to women in their 40s remains relatively small, their ranks have also increased by a third in recent years.

If you've lived for more than 35 years, you're probably aware that nothing in life is completely risk free. These days, pregnancy risks are very small to begin with, but they do increase slightly and gradually as you get older. However, the many benefits of starting a family at the time that's right for you can far outweigh any small risks (all of which can be reduced anyway, thanks to medical advancements).

The major reproductive risk faced by a woman in your age group is that she might not become pregnant at all because of decreased fertility. Once you've overcome that and become pregnant (congratulations!), you also face a somewhat greater chance of having a baby with Down syndrome. The inci-

Is 35 the Magic Number?

Just because you've already clocked in 35 years doesn't mean you'll necessarily need more or different testing than your younger pregnant pals. In fact, screening tests are recommended for all women, regardless of how many birthdays they've celebrated—and only those whose screens show a possible elevated risk need to consider more invasive prenatal diagnosis.

dence increases with mom's age: 1 in 1,250 for 25-year-old mothers, about 3 in 1,000 for 30-year-old mothers, 1 in about 300 for 35-year-old mothers, and 1 in 35 for 45-year-old mothers (you'll notice the risk gradually increases with age—it doesn't just spike at 35). It's speculated that this and other chromosomal abnormalities, though still relatively rare, are more common in older women because their eggs are older, too (every woman is born with a lifetime supply of eggs that age along with her), and have had more exposure to X-rays, drugs, infections, and so on. (It is now known, however, that the egg is not always responsible for such chromosomal abnormalities. An estimated minimum 25 percent of Down syndrome cases can be linked to a defect in an older father's sperm.)

A handful of other risks increase slightly with age. Being older, particularly over 40, means you might be more likely to develop high blood pressure (particularly if you're overweight), diabetes, or cardiovascular disease during pregnancy—but all of these conditions are more common in older groups in general, and all are usually controllable. Older mothers-to-be are also more subject to miscarriage (because of their older eggs), preeclampsia, and preterm labor. Labor and delivery, on average, are longer and slightly more likely to be complicated, with C-section and other forms of assisted delivery (such as vacuum extraction) more common. In some older women, a decrease in muscle tone and joint flexibility may make labor a little tougher—but for many others, especially those who are in excellent physical shape thanks to regular exercise routines and healthy eating, this isn't the case.

But in spite of these slightly increased risks, there's lots of good news for expectant moms over 35, too. Today's older mothers have more going for

them than ever before. Though Down syndrome isn't preventable, it can be identified in utero through a variety of screening and diagnostic tests. Even better news: Today's essentially noninvasive first-trimester screenings (see page 59), which are recommended to all pregnant women regardless of age, are much more accurate than in the past, which means they screen out moms who don't necessarily need to proceed to a more invasive diagnostic test (even moms-to-be over 35)—saving money and stress. Chronic conditions that are more common in older moms can be well controlled. Drugs and close medical supervision can sometimes forestall preterm labor. And medical breakthroughs continue to decrease risks in the birthing room.

But as much as medical science can do to help you have a safe pregnancy and a healthy baby, it's nothing compared to what you can do yourself through exercise, diet, and quality prenatal care. Just being older doesn't necessarily put you in a high-risk category, but an accumulation of many individual risks can. Eliminate or minimize as many risk factors as you can, and you'll be able to take years off your pregnancy profile—making your chances of delivering a healthy baby virtually as good as those of a younger mother. Maybe even better.

So relax, enjoy your pregnancy, and be reassured. There's never been a better time to be over 35 and expecting a baby.

The Father's Age

"I'm only 31, but my husband is over 50. Could his age affect our baby?"

Throughout most of history, it was believed that a father's responsibility in the reproductive process was limited to fertilization. Only during the twentieth century (too late to help those

Uninsured, Mama?

Having a baby these days can definitely be an expensive proposition—and that's before you even purchase onesie number one. Still, no expectant mother needs to go through pregnancy and childbirth without the prenatal care she and her baby need, even if she's uninsured. If you can't afford to pick up health insurance now, here are some other ways to find that care at a price you can afford:

■ Check online or in the phone book. Search under "Clinics" or "Health Care Centers." Most communities provide health services through organizations such as Planned Parenthood and at women's health centers. Many of these can provide some free care, and most will offer care on a sliding pay-what-you-can basis.

■ Turn to the government. If your income is low enough, you may qualify for Medicaid. Through this program, you'll be entitled to prenatal care. If you don't qualify for Medicaid, there are low-cost health insurance programs (that will cover your preg-

nancy as well as your child's health care after delivery) offered through the government. Ask at any clinic or call (877) KIDS-NOW or (877) 543-7669. If affording nutritious food is an issue—or will be once you're feeding another mouth—contact WIC (Women, Infants, and Children), a government program that provides pregnant and nursing mothers with food and nutrition counseling. For information, contact WIC, www.fns.usda.gov/wic; (703) 305-2746.

■ Call your local hospital. Some hospitals provide a certain amount of free or low-cost obstetrical care to women who need it. Childbirth classes may also be available at little or no cost to women who can't afford to pay full price for them.

■ As a last resort (and this really should be the very last resort), try the ER. If you experience a pregnancy problem or go into labor before you've been able to secure a practitioner, head to the ER of the nearest hospital immediately.

queens who lost their heads for failing to produce a male heir) was it discovered that a father's sperm holds the deciding genetic vote in determining his child's gender. And only in the last few decades have researchers begun to suspect that an older father's sperm might contribute to an increased risk of miscarriage or birth defects. Like the older mother's eggs, the older father's spermatocytes (undeveloped sperm) have had longer exposure to environmental hazards and might conceivably contain altered or damaged genes or chromosomes. In fact, researchers found that regardless of the mother's age, a couple's risk of

miscarriage increases as the dad's age increases. It also appears that there is an increase in the incidence of Down syndrome when the father is over 50 or 55 (regardless of how old the mother is), though the association is weaker than in the case of maternal age.

Still, the evidence remains inconclusive, mostly because the research involving older dads is still in its infancy. Despite what seems to be a small yet growing body of evidence to implicate paternal age as a factor in birth defects and miscarriages, genetic counselors do not recommend amniocentesis on the basis of a father's age alone. The screening tests that are now offered routinely to every mother-to-be, regardless of her age, should put your mind at ease. If your screening tests turn out normal, you can relax about your husband's age without having to go through amniocentesis.

Genetic Counseling

"I keep wondering if I might have a genetic problem and not know it. Should I get genetic counseling?"

Just about everyone carries at least one gene for a genetic disorder. But fortunately, because most disorders require a matched pair of genes, one from mom and one from dad, they're not likely to show up in their children. One or both parents can be tested for some of these disorders before or during pregnancy—but such testing usually makes sense only if there is a better-than-average possibility that both parents are carriers of a particular disorder. The clue is often ethnic or geographic. For example, it is recommended that all Caucasians be tested for cystic fibrosis (since a CF mutation is carried by about 1 in 25 Caucasians of European descent). Jewish couples whose ancestors came from Eastern Europe should be tested for Tay-Sachs, Canavan disease, and possibly for other disorders. Tay-Sachs has also been noted in other ethnic groups, including Louisiana Cajuns and French Canadians, so getting tested is something to consider if your family has these roots. Similarly, black couples should be tested for the sickle cell anemia trait, and those of Mediterranean and Asian descent for thalassemia (a hereditary form of anemia). In most cases, testing is recommended for one parent; testing the second parent becomes necessary only if the first tests positive.

Pregnancy and the Single Mother

Are you a single mom-to-be? Just because you don't have a partner doesn't mean you have to go it alone during pregnancy—and you shouldn't try. The kind of support you'll need can come from sources other than a partner. A good friend or a relative you feel close to and comfortable with can step in to hold your hand, emotionally and physically, throughout pregnancy. That person can, in many ways, play the partner role during the nine months and beyond—accompanying you to prenatal visits and childbirth education classes, lending an ear (and a shoulder) when you need to talk about your concerns and fears as well as your excited anticipation, helping you get both your home and life ready for the new arrival, and acting as coach, supporter, and advocate during labor and delivery. And since no one will know better what you're going through than another single mom, you might also consider joining (or starting) a support group for single mothers, or find an online support group (check out the single mom's message board at whattoexpect.com).

Diseases that can be passed on via a single gene from one carrier parent (hemophilia, for example) or by one affected parent (Huntington's disease) have usually turned up in the family before, though it may not be common knowledge. That's why it's important to keep family health history records and to try to dig up as many health details from your parents, grandparents, and other close relatives as you can when you're pregnant (or are trying to conceive).

Most expectant parents, happily, are at such low risk for transmitting genetic problems that they don't need to see a genetic counselor. In many cases, a prenatal practitioner will discuss with a couple the most common genetic issues, referring to a genetic counselor or a maternal-fetal medicine specialist those with a need for more expertise:

- Couples whose blood tests show they are carriers of a genetic disorder that they might pass on to their children.

- Parents who have already had one or more children with genetic birth defects.

- Couples who have experienced three or more consecutive miscarriages.

- Couples who know of a hereditary disorder on any branch of either of their family trees. In some cases (as with cystic fibrosis or certain thalassemias), doing DNA testing of the parents before pregnancy makes interpreting later testing of the fetus much easier.

- Couples in which one partner has a congenital defect (such as congenital heart disease).

- Pregnant women who have had positive screening tests for the presence of a fetal defect.

- Closely related couples; the risk of inherited disease in offspring is greatest when parents are related (for example, 1 in 9 for first cousins).

The best time to see a genetic counselor is before getting pregnant, or in the case of close relatives who intend to start a family, before getting married. A genetic counselor is trained to give couples the odds of their having a healthy child based on their genetic profiles and can guide them in deciding whether or not to have children. But it's not too late even after pregnancy is confirmed. The counselor can suggest appropriate prenatal testing based on the couple's genetic profile, and if testing uncovers a serious defect in the fetus, a genetic counselor can outline for the expectant parents all the options available and help them decide how to proceed. Genetic counseling has helped countless high-risk couples avoid the heartbreak of giving birth to children with serious problems, while helping them realize their dreams of having completely healthy babies.

Prenatal Diagnosis

Is it a boy or a girl? Will it have blond hair or brown? Green eyes or blue? Will it have mom's mouth and dad's dimples? Dad's voice and mom's knack for numbers (or the other way around)? Babies definitely keep their parents guessing (and placing friendly bets) long before they actually arrive—sometimes before they're conceived. But the one question that expectant parents wonder about the most is also the one they're most hesitant to speculate on or even talk about: "Will my baby be healthy?"

Until recently, that question could be answered only at birth. Today, it can be answered as early as the first trimester, through prenatal screening and diagnostic tests. Most expectant mothers undergo several screening tests during their 40 weeks—even those whose odds of having a baby with a defect are low (because of age, good nutrition, and excellent prenatal care). That's because such screening tests (from the combined and integrated screenings to the ultrasound and the quad screen) pose no risk to mom or baby but can provide a lot of beneficial reassurance.

Going one step further to definitive diagnostic tests (CVS, amnio, or more detailed ultrasound), however, isn't for everyone. Many parents—particularly those whose screening tests come back negative—can continue to play the waiting game, with the happy assurance that the chances are overwhelming that their babies are indeed completely healthy. But for those whose concerns represent more than normal expectant-parent jitters, the benefits of prenatal diagnosis can far outweigh the risks. Women who are good candidates for such testing include those who:

- Are over 35 (though an older mom with reassuring screening results may decide, after consultation with her practitioner, to skip the diagnostic tests).

- Have been exposed since conception to a substance or substances that they

fear might have been harmful to their developing baby. (Consultation with a physician can help determine whether prenatal diagnosis is warranted in a particular case.)

- Have a family history of genetic disease and/or have been shown to be carriers of such a disease.

- Have a genetic disorder themselves (such as cystic fibrosis or congenital heart disease).

- Have been exposed to infection (such as rubella or toxoplasmosis) that could cause a birth defect.

- Have had pregnancy losses previously, or have had babies with birth defects.

- Have tested positive on a prenatal screening test.

Why go through diagnostic tests if there's some risk involved? The best reason for prenatal diagnosis is the reassurance it almost always brings. The vast majority of babies whose possibly-at-risk moms undergo such testing will receive a perfect bill of health—which means that mom and dad can quit worrying and start enjoying their pregnancy.

First Trimester

First-Trimester Ultrasound

What is it? One of the simplest screening tests is the ultrasound. Using sound waves so high they can't be heard by the human ear, sonography allows visualization and "examination" of the fetus without X-rays. Though sonography tends to

be fairly accurate for most uses, in screening for birth defects the test can yield some false negatives (it seems as though everything is fine, but it's not) and some false positives (it looks as though there is a problem, but there really isn't).

A first-trimester ultrasound (usually a basic level 1 ultrasound) is performed in order to:

- Confirm the viability of a pregnancy

- Date a pregnancy

- Determine the number of fetuses

- Determine the cause of bleeding, if any

- Locate an IUD that was in place at the time of conception

- Locate the fetus prior to CVS or amniocentesis

- Assess the risk for chromosomal abnormality as part of a screening test

How is it done? Though ultrasound examination is often performed using a wand or transducer over the abdomen (transabdominal), during the first trimester a transvaginal exam may be preferred, especially early on. The procedures can last from 5 to 30 minutes and are painless, except for the discomfort of the full bladder necessary for the first-trimester transabdominal exam.

During either exam, you'll lie on your back. For the transabdominal, your bare abdomen is spread with a film of gel that will improve the conduction of sound. A transducer is then moved slowly over your belly. For the transvaginal, the transducer is inserted into your vagina. In both procedures, the instruments record echoes of sound waves as they bounce off parts of your baby and translate them into pictures on a viewing screen.

When is it done? Ultrasound is done anytime during the first trimester of pregnancy, depending on the reason for performing one. A gestational sac can be visualized on ultrasound as early as 4½ weeks after your last period; a heartbeat can be detected as early as 5 to 6 weeks (though it might not be detected that early in all cases). For information on second-trimester ultrasound, see page 66.

How safe is it? After many years of clinical use and study, no known risks and a great many benefits have been associated with the use of ultrasound. Many practitioners order ultrasound exams routinely, at least once in a woman's pregnancy. Still, it's generally recommended by most experts that ultrasound be used in pregnancy only when a valid indication exists.

First-Trimester Combined Screening

What is it? First-trimester combined screening involves both an ultrasound and a blood test. First the ultrasound measures a thin layer of fluid that accumulates in the back of the baby's neck, called nuchal translucency (NT). Increased fluid *may* indicate an increased risk of chromosomal abnormalities such as Down syndrome, congenital heart defects, and other genetic disorders.

Then the blood test measures for high levels of PAPP-A (pregnancy-associated plasma protein A) and hCG, two hormones produced by the fetus and passed into the mother's bloodstream. These levels, combined with the NT measurement and the mother's age, can provide a risk assessment for Down syndrome and trisomy 18.

A few medical centers also look for the absence of a nasal bone in the fetus during the ultrasound. Some studies have shown that the lack of a nasal bone during the first trimester may indicate a higher risk of Down syndrome, but other studies haven't backed that up, making this type of assessment somewhat controversial.

Though the first-trimester combined screening test can't give you the definite diagnosis you'd get from more invasive diagnostic tests, it can help you decide whether you want to undergo diagnostic testing. If your screening test shows that your baby may be at an increased risk of having a chromosomal defect, a diagnostic test such as chorionic villus sampling (CVS; see this page) or amniocentesis (see page 64) will be offered. If the screening test doesn't show an increased risk, your practitioner might recommend that you take the quad screen test in the second trimester (see page 63) to rule out neural tube defects. And because increased NT measurements are also associated with fetal heart defects, your practitioner might suggest a fetal echocardiogram at around 20 weeks to screen for heart defects if your levels are high. Increased NT measurements may also be linked to a very slightly higher risk of preterm labor, so you may be monitored for that as well.

When is it done? First-trimester combined screening is performed between 11 and 14 weeks of pregnancy.

How accurate is it? This screening test doesn't directly test for chromosomal problems, nor does it diagnose a specific condition. Rather, the results merely provide you with your baby's statistical likelihood of having a problem. An abnormal result on the combined screening test doesn't mean that your baby has a chromosomal problem, just that he or she has an increased risk of having one. In fact, most women who have an abnormal result on their screening test go on to have a perfectly normal and healthy child. At the same time, a normal result is not a guarantee that your baby is normal, but it does mean that it is very unlikely that your baby has a chromosomal defect.

The first-trimester combined screening can detect approximately 80 percent of Down syndrome and 80 percent of trisomy 18 problems.

How safe is it? Both the ultrasound and the blood test are painless (unless you count the needle prick for the blood test) and carry no risk to you or your baby. But there is one caveat. This type of screening test requires sophisticated ultrasound technology. To assure the best possible accuracy of the results, it should only be done with special equipment (a high-quality ultrasound machine) and by physicians and sonographers with special ongoing training. Keep in mind, too, that a risk of the test is that a false-positive (screen-positive) result may lead to follow-up procedures that present greater risk. Before you consider taking any action on the basis of prenatal screening, be sure an experienced physician or genetic counselor has evaluated the results. Get a second opinion if you have any doubts.

Chorionic Villus Sampling

What is it? Chorionic villus sampling (CVS) is a prenatal diagnostic test that involves taking a small tissue sample from the finger-like projections of the placenta called the chorionic villi and testing the sample to detect chromosomal abnormalities. At present, CVS is used to detect disorders such as Down syndrome, Tay-Sachs, sickle cell anemia, and most types of cystic fibrosis. CVS cannot test for neural tube and other anatomical defects. Testing for specific diseases (other than Down syndrome) is usually done only when there is a family history of the disease or the parents are known to be carriers. It is believed that CVS will eventually be able to detect over 1,000 disorders for which defective genes or chromosomes are responsible.

How is it done? CVS is most often performed in a hospital, though it can

---

It's a ... Surprise!

Diagnostic testing can determine your baby's gender. But unless it's a necessary part of the diagnosis, you'll have the option of either learning the results when you receive the CVS or amnio results (if you haven't already found out through ultrasound results) or waiting to find out the old-fashioned way, in the birthing room. Just make sure your practitioner knows about your decision ahead of time so your surprise won't be inadvertently spoiled.

---

also be performed in a doctor's office. Depending on the location of the placenta, the sample of cells is taken via the vagina and cervix (transcervical CVS) or via a needle inserted in the abdominal wall (transabdominal CVS). Neither method is entirely pain free; the discomfort can range from very mild to moderate. Some women experience cramping (similar to to menstrual cramps) when the sample is taken. Both methods take about 30 minutes, start to finish, though the actual withdrawal of cells takes no more than a minute or two.

In the transcervical procedure, while you lie on your back, a long thin tube is inserted through your vagina into your uterus. Guided by ultrasound imaging, the doctor positions the tube between the uterine lining and the chorion, the fetal membrane that will eventually form the fetal side of the placenta. A sample of the chorionic villi is then snipped or suctioned off for diagnostic study.

In the transabdominal procedure, you'll also lie tummy up. Ultrasound is used to determine the location of the placenta and to view the uterine walls. Then, while still under ultrasound guidance, a needle is inserted through your abdomen and the uterine wall to the edge of the placenta, and the cells to be studied are drawn up through the needle.

Because the chorionic villi are of fetal origin, examining them can give a clear picture of the genetic makeup of the developing fetus. Test results are available in one to two weeks.

When is it done? CVS is performed between the 10th and 13th weeks of pregnancy. Its main advantage is the fact that it can be performed in the first trimester and it can give results (and most often, reassurance) earlier in pregnancy than amniocentesis, which is usually performed after the 16th week. The earlier diagnosis is particularly helpful for those who might consider a therapeutic pregnancy termination if something is seriously wrong, since an earlier abortion is less complicated and traumatic.

How accurate is it? CVS is able to accurately detect chromosomal abnormalities 98 percent of the time.

How safe is it? CVS is safe and reliable, carrying a miscarriage rate of about 1 in 370. Choosing a testing center with a good safety record and waiting until right after your 10th week can reduce any risks associated with the procedure.

Some vaginal bleeding can occur after CVS and should not be a cause for concern, though it should be reported. You should also let your doctor know if the bleeding lasts for three days or longer. Since there is a very slight risk of infection with CVS, report any fever that occurs in the first few days following the procedure.

First and Second Trimester

Integrated Screening

What is it? Like the first-trimester combined screening, the integrated screening test involves both an ultrasound and blood test results, but in this case, the ultrasound (to measure NT) and a first blood test (to measure the concentration of PAPP-A) are performed during the first trimester, and a second blood test (to measure the same four markers in the blood as in the quad screen; see below) is performed during the second trimester. All three tests are integrated to give you the results. Like other screening tests, the integrated test doesn't directly test for chromosomal problems, nor does it diagnose a specific condition; rather, the results merely provide you with your baby's statistical likelihood of having a problem. Once you have that information, you can decide, together with your practitioner, whether you want to undergo diagnostic testing.

When is it done? The ultrasound is performed between the 10th and 14th weeks. The first blood test is done on the same day as the ultrasound, and the second blood test is done between 16 and 18 weeks. The results are reported to you after the second blood test.

How accurate is it? A test gathering and integrating information from both the first and second trimester of pregnancy is more effective than one that uses information from the first or second trimesters alone. With the integrated screening test, about 90 percent of Down syndrome cases and 80 to 85 percent of neural tube defects are detected.

How safe is it? Both the ultrasound and the blood tests are painless and carry no risk to the mom or her baby.

Second Trimester

Quad Screening

What is it? Quad screening is a blood test that measures the levels of four substances produced by the fetus and passed into the mother's bloodstream: alpha-fetoprotein (AFP), hCG, estriol, and inhibin-A. (Some doctors test only for three of the substances in a triple screen.) High levels of AFP may suggest the possibility (but by no means the probability) that a baby is at higher risk for a neural tube defect. Low levels of AFP and abnormal levels of the other markers may indicate that the developing baby may be at higher risk for a chromosomal abnormality, such as Down syndrome. The quad screening, like all screening tests, can't diagnose a birth defect; it can only indicate a higher risk. Any abnormal result simply means that further testing is needed.

Interestingly, studies indicate that women who receive abnormal results on their quad screen but receive normal results on follow-up testing such as amniocentesis *may* still be at very slightly increased risk of certain pregnancy complications, such as a small-for-gestational-age fetus, preterm delivery, or preeclampsia. If you receive results like this, ask your practitioner what steps you can take to reduce the chances of any potential complications later on, keeping in mind that the association between abnormal results and such complictions is very small to begin with.

When is it done? Quad screening is performed between weeks 14 and 22.

How accurate is it? The quad screen can detect an increased risk of the defects for approximately 85 percent of neural tube defects, nearly 80 percent of Down syndrome cases, and 80 percent of trisomy 18 problems. The false-positive rate for the independent quad screen is high. Only 1 or 2 out of 50 women with abnormally high readings eventually prove to have an affected fetus. In the other 48 or 49, further testing reveals that the reason the hormone levels are abnormal is that there is more than one fetus, the fetus is either a few weeks older or younger than originally thought, or the results of the test were just wrong. If the woman is carrying only one fetus and the ultrasound shows the dates are correct, an amniocentesis is offered as follow-up.

How safe is it? Because the quad screen requires only a blood sample, it is completely safe. The major risk of the test is that a positive result may lead to follow-up procedures that present greater risk. Before you consider taking any action on the basis of prenatal screening, be sure an experienced physician or genetic counselor has evaluated the results.

Amniocentesis

What is it? The fetal cells, chemicals, and microorganisms in the amniotic fluid surrounding the fetus provide a wide range of information about the growing baby inside you, such as genetic makeup, present condition, and level of maturity. Being able to extract and examine some of the fluid through amniocentesis has been one of the most important advances in prenatal diagnosis. It is offered when:

- Results of a screening test (the combined first-trimester screen, the integrated screen, triple or quad screen, or ultrasound) turn out to be abnormal, and evaluation of the amniotic fluid is necessary to determine whether or not there actually is a fetal abnormality.

- The mother is older (usually over age 35), primarily to determine if the fetus has Down syndrome (though an older mom with reassuring screening results may opt, in consultation with her practitioner, to skip amnio).

- The couple has already had a child with a chromosomal abnormality, such as Down syndrome, a metabolic disorder, or an enzyme deficiency such as cystic fibrosis (CF).

- The mother is a carrier of an X-linked genetic disorder, such as hemophilia (which she has a 50 percent chance of passing on to any son she bears).

- Both parents are carriers of an autosomal recessive inherited disorder, such as Tay-Sachs disease or sickle cell anemia, and thus have a 1 in 4 chance of bearing an affected child.

- Toxoplasmosis, fifth disease, cytomegalovirus, or other fetal infection is suspected.

- It is necessary to assess the maturity of the fetal lungs late in pregnancy (among the last organs ready to function on their own).

How is it done? While you lie on your back, your baby and the placenta are located via ultrasound, so the doctor will be able to steer clear of them during the procedure. It's possible that your abdomen will be numbed with an injection of a local anesthetic, but because this injection is as painful as the procedure itself, most practitioners skip it. A long, hollow needle is inserted through your abdominal wall into your uterus and a small amount of fluid is withdrawn from the sac that surrounds your fetus. (Don't worry—baby will produce more amniotic fluid to replace what's withdrawn.) The slight risk of accidentally pricking the fetus during this part of the procedure is further reduced by the use of simultaneous ultrasound guidance. The entire procedure—including prep time and ultrasound—will usually take about 30 minutes, start to finish (though the actual withdrawal of amniotic fluid takes no more than a minute or two). If you're Rh negative, you'll be given an injection of Rh-immune globulin (RhoGAM) after the amniocentesis to be sure the procedure does not result in Rh problems (see page 48).

When is it done? Diagnostic amniocentesis is usually performed between the 16th and 18th weeks of pregnancy, but occasionally as early as the 13th or 14th or as late as the 23rd or 24th week. Test results are usually back in 10 to 14 days. Some labs offer the FISH—fluorescent in situ hybridization—method, which quickly counts the number of certain chromosomes within cells. It can be used on an amniocentesis sample to get a faster result, often within a day or two (the Flash FISH offers results in just a couple of hours)—but since the result won't be complete, it's always followed by the usual chromosomal test in the lab. Amniocentesis can also be performed in the last trimester to assess the maturity of fetal lungs.

How accurate is it? Amniocentesis is more than 99 percent accurate in diagnosing—or ruling out, which is

far more likely—Down syndrome. (A normal FISH test is about 98 percent accurate.)

How safe is it? Amniocentesis is extremely safe; the risk that the procedure will result in a miscarriage is believed to be as low as 1 in 1,600. You may experience a few minutes to no more than a few hours of mild cramping after the procedure. Some doctors recommend resting for the remainder of the day; others don't. Rarely, slight vaginal bleeding or amniotic fluid leakage may be experienced. If you notice either, report it at once. The chances are very good that both the leakage and the spotting will stop after a few days, but bed rest and careful observation are usually recommended until it does.

A False Screen

You undergo screening tests for the reassurance you hope they'll provide, but unfortunately, what happens so often instead—particularly with the triple or quad screen—is a false positive (it seems things might not be okay when ultimately it turns out they're just fine). There goes the reassurance you were hoping to find—and here comes the needless anxiety and worry you were so hoping to avoid.

That's why it's so important to start off the screening process with an open discussion with your practitioner about the high rate of false positives and what it really means if you get one. What you'll hear is this reassuring news: More than 90 percent of moms who get that positive screen will end up having perfectly normal and healthy babies. Talk about positive!

How to Freak Out a Pregnant Woman

Happily, most ultrasound exams show that all is going (and growing) well with baby. But for some women, a level 2 ultrasound may go something like this: One minute you're starry-eyed as you gaze at the ultrasound screen, marveling at the miraculous image of your baby floating blissfully inside you. The next minute, the technician is calling for the doctor, who knocks you right off cloud nine and into a state of panic with a few frightening words: "We see something—a soft marker—that might indicate a problem."

But before you panic, it's important to gain some reassuring perspective. Though "soft markers" on an ultrasound (detected during 5 to 10 percent of second-trimester ultrasounds, depending on the marker) are subtle characteristics that may indicate an increased risk of a chromosomal problem (most often Down syndrome or trisomy 18), these characteristics are also found in plenty of babies who are perfectly healthy. In fact, very few babies who show these soft markers (such as choroid plexus cyst, echogenic foci, or pyelectasia, to name a few) actually end up having a chromosomal abnormality. Which means that in the majority of cases, these so-called abnormal findings don't indicate anything abnormal at all.

Your practitioner may suggest some more tests (like an amnio) to find out for sure, but in the meantime, take a deep breath and remember that sometimes technology—which can bring so much joy—can also bring unneeded worry.

Second-Trimester Ultrasound

What is it? Even if you had an ultrasound in your first trimester to date your pregnancy or as part of the combined or integrated screening test, you'll probably also get an ultrasound in your second trimester. This level 2, or "targeted," ultrasound is a much more detailed scan that focuses closely on fetal anatomy and can be used to check in on the growing fetus for a variety of other reasons as pregnancy progresses. It also can be a lot more fun to look at, because it gives a far clearer picture of your baby-to-be.

These days, as ultrasound images become ever sharper, even nonexperts (like parents) are able to tell a head from a bottom, and much more. During your level 2 ultrasound, and with the help of the technician or doctor, you may be able to spot your baby's beating heart; the curve of the spine; the face, arms, and legs. You may even catch sight of your baby sucking its thumb. Usually, the genitals can be seen and the sex surmised, although with less than 100 percent reliability and depending on baby's cooperation (if you'd like to keep the sex a surprise until delivery, make sure you let the doctor or technician know this in advance). In most cases, you'll be able to bring home a souvenir of your exam, a "photo" or a copy of the 3-D or 4-D digital video to show to friends and family.

When is it done? It is usually performed between 18 and 22 weeks.

How safe is it? No known risks and many benefits have been associated with the use of ultrasound. And many practitioners order ultrasound exams, at least once in a woman's pregnancy, often several times. Still, most experts advise that ultrasound be used in pregnancy only when a valid indication exists.

If a Problem Is Found

In the vast majority of cases, prenatal diagnosis yields the results that parents hope for—that all is well with their baby-to-be. But when the news isn't good—when something does turn out to be wrong with their baby—the information provided by such a heartbreaking diagnosis can still be valuable to parents. Teamed with expert genetic counseling, it can be used to make vital decisions about this and future pregnancies. Possible options include:

Continuing the pregnancy. This option is often chosen when the defect uncovered is one the couple feels that both they and the baby they're expecting can live with, or when the parents are opposed to abortion under any circumstance. Having some idea of what is to come allows parents to make preparations (both emotional and practical) for receiving a child with special needs into the family, or for coping with the inevitable loss of a child. Parents can also begin working through the reactions (denial, resentment, guilt) that can come with discovering their baby has a problem, rather than waiting until after delivery. They can learn about the particular problem in advance and prepare to ensure the best possible life for their child. Joining a support group—even one online—can help make coping somewhat easier.

Terminating the pregnancy. If testing suggests a defect that will be fatal or extremely disabling, and retesting and interpretation by a genetic counselor confirms the diagnosis, some parents opt to terminate the pregnancy. Should you decide to terminate, an autopsy, in which fetal tissue is carefully examined afterward, may be helpful in determining the chances that the abnormality will repeat in future pregnancies. Most couples, armed with this information and the guidance of a physician or genetic counselor, do try again, with the hope that the tests and the pregnancy will be completely normal next time around. And most often they are.

Prenatal treatment of the fetus. Treatment may consist of blood transfusion (as in Rh disease), shunts or surgery (to drain an obstructed bladder, for instance), or administration of enzymes or medication (such as steroids to speed lung development when a baby must be delivered early). As technology advances, more kinds of prenatal surgery, genetic manipulation, and other treatments may also become common.

Donating the organs. If diagnosis indicates that the fetal defects are not compatible with life, it may be possible to donate one or more healthy organs to an infant in need. Some parents find that this provides some consolation for their own loss. A maternal-fetal specialist or neonatologist may be able to provide helpful information in such a situation.

As far as prenatal diagnosis has come, it's still important to remember that it's far from infallible. Mistakes happen, even in the best labs and facilities, even with the most skilled professionals wielding the most high-tech equipment—with false positives being much more common than false negatives. That's why further testing and/or consultation with additional professionals should always be used to confirm a result that indicates there is something wrong with the fetus.

It's also important to keep in mind that for the vast majority of couples, it will never come to that. Most expectant mothers who undergo prenatal testing receive the diagnosis they're hoping for right from the start: All is well with their baby and their pregnancy.

Your Pregnancy Lifestyle

O F COURSE YOU'RE EXPECTING TO make some adjustments in your everyday life now that you're expecting (good-bye baby-tees, hello baby-on-board tees). But you might also be wondering just how drastically your lifestyle will have to change now that you're living for two. How about that predinner cocktail—will it have to wait until postdelivery? Those regular dips in the hot tub at the gym—are those washed up, too? Can you wipe your bathroom sink with that smelly (but effective) disinfectant? And what's that you heard about cat litter? Does being pregnant really mean you have to think twice about all those things you've never given a second thought to—from letting your best friend smoke in your living room to zapping your dinner in the microwave? In a few cases, you'll find, the answer is an emphatic yes (as in "no wine for me, thanks"). But in many others, your expectant self will be able to continue doing business—and pleasure—as usual, with maybe just a side of caution ("Honey, it's your turn to change the cat litter—for the next nine months!").

What You May Be Wondering About

Sports and Exercise

"Can I keep up with my regular exercise program now that I'm pregnant?"

In most cases, pregnancy doesn't mean giving up the sporting life; just remember that while you're carrying a new life, moderation makes sense. Most practitioners not only permit but encourage expectant moms whose pregnancies are progressing normally to continue their accustomed workout routines and athletic pursuits for as long as is practical—but with several caveats. Among the most important: Always check with your practitioner before continuing or beginning an exercise program, and never exercise to the point of fatigue. (See page 215 for more information.)

Caffeine

"I use coffee to keep me going all day. Do I have to give up caffeine while I'm pregnant?"

No need to surrender your Starbucks card entirely—though you may have to start pulling it out a little less often. Most evidence suggests that drinking up to approximately 200 mg of caffeine a day is safe during pregnancy. Depending on how you take your coffee (black or with lots of milk), that could mean limiting yourself to about two cups (give or take) a day. Which means you're good to go (and fuel your get-up-and-go) if you're a light to moderate coffee drinker—but that you'll have to reassess your intake if you've got a more serious java jones (five-shot lattes, twice a day, come to mind?).

Why go so low? Well, for one thing, you share those lattes—like everything you eat and drink when you're expecting—with your baby. Caffeine (found most famously in coffee but also available in other foods and beverages) does cross the placenta—though to what extent (and at what dose) it affects a fetus is not completely clear. The latest information indicates that heavier caffeine intake early in pregnancy slightly increases the risk of miscarriage.

And there's more to the caffeine story. Sure, it has impressive pick-me-up powers, but it also has equally notable diuretic powers, causing calcium and other key pregnancy nutrients to be washed out of your system before they can be thoroughly absorbed. Another downside to this diuretic effect: more frequent urination, which is the last thing a pregnant woman needs (you'll be peeing plenty on your own now that you're expecting). Need more motivation for cutting down? Caffeine's stimulating effects may exacerbate your mood swings, making them even more volatile and intense than they already are (or than they will be once your hormones rev into action). It can also prevent you from getting the rest your body's craving more than ever, especially if you drink it after noon. Plus excessive caffeine may interfere with the absorption of the iron both you and your baby need.

Different practitioners have different recommendations on caffeine consumption, so check in with yours for a bottom line on your favorite brew. When calculating your daily caffeine intake, keep in mind that it's not necessarily as easy as counting cups. Caffeine isn't just found in coffee—it's also in caffeinated soft drinks (too many Mountain Dews will have to be a Mountain Don't), coffee ice cream, tea, energy bars and drinks, and chocolate (though the amount varies from product to product). You'll need to know, too, that dark brews sold in coffeehouses contain far more caffeine than homemade; likewise, instant coffee contains less than drip does (see box, next page).

How do you cut down on a hefty caffeine habit (or cut it out altogether)? That depends on what's in the caffeine for you. If it's a part of your day (or many parts of your day—an eye-opener when you wake up, a companion on your way to work, a desktop fixture, an afternoon pick-me-up) that you're not anxious to part with, there's no need to. Just make your morning joes regular and your afternoons decaf. Or order your latte with mostly decaf shots instead of regular—or with less espresso and more milk (you'll get a bigger calcium bonus anyway).

If it's the lift you crave—and that your body has become accustomed to—cutting back will be a taller order (make that a Venti order). As any coffee lover is well aware, it's one thing to be motivated to cut back on or kick caffeine altogether and another thing to do it. Caffeine is addictive (that's where the craving comes in), and quitting—or even cutting

way back on—a heavy habit comes with its own set of withdrawal symptoms, including headache, irritability, fatigue, and lethargy. That's why it's a good idea to ease off heavy consumption gradually. Try cutting back a cup at a time, and give yourself a few days to adjust to the lower dose before cutting back by another cup. Another way to cut back: Take each cup half-caf, gradually going full decaf in more and more cups—until your total caffeine consumption is down to that two-a-day-or-less goal.

No matter what's been driving you to the coffee bar, cutting back on or kicking caffeine will be less of a drag (literally) if you follow these energizing solutions:

- Keep your blood sugar (and thus your energy level) up. You'll get a natural, longer-lasting boost from eating and snacking on healthy foods often, especially complex carbs and protein (a combo that will give you the lift that keeps on lifting).

- Get some pregnancy-appropriate exercise each day. Exercise also raises the energy roof, while releasing those feel-good endorphins. Adding fresh air to the exercise mix will give you an extra energy boost.

- Clock in enough sleep time. Getting the rest your body needs at night (which will probably be easier to do without all that caffeine keeping you wired) will help you feel more refreshed in the morning, even before you've filled your first mug.

Caffeine Counter

How much caffeine do you get per day? It may be more—or less—than you think (and more or less than that approximate target of 200 mg). Check out this handy list, so you can do the math before you belly up to the coffee bar:

- 1 cup brewed coffee (8 ounces) = 135 mg

- 1 cup instant coffee = 95 mg

- 1 cup decaf coffee = 5 mg

- 6 ounces caffe latte or cappuccino = 90 mg

- 1 ounce espresso = 90 mg

- 1 cup tea = 40 to 60 mg (green tea has less caffeine than black tea)

- 1 can of cola (12 ounces) = about 35 mg caffeine

- 1 can of diet cola = 45 mg

- 1 ounce milk chocolate = 6 mg

- 1 ounce dark chocolate = 20 mg

- 1 cup chocolate milk = 5 mg

- 8 ounces coffee ice cream = 40 to 80 mg

Drinking

"I had a couple of drinks at least a couple of times before I knew I was pregnant. Could the alcohol have harmed my baby?"

Wouldn't it be nice to get an instant message from your body alerting you the moment sperm and egg met up? ("Just wanted to let you know we have a baby on board—time to switch to Evian.") But since that biotechnology doesn't exist (not yet, at least), many moms-to-be are oblivious that baby making has begun until several weeks into their pregnancies. And in the meantime, they're apt to have done a thing or two they wouldn't have done if they'd only known. Like having a few, a few times too many. Which is why your concern is one of the most common ones brought to the first prenatal visit.

Fortunately, it's a concern that you can cross off the list. There's no evidence that a couple of drinks on a couple of occasions very early in pregnancy, when you didn't even know you were pregnant, can harm a developing embryo. So you—and all the other moms who didn't get the message right away—can relax.

That said, it's definitely time to change that drink order now. Although you've probably heard of some women who drank lightly during pregnancy—one glass of wine nightly, for instance—and delivered perfectly healthy babies, there's just no research to support that this is a completely safe bet. In fact, the Surgeon General, ACOG, and the American Academy of Pediatrics (AAP) advise that no amount of alcohol is safe for pregnant women. That recommendation—and the research behind it—also leads to this recommendation: Although you shouldn't worry about what you drank before you knew you were pregnant, it would be prudent to take a pass for the rest of your pregnancy. (You can also ask your own practitioner about what he or she recommends.)

Why such a strong edict from the medical community? It's to be on the safe side—always the best side to be on when you have a baby on board. Though nobody knows for sure whether there is a safe limit when it comes to alcohol con-

sumption during pregnancy (or whether that limit would be different in different women), it is known that alcohol enters the fetal bloodstream in about the same concentrations present in the expectant mother's blood. In other words, a pregnant woman never drinks alone—she shares each glass of wine, each beer, each cocktail equally with her baby. Since it takes the fetus twice as long as its mother to eliminate the alcohol from its system, the baby can be at the point of passing out when the mother is just pleasantly buzzed.

Heavier drinking (generally considered to be the consumption of five or six drinks of wine, beer, or liquor a day) throughout pregnancy can result not only in many serious obstetrical complications but also in fetal alcohol syndrome (FAS). Described as "the hangover that lasts a lifetime," this condition produces infants who are born undersized, usually mentally deficient, with multiple deformities (particularly of the head and face, limbs, heart, and central nervous system) and a high mortality rate. Later, those who survive display vision, learning, behavioral, and social problems, and they generally lack the ability to make sound judgments. They are also more likely to end up with a drinking problem of their own by the time they reach 21. The sooner a heavy drinker stops drinking during pregnancy, the less risk to her baby.

The risks of continued drinking are definitely dose related: The more you drink, the more potential danger to your baby. But even moderate consumption (one to two drinks daily or occasional heavy bingeing on five or more drinks), if it occurs throughout pregnancy, is related to a variety of serious problems, including increased risk of miscarriage, labor and delivery complications, low birthweight, stillbirth, abnormal growth, and developmental and low IQ problems in childhood. Such drinking has also been linked to the somewhat more subtle fetal alcohol effect (FAE), characterized by numerous developmental and behavioral problems.

Passing up a drink during pregnancy is as easily done as said for some women, especially those who develop an aversion to alcohol (its taste and its smell) in early pregnancy, which sometimes lingers through delivery. For others, particularly those who are accustomed to unwinding with a Cosmo at the end of the day or to sipping a glass of red with dinner, abstinence may require a concerted effort and may include a lifestyle change. If you drink to relax, for example, try substituting other methods of relaxation: music, warm baths, massage, exercise, or reading. If drinking is part of a daily ritual that you don't want to give up, try a Virgin Mary (a Bloody Mary without the vodka) at brunch, sparkling juice or nonalcoholic beer at dinner, or a juice spritzer (half juice, half sparkling water, with a twist)—served at the usual time, in the usual glasses (unless, of course, these look-alike beverages trigger a yen for the real stuff). If your spouse joins you on the wagon (at least while in your company), the ride will be considerably smoother.

If you're having trouble giving up alcohol, ask your practitioner for help and for a referral to a program that can help you quit.

Smoking

"I've been smoking cigarettes for 10 years. Will this hurt my baby?"

Happily, there's no clear evidence that any smoking you've done prior to pregnancy—even if it's been for 10 or more years—will harm a developing fetus. But it's well documented (as well as plastered on cigarette packs) that smoking during pregnancy, particularly beyond

---

(Don't) Put That in Your Pipe

Your baby will thank you, also, for not smoking cigars and pipes—and for avoiding situations where they're being smoked. Because they aren't inhaled, cigars and pipes release even more smoke into the air than cigarettes do, which makes them even more potentially harmful to your baby. Want to announce your expected pride and joy with something safe and festive? Pass out chocolate cigars instead.

---

the third month, isn't just hazardous to your health—but to your baby's, too.

In effect, when you smoke, your fetus is confined in a smoke-filled womb. Its heartbeat speeds and, worst of all, due to insufficient oxygen, it can't grow and thrive as it should.

The results can be devastating. Smoking can increase the risk of a wide variety of pregnancy complications, including (among the more serious of these) ectopic pregnancy, abnormal placental implantation, premature placental detachment, premature rupture of the membranes, and possibly early delivery.

There is also strong evidence that a baby's development in utero is adversely and directly affected by an expectant mother's smoking. The most widespread risks for babies of smokers are low birthweight, shorter length and smaller head circumference, as well as cleft palate or cleft lip and heart defects. And being born too small is the major cause of infant illness and perinatal death (those that occur just before, during, or after birth).

There are other potential risks as well. Babies of smokers are more likely to die from SIDS (sudden infant death syndrome). They are also more prone to apnea (breathing lapses) and, in general, they aren't as healthy at birth as babies of nonsmokers, with three-pack-a-day maternal smoking associated with a quadrupled risk of low Apgar scores (the standard scale used to evaluate an infant's condition at birth). And evidence indicates that, on average, these children will suffer long-term physical and intellectual deficits, especially if parents continue to smoke around them. They are particularly prone to a lowered immune system, respiratory diseases, ear infections, colic, TB, food allergies, asthma, short stature, and problems in school, including attention deficit hyperactivity disorder (ADHD). Studies also show that pregnant women who smoke are more likely to have children who are abnormally aggressive as toddlers and who continue to have behavioral problems into adulthood. Children of mothers who smoked while pregnant are hospitalized more often in their first year of life than children of mothers who did not smoke while pregnant. These children are also more likely to grow up to be smokers themselves.

The effects of tobacco use, like those of alcohol use, are dose related: Tobacco use reduces the birthweight of babies in direct proportion to the number of cigarettes smoked, with a pack-a-day smoker 30 percent more likely to give birth to a low-birthweight child than a nonsmoker. So cutting down on the number of cigarettes you smoke may help some. But cutting down can be misleading because a smoker often compensates by taking more frequent and deeper puffs and smoking more of each cigarette. This can also happen when she tries to reduce the risk by using low-tar or low-nicotine cigarettes.

An Early Baby Present

There are no sure things when it comes to making a baby, but there are plenty of ways of improving your chances of having the best outcome possible: an uncomplicated pregnancy and delivery, and a perfectly healthy, full-term bundle of joy. And giving up smoking and drinking definitely tops the list.

Of course, there's the possibility that you can have that happy outcome even if you smoke or drink your way through pregnancy (or even smoke or drink lightly but regularly)—after all, everybody's heard of women who have done both and delivered healthy babies, right on time. But there's also the chance—and depending on how much smoking or drinking you do, a very significant risk—that you and your baby wouldn't be that lucky. Consider that different mothers and different babies are affected differently by pregnancy smoking and drinking (and there's no way to predict how you and your baby will be affected). Consider, too, that some of the deficits—physical and intellectual—linked to maternal smoking and drinking don't always show up at birth but often years later (a seemingly healthy infant can grow into a child who is often sick, who is hyperactive, or who has trouble learning).

Giving up pregnancy-unfriendly habits like drinking and smoking isn't always easy—and sometimes it's a real struggle. But giving your baby the very best chances of being born healthy is definitely the very best gift you can give.

Breaking the Smoking Habit

Congratulations—you've decided to give your baby a smoke-free environment, in utero and out. Making that commitment is the first and most important step. Realistically, however—as you probably already know if you've tried quitting before—it's not the most difficult step. Actually quitting is. But with a lot of determination and a little help from the following tips, you *can* do it.

Identify your motivations for quitting. When you're pregnant, that's easy. You've never had a more motivating reason.

Choose your method of withdrawal. Do you want to go cold turkey or taper off? Either way, pick a "last day" that isn't far off. Plan a full schedule of fun and distracting activities for that date—those you don't associate with smoking (in places, preferably, that don't allow smoking).

Identify your motivations for smoking. For example, do you smoke for pleasure, stimulation, or relaxation? To reduce tension or frustration? To have something in your hand or mouth? To satisfy a craving? Perhaps you smoke out of habit, lighting up without thinking about it. Once you understand your motivations, it'll help you find substitutes:

- If you smoke mainly to keep your hands busy, try playing with a pencil, beads, or a straw. Knit, play Sudoku on the computer, squeeze a stress ball, catch up on your e-mail, play video games, paint, doodle, do a crossword puzzle—anything that might make you forget to reach for a cigarette.

- If you smoke for oral gratification, try a substitute: a toothpick, gum, raw vegetables, popcorn, a lollipop or hard candy.

- If you smoke for stimulation, try to get your lift from a brisk walk, a workout session at the gym, an absorbing book, a long chat with a friend.

- If you smoke to reduce tension and relax, try exercise instead. Or relaxation techniques. Or listening to soothing music. Or a long walk. Or a massage. Or making love.

- If you smoke for pleasure, seek pleasure in other pursuits, preferably in no-smoke situations. Go to a movie, visit baby boutiques, tour a favorite museum, attend a concert or a play, have dinner with a friend who's a nonsmoker. Or try something more active, like a prenatal fitness class.

But the news isn't all bad. Some studies show that women who quit smoking early in pregnancy—no later than the third month—can eliminate all of the associated risks. For some smoking women, quitting will never be easier than in early pregnancy when they might develop a sudden distaste for cigarettes—probably the warning of an intuitive body. Sooner is better, but quitting even in the last month can help preserve oxygen flow to the baby during delivery.

If you're concerned that quitting will cause you to gain extra weight, keep in mind that although there is no evidence that smoking actually keeps weight down (many smokers are overweight, after all), it is true that some smokers gain weight while in the process of quitting. Interestingly enough, those who gain some

■ If you smoke out of habit, avoid the settings in which you habitually smoke and friends who smoke; frequent places with no-smoking rules instead.

■ If you associate smoking with a particular beverage, food, or meal, avoid the food or beverage, or eat the meal in a different location. (Say you smoke with breakfast but you never smoke in bed. Have breakfast in bed for a few days. You always smoke with your coffee? Have that latte in the coffeehouse, where smoking's not on the menu.)

■ When you feel the urge to smoke, take several deep breaths with a pause between each. Hold the last breath while you strike a match. Exhale slowly, blowing out the match. Pretend it was a cigarette and crush it out.

If you do slip up and have a cigarette, put it behind you. Don't give a second thought to the cigarette you smoked—think instead about all the ones you passed up. Get right back on your program, knowing that every cigarette you don't smoke is going to help your baby.

Try to look at smoking as nonnegotiable. When you were a smoker, you couldn't smoke in theaters, subways, at the mall, in many restaurants, and probably at your workplace. That was that. Now try telling yourself that you can't smoke, period—and that's that.

Let your baby inspire you. Post copies of your baby's ultrasound picture everywhere you might be tempted to smoke (make it your screensaver, frame it on the kitchen table, tape it on your dashboard, carry one in your bag). No ultrasound yet? Post pictures of adorable babies that you've cut out from magazines.

Get some support. There's plenty of help for smokers who want to quit. Look into hypnosis, acupuncture, and relaxation techniques, which have made quitters out of many smokers. If you're comfortable with a group approach to quitting, consider programs run by Nicotine Anonymous (misery often loves company—and support), the American Lung Association, the American Cancer Society, and SmokEnders, which have helped millions of smokers break the habit. Or seek support online from other pregnant women who are trying to call it quits.

If at first you don't succeed, try, try again. Nicotine is a powerful drug, and giving it up isn't easy, but it can be done. Many smokers don't succeed the first time they try quitting, yet they do if they keep trying. So don't beat yourself up when you slip up—pat yourself on the back for your efforts, and then up your efforts. You can do it!

Note: Using nicotine patches, lozenges, or gums during pregnancy is risky and not recommended.

weight while trying to break the smoking habit are more likely to succeed—and they find it fairly easy to drop those few pounds later. Trying to diet while trying to quit usually leads to failure in both arenas. What's more, dieting while growing a baby is never a good idea. So though you should definitely pack away the cigarettes for good, don't worry if you start packing on a few more pounds than you otherwise

would have. There's never been a better reason for both.

Since nicotine is an addictive drug, most people experience withdrawal symptoms when they quit smoking, though the symptoms and their intensity vary from person to person. Besides the obvious craving for tobacco, some of the most common symptoms are irritability, anxiety, restlessness, tingling or numbness in the hands and feet, lightheadedness, fatigue, and sleep and gastrointestinal disturbances. Some people also find that both physical and mental performance are impaired at first. Most find that they initially cough more, rather than less, because their bodies are suddenly better able to bring up all the secretions that have accumulated in the lungs.

To try to slow the release of nicotine and the jitteriness that may result, avoid caffeine, which can add to the jitters. Get plenty of rest (to counter fatigue) and exercise (to replace the kick you used to get from nicotine). Avoid activities that require a lot of focus and concentration if you find you're in something of a fog, but keep busy by doing mindless tasks. Hanging out wherever smoking is prohibited by your state laws may also help. If you experience serious depression as part of withdrawal, talk to your practitioner immediately.

The worst effects of withdrawal will last a few days to a few weeks. The benefits, however, will last a lifetime—for you and your baby. See box, previous page, for more tips on how to quit.

Secondhand Smoke

"I don't smoke, but my husband does. Will this hurt our baby?"

Smoking doesn't affect just the smoker. It affects everyone around him, including a developing fetus whose mother happens to be nearby. So if your spouse (or anyone else you spend time with) smokes, your baby's body is going to pick up nearly as much contamination from tobacco smoke by-products as if you were lighting up.

If your spouse says he can't quit smoking, ask him to at least do all his smoking out of the house, away from you and the baby (but remember that smoke and its by-products will stick to

his clothes and skin, which means you'll still get some exposure to them). Quitting, of course, would be better, not just for his own health, but also for the baby's long-term well-being. Parental smoking—mother's or father's—increases the risk of SIDS in infancy, of respiratory problems at all ages, and of damage to the lungs even into adulthood. And it ups the chances that your children will become smokers one day.

You probably won't be able to get friends and other relatives to kick the habit, but you may be able to get them to curb their smoking around you (otherwise, you'll have to spend less time around them). Keeping smoking coworkers out of your breathing space will be easier to do if there are laws protecting nonsmokers in your workplace (many states have such laws). If the law isn't on your side, try tactful persuasion—show them this section on the dangers of secondhand smoke to a fetus. If that fails, try to get a regulation passed where you work that limits smoking to certain areas, such as a lounge, and prohibits smoking in the vicinity of nonsmokers. If all else fails, try to move your work space for the duration of your pregnancy.

Marijuana Use

"I smoke pot occasionally—basically only socially—and have for years. Could this have caused harm to the baby I'm now carrying? And is smoking pot during pregnancy dangerous?"

You can safely put past pot behind you. While it's usually recommended that couples trying to conceive pass on pot because it can interfere with conception, you're already pregnant—so that won't be a problem for you. And there's no present evidence that the marijuana you've smoked before you conceived will harm your fetus.

But now that you're pregnant, it's time to get off the pot. All the research isn't in yet, and the research that has been done so far isn't the most helpful kind. That's because it's hard to study marijuana use—like many lifestyle choices—in a vacuum. Often those who smoke pot during pregnancy are also drinking alcohol, smoking cigarettes, or using other drugs, making the data inconclusive (is it the pot or the beer or the cigarettes that resulted in a poor fetal outcome?). Other times, pregnant women who smoke marijuana may have less than optimal prenatal care, so it's hard to know whether a bad outcome came from the pot or the lack of prenatal care. What is known so far about marijuana use during pregnancy is that the drug passes through the placenta, which means that when you smoke pot, you're sharing it with your unborn baby. Some studies show that marijuana use is associated with poor fetal growth and babies born small for gestational age; other studies show no such relationship. Still other studies have shown even more negative effects—from tremors and withdrawal-like crying during the newborn period to attention, learning, and behavioral problems later on in childhood.

With no sure proof that it's safe to smoke pot during pregnancy—and some evidence that suggests it may be quite harmful—it's wise to treat marijuana as you would any other drug during pregnancy: Just say no.

If you have already smoked early in your pregnancy, don't worry. But if you're tempted to continue using it, try some of the suggestions for quitting tobacco (and alcohol)—kicking one addiction is similar to kicking another. Focus especially on healthy forms of relaxation that'll net you that natural high (yoga, meditation, massage, even endorphin-releasing exercise). If you can't seem to stop smoking pot,

speak to your practitioner or seek other professional help as soon as possible.

Cocaine and Other Drug Use

"I did some cocaine a week before I found out I was pregnant. Now I'm worried about what that could have done to my baby."

Don't worry about past cocaine use; just make sure it was your last. On the upside: A single use of cocaine before you found out you were pregnant isn't likely to have had any effect. On the downside: Continuing to use it during pregnancy could be dangerous. How dangerous isn't quite clear. Studies on cocaine use during pregnancy aren't that easy to interpret, mostly because cocaine users are often also smokers—which means that it's difficult to separate the probable negative effects of cocaine use from the documented negative effects of smoking. What numerous studies have shown is that cocaine not only crosses the placenta once it develops, but it can damage it, reducing blood flow to the fetus and restricting fetal growth, particularly that of the baby's head. It is also believed to lead to birth defects, miscarriage, premature labor, low birthweight; jitteriness and withdrawal-like crying in the newborn; as well as numerous long-term problems for a child, including neurological and behavioral problems (such as difficulty with impulse control, with paying attention, and with responding to others), motor development deficits, and possibly lower IQ scores later on in childhood. Certainly, the more often an expectant mother uses cocaine, the greater the risk to her baby.

Tell your practitioner about any cocaine use since you've conceived. As with every aspect of your medical history, the more your doctor or midwife knows, the better care you and your baby will receive. If you have any difficulty giving up cocaine entirely, seek professional help immediately.

Pregnant women who use drugs of any kind—other than those that have been prescribed by a physician who knows they are pregnant—are putting their babies at risk. Every known illicit drug (including heroin, meth, crack, Ecstasy, "ice," LSD, and PCP) and many prescription drugs that are often abused (including narcotics, tranquilizers, sedatives, and diet pills) can, with continued use, cause serious harm to a developing fetus and/or to your pregnancy. Check with your practitioner or another knowledgeable doctor about any drugs you've used during pregnancy. Then, if you are still using drugs, get professional support (from a certified addiction counselor, an addictionologist, or a treatment center) to help you quit now. Enrolling in a drug-free-pregnancy program now can make a tremendous difference in the outcome of your pregnancy.

Cell Phones

"I spend hours a day on my cell phone. Could this have any effect on my baby?"

Look who's talking (on the cell phone): practically everyone. And luckily, there's no need to put your cell out of service now that you're talking for two. No pregnancy risks have ever been suggested from cell phone use. And there are plenty of good reasons to keep connected to your cell phone—it can allow you to be available for that call from the doctor or midwife you can't wait for at home, to make consultation appointments with pediatricians while you're waiting at the obstetrician's, to alert a spouse at the first signs of labor when you're nowhere near a landline.

A cell phone may also allow you to be more flexible in your workday and in the amount of time spent chained to a desk (which might result in more time for needed rest and relaxation or baby preparations).

That said, cell phones aren't completely risk free. Driving while talking on a handheld cell phone is unsafe—at any speed and under any circumstances (and illegal in some areas)—particularly when the hormone-induced fog of pregnancy leaves you more easily distracted than usual. Even a hands-free phone conversation can be risky if it takes your attention off the road. Play it smart and pull over to a safe area before placing your calls.

Microwaves

"I use my microwave practically every day to heat up food or even cook. Is microwave exposure safe during pregnancy?"

A microwave oven can be a mother-to-be's best friend, helping to make healthy eating-on-the-run possible—with a minimum of effort and cooking odor. And happily, all the research indicates that microwaves are completely safe to use during pregnancy (and at all other times). Two sensible precautions: Use only cookware that is specifically manufactured for use in the microwave, and don't let plastic wrap touch foods during microwaving.

Hot Tubs and Saunas

"We have a hot tub. Is it safe for me to use it while I'm pregnant?"

You won't have to switch to cold showers, but it's probably a good idea to stay out of the hot tub. Anything that raises the body temperature over

102°F and keeps it there for a while—whether it's a soak in a hot tub or an extremely hot bath, or an overzealous workout in hot weather—is potentially hazardous to the developing embryo or fetus, particularly in the early months. Some studies have shown that a hot tub doesn't raise a woman's temperature to dangerous levels immediately—it takes at least 10 minutes (longer if the shoulders and arms are not submerged or if the water is 102°F or less). But because individual responses and circumstances vary, play it safe by keeping your belly out of the hot tub. Feel free, however, to soak your feet.

If you've already had some brief dips in the hot tub, there is probably no cause for concern. Most women spontaneously get out of a hot tub before their body temperatures reach 102°F because they become uncomfortable. It's likely you did, too. If you are concerned, however, speak to your practitioner about the possibility of having an ultrasound exam or other prenatal test to help put your mind at ease.

Lengthy stays in the sauna or steam room aren't smart, either. A pregnant woman is at greater risk for dehydration, dizziness, and lower blood pressure in general, and these are all symptoms that may be exacerbated by such extreme heat. And as with a hot tub, pregnant women should avoid anything that might potentially raise their body temperatures.

For more information on the safety of other types of spa treatments (massage, aromatherapy, and so on), see page 147.

The Family Cat

"I have two cats at home. I've heard that cats carry a disease that can harm a fetus. Do I have to get rid of my pets?"

Is Hot Stuff Not So Hot?

Considering cuddling up with an electric blanket when the winter chill sets in? Or easing that achy-breaky back with a heating pad? Too much heat isn't so hot when you're pregnant, since it may raise your body temperature excessively. So cuddle up to your sweetie instead of that electric blanket (or if his tootsies are as icy as yours, invest in a down comforter, push up the thermostat, or heat the bed with an electric blanket and then turn it off before you turn in). Still feeling the chill? Keep in mind that as the months pass, you'll probably be keeping yourself so warm—thanks to a pregnancy-boosted metabolism—that you'll be kicking off all your covers anyway.

As for that heating pad, wrap it in a towel before you apply it to your back, belly, or shoulders to reduce the heat it passes along (an ankle or knee can take the heat), keep it at the lowest setting, limit applications to 15 minutes, and avoid sleeping with it. Already spent some time under that electric blanket or heating pad? Not to worry—there's no proven risk.

Don't send your feline friends packing. Since you've lived with them for a while, the chances are pretty good that you've already contracted the cat-related disease toxoplasmosis and have developed an immunity to it. It's estimated that up to 40 percent of the American population has been exposed, and the rates of exposure are much higher among people who have cats that spend time outdoors, as well as among people who frequently eat raw meat or drink unpasteurized milk, both of which can also harbor and transmit the infection. If you weren't tested prenatally to see if you were immune, it's not likely you will be tested now, unless you show symptoms of the disease (though some practitioners run regular tests on all pregnant women and others test only those who live with cats). If you were tested prenatally and were not immune, or if you're not sure whether you are immune or not, take the following precautions to avoid infection:

- Have your cats tested by a veterinarian to see if they have an active infection. If one or more do, board them at a kennel or ask a friend to care for them for at least six weeks, the period during which the infection is transmissible. If they are free of infection, keep them that way by not allowing them to eat raw meat, roam outdoors, hunt mice or birds (which can transmit toxoplasmosis to cats), or hang out with other cats.

- Have someone else handle the litter box. If you must do it yourself, use disposable gloves and wash your hands when you're finished, as well as after you touch your cats. The litter should be changed daily.

- Wear gloves when gardening. Don't garden in soil in which cats may have deposited feces. If you have children, don't allow them to play in sand that may have been used by cats or other animals.

- Wash fruits and vegetables, especially those grown in home gardens, rinsing very thoroughly, and/or peel or cook them.

- Don't eat raw or undercooked meat or unpasteurized milk. In restaurants, order meat well done.

- Wash your hands thoroughly after handling raw meats.

Some practitioners are urging routine testing before conception or in very early pregnancy for all women, so that those who test positive can relax, knowing they are immune, and those who test negative can take the necessary precautions to prevent infection. However, public health officials believe the financial cost of such testing outweighs the benefit it may provide. Check with your practitioner to see what he or she recommends.

Household Hazards

"How much do I really have to worry about household hazards like cleaning products and bug sprays? And what about tap water—is it safe to drink it while I'm pregnant?"

A little perspective goes a long way when you're expecting. Sure, you've read or heard that cleaning products, insecticides, drinking water, and other substances around the house can be dangerous to live with, especially when you're living for two. But the fact is that your home is probably a very safe place for you and your baby to hang out—especially if you couple a little caution with a lot of common sense. Here's what you need to know about so-called household hazards:

Household cleaning products. Mopping your kitchen floor or polishing your dining room table may be tough on your pregnant back, but it's not tough on your pregnancy. Still, it makes sense to clean with care when you're expecting. Let your nose and the following tips be your guide:

- If the product has a strong odor or fumes, don't breathe it in directly. Use it in an area with plenty of ventilation, or don't use it at all (what better excuse for getting your spouse to scrub the toilet?).

- Never (even when you're not pregnant) mix ammonia with chlorine-based products; the combination produces deadly fumes.

- Try to avoid using products such as oven cleaners and dry-cleaning fluids whose labels are plastered with warnings about toxicity.

- Wear rubber gloves when you're using a really strong product. Not only will this spare your hands a lot of wear and tear, it'll prevent the absorption of chemicals through the skin.

Lead. Exposure to lead isn't just potentially harmful to small children but to pregnant women and their fetuses as well. Fortunately, it's also pretty easy to avoid. Here's how:

- Since drinking water is a common source of lead, be sure yours is lead free (see below).

- Old paint is a major source of lead. If your home dates back to 1955 or earlier and layers of paint are to be removed for any reason, stay away from the house while the work is being done. If you find paint is flaking in an older home, or if you have a piece of old painted furniture that's flaking, see about having the walls or furniture repainted to contain the flaking lead paints, or have the old paint removed—again, stay away while the job is being done.

- Flea market fan? You might want to know that lead can also be leached from older earthenware, pottery, and china. If you have pitchers or dishes that are home-crafted, imported, antique, or just plain old (the FDA did

not set limits on lead in dishes until 1971), don't use them for serving food or beverages, particularly those that are acidic (citrus, vinegar, tomatoes, wine, soft drinks).

Tap water. It's still the best drink in the house—and in most houses, water is completely safe and drinkable straight from the tap. To be sure that when you fill a glass of water you'll be drinking to your—and your baby's—good health, do the following:

- Check with your local Environmental Protection Agency (EPA) or health department about the purity and safety of community drinking water or a well, if that is the source of your tap water (go to epa.gov/safewater/dwinfo/index.html). Or check with the EPA Water Safety Hotline at (800) 426-4791 or online at scorecard.org. If there is a possibility that the quality of your water might differ from the rest of the community's (because of pipe deterioration, because your home borders on a waste disposal area, or because of odd taste or color), arrange to have it tested. Your local EPA or health department can tell you how.

- If your tap water fails the test, invest in a filter (what kind depends on what turns up in your water) or use bottled water for drinking and cooking. Be aware, however, that bottled waters are not automatically free of impurities; some contain more than tap water, and some are bottled directly from the tap (talk about throwing money down the drain). Many bottled waters also don't contain fluoride, an important mineral, especially for growing teeth (your baby's). To check the purity of a particular brand, contact the National Sanitation Foundation at (800) 673-6275 or nsf.org. Avoid distilled waters (from which beneficial minerals have been removed).

- If you suspect lead in your water, or if testing reveals high levels, changing the plumbing would be the ideal solution, but this is not always feasible. To reduce the levels of lead in the water you drink, use only cold water for drinking and cooking (hot leaches more lead from the pipes), and run the cold-water tap for about five minutes in the morning (as well as anytime the water has been off for six hours or more) before using it. You can tell that lead-free fresh water from the street pipes has reached your faucet when the water has gone from cold to warmer to cold again.

- If your water smells and/or tastes like chlorine, boiling it or letting it stand, uncovered, for 24 hours will evaporate much of the chemical.

Pesticides. Can't live with roaches, ants, and other yucky insects? Living with them, of course, often means eliminating them through the use of chemical pesticides. Fortunately, pest control and pregnancy can be completely compatible, with a few precautions. If your neighborhood is being sprayed, avoid hanging around outside for long periods until the chemical odors have dissipated, usually about two to three days. When indoors, keep the windows closed. If spraying for roaches or other insects is necessary in your apartment or house, be sure all closets and kitchen cabinets are tightly closed (so the chemicals don't seep in and settle on dishes and food) and all food-preparation surfaces are covered. Ventilate with open windows until the fumes have dissipated. Once the spray has settled, make sure food-preparation surfaces in or near the sprayed area have been thoroughly wiped down.

Whenever possible, try to take a natural approach to pest control. Pull weeds instead of spraying them. Eliminate some pests from garden and houseplants by spraying with a forceful stream from the garden hose or with a biodegradable insecticidal soap mixture (the procedure may need to be repeated several times to be effective). Invest in an infantry of ladybugs or other beneficial predators (available from some garden supply houses) that like to feed on the bugs that are bugging you.

Inside the house, use "motel" or other types of traps, strategically placed in heavy bug traffic areas, to get rid of roaches and ants; use cedar blocks instead of mothballs in clothes closets; and check an environmentally friendly store or catalog for nontoxic pesticides. If you have young children or pets, keep all traps and pesticide products out of their reach. Even so-called natural pesticides, including boric acid, can be toxic when ingested or inhaled, and they can be irritating to the eyes. For more information on natural pest control, contact your regional Cooperative Extension Service or a local environmental group. You may even have a "green" exterminator in your neighborhood.

Also keep in mind that brief, indirect exposure to insecticides or herbicides isn't likely to be harmful. What does increase the risk is frequent, long-term exposure, the kind that working daily around such chemicals (as in a factory or heavily sprayed field) would involve.

Paint fumes. In the entire animal kingdom, the period before birth (or egg laying) is spent in hectic preparation for the arrival of the new offspring. Birds feather their nests, squirrels line their tree-trunk homes with leaves and twigs, and human mothers and fathers sift madly through online design catalogues. And almost invariably, plans involve painting the

The Green Solution

Looking for a way to breathe easier about the air you're breathing at home? Go green, filling your living space with living plants. Plants have the ability to absorb assorted pollutants in the air while adding oxygen to the indoor environment. In making your selections, however, be sure to avoid plants that are toxic when ingested, such as philodendron or English ivy. You won't likely be munching on shrubbery, but the same can't necessarily be said for your baby once he or she begins crawling around the house.

---

baby's room (once you can settle on the color, that is). Fortunately, today's paints don't contain lead or mercury and are safe to use when you're pregnant. Still, there are plenty of good reasons why you should pass the paintbrush to someone else—even if you're trying desperately to keep busy in those last weeks of waiting. The repetitive motion of painting can be a strain on back muscles already under pressure from the extra weight of pregnancy. In addition, balancing on ladder tops is precarious at the least, and paint odors (though not harmful) can offend the pregnant nose and bring on a bout of nausea.

While the painting is being done, try to arrange to be out of the house. Whether you're there or not, keep windows open for ventilation. Avoid exposure to paint removers entirely, because they are highly toxic, and steer clear of the paint-removing process (whether chemicals or sanders are used), particularly if the paint that's being removed is older and might contain mercury or lead.

Air Pollution

"Can city air pollution hurt my baby?"

Take a deep breath. Ordinary breathing in the big city is a lot safer than you'd think. After all, millions of women live and breathe in major cities across the nation and give birth to millions of healthy babies. Still, it's always sensible to avoid extraordinarily high doses of most air pollutants. Here's how:

- Avoid smoke-filled rooms. Since tobacco smoke is one pollutant that's known to hurt the fetus, ask family, guests in your home, and coworkers not to smoke near you. That goes for cigars and pipes, too, because they release even more smoke into the air than cigarettes do.

- Have the exhaust system on your car checked to be sure there is no leakage of noxious fumes and the exhaust pipe isn't rusting away. Never start your car in the garage with the garage door closed; keep the tailgate on an SUV or minivan closed when the engine is running; keep your car's outside air vent closed when driving in heavy traffic.

- If there is a pollution alert in your area, stay indoors as much as you can, with the windows closed and the air conditioner, if you have one, running. Follow any other instructions given by health officials for residents who are at special risk. If you want to work out, go to the gym or go for a long walk at an indoor mall.

- Don't run, walk, or bicycle along congested highways, no matter what the weather, since you breathe in more air—and pollution—when you're active. Instead, choose a route through a park or a residential area with little traffic and a lot of trees. Trees, like indoor greenery, help to keep the air clean.

- Make sure fireplaces, gas stoves, and wood-burning stoves in your home are vented properly. Also, make sure the fireplace flue is open before lighting a fire.

- Try the Green Solution (see previous page). Plants, and the air-purification properties that they provide, can help you breathe easier both inside your home and out.

Domestic Violence

Protecting her baby from harm is every expectant mother's most basic instinct. But sadly, some women can't even protect themselves during pregnancy. That's because they're victims of domestic violence.

Domestic violence can strike at any time, but it's especially common during pregnancy. While having a baby brings out a new (or renewed) tenderness in many relationships, it rocks others, sometimes triggering unexpectedly negative emotions in a woman's partner (from anger to jealousy to a feeling of being trapped), particularly if the pregnancy wasn't planned. In some cases, unfortunately, those emotions play out in the form of violence against both the mother and her unborn baby.

Surprisingly, domestic violence is the leading cause of death among pregnant women, killing more often than pregnancy complications or car crashes. Even without the homicides, the statistics are just as alarming: Nearly 20 percent of women experience violence at the hands of their partners during pregnancy. This means, statistically, that pregnant women are twice as likely to experience physical abuse during their nine months than experience a preterm birth or preeclampsia.

Domestic abuse (emotional and physical) against pregnant women carries more than just the immediate risk of injury to the mother-to-be and her baby (such as uterine rupture or hemorrhaging). Being battered during pregnancy can lead to numerous negative health consequences for the mom-to-be, including poor nutrition, poor prenatal care, substance abuse, and so on. Its effects on the pregnancy can also include stillbirth or miscarriage, preterm labor, premature rupture of the membranes, or low birthweight. And once a baby is born into a physically abusive household, he or she can easily become a victim of direct violence as well.

Abused women come from all backgrounds and socioeconomic areas, every age, every race and ethnicity, and every educational level. If you're the victim of domestic violence, remember that it is not your fault. You have done nothing wrong. If you are in an abusive relationship, don't wait—get help now. Without intervention, the violence will only get worse. Keep in mind that if you're not safe in your relationship, your child won't be safe either.

Talk to your practitioner, tell your trusted friends and family, and call a local domestic violence hotline. Many states have programs that can help you with shelter, clothing, and prenatal care. Check out The Safety Zone, thesafetyzone.org; Violence Against Women, 4woman.gov/violence/index .cfm; Family Violence Prevention Fund, endabuse.org; National Coalition Against Domestic Violence, ncadv.org; or call the National Domestic Violence Hotline at (800) 799-7233.

If you are in immediate danger, call 911.

Complementary and Alternative Medicine

The days when alternative medicine was about as welcome in traditional medical practice as old wives' tales (and regarded with about as much credibility) are over. Today, these seemingly unrelated branches of healing are no longer considered incompatible; in fact, more and more practitioners in both consider them complementary. Which is why complementary and alternative medicine (CAM) is more and more likely to find a place—in some form—in your life and the life of your family.

The practitioners who practice complementary medicine take a broad view of health and well-being, examining and integrating the nutritional, emotional, and spiritual influences, as well as the physical ones. CAM also emphasizes the body's ability to heal itself—with a little help from some natural friends, including herbs, physical manipulation, the spirit, and the mind.

Since pregnancy is not an illness but rather a normal part of life, it would seem that CAM might make a natural addition to traditional obstetrical care. And for an increasing number of women and their health care providers, it has. A variety of CAM practices are currently being used in pregnancy, labor, and delivery, with varying degrees of success, including the following:

Acupuncture. The Chinese have known for thousands of years that acupuncture can be used to relieve a number of pregnancy symptoms—but it's only recently that the traditional obstetrical community has started to catch on. Scientific studies now back up the ancient wisdom; researchers have found that acupuncture triggers the release of several brain chemicals, including endorphins, which block pain signals. How is it done? An acupuncturist inserts dozens of thin needles at prescribed points along invisible paths (or meridians) on the body. According to ancient tradition, the paths are the channels through which chi, the body's life force, flows. Researchers have found that the points correspond to deep-seated nerves, so that when the needles are twirled (or electrically stimulated, in a procedure known as electropuncture), the nerves are activated, leading to the release of endorphins—and relief from back pain, nausea, and other symptoms, including pregnancy depression. Acupuncture may also be used during labor to relieve pain, as well as to help speed progress along. For those finding conception elusive, acupuncture may help with fertility issues.

Acupressure. Acupressure—or shiatsu—works on the same principle as acupuncture, except that instead of getting poked with needles, your practitioner will use thumb or finger pressure, or will apply firm pressure with small beads, to stimulate the points. Pressure on a certain point just above your inner wrist can ease nausea (which is why Sea-Bands can also work; see page 134). Acupressure on the center of the ball of the foot is said to help back labor. There are several acupressure points that are said to induce contractions (such as those in the ankle)—which is why they should be avoided until term (at which point, impatient moms-to-be might want to give them a try—at the hands of a professional, that is).

Biofeedback. Biofeedback is a method that helps patients learn how to control their biological responses to physical pain or emotional stress, and it can be used safely to relieve a variety of pregnancy symptoms, including headache, backache, and other pains, plus insomnia and possibly morning sickness. Biofeedback can also be used to lower blood pressure and combat depression, anxiety, and stress.

Chiropractic medicine. This therapy uses physical manipulation of the spine and other joints to enable nerve impulses to move freely through an aligned body, encouraging the body's natural ability to heal. Chiropractic medicine can help pregnant women battle nausea; back, neck, or joint pain; and sciatica (plus other types of pain), as well as help relieve postpartum pain. Be sure any chiropractic practitioner you see during pregnancy is familiar with caring for expectant women, using tables that adjust for a pregnant woman's body and using techniques that avoid pressure on the abdominal area.

Massage. Massage can help relieve some of pregnancy's discomforts, including heartburn, nausea (but only in some women; others may be more nauseated by massage), headaches, backache, and sciatica, while preparing muscles for childbirth. It can also be used during labor and delivery to relax muscles between contractions and reduce the pain of back labor. What's more, it's a great way to reduce stress and relax. Just make sure you're being massaged by someone who's trained in the art of prenatal massage (not all massage therapists are); see page 147 for more.

Reflexology. Similar to acupressure, reflexology is a therapy in which pressure is applied to specific areas of the feet, hands, and ears to relieve a variety of aches and pains, as well as to stimulate labor and reduce the pain of contrac-

tions. Because applying pressure to certain areas on or near the feet and on the hands can trigger contractions, it's very important that the reflexologist you visit be well trained and aware of your pregnancy, and that he or she avoids these areas before term (afterward, again, they could be just the ticket to bring on a long-awaited labor).

Hydrotherapy. This therapeutic use of warm water (usually in a whirlpool tub) is used in many hospitals and birthing centers to help relax a laboring woman and reduce her discomfort. Some women choose to give birth in water; see page 24.

Aromatherapy. Scented oils are used to heal body, mind, and spirit and are utilized by some practitioners during pregnancy; however, most experts advise caution, since certain aromas (in this concentrated form) may pose a risk to pregnant women; see page 147.

Meditation, visualization, and relaxation techniques. All of these can help a woman safely through a variety of physical and emotional stresses during pregnancy, from the miseries of morning sickness to the pain of labor and delivery. They can work wonders on general expectant mom anxiety, too; see page 142 for a relaxation exercise you can try.

Hypnotherapy. Hypnosis may be useful in relieving pregnancy symptoms (from nausea to headaches), reducing stress and easing insomnia, turning a breech birth (in conjunction with the more traditional external cephalic version), holding off preterm labor, and providing pain management during labor and delivery (hypnobirthing). It works by getting you deeply relaxed—and in the case of pain management, so relaxed that you're unaware of any discomfort. Keep in mind that hypnosis isn't for everyone; about 25 percent of the population is highly resistant to hypnotic suggestion, and many more aren't suggestive enough to use it for effective pain relief. Make sure any hypnotherapist you use is certified and experienced in pregnancy therapies. For more on hypnobirthing, see page 306.

Moxibustion. This alternative medicine technique combines acupuncture with heat (in the form of smoldering mugwort, an herb) to gradually help turn a breech baby. If you're interested in trying moxibustion to turn your breech baby, look for a practitioner who's experienced in the technique (not all acupuncturists are).

Herbal remedies. "Botanicals" have been used since humankind first began looking for relief from ailments, and they are today used by some practitioners to relieve pregnancy symptoms. Most experts, however, do not recommend herbal remedies for pregnant women because adequate studies on safety have not yet been done.

Clearly, CAM is making an impact in obstetrics. Even the most traditional ob-gyns are realizing that it's a holistic force to be reckoned with, and one to begin incorporating into ob-business as usual. But in making CAM a part of your pregnancy, it's wise to proceed with prudence and with these caveats in mind:

- Make sure your traditional ob-gyn or midwife is aware that you're seeking a CAM treatment, so your care is truly complementary. Keeping your entire prenatal team in the know is important for your safety and that of your baby.

- Complementary medications (such as homeopathic and herbal preparations) are not tested or approved by the FDA. Because they haven't been thoroughly tested—as FDA-approved drugs are—their safety hasn't been clinically established. Which is not to say that there aren't complementary medications that are safe to use in pregnancy and possibly very beneficial, just that there is no official system in place to determine those that are and those that aren't. Until more is known, it makes sense to avoid taking any homeopathic, herbal medication, dietary supplement, or aromatherapy treatment unless it has been specifically prescribed by a traditional practitioner who is knowledgeable in CAM and who knows you're pregnant. (This is also true once the baby is born if you are breastfeeding.)

- Complementary procedures that are usually benign—or even beneficial— for the nonpregnant may not be safe during pregnancy. From therapeutic massage to chiropractic maneuvers, special precautions must be observed when a patient is pregnant.

- CAM can still be strong medicine. Depending on how it's used, this potency can be therapeutic or it can be hazardous. Keep in mind that "natural" is not synonymous with "safe" any more than "chemical" is synonymous with "dangerous." Have your practitioner help you navigate through the potential pitfalls and steer you toward CAM practices that can help—not hurt—when you're expecting.

CHAPTER 5

Nine Months of Eating Well

THERE'S A TINY NEW BEING DEVEL-oping inside of you—a baby in the making. Adorable little fingers and toes are sprouting, eyes and ears are forming, brain cells are rapidly growing. And before you know it, the speck of a fetus inside of you will come to resemble the baby of your dreams: fully equipped and suitable for cuddling.

Not surprisingly, a lot goes into making a baby. Happily for babies and the parents who love them, nature's incredibly good at what it does. Which means that the chances that your baby will be born not only perfectly cute, but perfectly healthy, are already excellent. What's more, there's something you can do to help make those excellent chances even better—while helping yourself to a healthier and more comfortable pregnancy. It's something that's relatively easy to do (except maybe when you're feeling queasy)—and something that you probably already do at least three times a day. Yes, you guessed it: eating. But the challenge during pregnancy isn't just to eat (though that may be challenge enough during those early months)—it's to eat as well as you can. Think of it this way. Eating well when you're expecting is one of the first and best gifts you can give to your soon-to-arrive bundle of joy—and it's a gift that can keep on giving, handing out not just a healthier start in life but a healthier lifetime.

The Pregnancy Diet is an eating plan dedicated to baby's good health—and yours. What's in it for your baby? Among many other impressive benefits, a bet-ter chance for a bouncing birth weight, improved brain development, reduced risk for certain birth defects—and as a bonus, believe it or not, better eating hab-its as baby grows to be a potentially picky preschooler (a perk you'll really appreci-ate when broccoli's on the dinner menu). It may even make it more likely that your child will grow to be a healthier adult.

And your baby's not the only one who's likely to benefit. The Pregnancy Diet can also increase the chances that you'll have a safe pregnancy (some complications, such as anemia, gestational diabetes, and preeclampsia, are less common among women who eat well); a comfortable pregnancy (a sensibly selected diet can minimize morning sickness, fatigue, constipation, and a host of other pregnancy symptoms); a balanced emotional state (good nutrition can help moderate those crazy mood swings); a timely labor and delivery (in general, women who eat regularly and well are less likely to deliver too early); and a speedier postpartum recovery (a well-nourished body can bounce back faster and more easily, and weight that's been gained at a sensible rate can be shed more quickly). For more on the many benefits of a healthy diet during pregnancy, see *What to Expect: Eating Well When You're Expecting.*

Luckily, scoring those benefits is a piece of (carrot) cake, especially if you're already eating pretty well, and even if you're not (you'll just have to be a little more selective before bringing fork to mouth). That's because the Pregnancy Diet isn't all that different from the average healthy diet. While a few modifications have been made for the pregnant set (not surprisingly, baby making requires more calories and more of certain nutrients), the foundation is the same: a good, balanced mix of lean protein and calcium, whole grains, a rainbow of fruits and vegetables, and healthy fats. Sound familiar? It should—after all, it's what sensible folks in the nutrition field have been touting for years.

And here's some more good news. Even if you're coming to your pregnancy (and bellying up to the table) with less than ideal eating habits, changing them to follow the Pregnancy Diet won't be

Have It Your Way

Have your doubts about diets? Not a fan of eating plans? Just don't like being told what to eat—or how much? No problem. The Pregnancy Diet is one way to feed yourself and your baby well, but it definitely isn't the only way. A balanced, healthy diet—one that includes plenty of protein, whole grains, and fruits and vegetables, plus about 300 extra calories a day—will get the job done, too. So if you'd rather not keep track—don't. Eat well, your way!

that tough, especially if you're committed to making the changes. There are healthy alternatives for almost every less healthy food and beverage you've ever brought to your lips (see box, next page), which means there are nourishing ways to have your cake (and cookies and chips and even fast food) and eat it, too. Plus, there are countless ways to sneak crucial vitamins and minerals into recipes and favorite dishes—which means that you can eat well when you're expecting without your taste buds being the wiser.

There is a very important point to keep in mind as you embark on making a diet change for the better: What's presented in this chapter is the ideal, the best possible plan for eating well when you're expecting. Something you should strive for, certainly, but nothing you should stress over (especially early in pregnancy, when your appetite for healthy foods may face a smorgasbord of suppressive symptoms—from nausea to food aversions). Maybe you'll choose to follow the diet closely, at least most of the time. Or you'll follow it loosely, all of the time. But even if your allegiance remains to burgers and fries, you'll still

---

Try These Instead

L ooking for healthy alternatives to your not-so-healthy favorite foods? Here are some ideas to get you started:

Instead of . . .	Try . . .
Potato chips	Soy chips
A bag of M&M's	Trail mix (with a few M&M's)
Before-dinner pretzels	Before-dinner edamame
Fried chicken	Grilled chicken
Hot fudge sundae	Frozen yogurt with fruit and granola
Taco chips and cheese sauce	Veggies and cheese sauce
French fries	Roasted sweet potato chips
Anything on white bread	Anything on whole wheat
A soft drink	A fruit smoothie
Sugar cookies	Whole-grain Fig Newtons

---

pick up in the pages that follow at least a few pointers that will help nourish you and your baby better during the next nine months (salad with that burger?).

Nine Basic Principles for Nine Months of Healthy Eating

Bites count. Chew on this: You've got nine months' worth of meals and snacks (and nibbles and noshes) ahead of you—each one of them an opportunity to feed your baby well before he or she is even born. So open wide, but think first. Try to make your pregnancy bites count by choosing them (at least most of the time) with baby in mind. Remember that each bite during the day is an opportunity to feed that growing baby of yours healthy nutrients.

All calories are not created equal. Choose your calories with care, selecting quality

over quantity when you can. It may seem obvious—and inherently unfair—but those 200 calories in a doughnut are not equal to the 200 calories in a whole-grain raisin-bran muffin. Nor are the 100 calories in 10 potato chips equal to the 100 calories in a baked potato served in its skin. Your baby will benefit a lot more from 2,000 nutrient-rich calories daily than from 2,000 mostly empty ones. And your body will show the benefits postpartum as well.

Starve yourself, starve your baby. Just as you wouldn't consider starving your baby after it's born, don't consider starving it when it's at home in your uterus. A fetus can't thrive by living off your flesh, no matter how much you're sporting. It needs regular nourishment at regular intervals—and as the sole caterer of your uterine café, only you can provide it. Even if you're not hungry, your baby is. So try not to skip meals. In fact, eating frequently may be the best route to a well-nourished fetus. Research shows that mothers who eat at least five times a day (three meals plus two snacks or six mini meals, for instance) are more likely to carry to term. Of course, that's easier said than done, especially if you've been too busy hugging the toilet to even think about eating. And what if your heart-burn has made eating a pain—literally? You'll find plenty of tips on how to eat around these pregnancy inconveniences on pages 130 and 153.

Efficiency is effective. Think it's impossible to fill each of the Daily Dozen requirements (see page 93) each and every day (let's see, six whole-grains means one every four hours . . .)? Worried that even if you do manage to eat it all, you'll end up looking like a pregnant blimp? Think and worry no more. Instead, become an efficiency expert. Get more nutritional bang for your buck by choosing foods that are lightweights when it comes to calories, heavy hitters when it comes to nutrients. Need an example? Eating a cup of pistachio nuts at 715 calories (about 25 percent of your daily allotment) is a considerably less efficient way of netting a 25-gram protein serving than eating a 4-ounce turkey burger, at 250 calories. Another efficiency case in point: Eating a cup and a half of ice cream (about 500 calories; more if you've chosen the really good stuff) is a fun but far less efficient way of scoring a 300-mg calcium serving than eating a cup of nonfat frozen yogurt (still fun, but only about 300 calories). Because fat has more than twice as many calories per gram as either proteins or carbohydrates, opting often for lower-fat foods will step up your nutritional efficiency. Choose lean meats over fatty ones, fat-free or low-fat milk and dairy products over full-fat versions, grilled or broiled foods over fried. Spread butter lightly; use a tablespoon of olive oil for sautéing, not a quarter of a cup. Another

trick of the efficient-eating trade: Select foods that are overachievers in more than one Daily Dozen category, thus filling two or more requirements at once.

Efficiency is important, too, if you're having trouble gaining enough weight. To start tipping the scale toward a healthier weight gain, choose foods that are dense in nutrients and calo-ries—avocados, nuts, and dried fruits, for instance—that can fill you and your baby out without filling you up too much.

Carbohydrates are a complex issue. Some women, concerned about gaining too much weight during pregnancy, mistakenly drop carbohydrates from their diets like so many hot potatoes. There's no doubt that refined carbs (like white bread, crackers, and pretzels; white rice; refined cereals, cakes, and cookies) are nutritional slackers. But unrefined (com-plex) carbohydrates (whole-grain breads and cereals, brown rice, fresh fruits and vegetables, dried beans and peas, and, of course, hot potatoes in their skins) sup-ply essential B vitamins, trace minerals,

The Six-Meal Solution

Too bloated, queasy, heart-burned, or constipated (or all four) to contemplate a full meal? No matter what tummy troubles are getting you down (or keeping food from staying down), you'll find it easier to spread your Daily Dozen (see page 93) into five or six mini meals instead of three squares. A grazing approach keeps your blood sugar level, so you'll get an energy boost, too (and who couldn't use that?). And you'll have fewer headaches—and fewer wild mood swings.

protein, and important fiber. They're good not only for your baby, but also for you (they'll help keep nausea and constipation in check). And because they are filling and fiber-rich but not fattening, they'll help keep your weight gain in check, too. Recent research suggests yet another bonus for complex car-bohydrate consumers: Eating plenty of fiber may reduce the risk of developing gestational diabetes. Be careful to move from a low-fiber diet to a high-fiber diet slowly to avoid possible stomach upset (too much fiber too fast can pump you up with too much gas).

Sweet nothings are exactly that. There's no gentle way to put this: Sugar calories, sadly, are empty calories. And though empty calories are fine once in a while—even when you're pregnant—they tend to add up a lot more quickly than you'd think, leaving less room in your diet for nutritionally substantial calories. In addition, researchers are finding that sugar may not only be void of value, but in excessive amounts may potentially be harmful. Studies have suggested that in addition to contributing to obesity, heavy sugar consumption may be linked to tooth decay, diabetes, heart disease, and colon cancer. Perhaps sugar's biggest shortcoming, however, is that large quantities are often found in foods and drinks that are, on the whole, nutritional underachievers (candy and soda come to mind).

Refined sugar goes by many names on the supermarket shelves, including corn syrup and dehydrated cane juice. Honey, an unrefined sugar, has a nutritional edge because it contains disease-fighting antioxidants. Plus, it is more likely to find its way into more nutritious foods—particularly those whole-grain ones you'd find in the health food sections of your market. Try to limit your intake of all forms of sugar, however, since the calories you save can be spent on foods that pack a much more wholesome punch.

For delicious and nutritious sweetness, substitute fruit, dried fruit, and fruit juice concentrates for sugar when you can. Besides being sweet, they contain vitamins, trace minerals, and valuable

No More Guilt

Willpower has its place, particularly while you're trying to eat well for two. Still, everyone needs to give in to temptation now and then, without feeling guilty about it. So lose the guilt, hold the deprivation, and allow yourself a treat every once in a while—something that doesn't add appreciably to your nutritional bottom line but makes your taste buds jump for joy: a blueberry muffin that's probably more sugar than blueberries but is also off-the-charts yummy, a double scoop of cookies-and-cream (when frozen yogurt just doesn't cut it), the fast-food burger you've been craving like crazy. And when you say "yes" to that occasional frosted brownie or candy bar, serve it up without a side of remorse.

But when venturing down the path of least nutritious, try to pump it up—add a slice of banana and some nuts to your ice-cream sundae; choose a candy bar that's filled with almonds; order your burger with cheese and tomato (and maybe a side salad). Keeping portions of these foods small is another good strategy: Share that serving of onion rings; take a slender slice of pecan pie instead of a hefty slab. And remember to stop before you get too carried away; otherwise, you might just begin to feel that guilt after all.

phytochemicals (plant chemicals that may help the body defend itself against disease and aging), all absent in sugar. You can also find sweet revenge in the calorie-free sugar substitutes that appear to be safe for pregnancy use (see page 111).

Good foods remember where they came from. Nature knows a thing or two about nutrition. So it's not surprising that the most nutritious foods are often the ones that haven't strayed far from their natural state. Choose fresh vegetables and fruits when they're in season, or fresh-frozen or canned when fresh are unavailable or you don't have time to prepare them (look for ones that don't have added sugar, salt, or fat). And speaking of preparation, less is more when it comes to nutrients. Try to eat some raw vegetables and fruit every day, and when you're cooking, opt for steaming or a light stir-fry, so more vitamins and minerals will be retained.

And there's more nutritional know-how in nature's model. Avoid processed foods; not only have they picked up a lot of chemicals, fat, sugar, and salt on the assembly line, but they're frequently low in nutrition. Choose fresh roasted turkey breast over smoked turkey, macaroni and cheese made with whole-grain macaroni and natural cheese over that bright orange variety, fresh oatmeal made from rolled oats over the lower-fiber and super sugary instant varieties.

Healthy eating begins at home. Let's face it. It isn't easy to nibble on fresh fruit when your darling husband's diving headfirst into a half-gallon of ice cream—right next to you on the sofa. Or to reach for the soy chips when he's filled the cabinets with those orange cheese balls you can't resist. So enlist him—and other family members—in making your home a healthy food zone. Make whole wheat your house bread,

stock your freezer with frozen yogurt, and ban the unhealthy snacks you can't help attacking when they're within reach. And don't stop after delivery. Research associates a good diet not only with a better pregnancy outcome but with a lower risk of many diseases, including adult-onset diabetes and cancer. Which means the family that eats well together is more likely to stay healthy together.

Bad habits can sabotage a good diet. Eating well is only part of the healthy prenatal picture. The best pregnancy diet in the world can be undermined by alcohol, tobacco, and other unsafe drugs. If you haven't done so already, change your other lifestyle habits to match.

The Pregnancy Daily Dozen

Calories. Technically, a pregnant woman is eating for two (rejoice, food lovers). But it's important to remember that one of the two is a tiny developing fetus whose caloric needs are significantly lower than mom's—a mere 300 on average a day, more or less (sorry, food lovers). So, if you're of average weight, you now need only about an average of 300 calories more than you used to eat prepregnancy—the equivalent of two glasses of skim milk and a bowl of oatmeal (not exactly the all-you-can-eat sundae bar you were envisioning). Pretty easy to spend (or overspend), given the extra nutritional requirements of pregnancy. What's more, during the first trimester you probably don't need any extra calories at all (that baby you're growing is only pea size), unless you're trying to compensate for starting out underweight. By the time your metabolism speeds up during the second trimester, you can aim for 300 to 350 extra calories. Later in pregnancy (when your baby is much bigger) you may even need more, or upward of about 500 extra calories a day.

Eating more calories than you and your baby need isn't only unnecessary, it isn't smart—and can lead to excessive weight gain. Eating too few calories, on the other hand, is not only unwise but also potentially dangerous as pregnancy progresses; women who don't take in enough calories during the second and third trimesters can seriously slow the growth of their babies.

There are four exceptions to this basic formula—and if any apply to you, it's even more important to discuss your caloric needs with your practitioner. If you're overweight, you can possibly do with fewer calories, as long as you have the right nutritional guidance. If you're seriously underweight, you'll need more calories so you can catch up weightwise. If you're a teen, you're still growing yourself, which means you have unique nutritional needs. And if you're carrying multiples, you'll have to add about 300 calories for each additional baby.

While calories count during pregnancy, keep in mind that they don't have to be literally counted. Instead of adding them up at every meal, step on a reliable scale every once in a while (once a week if you're really curious, once every two to three weeks if you're more scalephobic) to check your progress. Weigh yourself at the same time of day, either naked or wearing the same clothing (or clothing that weighs about the same), so that your calculations won't be thrown off by a heavy meal one week or heavy jeans the next. If your weight gain is going according to schedule (an average of about one pound a week in the second and third trimesters), you're getting the right number of calories. If it's less than that, you're getting too few; if it's

Count 'Em Once, Count 'Em Twice

Many of your favorite foods fill more than one Daily Dozen requirement in each serving, giving you two for the caloric price of one. Case in point: A slice of cantaloupe nets a Green Leafy and a Vitamin C in one delicious package. One cup of yogurt yields 1 Calcium serving and half a Protein serving. Use such overlappers as often as you can to save yourself calories and stomach space.

more than that, you're getting too many. Maintain or adjust your food intake as necessary, but be careful not to cut out nutrients you need along with calories.

Protein foods: 3 servings daily. How does your baby grow? Using, among other nutrients, the amino acids (the building blocks of human cells) from the protein you eat each day. Because your baby's cells are multiplying rapidly, protein is an extremely crucial component of your pregnancy diet. Aim to have about 75 grams of protein every day. If that sounds like a lot, keep in mind that most Americans (including you, most likely) consume at least that much daily without even trying, and those on high-protein diets pack away a lot more. To get your share of protein, all you have to do is eat a total of three servings of Protein foods from the list that follows. When tallying your Protein servings, don't forget to count the protein found in many high-calcium foods: a glass of milk and an ounce of cheese each provide a third of a Protein serving; a cup of yogurt equals half a serving. Whole grains and legumes contribute protein, too.

Every day have three of the following (each is 1 Protein serving, or about 25 grams of protein), or a combination equivalent to three servings. Keep in mind that most of the dairy options also fill calcium requirements, which make them especially efficient choices.

24 ounces (three 8-ounce glasses) of milk or buttermilk

1 cup cottage cheese

2 cups yogurt

3 ounces (¾ cup grated) cheese

4 large whole eggs

7 large egg whites

3½ ounces (drained) canned tuna or sardines

4 ounces (drained) canned salmon

4 ounces cooked shellfish, such as shelled shrimp, lobster, clams, or mussels

4 ounces (before cooking) fresh fish

4 ounces (before cooking) skinless chicken, turkey, duck, or other poultry

4 ounces (before cooking) lean beef, lamb, veal, pork, or buffalo

Calcium foods: 4 servings daily. Back in elementary school, you probably learned that growing children need plenty of calcium for strong bones and teeth. Well, so do growing fetuses on their way to becoming growing children. Calcium is also vital for muscle, heart, and nerve development, blood clotting, and enzyme activity. But it's not only your baby who stands to lose when you don't get enough calcium. If incoming supplies aren't keeping up, your baby-making factory will tap into the calcium in your own bones to help meet its quota, setting you up for osteoporosis later in life. So do your best to get your four servings of calcium-rich foods a day.

Can't stomach the idea—or the taste—of four glasses of milk each day? Luckily, calcium doesn't have to be served in glasses at all. It can be served up as a cup of yogurt or a piece of cheese. It can be enjoyed in smoothies, soups, casseroles, cereals, dips, sauces, desserts, and more.

For those who can't tolerate or don't eat dairy products at all, calcium also comes in nondairy form. A glass of calcium-fortified orange juice, for instance, efficiently provides a serving of Calcium and Vitamin C; 4 ounces of canned salmon with bones provides both a serving of Calcium and Protein; one portion of cooked greens yields not only a Green Leafy and a Vitamin C serving, but a bonus of calcium. For women who are vegans or lactose-intolerant, or who for other reasons cannot be sure they're getting enough calcium in their diets, a calcium supplement (one that includes vitamin D as well) may be recommended.

Aim for four servings of calcium-rich foods each day, or any combination of them that is equivalent to four servings (so don't forget to count that half cup of yogurt, that sprinkle of cheese). Each serving listed below contains about 300 mg of calcium (you need a total of about 1,200 mg a day), and many also fill your protein requirements:

¼ cup grated cheese

1 ounce hard cheese

½ cup pasteurized ricotta cheese

1 cup milk or buttermilk

5 ounces calcium-added milk (shake well before serving)

⅓ cup nonfat dry milk (enough to make 1 cup liquid)

1 cup yogurt

1½ cups frozen yogurt

1 cup calcium-fortified juice (shake well before serving)

4 ounces canned salmon with bones

Vegetarian Proteins

Good news for vegans: You don't have to combine to conquer vegetarian proteins, as long as you have some of each type (legumes, grains, and seeds and nuts) every day. To be sure you are getting a full protein serving at each meal, double or choose two half servings listed below. And keep in mind that many of these foods fulfill the requirements for Whole Grains and Legumes as well as Protein.

The following selections are nutritious foods for all pregnant women—you don't have to be a vegetarian to tap into them and count them in your daily total. In fact, many may be soothing protein alternatives when early-pregnancy queasiness and aversions push meat off the menu.

Legumes (half Protein servings)

¾ cup cooked beans, lentils, split peas, or chickpeas (garbanzos)

½ cup cooked edamame

¾ cup green garden peas

1½ ounces peanuts

3 tablespoons peanut butter

¼ cup miso

4 ounces tofu (bean curd)

3 ounces tempeh

1½ cups soy milk*

3 ounces soy cheese*

½ cup vegetarian "ground beef"*

1 large vegetarian "hot dog" or "burger"*

1 ounce (before cooking) soy or high-protein pasta

Grains (half Protein servings)

3 ounces (before cooking) whole-wheat pasta

⅓ cup wheat germ

¾ cup oat bran

1 cup uncooked (2 cups cooked) oats

2 cups (approximately) whole-grain ready-to-eat cereal*

½ cup uncooked (1½ cups cooked) couscous, bulgur, or buckwheat

½ cup uncooked quinoa

4 slices whole-grain bread

2 whole-wheat pitas or English muffins

Nuts and Seeds (half Protein servings)

3 ounces nuts, such as walnuts, pecans, or almonds

2 ounces sesame, sunflower, or pumpkin seeds

½ cup ground flaxseed

*Protein content varies widely, so check labels for 12 to 15 grams protein per half serving.

3 ounces canned sardines with bones

3 tablespoons ground sesame seeds

1 cup cooked greens, such as collards or turnips

1½ cups cooked Chinese cabbage (bok choy)

1½ cups cooked edamame

1¾ tablespoons blackstrap molasses

You'll also score a calcium bonus by eating cottage cheese, tofu, dried figs, almonds, broccoli, spinach, dried beans, and flaxseed.

Vitamin C foods: 3 servings daily. You and baby both need vitamin C for tissue repair, wound healing, and various other metabolic (nutrient-utilizing) processes. Your baby also needs it for proper growth and for the development of strong bones and teeth. Vitamin C is a nutrient the body can't store, so a fresh supply is needed every day. Lucky for you, vitamin C usually comes from foods that naturally taste good. As you can see from the list of Vitamin C foods below, the old standby orange juice (good as it is) is far from the only, or even the best, source of this essential vitamin.

Aim for at least 3 Vitamin C servings every day. (Fruit fanatic? Help yourself to more.) Your body can't store this vitamin, so try not to skip a day. Keep in mind that many Vitamin C foods also fill the requirement for Green Leafy and Yellow Vegetables and Yellow Fruit.

½ medium-size grapefruit

½ cup grapefruit juice

½ medium-size orange

½ cup orange juice

2 tablespoons orange, white grape, or other fortified juice concentrate

¼ cup lemon juice

½ medium-size mango

¼ medium-size papaya

⅛ small cantaloupe or honeydew (½ cup cubed)

⅓ cup strawberries

⅔ cup blackberries or raspberries

½ medium-size kiwi

½ cup diced fresh pineapple

2 cups diced watermelon

¼ medium-size red, yellow, or orange bell pepper

½ medium-size green bell pepper

½ cup raw or cooked broccoli

1 medium-size tomato

¾ cup tomato juice

½ cup vegetable juice

½ cup raw or cooked cauliflower

½ cup cooked kale

1 packed cup raw spinach, or ½ cup cooked

¾ cup cooked collard, mustard, or turnip greens

2 cups romaine lettuce

¾ cup shredded raw red cabbage

1 sweet potato or baking potato, baked in skin

1 cup cooked edamame

Green Leafy and Yellow Vegetables and Yellow Fruits: 3 to 4 servings daily. These bunny favorites supply the vitamin A, in the form of beta-carotene, that is vital for cell growth (your baby's cells are multiplying at a fantastic rate), healthy skin, bones, and eyes. The green leafies and yellows also deliver doses of other essential carotenoids and vitamins (vitamin E, riboflavin, folic acid, and other B vitamins), numerous minerals (many green leafies provide a good deal of calcium as well as trace minerals), disease-fighting phytochemicals, and constipation-fighting fiber. A bountiful selection of green leafy and yellow vegetables and yellow fruit can be found in the list that follows. Those with an anti-vegetable agenda may be pleasantly surprised to

Can't Find Your Favorite?

Is your favorite fruit, grain, or protein food nowhere to be found on these lists? That doesn't mean it doesn't rate nutritionally. For reasons of space, only the more common foods are listed. There are longer food lists in *What to Expect: Eating Well When You're Expecting,* and even longer ones on the USDA National Nutrient Database: nal .usda.gov/fnic/foodcomp/search/.

discover that broccoli and spinach are not the only sources of vitamin A and that, in fact, the vitamin comes packaged in some of nature's most tempting sweet offerings—dried apricots, yellow peaches, cantaloupe, and mangoes, for example. And those who like to drink their vegetables may be happy to know that they can count a glass of vegetable juice, a bowl of carrot soup, or a mango smoothie toward their daily Green Leafy and Yellow allowance.

Try to eat at least three to four servings a day. If possible, aim to have some yellow and some green daily (and eat some raw for extra fiber). Remember, many of these foods also fill a Vitamin C requirement.

⅛ cantaloupe (½ cup cubed)

2 large fresh apricots or 6 dried apricot halves

½ medium-size mango

¼ medium-size papaya

1 large nectarine or yellow peach

1 small persimmon

¾ cup pink grapefruit juice

1 pink or ruby red grapefruit

1 clementine

½ carrot (¼ cup grated)

½ cup raw or cooked broccoli pieces

1 cup coleslaw mix

¼ cup cooked collard greens, Swiss chard, or kale

1 packed cup green leafy lettuce, such as romaine, arugula, or red or green leaf

1 packed cup raw spinach, or ½ cup cooked

¼ cup cooked winter squash

½ small sweet potato or yam

2 medium-size tomatoes

½ medium-size red bell pepper

¼ cup chopped parsley

Other fruits and vegetables: 1 to 2 servings daily. In addition to produce rich in vitamin C and beta-carotene (vitamin A), aim to eat at least one or two "other" types of fruit or vegetable daily. While "Others" were once considered nutritional B-listers, they're now getting a second look. Turns out they're rich not only in minerals, such as potassium and magnesium, that are vital to good pregnancy health, but also in an impressive host of other up-and-coming trace minerals. Many also have phytochemicals and antioxidants in abundance (particularly those that sport the colors of the rainbow, so pick produce that's brightly hued for the biggest nutritional return). From that apple a day to those headline-making blueberries and pomegranates, "Others" are definitely worthy of a spot in your daily diet.

You're sure to find plenty of "Others" among your favorite fruits and vegetables. Round out your produce picks with one to two from this list daily:

1 medium-size apple

½ cup apple juice or applesauce

½ cup pomegranate juice

2 tablespoons apple juice concentrate

1 medium-size banana

½ cup pitted fresh cherries

¼ cup cooked cranberries

1 medium-size white peach

1 medium-size pear or 2 dried halves

½ cup unsweetened pineapple juice

2 small plums

½ cup blueberries

½ medium-size avocado

½ cup cooked green beans

½ cup fresh raw mushrooms

½ cup cooked okra

½ cup sliced onion

½ cup cooked parsnips

½ cup cooked zucchini

1 small ear cooked sweet corn

1 cup shredded iceberg lettuce

½ cup green garden peas or snow peas

Whole Grains and Legumes: 6 or more servings a day. There are plenty of reasons to go with the grain. Whole grains (whole wheat, oats, rye, barley, corn, rice, millet, wheat berries, buckwheat, bulgur, quinoa, and so on) and legumes (peas, beans, and peanuts) are packed with nutrients, particularly the B vitamins (except for vitamin B_{12}, found only in animal products) that are needed for just about every part of your baby's body. These concentrated complex carbohydrates are also rich in iron and trace minerals, such as zinc, selenium, and magnesium, which are very important in pregnancy. An added plus: Starchy foods may also help reduce morning sickness. Though these selections have many nutrients in common, each has its own strengths. To get the maximum benefit, include a variety of whole grains and legumes in your diet. Be adventurous: Coat your fish or chicken with whole-wheat bread crumbs seasoned with herbs and Parmesan cheese. Try quinoa (a tasty high-protein grain) as a side dish, or add bulgur or wheat berries to a wild-rice pilaf. Use oats in your favorite cookie recipe. Substitute navy beans for limas in your soup. And though you'll likely sometimes eat them, remember that refined grains just don't stack up nutritionally. Even if they're "enriched," they are still lacking in fiber, in protein, and in more than a dozen vitamins and trace minerals that are found in the original whole grain.

Aim for six or more from this list every day. Don't forget that many also contribute toward your protein requirement, often significantly.

White Whole Wheat

Not a whole-hearted fan of whole wheat—or craving the comfort of white during your queasy days? There's a new bread in town that might be just the ticket. "White wheat" breads are made with naturally white wheat, which has a milder, sweeter taste than the red wheat that whole wheat's made from. Is white whole wheat the best thing since sliced bread? Well, maybe not exactly. It's definitely healthier than white, but since it's processed, some nutrients are still lost on the assembly line—which means that whole wheat's still top shelf nutritionally. Still, if your cravings—or queasiness—are sending you reaching for the white, "white wheat" is definitely the best one to reach for. Also, if you're baking, look for it in flour form for less dense results than regular whole wheat.

1 slice whole-wheat, whole-rye, or other whole-grain or soy bread

½ whole-wheat pita, roll, bagel, 12-inch wrap, tortilla, or English muffin

1 cup cooked whole-grain cereal, such as oatmeal or Wheatena

1 cup whole-grain ready-to-eat cereal (serving sizes vary, so check labels)

½ cup granola

2 tablespoons wheat germ

½ cup cooked brown or wild rice

½ cup cooked millet, bulgur, couscous, kasha (buckwheat groats), barley, or quinoa

1 ounce (before cooking) whole-grain or soy pasta

½ cup cooked beans, lentils, split peas, or edamame

2 cups air-popped popcorn

1 ounce whole-grain crackers or soy crisps

¼ cup whole-grain or soy flour

Iron-rich foods: some daily. Since large amounts of iron are essential for the developing blood supply of the fetus and for your own expanding blood supply, you'll need to pump up your iron intake during these nine months. Get as much of your iron as you can from your diet (see the list below). Eating foods rich in vitamin C at the same sitting as Iron-rich foods will increase the absorption of the mineral by your body.

Because it's sometimes difficult to fill the pregnancy iron requirement through diet alone, your practitioner may recommend that you take a daily iron supplement in addition to your prenatal vitamins from the 20th week on, or whenever routine testing shows an iron shortfall. To enhance the absorption of the iron in the supplement, take it between meals with a fruit juice rich in vitamin C (caffeinated beverages, antacids, high-fiber foods, and high-calcium foods can interfere with iron absorption).

Small amounts of iron are found in most of the fruits, vegetables, grains, and meats you eat every day. But try to have some of the following higher-iron-content foods daily, along with your supplement. Again, many Iron-rich foods also fill other requirements at the same time.

Beef, buffalo, duck, turkey

Cooked clams, oysters, mussels, and shrimp

Sardines

Baked potato with skin

Spinach, collard, kale, and turnip greens

Seaweed

Pumpkin seeds

Oat bran

Barley, bulgur, quinoa

Beans and peas

Edamame and soy products

Blackstrap molasses

Dried fruit

Fats and high-fat foods: approximately 4 servings daily (depending on your weight gain). As you're probably all too aware, the requirement for fat is definitely not only the easiest to fill, it's also the easiest to overfill. And though there's no harm—and probably some benefit—in having a couple of extra Green Leafies or Vitamin C foods, excess Fat servings could spell excess pounds. Still, though keeping fat intake moderate is a good idea, eliminating all fat from your diet is a dangerous one. Fat is vital to your developing baby; the essential fatty acids in them are just that—essential. Especially beneficial in the third trimester are omega-3 fatty acids (see box, opposite).

A Little Fat Goes a Long Way

Trying to keep those calories down by skipping the dressing on your salad or the oil in your stir-fry? You'd be getting an "A" for willpower—but less "vitamin A" in your veggies. Research shows that many of the nutrients found in vegetables aren't well absorbed by the body if not accompanied by a side of fat. So make a point of including a little fat (keep in mind that a little goes a long way) with your veggies: Enjoy oil with your stir-fry, a sprinkle of nuts on your broccoli, and dressing with your salad.

The Good Fat Facts

Are you fat phobic (especially since pregnancy put you on the weight gain fast track)? Fear not your fat—just choose the right ones. After all, not all fats are created equal. Some fats are good ones—and they're especially good (make that great) when you're expecting. Omega-3 fatty acids, most notably DHA, are the best addition you can make to your diet when you're eating for two. That's because DHA is essential for proper brain growth and eye development in fetuses and young babies. In fact, researchers have found that toddlers whose moms consumed plenty of DHA during pregnancy had better hand-eye coordination than their peers. Getting enough of this vital baby brain fuel in your diet is especially important during the last three months (when your baby's brain grows at a phenomenal pace) and while you're nursing (the DHA content of a baby's brain triples during the first three months of life).

And what's good for the expected is also good for the expecting. For you, getting enough DHA may mean moderated mood swings and a lowered risk of preterm labor and postpartum depression. Another postpartum perk? Getting enough DHA when you're expecting means you're more likely to have a baby with better sleep habits. Luckily, DHA is found in plenty of foods you probably already eat—and like to eat: salmon (choose wild when you can) and other oily fish, such as sardines; walnuts; DHA-rich eggs (sometimes called omega-3 eggs); arugula; crab and shrimp; flaxseed; and even chicken. You can also ask your practitioner about pregnancy-safe DHA supplements. Some prenatal supplements contain some DHA.

Keep track of your fat intake; fill your daily quota but try not to overfill it. And in keeping track, don't forget that the fat used in cooking and preparing foods counts, too. If you've fried your eggs in ½ tablespoon of butter (a half serving) and tossed your cole slaw with a tablespoon of mayonnaise (one serving), include the one and a half servings in your daily tally.

If you're not gaining enough weight, and increasing your intake of other nutritious foods hasn't done the trick, try adding an extra Fat serving each day; the concentrated calories it provides may help you hit your optimum weight gain stride. If you're gaining too quickly, you can cut back by one or two servings.

The foods in this list are comprised completely (or mostly) of fat. They certainly won't be the only source of fat in your diet (foods such as cream sauces, full-fat cheeses and yogurts, and nuts and seeds are all high in fat), but they're the only ones you need to keep track of. If your weight gain is on target, aim for about four full (about 14 grams each) or eight half (about 7 grams each) servings of fat each day. If not, consider adjusting your fat intake up or down.

1 tablespoon oil, such as vegetable, olive, canola, or sesame

1 tablespoon regular butter or margarine

1 tablespoon regular mayonnaise

2 tablespoons regular salad dressing

2 tablespoons heavy or whipping cream

¼ cup half-and-half

¼ cup whipped cream

¼ cup sour cream

2 tablespoons regular cream cheese

2 tablespoons peanut or almond butter

Salty foods: in moderation. At one time, the medical establishment prescribed restricting salt during pregnancy because it contributed to water retention and swelling. Now it's believed that some increase in body fluids in pregnancy is necessary and normal, and a moderate amount of sodium is needed to maintain adequate fluid levels. In fact, sodium deprivation can be harmful to the fetus. Still, very large quantities of salt and very salty foods (such as those pickles you can't stop eating, soy sauce by the gallon on your stir-fry, and potato chips by the bagful), especially if they're consumed frequently, aren't good for anyone, pregnant or not. High sodium intake is closely linked to high blood pressure, a condition that can cause complications in pregnancy, labor, and delivery. As a general rule, salt only lightly—or don't salt at all—during cooking; salt your food to taste at the table instead. Have a pickle when you crave it, but try to stop at one or two instead of eating half the jar. And, unless your practitioner recommends otherwise (because you are hyperthyroid, for example), use iodized salt to be sure you meet the increased need for iodine in pregnancy.

Fluids: at least eight 8-ounce glasses daily. You're not only eating for two, you're drinking for two. Your baby's body, like yours, is composed mostly of fluids. As that little body grows, so does its demand for fluids. Your body needs fluids more than ever, too, since pregnancy pumps up fluid volume significantly. If you've always been one of those people who goes through the day with barely a sip, now's the time to tap into fluids. Water helps keep your skin soft, eases constipation, rids your body of toxins and waste products (and baby's, too), and reduces excessive swelling and the risk of urinary tract infection and preterm labor. Be sure to get at least

8 glasses a day—more if you're retaining a lot of fluid (paradoxically, a plentiful fluid intake can flush out excess fluids), if you're exercising a lot, or if it's very hot. Try not to do your drinking just before meals, though, or you might end up too full to eat.

Of course, not all your fluids have to come from the tap (or from the water cooler). You can count milk (which is two-thirds water), fruit and vegetable juices, soups, decaffeinated coffee or tea (hot or iced), and bottled plain and sparkling waters. Cutting fruit juice with sparkling water (half and half) will keep you from pouring on too many calories. Fruit and vegetables count, too (five servings of produce net two fluid servings).

Prenatal vitamin supplements: a pregnancy formula taken daily. With all the nutrients already prepacked into the Daily Dozen (or any healthy diet), why would you need to add a prenatal vitamin to the mix? Couldn't you fill all of your requirements by filling yourself with the right foods? Well, you probably could—that is, if you lived in a laboratory where your food was precisely prepared and measured to calculate an adequate daily intake, if you never ate on the run, had to work through lunch, or felt too sick to eat. In the real world—the one you most likely live in— a prenatal supplement provides extra health insurance for you and your baby, covering those nutritional bases when your diet doesn't. And that's why one is recommended daily.

Still, a supplement is just a supplement. No pill, no matter how complete, can replace a good diet. It's best if most of your vitamins and minerals come from foods, because that's the way nutrients can be most effectively utilized. Fresh foods contain not only nutrients that we know about and can be synthesized in a pill, but probably lots of others that are as yet undiscovered. Food also supplies fiber and water (fruits and vegetables are loaded with both) and important calories and protein, none of which comes efficiently packaged in a pill.

But don't think that because a little is good, a lot is better. Vitamins and minerals at high doses act as drugs in the body and should be treated as drugs, especially by expectant moms; a few, such as vitamins A and D, are toxic at levels not much beyond the rec-

ommended dietary allowance (RDAs are now called DRIs, dietary reference intakes, or DVs, daily values). Any supplementation beyond the DRI should be taken only under medical supervision. The same goes for herbal and other supplements. As for vitamins and minerals you can get from your diet, you can't overdo the nutrients by piling up your plate at the salad bar—so no need to hold back when the carrots call or the broccoli beckons.

What's in a Pill?

What's in a prenatal pill? That depends on which one you're taking. Since there aren't any standards set for prenatal supplements, formulas vary. Chances are your practitioner will prescribe or recommend a supplement, which will take the guesswork (and homework) out of choosing a formula yourself. If you're facing the pharmacy shelves without a recommendation, get ready to do some reading, and to look for a formula that contains:

- No more than 4,000 IU (800 mcg) of vitamin A; amounts over 10,000 IU could be toxic. Many manufacturers have reduced the amount of vitamin A in their vitamin supplements or have replaced it with beta-carotene, a much safer source of vitamin A.

- At least 400 to 600 mcg of folic acid (folate)

- 250 mg of calcium. If you're not getting enough calcium in your diet, you will need additional supplementation to reach the 1,200 mg needed during pregnancy. Do not take more than 250 mg of calcium at the same time as supplementary iron because these minerals interfere with iron

absorption. Take any larger doses at least two hours before or after your iron supplement.

- 30 mg iron

- 50 to 80 mg vitamin C

- 15 mg zinc

- 2 mg copper

- 2 mg vitamin B_6

- Not more than 500 mcg vitamin D

- Approximately the DRI for vitamin E (15 mg), thiamin (1.4 mg), riboflavin (1.4 mg), niacin (18 mg), and vitamin B_{12} (2.6 mg). Most prenatal supplements contain two to three times the DRI of these. There are no known harmful effects from such doses.

- Some preparations may also contain magnesium, fluoride, biotin, phosphorus, pantothenic acid, extra B_6 (to combat queasiness), ginger (ditto), and/or baby brain–boosting DHA.

Also important: Scan for ingredients that shouldn't be in your prenatal supplement, such as herbs. When in doubt, ask your practitioner.

What You May Be Wondering About

Milk-Free Mom

"I can't tolerate milk, and drinking four cups a day would really make me uncomfortable. But don't babies need milk?"

It's not milk your baby needs, it's calcium. Since milk is one of nature's finest and most convenient sources of calcium in the American diet, it's the one most often recommended for filling the greatly increased requirement during pregnancy. But if milk leaves you with more than a sour taste in your mouth and a mustache above your lip (got gas?), you probably think twice before reaching for that glass of the white stuff. Fortunately, you don't have to suffer so your baby can grow healthy teeth and bones. If you're lactose intolerant or just don't have a taste for milk, plenty of substitutes are available that fill the nutritional bill just as well.

Even if milk turns your tummy, you still might be able to tolerate some kinds of dairy products, such as hard cheeses, fully processed yogurts (choose ones with active cultures, which actually help your digestion), and lactose-free milk, in which all of the lactose has been converted to a more easily digested form. Another advantage of using lactose-free milk products: Some are fortified with extra calcium. Check labels and choose one that is. Taking a lactase tablet before ingesting milk or milk products, or adding lactase drops or tablets to your milk, can also minimize or eliminate dairy-induced tummy troubles.

Even if you've been lactose intolerant for years, you may discover that you're able to handle some dairy products during the second and third trimes-

ters, when fetal needs for calcium are the greatest. If that's so, don't overdo it; try to stick primarily to products that are less likely to provoke a reaction.

If you can't handle any dairy products or are allergic to them, you can still get all the calcium your baby requires by drinking calcium-fortified juices and eating the nondairy foods listed under Calcium foods on page 95.

If your problem with milk isn't physiological but just a matter of taste, try some of the dairy or nondairy calcium-

Pasteurized, Please

When it was invented by French scientist Louis Pasteur in the mid-1800s, pasteurization was the greatest thing to happen to dairy products since cows. And it still is, particularly as far as pregnant women are concerned. To protect yourself and your baby from hazardous bacterial infections, such as listeria, make sure all the milk you drink is pasteurized, and all the cheeses and other dairy products you eat are made from pasteurized milk ("raw milk" cheeses are not). Juice, which can contain *E. coli* and other dangerous bacteria when it's raw, should also always be purchased pasteurized. Even eggs now come pasteurized (which eliminates the risk of salmonella without changing taste or nutrition). It's unclear whether flash pasteurization, a fast method, is safe enough when you're expecting, so until more is known, stick to products that have undergone conventional pasteurization.

rich alternatives. There are bound to be plenty that your taste buds can embrace. Or disguise your milk in cereal, soups, and smoothies.

If you can't seem to get enough calcium into your diet, ask your practitioner to recommend a calcium supplement (there are plenty of chewable varieties that are sweet revenge for those who find a pill hard to swallow). You'll also need to be sure that you're getting enough vitamin D (which is added to cow's milk). Many calcium supplements include vitamin D (which actually boosts absorption of calcium), and you'll also be getting some in your prenatal supplement.

A Red-Meat-Free Diet

"I eat chicken and fish but no red meat. Will my baby get all the necessary nutrients without it?"

Your baby won't have a beef with your red-meat-free diet. Fish and lean poultry, in fact, give you more baby-building protein and less fat for your calories than beef, pork, lamb, and organ meats—making them more efficient pregnancy choices. They're also rich sources, like red meat, of many of the B vitamins your baby needs. The only nutrient poultry and fish can't always compete for with meat is iron (duck, turkey, and shellfish are iron-rich exceptions), but there are plenty of other sources of this essential mineral, which is also easy to take in supplement form.

A Vegetarian Diet

"I'm a vegetarian and in perfect health. But everyone says that I have to eat animal products to have a healthy baby. Is this true?"

Vegetarians of every variety can have healthy babies without compromising their dietary principles—they just have to be a little more careful in planning their diets than meat-eating mothers-to-be. When choosing your meat-free menus, make sure you get all of the following:

Enough protein. For the ovo-lacto vegetarian, who eats eggs and milk products, getting enough protein is as easy as getting enough of these dairy-case favorites. If you're a vegan (a vegetarian who eats neither milk nor eggs), you may find you'll need to work a little harder in the protein department, turning to ample quantities of dried beans, peas, lentils, tofu, and other soy products (see page 96 for more vegetarian proteins).

Enough calcium. This is no tall order for the vegetarian who eats dairy products, but it can be trickier for those who don't. Luckily, dairy products are the most obvious but not the only sources of calcium. Calcium-fortified juices offer as much calcium as milk, ounce for ounce (just make sure you shake them before using). Other nondairy dietary sources of calcium include dark leafy green vegetables, sesame seeds, almonds, and many soy products (such as soy milk, soy cheese, tofu, and tempeh). For added insurance, vegans should probably also take a calcium supplement; check with your practitioner for a recommendation.

Vitamin B_{12}. Though B_{12} deficiencies are rare, vegetarians, particularly vegans, often don't get enough of this vitamin because it is found only in animal foods. So be certain to take supplemental B_{12}, as well as folic acid and iron (ask your practitioner if you need more B_{12} than what's provided in your prenatal vitamin). Other dietary sources include B_{12}-fortified soy milk, fortified cereals, nutritional yeast, and fortified meat substitutes.

Vitamin D. This important vitamin is produced by your skin when you're exposed to sunlight. But since spending lots of time in the sun is no longer considered a good health or beauty bet, relying on this source of vitamin D isn't smart (especially for women with dark skin, who can't absorb as much from the sunlight anyway). To ensure adequate intake of vitamin D, federal law requires that milk be fortified with 400 mg of vitamin D per quart. If you don't drink cow's milk, be sure there is enough vitamin D added to the soy milk you drink or in the pregnancy supplement you are taking. Breads and cereals are also fortified with it.

Low-Carb Diets

"I've been on a low-carb/high-protein diet to lose weight. Can I continue the diet while I'm pregnant?"

Here's the low-down on low-carb: When you're expecting, low isn't the way to go. Going low on any essential nutrient, in fact, isn't smart when you're expecting. Your highest pregnancy priority: getting a balance of all of the best baby-making ingredients, including carbs. As popular as they are, diets that limit carbohydrates (including fruits, vegetables, and grains) limit the nutrients—especially folic acid—that growing fetuses need. And what's bad for baby can also be bad for mom: Skimp on complex carbohydrates and you'll be skimping on constipation-fighting fiber, plus all the B vitamins known to battle morning sickness and pregnancy-unsettled skin.

Another important point: Pregnancy is a time for healthy eating, not for dieting. So shelve those weight-loss books (at least until after you deliver) and stay well-balanced for a well-fed baby.

Cholesterol Concerns

"My husband and I are very careful about our diets, and we limit the cholesterol we eat. Should I keep doing this while I'm pregnant?"

Tired of hearing about all the things you can't have, shouldn't have, or need to cut back on now that you're pregnant? Then this bulletin should cheer you up: Cholesterol doesn't have to be off the table when you're expecting. Pregnant women, and to a lesser extent nonpregnant women of childbearing age, are protected to a certain degree against the artery-clogging effects of cholesterol—putting them in an enviable position as far as bacon, egg, and burger lovers are concerned. In fact, cholesterol is necessary for fetal development, so much so that the mother's body automatically increases its production, raising blood cholesterol levels by anywhere from 25 to 40 percent. Though you don't have to eat a high-cholesterol diet to help your body step up production, you can feel free to indulge a bit (unless your practitioner advised you otherwise). Scramble some eggs for breakfast (choose omega-3 eggs for the best fat benefits), use cheese to meet your calcium requirement, and bite into that burger, all without guilt.

Junk Food Junkie

"I'm addicted to junk foods like doughnuts, chips, and fast food. I know I should be eating healthier—and I really want to—but I'm not sure I can change my habits."

Ready to junk the junk food? Getting motivated to change your eating habits is the first and most important step—so congratulate yourself on taking it. Actually making the changes will involve some serious effort—but the effort will be seriously worth it. Here are several ways to make your withdrawal from your junk food habit almost as painless as it is worthwhile:

Move your meals. If the coffee crumble calls when you breakfast at your desk, fill up on a better breakfast at home (one that's packed with the blood-sugar stabilizing, stick-with-you combo of complex carbs and protein, like oatmeal, will actually help you fight those junk food cravings when they strike later on). If you know you can't resist the golden fries once you pass through the Golden Arches, don't go there—literally. Order in a healthy sandwich from the local deli—or head to that wrap place that doesn't fry anything.

Plan, plan, and plan some more. Planning for meals and snacks ahead of time (instead of grabbing what's easiest or nearest, like that package of cheese crackers from the vending machine) will keep you eating well throughout your pregnancy. So pack those brown bags. Keep a handy supply of takeout menus from restaurants that offer healthy options, so a nourishing meal's always just a phone call away (and place your order before hunger strikes). Stock your home, workplace, bag, and car with wholesome but satisfying snacks: fresh fruit, trail mix, soy chips, whole-grain granola bars and crackers, individual-size yogurts or smoothies, string cheese or wedges. So that the soda won't speak to you next time you get thirsty, keep water at the ready.

Don't test temptation. Keep candy, chips, cookies, and sugar-sweetened soft drinks out of the house so they'll be out of reach (if not out of mind). Step away from the pastry case before

that Danish makes eye contact with you. Drive the long way home from the office if it means you won't drive by the drive-through.

Make substitutions. Crave a Krispy Kreme with your morning coffee? Dunk a bran muffin instead. The midnight munchies have you digging for Doritos? Settle for the baked tortilla chips (that you were smart enough to stock up on at the market last time), dipped in salsa for more flavor and a healthy helping of vitamin C. Is your sweet tooth aching for ice cream? Stop by the juice bar for a thick, creamy, sweet fruit smoothie instead.

Keep baby on your mind. Your baby eats what you eat, but that's sometimes hard to keep in mind (especially when the smell of a cinnamon bun tries to seduce you at the mall). If you find it helps keep baby-feeding front of brain, put pictures of cute well-fed babies wherever you might need a little inspiration (and a lot of willpower). Keep one on your desk, in your wallet, in your car (so when you're tempted to veer into the drive-through, you'll drive by instead).

Know your limits. Some junk food junkies can handle a once-in-a-while approach to indulging their cravings, others can't (and you know who you are). If enough junk food is never enough for you—if a snack-size candy bar leads to king-size, if a single doughnut leads to a dozen, if you know you'll polish off the whole bag of chips once you tear it open—you might have an easier time quitting your habit cold turkey then trying to moderate it.

Remember that good habits can last a lifetime, too. Once you've put the effort into developing healthier eating habits, you might want to consider keeping them. Continuing to eat well after delivery will give you more of the energy you'll need to fuel your

---

Shortcuts to Healthy Eating

Healthy food can be fast food, too. Here's how:

- If you're always on the run, remember that it takes no more time to make a roast turkey, cheese, lettuce, and tomato sandwich to take to work (or to order one at the deli) than it does to stand in line for a burger.

- If the prospect of preparing a real dinner every night seems overwhelming, cook enough for two or three dinners at one time and give yourself alternate nights off.

- Keep it simple when you're cooking healthy. For a quick meal, broil a fish fillet and top it with your favorite jarred salsa, a little chopped avocado, and a squeeze of fresh lime juice. Layer tomato sauce and mozzarella cheese on a cooked boneless chicken breast, and then run it under the broiler. Or scramble some eggs and wrap them in a corn tortilla along with shredded cheddar and some microwave-steamed vegetables.

- When you don't have time to start from scratch (when do you ever?), turn to canned beans, soups, frozen or packaged ready-to-prepare healthy entrees, frozen vegetables, or the fresh prewashed veggies sold in supermarket produce sections (the ones you can microwave in the bag are especially convenient).

---

new-mom lifestyle. Plus it'll make it more likely that your baby will grow up with a taste for the healthier things in life.

Eating Out

"I try hard to stay on a healthy diet, but I eat out so often, it seems impossible."

For many pregnant women, it isn't substituting mineral water for martinis that poses a challenge at the restaurant table; it's trying to put together a meal that's baby friendly and doesn't break the calorie bank. With those goals in mind, and the following suggestions, it's easy to take the Pregnancy Diet out to lunch or dinner.

- Look for whole grains before you leap into the bread basket. If there aren't any in the basket, ask if there are any in the kitchen. If not, try not to fill up too much on the white stuff. Go easy, too, on the butter you spread on your bread and rolls, as well as the olive oil you dip them into. There will probably be plenty of other sources of fat in your restaurant meal—dressing on the salad, butter or olive oil on the vegetables—and, as always, fat adds up quickly.

- Go for a green salad as a first course. Other good first-course choices include shrimp cocktail, steamed seafood, grilled vegetables, or soup.

- If soup's on, look to ones with a vegetable base (particularly sweet potato, carrot, winter squash, or tomato). Lentil or bean soups pack a protein punch, too. In fact, a large bowl may eat like a meal, especially if you toss some grated cheese on top. Generally steer clear of cream soups, and take Manhattan-style when it comes to clam chowder.

- Make the most of your main. Get your protein—fish, seafood, chicken breast, or beef—the lean way (good words to look for: grilled, broiled, steamed, and poached). If everything comes heavily sauced, ask for yours on the side. And don't shy away from special requests (chefs are used to them; plus, it's hard to turn down a pregnant woman). Ask if that chicken breast can be broiled plain, instead of breaded and pan-seared or if the snapper can be grilled instead of fried. If you're a vegetarian, scan the menu for tofu, beans and peas, cheeses, and combinations of these. Vegetable lasagna, for example, might be a good choice in an Italian restaurant, bean curd and vegetables in a Chinese one.

- Be selective on the side, scouting for baked white or sweet potatoes, brown or wild rice, legumes (beans and peas), and fresh vegetables.

- Consider a fruity finish to your restaurant meal (fresh berries can be surprisingly satisfying). Fruit alone doesn't cut it (at least not all the time)? Add whipped cream, sorbet, or ice cream. Craving serious sweets? Join the "two spoons" club and share a decadent dessert with others at your table.

Reading Labels

"I'm eager to eat well, but it's difficult to figure out what's in the products I buy. I just can't make sense out of the labels."

Labels aren't designed to help you as much as to sell you. Keep this in mind when filling your shopping cart, and learn to read the small print, especially the ingredients list and the nutrition label (which *is* designed to help you).

The ingredients listing will tell you, in order of predominance (with the first ingredient the most plentiful and the last the least), exactly what's in a product. A quick look will tell you whether the major ingredient in a cereal is a refined grain or a whole grain. It will also tell you when a product is high in sugar, salt, fat, or additives. For example, when sugar is listed near the top of the ingredients list or when it appears in several different forms on a list (corn syrup, honey, and sugar), you know the product is chock-full of sugar.

Checking the grams of sugar on the label will not be useful until the FDA orders that the grams of "added sugar" be separated from the grams of "naturally occurring sugar" (those found in the raisin part of the raisin bran you're considering, for instance). Though the number of grams of sugar on the present label may be the same on a container of orange juice and a container of fruit drink, they aren't equivalent. It's like comparing oranges and corn syrup: The real OJ gets its naturally occurring sugar from fruit; the fruit drink contains added sugar.

Nutrition labels, which appear on most packaged products on your grocer's shelves, can be particularly valuable for a pregnant woman counting her protein and watching her calories, since they provide the grams of the former and the number of the latter in each serving. The listing of percentages of the government's recommended dietary allowance (called DRIs), however, is less useful because the DRI for pregnant women is different than the DRI used on package labels. Still, a food that scores high in a wide variety of nutrients is a good product to drop into your cart.

While it's important to pay attention to the small print, it's sometimes just as important to ignore the large print. When a box of English muffins boasts, "Made with whole wheat, bran, and honey," reading the small print may reveal that the major ingredient (first on the list) is white, not whole wheat, flour, that the muffins contain barely any bran (it's near the bottom of the ingredients

You Can't Tell a Fruit by Its Cover

When it comes to nutrition, the darker the color of most fruits and vegetables, the more vitamins and minerals (especially vitamin A) you'll be able to harvest from them. But keep in mind that it's the color inside—not outside—that signals good nutrition. So while cucumbers (dark on the outside, pale on the inside) are lightweights in that department, cantaloupes (pale on the outside, dark on the inside) are standouts.

list), and that there's a lot more white sugar (it's high on the list) than honey (it's low).

"Enriched" and "fortified" are also banners to be wary of. Adding a few vitamins to a not-so-good food doesn't make it a good food. You'd be much better off with a bowl of oatmeal, which comes by its nutrients naturally, than with a refined cereal that contains 12 grams of added sugar and a few pennies' worth of tossed-in vitamins and minerals.

Sushi Safety

"Sushi is my favorite food, but I heard you're not supposed to eat it while you're pregnant. Is that true?"

Sorry to say, sushi and sashimi will have to go the way of sake (the Japanese wine often served with them) during pregnancy—which is to say, they're off the table. Same holds true for raw oysters and clams, ceviche, fish tartares or carpaccios, and other raw or barely cooked fish and shellfish. That's because when seafood isn't cooked, there's a slight chance that it can make you sick (something you definitely don't want to be when you're pregnant). But that doesn't mean you have to steer clear of your favorite Japanese restaurants. Plenty of other options exist there, even at the sushi bar. Rolls that contain cooked fish or seafood and/or vegetables are, in fact, healthy options. (But don't worry about any raw fish you've eaten up to this point.)

Hot Stuff

"I love spicy food—the hotter, the better. Is it safe to eat it while I'm pregnant?"

Hot mamas-to-be can continue to challenge their taste buds with four-alarm chilis, salsas, and stir-fries—as long as you can tolerate the almost inevitable heartburn and indigestion that follow. There's no risk from spicy foods during pregnancy, and, in fact, since peppers of all kinds (including hot ones) are packed with vitamin C, many of these foods are extra nutritious. So enjoy—just make sure you save room for Tums.

Spoiled Food

"I ate a container of yogurt this morning without realizing that it had expired a week ago. It didn't taste spoiled, but should I worry?"

No need to cry over spoiled milk . . . or yogurt. Though eating dairy products that have recently "expired" is never a particularly good idea, it's rarely a dangerous one. If you haven't shown any ill effects from your post-date snack (symptoms of food poisoning usually occur within eight hours), there's obviously no harm done. Besides, food poisoning is an unlikely possibility if the yogurt had been refrigerated continuously. In the future, however, check dates more carefully before you buy or eat perishables, and, of course, never eat foods that appear to have developed mold. For more on food safety, see the box on page 116.

"I got food poisoning from something I ate last night, and I've been throwing up. Will that hurt my baby?"

You're much more likely to suffer from the food poisoning than your baby is. The major risk—for you and your baby—is that you'll become dehydrated from vomiting and diarrhea. So make sure you get plenty of fluids (which are more important in the short term than solids) to replace those that you're losing. And contact your practitioner if your diarrhea is severe and/or your stools contain blood or mucus. See page 501 for more on stomach bugs.

Sugar Substitutes

"I'm trying not to gain too much weight, but I love sweets. Can I use sugar substitutes?"

It sounds like a sweet deal, but the truth is that sugar substitutes are a mixed bag for expectant moms. Though most are probably safe, some research is still inconclusive. Here's how sugar substitutes stack up at the moment:

Sucralose (Splenda). Made from sugar, but chemically converted to a form that's not absorbable by the body, sucralose appears right now to be the best bet for pregnant women seeking sweetness with no calories and little aftertaste. You can sweeten your coffee or tea with sucralose, and use it in cooking and baking (unlike other sugar substitutes, it doesn't lose its sweetness when heated), or buy products that have been sweetened with it (including drinks, yogurts, candy, and ice cream). Keep in mind that moder-

ation's probably smart. Even though it seems to be safe, the product is relatively new, and no long-term data are available to confirm that.

Aspartame (Equal, NutraSweet). Aspartame is used in beverages, yogurt, and frozen desserts but not in baked goods or cooked foods (the sweetness doesn't survive when heated for long periods). The jury is still out on the safety of this widely used sugar substitute. Many practitioners consider it harmless and will okay light or moderate use in pregnancy. Others are less convinced of its safety and suggest that, until more is known, pregnant women be cautious in their use of this sweetener. Check with your practitioner for his or her aspartame bottom line. (Women with PKU must limit their intake of phenylalanine and are advised never to use aspartame.)

Saccharin. Not much research has been done on saccharin use in human pregnancy, but animal studies show an increase in cancer in the offspring of pregnant animals who ingest large quantities of the chemical. Whether a similar risk exists for human offspring is unclear (especially because animal studies don't always correlate well to human reality—after all, you're not pregnant with a baby rat). Still, combined with the fact that the sweetener crosses the placenta in humans and is eliminated very slowly from fetal tissues, most practitioners advise minimizing its use during pregnancy. Don't worry, however, about saccharin you had before finding out that you were pregnant because, again, there are no documented risks.

Acesulfame-K (Sunett). This sweetener, 200 times sweeter than sugar, is approved for use in baked goods, gelatin desserts, chewing gum, and soft drinks. The FDA says it's okay to use in moderation during pregnancy, but since few studies have been done to prove its safety, ask your practitioner what he or she thinks before gobbling the stuff up.

Sorbitol. This is a relative of sugar found naturally in many fruits and berries. With half the sweetness of sugar, it is used in a wide range of foods and beverages and is safe for use in pregnancy in moderate amounts. But it does present a problem in large doses: Too much can cause bloating, gas pains, and diarrhea—a trio no pregnant woman needs.

Mannitol. Less sweet than sugar, mannitol is poorly absorbed by the body and thus provides fewer calories than sugar (but more than other sugar substitutes). Like sorbitol, it is safe in modest amounts, but large quantities can cause gastrointestinal unrest.

Xylitol. This sugar alcohol, which is produced as a sugar substitute from plants (but is also naturally occurring in many fruits and vegetables and is even created by the body during normal metabolism), is found in chewing gum, toothpaste, candies, and some foods. One of its benefits is that it can prevent tooth decay (which is why chewing gum made with xylitol can be a very good thing). Xylitol has 40 percent fewer calories than sugar and is considered safe during pregnancy in moderation (so in other words, it's fine to chew one pack of xylitol gum— but you might not want to chew five).

Stevia. Derived from a South American shrub, stevia has not been approved by the FDA as a sweetener (it's considered a dietary supplement). No clear research proves stevia is safe during pregnancy, so before you dip into this sweetner, check with your practitioner for his or her recommendation.

Lactose. This milk sugar is one sixth as sweet as table sugar and adds light sweetening to foods. For those who are lactose-intolerant, it can cause uncomfortable symptoms; otherwise it's safe.

Honey. Everyone's all abuzz about honey these days because of its high levels of antioxidants (darker varieties, such as buckwheat honey, are the richest in antioxidants). But it's not all sweet news. Though it's a good substitute for sugar, honey is definitely not low-cal. It's got 19 more calories per tablespoon than sugar does. How's that for sticky?

Fruit juice concentrates. Unquestionably nutritious, fruit juice concentrates, such as white grape and apple, are a safe (if not low-calorie) sweetener to turn to during pregnancy. They're surprisingly versatile in the kitchen (you can substitute them for the sugar in many recipes) and they're readily available in frozen form at the supermarket. Look for them in a host of commercial products, too, from jams and jellies to whole-grain cookies, muffins, cereals, and granola bars, to pop-up toaster pastries, yogurt, and sparkling sodas. Unlike most products sweetened with sugar or other sugar substitutes, the majority of fruit-juice-sweetened products are made with nutritious ingredients, such as whole-grain flour and healthy fats. How sweet it is.

Herbal Tea

"I drink a lot of herbal tea. Is it safe to keep drinking it while I'm pregnant?"

Should you take (herbal) tea for two? Unfortunately, since the effect of herbs in pregnancy has not been well researched, there's no definitive answer to that question yet. Some herbal teas are probably safe, some probably not—and some, such as red raspberry leaf, taken in very large amounts (more than four 8-ounce cups a day), are thought to trigger contractions (good if you're 40 weeks and impatient, not good if you haven't reached term). Until more is known, the FDA has urged caution on the use of most herbal teas in pregnancy and during lactation. And though many women have drunk lots of herbal teas throughout pregnancy without a problem, it is probably safest to stay away from, or at least limit, herbal teas while you're expecting—unless they've been specifically recommended or cleared by your practitioner. Check with your practitioner for a list of which herbs he or she believes are safe and which are pregnancy no-no's.

To make sure you're not brewing up trouble (and an herb your practitioner hasn't cleared) with your next cup of tea, read labels carefully; some brews that seem from their names to be fruit based also contain a variety of herbs. Stick to regular (black) tea that comes flavored, or mix up your own by adding any of the following to boiling water or regular tea: orange, apple, pineapple, or other fruit juice; slices of lemon, lime, orange, apple, pear, or other fruit; mint leaves, cinnamon, nutmeg, cloves, or ginger (a great alleviator of the queasies). Chamomile is also considered safe in small amounts during pregnancy and can be soothing to a pregnancy-unsettled tummy. The jury's still out on green tea, which can decrease the effectiveness of folic acid, that vital pregnancy vitamin—so if you're a green tea drinker, drink in moderation. And never brew a homemade tea from a plant growing in your backyard, unless you are absolutely certain what it is and that it's safe for use during pregnancy.

Chemicals in Foods

"With additives in packaged foods, pesticides on vegetables, PCBs and mercury in fish, antibiotics in meat, and nitrates in hot dogs, is there anything I can safely eat during pregnancy?"

Take heart—and take it easy. You don't have to go crazy (or hungry) to protect your baby from food hazards. In spite of anything you might have read and heard, very few substances found in food have been absolutely proven harmful to the unborn.

Still, it's smart to reduce risk whenever you can—particularly when you're reducing risk for two. And it's not that difficult to do, especially these days. To feed yourself and your baby as safely as you can, use the following as a guide to help you decide what to drop into your shopping cart and what to pass up:

■ Choose your foods from the Pregnancy Diet. Because it steers away from processed foods, it steers you clear of many questionable and unsafe substances. It also supplies Green Leafies and Yellows, rich in protective beta-carotene, as well as other fruits and vegetables rich in phytochemicals, which may counteract the effects of toxins in food.

■ Whenever possible, cook from scratch with fresh ingredients or use frozen or packaged organic ready-to-eat foods. You'll avoid many questionable additives found in processed foods, and your meals will be more nutritious, too.

■ Go as natural as you can, when you can. Whenever you have a choice (and you won't always), choose foods that are free of artificial additives (colorings, flavorings, and preservatives). Read labels to screen for foods that are either additive free or use natural additives (a cheddar cheese cracker that gets its orange hue from annatto, instead of red dye #40, and its flavor from real cheese, instead of artificial cheese flavoring). Keep in mind that although some artificial additives are considered safe, others are of questionable safety, and many are used to enhance foods that aren't very nutritious to start with. (For a listing of questionable and safe additives, go to cspinet.org/reports/chemcuisine .htm).

- Generally avoid foods preserved with nitrates and nitrites (or sodium nitrates), including hot dogs, salami, bologna, and smoked fish and meats. Look for those brands (you'll find plenty in the market these days) that do not include these preservatives.

- Fish is a great source of lean protein, as well as baby brain–building omega-3 fatty acids, two good reasons to keep it on your pregnancy menu—or even to consider adding it (aversions allowing) if you've never been a fish eater before. And in fact, research has shown brain benefits for babies whose moms eat lots of fish when they're expecting. So go fish, by all means, but fish selectively, sticking to those varieties that are considered safe. According to the EPA and other experts, it's smart to avoid shark, swordfish, king mackerel, tilefish, and tuna steaks. These large fish can contain high levels of methylmercury, a chemical that in large, accumulated doses can possibly be harmful to a fetus's developing nervous system. Don't worry if you've already enjoyed a serving or two of swordfish—any risks would apply to regular consumption—just skip these fish from now on. Also limit your consumption of canned tuna (chunk light tuna contains less mercury

than white) and freshwater fish caught by recreational fishers to an average of 6 ounces (cooked weight) per week; commercially caught fish usually has lower levels of contaminants, so you can safely eat more. Steer clear of fish from waters that are contaminated (with sewage or industrial runoff, for example) or tropical fish, such as grouper, amberjack, and mahimahi (which sometimes contain toxins). Fortunately, that leaves plenty of fish in the sea to enjoy safely and often (an average of 12 ounces of cooked fish per week is considered safe according to government guidelines). Choose from salmon (wild caught is best), sole, flounder, haddock, tilapia, halibut, ocean perch, pollack, cod, and trout, as well as other smaller ocean fish (anchovies, sardines, and herring are not only safe, but also loaded with omega-3) and seafood of all kinds. Remember, all fish and seafood should be well cooked. For the latest information on fish safety, contact the FDA at (888) SAFE-FOOD (723-3366) or cfsan.fda.gov or the EPA at epa.gov/ost/fish.

- Choose lean cuts of meat and remove visible fat before cooking, since chemicals that livestock ingest tend to concentrate in the fat of the animal. With poultry, remove both the fat and the skin to minimize chemical intake. And don't eat organ meats (such as liver and kidneys) very often, for the same reason.

- When it's available and your budget permits, buy meat and poultry that has been raised organically (or grassfed), without hormones or antibiotics (remember, you eat what your dinner ate). Choose organic dairy products and eggs, when possible, for the same reason. Free-range chickens (and eggs) are not only less likely to be contaminated with chemicals, they are also less

Something's Cooking

You can find recipes that put it all together in *What to Expect: Eating Well When You're Expecting.*

likely to carry such infections as salmonella because the birds are not kept in cramped, disease-breeding quarters. And here's a plus when it comes to grass-fed beef: It's likely to be lower in calories and fat, higher in protein, and a rich source of those baby-friendly omega-3 fatty acids.

- Buy organic produce when possible and practical. Produce that is certified organic usually is as close as possible to being free of all chemical residues. Transitional produce may still contain some residues from soil contamination but should be safer than conventionally grown produce. If organic produce is available locally and you can afford the premium price, make it your choice—just keep in mind as you load up your shopping cart that organic produce will have a much shorter shelf life (same goes for organic poultry and meats). If price is an object, pick organic selectively (see box).

- As a precaution, give all vegetables and fruits a bath. Washing produce thoroughly is important no matter what (even organic produce can wear a coating of bacteria), but it's key to removing chemical pesticides your fruits and veggies may have picked up in the field. Water will wash off some, but a dip in or a spray with produce wash will take off much more (rinse thoroughly afterward). Scrub skins when possible and practical to remove surface chemical residues, especially when a vegetable has a waxy coating (as cucumbers and sometimes tomatoes, apples, peppers, and eggplant do). Peel skins that still seem "coated" after washing.

- Favor domestic produce. Imported (and foods made from such produce) often contain higher levels of pesticides than U.S.-grown equivalents because

Pick and Choose Organic

Spending the big bucks on organic produce isn't always worth it. Here's the lowdown on when to spring for the organic and when it's safe to stick with conventional:

Best to buy organic (because even after washing, these foods still carry higher levels of pesticide residue than others): Apples, cherries, grapes, peaches, nectarines, pears, raspberries, strawberries, bell peppers, celery, potatoes, and spinach.

No need to go organic on these foods (because these products generally don't contain pesticide residue on them): Bananas, kiwi, mango, papaya, pineapples, asparagus, avocado, broccoli, cauliflower, corn, onions, and peas.

Consider organic for milk, beef, and poultry because they won't contain antibiotics or hormones, though they will cost more. Don't bother with so-called organic fish. There are no USDA organic certification standards for seafood (which means producers are making their own claims about why it's organic).

pesticide regulation in other countries is often lax or nonexistent.

- Go local. Locally grown produce is likely to contain more nutrients (it's fresh from the field) and possibly sport less pesticide residue. Many of the growers at your local farmers' market may grow without pesticides (or with very little), even if their products aren't marked "organic." That's because certification is too expensive for some small growers to afford.

- Vary your diet. Variety ensures not only a more interesting eating experience

Eating Safe for Two

Worried about the pesticides your peach picked up in South America? That's sensible, especially because you're trying to eat safely for two. But what about the sponge you're about to wipe that peach down with (the one that's been hanging around your sink for the last three weeks)? Have you thought about what that might have picked up lately? And the cutting board you were planning to slice your peach on—isn't that the same one you diced that raw chicken on last night before you tossed it into the stir-fry? Here's a food safety reality check: A more immediate—and proven—threat than the chemicals in your food are the little organisms, bacteria and parasites, that can contaminate it. It's not a pretty picture (or one that's visible without the help of a microscope), but these nasty bugs can cause anything from mild stomach upset to severe illness. To make sure that the worst thing you'll pick up from your next meal is a little heartburn (the last thing an expectant mom needs is another reason for gastrointestinal upset), shop, prepare, and eat with care:

- When in doubt, throw it out. Make this your mantra of safe eating. It applies to any food you even suspect might be spoiled. Read and abide by freshness dates on food packages.

- When food shopping, avoid fish, meat, and eggs that are not well refrigerated or kept on ice. Steer clear of jars that are leaky or don't "pop" when you open them and cans that are rusty or seem swollen or otherwise misshapen. Wash can tops before opening (and wash your can opener frequently in hot soapy water or in the dishwasher).

- Wash your hands before handling food and after touching raw meat, fish, or eggs. If you have a cut on your hand, wear rubber or plastic gloves while you prepare food, and remember, unless they're disposable, the gloves need to be washed as often as your bare hands.

- Keep kitchen counters and sinks clean. Same goes for cutting boards (wash with soap and hot water or in the dishwasher). Wash dishcloths frequently and keep sponges clean (replace them often, wash them in the dishwasher each night, or periodically pop dampened ones into the microwave for a couple of minutes); they can harbor bacteria.

- Serve hot foods hot, cold foods cold. Leftovers should be refrigerated quickly and heated until steaming before reusing. (Toss perishable foods that have been left out for more than two hours.) Don't eat frozen foods that have been thawed and then refrozen.

- Measure the fridge interior temperature with a refrigerator thermometer and be sure it stays at 41°F or less. Ideally, the freezer should be at 0°F, though many freezers are not designed to meet that requirement; don't worry if yours isn't.

and better nutrition but also better chances of avoiding excessive exposure to any one chemical. Switch between broccoli, kale, and carrots, for instance; melon, peaches, and strawberries; salmon, halibut, and sole; cereals made from whole wheat, corn, and oats.

- Thaw foods in the refrigerator, time permitting. If you're in a rush, thaw food in a watertight plastic bag submerged in cold water (and change it every 30 minutes). Never thaw foods at room temperature.

- Marinate meat, fish, or poultry in the refrigerator, not on the counter. Discard the marinade after use, because it contains potentially hazardous bacteria. If you'd like to use the marinade as a dip or sauce, or to baste with, reserve a portion for that purpose before you add the meat, poultry, or fish. Use a new spoon or brush each time you baste to avoid recontaminating the marinade, or just cook for a few more minutes after the last basting.

- Don't eat raw or undercooked meats, poultry, fish, or shellfish while you're expecting. Always cook meats and fish to medium (to 160°F) and poultry thoroughly (to 165°F). In general, place the thermometer in the thickest part of the food, away from bone, fat, or gristle. In poultry, place it in the dark meat.

- Don't eat eggs that are runny (prefer well-scrambled to sunny-side up), and if you're mixing a batter that contains raw eggs, resist the urge to lick the spoon (or your fingers). The exception to this rule: eggs that are pasteurized, since this process effectively eliminates the risk of salmonella poisoning.

- Wash raw vegetables thoroughly (especially if they won't be cooked before eating). Those fresh blueber-ries from the farmers' market might have been grown organically—but that doesn't mean they're not sporting a layer of bacteria.

- Avoid alfalfa and other sprouts, which are often contaminated with bacteria.

- Stick to pasteurized dairy products, and make sure those that you use have been refrigerated continuously. Soft cheeses, such as imported feta, Brie, blue cheeses, and soft Mexican-style cheese made from unpasteurized milk, can be contaminated with listeria (see page 501) and should be avoided by pregnant women, unless heated until bubbly. Domestic cheese is almost always pasteurized except for those made from "raw milk."

- Hot dogs, deli meats, and cold-smoked seafood can also be contaminated. As a precaution, even ready-cooked meats or smoked fish should be heated to steaming before eating (use them in casseroles).

- Juice should be fully pasteurized, too. Avoid unpasteurized or flash pasteurized juice or cider, whether it's bought at a health food store or a roadside stand. If you're not sure whether a juice is pasteurized, don't drink it.

- When eating out, avoid establishments that seem to ignore basic sanitation rules. Some signs are pretty obvious: Perishable foods are kept at room temperature, the bathrooms are unclean, it's open season for flies, and so on.

- Drive yourself to the health food market, but don't drive yourself crazy. Though it's smart to try to avoid theoretical hazards in food, making your life stressful in the pursuit of a natural meal isn't necessary. Do the best you can—and then sit back, eat well, and relax.

PART 2

Nine Months & Counting

From Conception to Delivery

CHAPTER 6

The
First
Month

Approximately 1 to 4 Weeks

ONGRATULATIONS, AND WELCOME to your pregnancy! Though you almost certainly don't look pregnant yet, chances are you're already starting to feel it. Whether it's just tender breasts and a little fatigue you're experiencing, or every early pregnancy symptom in the book (and then some), your body is gearing up for the months of baby making to come. As the weeks pass, you'll notice changes in parts of your body you'd expect (like your belly), as well as places you wouldn't expect (your feet and your eyes). You'll also notice changes in the way you live—and look at—life. But try not to think (or read) too far ahead. For now, just sit back, relax, and enjoy the beginning of one of the most exciting and rewarding adventures of your life.

Your Baby This Month

Week 1 The countdown to baby begins this week. Only thing is, there's no baby in sight—or inside. So why call this week 1 of pregnancy if you're not even pregnant? Here's why. It's extremely hard to pinpoint the precise moment when sperm meets egg (sperm from your partner can hang out in your body for several days before your egg comes out to greet it, and your egg can be kept waiting for a day for the sperm to make their appearance).

What isn't hard to pinpoint, however, is the first day of your last menstrual period (LMP, which you're having right now—so mark the calendar), allowing your practitioner to use that as the standard starting line for your 40-week pregnancy. The upshot of this dating system (besides a lot of potential for confusion)? You get to clock in two weeks of your 40 weeks of pregnancy before you even get pregnant (how's that for a head start?).

Week 2 Nope, still no baby yet. But your body isn't taking a break this week. In fact, it's working hard gearing up for the big O—ovulation. The lining of your uterus is thickening (feathering its nest for the arrival of the fertilized egg) and your ovarian follicles are maturing—some faster than others—until one becomes the dominant one, destined for ovulation. And waiting in that dominant follicle is an anxious egg (or two, if you're about to conceive fraternal twins) with your baby's name on it—ready to burst out and begin its journey from single cell to bouncing boy or girl. But first it will have to make a journey down your fallopian tube in search of Mr. Right—the lucky sperm that will seal the deal.

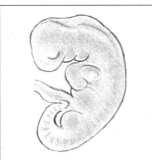
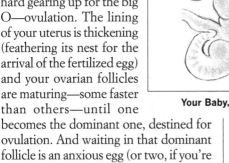

Your Baby, Month 1

Week 3 Congratulations—you've conceived! Which means your soon-to-be baby has started its miraculous transformation from single cell to fully formed baby boy or girl ready for cuddles and kisses. Within hours after sperm meets egg, the fertilized cell (aka zygote) divides, and then continues to divide (and divide). Within days, your baby-to-be has turned into a microscopic ball of cells, around one fifth the size of the period at the end of this sentence. The blastocyst—as it is now known (though you'll almost certainly come up with a cuter name soon)—begins its journey from your fallopian tube to your waiting uterus. Only 8½ more months—give or take—to go!

Week 4 It's implantation time! That ball of cells that you'll soon call baby—though it's now called embryo—has reached your uterus and is snuggling into the uterine lining where it'll stay connected to you until delivery. Once firmly in place, the ball of cells undergoes the great divide—

splitting into two groups. Half will become your son or daughter, while the other half will become the placenta, your baby's lifeline during his or her uterine stay. And even though it's just a ball of cells right now (no bigger than a poppy seed, actually, but a lot sweeter), don't underestimate your little embryo—he or she has already come a long way since those blastocyst days. The amniotic sac—otherwise known as the bag of waters—is forming, as is the yolk sac, which will later be incorporated into your baby's developing digestive tract. Each layer of the embryo—it has three now—is beginning to grow into specialized parts of the body. The inner layer, known as the endoderm, will develop into your baby's digestive system, liver, and lungs. The middle layer, called the mesoderm, will soon be your baby's heart, sex organs, bones, kidneys, and muscles. The outer layer, or ectoderm, will eventually form your baby's nervous system, hair, skin, and eyes.

Make the Pregnancy Connection

Log on to whattoexpect.com—your interactive pregnancy companion. Just fill in your due date, and you'll get weekly reports on your baby's growth and development, plus access to useful tools like the Pregnancy Planner and Baby Name Finder. Connect with other moms on the message boards, create your own blogs and profile pages, and make new friends!

Pregnancy Timetable

Though most women count their pregnancies in months, your doctor or midwife will do the calculations in weeks. And that's where things can get a little tricky. The average pregnancy lasts 40 weeks, but because counting begins from the first day of your last menstrual period (LMP)—and ovulation and conception don't take place until two weeks after that (if your periods are regular)—you actually become pregnant in week 3 of your pregnancy. In other words, you've already clocked two weeks by the time sperm meets egg. This may sound very confusing, but as your pregnancy progresses and you experience preg-

nancy milestones traditionally marked by weeks (baby's heartbeat heard with Doppler around 10 weeks; the top of the uterus reaches your belly button at 20 weeks), you'll start to make sense of the weekly calendar.

Though this book is organized in chapters by month, corresponding weeks are also provided. Weeks 1 to 13 (approximately) make up the first trimester and include months 1 to 3; weeks 14 to 27 (approximately) comprise the second trimester and include months 4 to 6; and weeks 28 to 40 (approximately) are the third trimester and include months 7 to 9.

What You May Be Feeling

While it's true that pregnancy has its share of wonderful moments and experiences to cherish, it also has a boatload (make that a bloatload) of less

Symptoms? Starting Soon

Most early pregnancy symptoms begin making their appearance around week 6, but every woman—and every pregnancy—is different, so many may begin earlier or later for you (or not at all, if you're lucky). If you're experiencing something that's not on this list or in this chapter, look ahead to the next chapters or check it out in the index.

than fabulous symptoms. Some you're probably expecting to have (like that queasy feeling that might already be settling in). Others you'd probably never expect (like drooling—who knew?). Many you'll probably not discuss in public (and will try your best not to do in public, like passing gas), and many you'll probably try to forget (which you might, by the way, since forgetfulness is another pregnancy symptom).

Here are a couple of things to keep in mind about these and other pregnancy symptoms. First, because every woman and every pregnancy is different, few pregnancy symptoms are universal. So while your sister or best friend might have sailed through her pregnancy without a single nauseous moment, you might be spending every morning (and afternoon and evening) hovering over the toilet. Second, the symptoms that follow are a good sampling of what you might expect to experience (though you almost certainly, thankfully, won't experience them all—at least not all at once), but there are plenty more where these came from. Chances are just about every weird and wacky sensation you feel during the next nine months (both the physical ones and the emotional ones) will be normal for pregnancy, and normal for you. But if a symptom ever leaves you with a nagging doubt (can this really be normal?), always check it out with your practitioner, just to be sure.

Though it's unlikely that you'll even know you're expecting this month (at least not until the very end of the month), you might begin noticing something's up—even this early on. Here's what you might experience this month:

Physically

- Possible staining or spotting when the fertilized egg implants in your uterus, around five to ten days after conception (fewer than 30 percent of women experience such so-called implantation bleeding)

- Breast changes (possibly more pronounced if you typically have breast changes before your period, and possibly somewhat less pronounced if you've had babies before): fullness, heaviness, tenderness, tingling, darkening of the areolas (the pigmented area around your nipples)

- Bloating, flatulence

- Fatigue, lack of energy, sleepiness

- More frequent urination than usual

- Beginnings of nausea, with or without vomiting (though most women don't start feeling queasy until around six

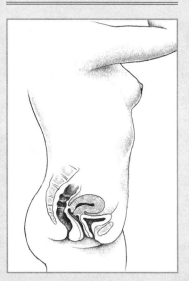

A Look Inside

There's definitely no way to tell this book by its cover yet. Though you may recognize a few physical changes in yourself—your breasts may be a little fuller, your tummy a tad rounder (though that's from bloat, not baby)—no one else is likely to have noticed. Make sure you take a good look at your waist: It may be the last time you'll see it for many months to come.

weeks of pregnancy), and/or excess saliva

- Increased sensitivity to smells

Emotionally

- Emotional ups and downs (like amped-up PMS), which may include mood swings, irritability, irrationality, inexplicable weepiness

- Anxiousness while waiting for the right time to take a home pregnancy test

What You Can Expect at Your First Prenatal Visit

Your first prenatal visit probably will be the longest you'll have during your pregnancy—and definitely will be the most comprehensive. Not only will there be more tests, procedures (including several that will be performed only at this visit), and data gathering (in the form of a complete medical history), but there will be more time spent on questions (questions you have for the practitioner, questions he or she will have for you) and answers. There will also be plenty of advice to take in—on everything from what you should be eating (and not eating) to what supplements you should be taking (and not taking) to whether (and how) you should be exercising. So be sure to come equipped with a list of the questions and concerns that have already come up, as well as with a pen and notebook (or *The What to Expect Pregnancy Journal and Organizer*).

One practitioner's routine may vary slightly from another's. In general, the exam will include:

Confirmation of your pregnancy. Your practitioner will check the following: the pregnancy symptoms you are experiencing; the date of your LMP to determine your estimated date of delivery (EDD), or due date (see page 20); your cervix and uterus for signs and approximate age of the pregnancy. A pregnancy test (urine and blood) will most likely be performed. Many practitioners also do an early ultrasound, which is the most accurate way of dating a pregnancy.

A complete history. To give you the best care possible, your practitioner will want to know a lot about you. Come prepared by checking records at home or calling your primary care doctor to refresh your memory on the following: your personal medical history (chronic illness, previous major illness or surgery, known allergies, including drug allergies); nutritional supplements (vitamins, minerals, herbal, and so on) or medications (over-the-counter, prescription) you are presently taking or have taken since conception; your family medical history (genetic disorders, chronic diseases, unusual pregnancy outcomes); your gynecological history (age at first period, usual length of your cycle, duration and regularity of periods); your obstetrical history (past live births, miscarriages, abortions), as well as the course of past pregnancies, labors, and deliveries. Your practitioner will also ask questions about your social history (such as your age and occupation) and about your lifestyle habits (what you typically eat, whether you exercise, drink, smoke, or use recreational drugs) and other factors in your personal life that might affect your pregnancy (information about the baby's father, information on your ethnicity).

A complete physical examination. This may include assessment of your general health through examination of heart, lungs, breasts, abdomen; measurement of your blood pressure to serve as a baseline reading for comparison at future visits; notation of your height and your weight (prepregnancy and present, if they're already different); a look at your arms and legs for varicose veins and swelling to serve as a baseline for comparison at future visits; examination of external genitalia and of your vagina and cervix (with a speculum in place, as when you get a Pap smear); examination

The Wholly Healthy Pregnancy

Not surprisingly, getting regular medical care in the form of prenatal visits makes a big difference in the outcome of your pregnancy. Women who see a practitioner regularly during pregnancy have healthier babies, and they are less likely to deliver prematurely and to have other serious pregnancy-related problems.

But though your health care should begin with your belly when you're expecting, it shouldn't end there. It'll probably be easy to remember to see your prenatal practitioner regularly (it's worth it just to hear the baby's heartbeat!), but will you remember to take care of the rest of you, even the less apparently pregnant parts?

To keep yourself wholly healthy during your whole nine months, stay on top of all your health care maintenance. Pay a visit to your dentist for a cleaning and a checkup; most dental work, particularly the preventive kind, can be done safely during pregnancy and may actually prevent pregnancy complications. Check in with your internist, family physician, or specialist if you have any chronic conditions or other medical problems that will need monitoring (make sure your pregnancy practitioner's in the loop about other care you're receiving). And see your allergist, if necessary. You probably won't begin a course of allergy shots now, but you may need to look into different treatment options now that you're breathing for two.

If new medical problems come up while you're expecting, don't ignore them, even if you're already in over your head with pregnancy-related symptoms. Check any issue out (even ones that seem relatively innocuous—a persistent sore throat or a chronic headache) with an appropriate physician. Your baby needs a wholly healthy mother.

---

of your pelvic organs bimanually (with one hand in the vagina and one on the abdomen) and also possibly through the rectum and vagina; assessment of the size and shape of the bony pelvis (through which your baby will eventually try to exit).

A battery of tests. Some tests are routine for every pregnant woman; some are routine in some areas of the country, or with some practitioners and not others; some are performed only when circumstances warrant. The most common prenatal tests given at the first visit include:

- A blood test to determine blood type and Rh status, hCG levels, and to check for anemia.

- Urinalysis to screen for glucose (sugar), protein, white blood cells, blood, and bacteria.

- Blood screens to determine antibody titer (levels) and immunity to such diseases as rubella.

- Tests to disclose the presence of infections such as syphilis, gonorrhea, hepatitis B, chlamydia, and, very often, HIV.

- A Pap smear for the detection of abnormal cervical cells.

Depending on your particular situation, and if appropriate, you may also receive:

- Genetic tests for cystic fibrosis, sickle

cell anemia, Tay-Sachs, or other genetic diseases.

- A blood sugar level test to check for any tendency toward diabetes, especially if you have a family history of diabetes, have high blood pressure, have previously had an excessively large baby or one with birth defects,

or gained excessive weight with an earlier pregnancy. (All women receive a glucose screening test for gestational diabetes at around 28 weeks; see page 297.)

An opportunity for discussion. Here's the time to bring out that list of questions and concerns.

What You May Be Wondering About

Breaking the News

"When should we tell friends and family that we are expecting?"

This is one question only you can answer. Some expectant parents can't wait to tell everyone they know (not to mention a fair number of strangers) the good news. Others tell only selectively at first, starting with those nearest and dearest (close relatives and

friends, perhaps), and waiting until their condition is obvious before making the pregnancy common knowledge. Still others decide they'd rather put off issuing any announcements until the first trimester has been successfully completed or until prenatal testing has been finished up.

So talk it over, and do what feels most comfortable. Just remember: In spreading the good news, don't forget to take the time to savor it as a twosome.

For tips on when to break the news at work, see page 188.

For the Other Pregnant Half

There isn't a page in this book that isn't intended for both expectant mothers and fathers. As a father-to-be, you'll gain plenty of insight into the pregnancy experience (as well as make some sense out of those crazy symptoms your spouse has been complaining about) by reading along with her, month by month. But because you're likely to have some questions and concerns that are uniquely yours, there's a chapter dedicated to you—the other pregnant half. See Chapter 19: Fathers Are Expectant, Too.

Vitamin Supplements

"Should I be taking vitamins?"

Virtually no one gets a nutritionally perfect diet every day, especially early in pregnancy, when round-the-clock morning sickness is a common appetite suppressant, or when the little nutrition some women manage to get down often doesn't stay down (sound familiar?). Though a daily vitamin supplement can't take the place of a good prenatal diet, it can serve as some dietary insurance, guaranteeing that your baby won't be cheated if you don't always hit the nutritional mark you're aiming for, especially during the early months when so much of your baby's most crucial construction occurs.

And there are other good reasons to take your vitamins. For one thing, studies show that women who take a vitamin supplement containing folic acid during the first months of pregnancy (and even prior to pregnancy) significantly reduce the risk of neural tube defects (such as spina bifida) in their babies, as well as help prevent preterm birth. For another, research has shown that taking a supplement containing at least 10 mg of vitamin B_6 before and during early pregnancy can minimize morning sickness (and who needs a better reason than that?).

Good formulations designed especially for expectant mothers are available by prescription or over-the-counter. (Ask your practitioner for a recommendation and see page 103 for details on what the supplement should contain.) Don't take any kind of dietary supplements other than such a prenatal formula without your practitioner's approval.

Some women find that taking the typical horse-size prenatal supplement increases nausea, especially early in pregnancy. Switching vitamin formulas or pill types may help, as may taking your pill with food (unless you usually throw up after eating) or taking it during the time of day when you're least likely to be nauseous. A coated pill is often easier to tolerate, as well as easier to swallow. If even that bothers you, you might consider a chewable supplement or a slow-release one. If your nausea is particularly bad, look for a formulation that's higher in vitamin B_6 (ginger is another good addition for the queasy set). But be sure any formula you select approximates the requirements for supplements designed for pregnancy and doesn't contain any extras that might not be safe (such as herbs). If your practitioner prescribed your supplement, check with him or her before switching.

In some women, the iron in a prenatal vitamin causes constipation or diarrhea. Again, switching formulas may bring relief. Taking a pregnancy supplement without iron and a separate iron preparation (your doctor can recommend one that dissolves in the intestines rather than in the more sensitive stomach—or one that is a slow release) may also relieve symptoms.

"I eat a lot of cereals and breads that are enriched. If I'm also taking a prenatal supplement, will I be taking in too many vitamins and minerals?"

You can get too much of a good thing, but not usually this way. Taking a prenatal vitamin along with the average diet, which includes plenty of enriched and fortified products, isn't likely to lead to excessive intake of vitamins and minerals. To take in that many nutrients, you'd have to be adding other supplements beyond the prenatal ones—which an expectant mother should never do unless advised by a physician who knows that she's pregnant. It's wise, however, to be wary of any foods (or drinks) that are fortified with more than the recommended daily allowance of vitamins A, D, E, and K, because these can be toxic in large amounts. Most other vitamins and minerals are water-soluble, which means any excesses that the body can't use are simply excreted in the urine. Which is, by the way, the reason why supplement-crazy Americans are said to have the most expensive urine in the world.

Fatigue

"Now that I'm pregnant, I'm tired all the time. Sometimes I feel as if I won't even be able to get through the day!"

Can't lift your head off the pillow each morning? Dragging your feet all day? Can't wait to crawl into bed as soon as you arrive home at night? If it seems like your get-up-and-go has left the building—and doesn't plan to be back anytime soon—it's not surprising. After all, you're pregnant. And even though there might not be any evidence on the outside that you're busily building a baby, plenty of exhausting work is going on inside. In some ways, your pregnant body is working harder when you're resting than a nonpregnant body is when running a marathon—only you're not aware of the exertion.

So what exactly is your body up to? For one thing, it's manufacturing your baby's life-support system, the placenta, which won't be completed until the end of the first trimester. For another, your body's hormone levels have increased significantly, you're producing more blood, your heart rate is up, your blood sugar is down, your metabolism is burning energy overtime (even when you're lying down), and you're using up more nutrients and water. And if that's not enough to wear you out, just toss into the enervating equation all the other physical and emotional demands of pregnancy that your body is adjusting to. Add it all up, and it's no wonder you feel as if you're competing in a triathlon each day—and coming in dead last (or at least, dead tired).

Happily, there is some relief headed your way—eventually. Once the herculean task of manufacturing the placenta is complete (around the fourth month) and your body has adjusted to the hormonal and emotional changes pregnancy brings, you'll feel a little peppier.

In the meantime, keep in mind that fatigue is a sensible signal from your body that you need to take it easier these days. So listen up, and get the rest your body needs. You may also be able to recapture some of that get-up-and-go with some of the following tips:

Baby yourself. If you're a first-time expectant mother, enjoy what will probably be your last chance for a long while to focus on taking care of yourself without feeling guilty. If you already have one or more children at home, you will have to divide your focus (see next page). But either way, this is not a time to strive for supermom-to-be status. Getting adequate rest is more important than keeping your house spotless or serving four-star dinners. Let the dishes wait until later, and turn the other way as the dust bunnies breed under your dining table. Order your groceries (and anything else you can think of) online instead of dragging yourself to the stores. Be a regular on the take-out circuit. Don't book activities—or take care of chores—that aren't essential. Never been a slacker? There's never been a better time to try it on for size.

Let others baby you. You're doing enough heavy lifting these days, so make sure your spouse is doing his fair share (right now, that should be more than half) of household chores, including laundry and grocery shopping. Accept your mother-in-law's offer to vacuum and dust the house when she's visiting. Have a pal pick up some essentials for you while she's going on a shopping run anyway. That way, you might actually have enough energy left to drag yourself out for a walk (before you drag yourself into bed).

Chill out more. Exhausted once the day's over? Spend evenings chilling out (preferably with your feet up) instead of stepping out. And don't wait until nightfall to take it easy. If you can squeeze in an afternoon nap, by all means go for it. If you can't sleep, lie down with a good book. If you're a working mom-to-be, a nap at the office may not be an option, of course, unless you have a flexible schedule and access to a comfortable sofa, but putting your feet up at your desk or on the sofa in the ladies' room during breaks and lunch hours may be possible. (If you choose to rest at lunch hour, make sure you make time to eat, too.)

Be a slacker mom. Have other kids? Fatigue may be more pronounced, for obvious reasons (you have less time to rest, more demands on your body). Or it may be less noticeable, since you're already accustomed to exhaustion—or too busy to pay attention to it. Either way, it's not easy babying yourself when you have other babies (and older children) clamoring for your attention. But try. Explain to them that growing a baby is hard work and it's leaving you beat. Ask for their help around the house, and their help in letting you get more rest. Instead of running around playgrounds during the day and chasing children at night, spend more time at quiet pursuits—reading, doing puzzles, being the patient in a game of "hospital" (you'll get to lie down), watching DVDs. Napping when you're mothering full-time may also be difficult, but if you can time your rest with the children's naptime (if they still nap), you may be able to swing it.

Get some more sleep. It may be stating the obvious, but just in case: Getting even an hour more sleep at night can pick you up come morning. Skip the *Late Show* and turn in earlier; ask your spouse to fix breakfast so you can turn out later. But don't overdo. Too many z's can actually leave you feeling even more exhausted.

Eat well. To keep your energy up, you need a steady supply of premium fuel.

Make sure you're getting enough calories each day (which may be easier said than done if morning sickness has you down—but is definitely worth the effort), and focus on long-lasting energy boosters, such as protein, complex carbohydrates, and iron-rich foods. Caffeine or sugar (or both) may seem like the perfect quick fix for an energy slump, but they're not. Though that candy bar or those jolt-in-a-can energy drinks might pick you up briefly, that blood sugar high will be followed by a free-falling crash, leaving you more beat than ever. (Plus, some canned energy drinks may contain dietary supplements that aren't safe for pregnancy use.)

Eat often. Like so many other pregnancy symptoms, fatigue responds well to the Six-Meal Solution (see page 91). Keeping your blood sugar on an even keel will help keep your energy steady, too—so resist meal skipping, and opt for frequent mini meals and snacks (the sustaining kind, comprised of protein and complex carbs).

Take a hike. Or a slow jog. Or a stroll to the grocery store. Or do a pregnancy exercise or yoga routine. Sure, the couch has never looked more inviting—but paradoxically, too much rest and not enough activity can heighten fatigue. Even a little exercise can be more rejuvenating than a sofa break. Just don't overdo it—you want to finish up your workout feeling energized, not enervated—and be sure to follow the guidelines starting on page 218.

Though fatigue will probably ease up by month 4, you can expect it to return in the last trimester (could it be nature's way of preparing you for the long sleepless nights you'll encounter once the baby has arrived?).

Morning Sickness

"I haven't had any morning sickness. Can I still be pregnant?"

Morning sickness, like a craving for pickles and ice cream, is one of those truisms about pregnancy that isn't necessarily true. Studies show that nearly three quarters of all expectant women experience the nausea and vomiting associated with morning sickness, which means that a little more than 25 percent of moms-to-be don't. If you're among those who never have a nauseous moment, or who feel only occasionally or mildly queasy, you can consider yourself not only pregnant but also lucky.

"My morning sickness lasts all day. I'm afraid that I'm not keeping down enough food to nourish my baby."

Welcome to the queasy club—a club that up to 75 percent of pregnant women belong to. Happily, though you and all the other miserable members are definitely feeling the effects of morning sickness—a misnamed malady, as you've already noticed, since it can strike morning, noon, night, or all three—your baby almost definitely isn't. That's because your baby's nutritional needs are minuscule right now, just like your baby (who's not even the size of a pea yet). Even women who have such a hard time keeping food down that they actu-

Your Nose Knows

Have you noticed, now that you're expecting, that you can smell what's on the menu before you even set foot in the restaurant? That heightened sense of smell you're experiencing is actually a very real side effect of pregnancy, caused by hormones (in this case estrogen) that magnify every little scent that wafts your way. What's worse, this bloodhound syndrome can also ramp up morning sickness symptoms. Smell trouble? Here are some strategies you can try to give your poor nose a break:

- If you can't stand the smell, get out of the kitchen. Or the restaurant. Or the perfume aisle of the department store. Or anywhere odors that sicken you hang out.

- Open your windows whenever possible to banish cooking or musty odors. Or run the exhaust fan on the stove.

- Wash your clothes more often than usual, since fibers tend to hold on to odors. Use unscented detergent and

softener, though, if the scented ones bother you (same goes for all your cleaning supplies).

- Switch to unscented or lightly scented toiletries.

- Ask those who are regularly within sniffing distance of you (and who you know well enough to ask) to be extra considerate of your sensitive smell status. Get your spouse to wash up, change his clothes, and brush his teeth after stopping for a chili cheeseburger. Request that friends and coworkers go easy on the perfume when they're with you. And, of course, avoid people who are smoking.

- Try to surround yourself with those scents (if there are any) that actually make you feel better. Mint, lemon, ginger, and cinnamon are more likely to be soothing, especially if you're queasy, though some expectant moms suddenly embrace smells that invoke infants, such as baby powder.

ally lose weight during the first trimester aren't hurting their babies, as long as they make up for the lost weight in later months. Which is usually pretty easy to do because the nausea and vomiting of morning sickness don't generally linger much beyond the 12th to 14th week. (An occasional expectant mom continues to experience symptoms into the second trimester, and a very few, particularly those expecting multiples, may suffer some well into the third.)

What causes morning sickness? No one knows for sure, but there's no shortage of theories, among them the high level of the pregnancy hormone hCG in the blood in the first trimester, elevated estrogen levels, gastroesophageal reflux (GER), the relative relaxation of muscle tissue in the digestive tract (which makes digestion less efficient), and the enhanced sense of smell that pregnant women develop.

Not all pregnant women experience morning sickness the same way. Some have only occasional queasy moments, others feel queasy round the clock but never vomit, others vomit once in a while, and still others vomit frequently. There are probably several reasons for these variations:

Hormone levels. Higher-than-average levels (as when a woman is carrying multiple fetuses) can increase morning sickness; lower levels may minimize or eliminate it (though women with normal hormone levels may also experience little or no morning sickness).

Sensitivity. Some brains have a nausea command post that's more sensitive than others, which means they're more likely to respond to hormones and other triggers of pregnancy queasiness. If you have a sensitive command center (you always get carsick or seasick, for instance), you're more likely to have more severe nausea and vomiting

in pregnancy. Never have a queasy day ordinarily? You're less likely to have lots of them when you're expecting.

Stress. It's well known that emotional stress can trigger gastrointestinal upset, so it's not surprising that symptoms of morning sickness tend to worsen when stress strikes.

Fatigue. Physical or mental fatigue can also exacerbate the symptoms of morning sickness (conversely, severe morning sickness can increase fatigue).

First-time pregnancy status. Morning sickness is more common and tends to be more severe in first pregnancies, which supports the idea that both physical and emotional factors may be involved. Physically, the novice pregnant body is less prepared for the onslaught of hormones and other changes it's experiencing than one that's been there, done that. Emotionally, first timers are more likely to be subject to the kinds of anxieties and fears that can turn a stomach—while women in subsequent pregnancies may be distracted from their nausea by the demands of caring for older children. (Generalities never hold true for every expectant mom, though, and some women are queasier in subsequent pregnancies than they were in their first.)

No matter the cause (and does it really matter when you're upchucking for the third time today?), the effect of morning sickness is the same: pure misery. Though there is no sure cure for the queasies but the passing of time, there are ways of minimizing the misery while you're waiting for a less nauseous day to dawn:

- Eat early. Morning sickness doesn't wait for you to get up in the morning. In fact, nausea's most likely to strike when you're running on empty, as you are after a long night's sleep. That's because when you haven't eaten in a while, the acids churning around inside your empty tummy have nothing to digest but your stomach lining—which, not surprisingly, increases queasiness. To head off heaving, don't even consider getting out of bed in the morning without reaching for a nibble (crackers or rice cakes, dry cereal, a handful of trail mix) that you stashed on your nightstand the night before. Keeping nibbles next to the bed also means you don't have to get up for them if you wake up hungry in the middle of the night. It's a good idea to have a bite when you rise for those midnight bathroom runs, too, just so your stomach stays a little bit full all night long.

- Eat late. Eating a light snack high in protein and complex carbs (a muffin and a glass of milk, string cheese and a few dried apricots) just before you go to sleep will help ensure a happier tummy when you wake up.

- Eat light. A stuffed tummy is just as susceptible to queasiness as an empty one. Overloading—even when you feel hungry—can lead to upchucking.

- Eat often. One of the best ways to keep nausea at bay is to keep your blood sugar at an even keel—and your stomach a little filled—all the time. To head off an attack of the queasies, join the graze craze. Eat small, frequent meals—six mini meals a day is ideal—instead of three large ones. Don't leave home without a stash of snacks that your tummy can handle (dried fruit and nuts, granola bars, dry cereal, crackers, soy chips, or pretzels).

- Eat well. A diet high in protein and complex carbohydrates can help combat queasiness. General good nutrition may help, too, so eat as well as

you can (given the circumstances, that might not always be so easy).

- Eat what you can. So the eating well thing isn't working out so well for you? Right now, getting anything in your tummy—and keeping it there—should be your priority. There will be plenty of time later on in your pregnancy for eating a balanced diet. For the queasy moment, eat whatever gets you through the day (and night), even if it's nothing but ice pops and gingersnaps. If you can manage to make them real fruit ice pops and whole-grain gingersnaps, great. If you can't, that's fine, too.

- Drink up. In the short term, getting enough fluids is more important than getting enough solids—particularly if you're losing lots of liquids through vomiting. If you're finding liquids are easier to get down when you're feeling green, use them to get your nutrients. Drink your vitamins and minerals in soothing smoothies, soups, and juices. If you find fluids make you queasier, eat solids with a high water content, such as fresh fruits and vegetables—particularly lettuce, melons, and citrus fruits. Some women find that drinking and eating at the same sitting puts too much strain on their digestive tract; if this is true for you, try taking your fluids between meals.

- Get chilly. Experiment with temperature, too. Many women find icy cold fluids and foods are easier to get down. Others favor warm ones (melted cheese sandwiches instead of cold ones).

- Switch off. Often, what starts out as a comfort food (it's the only thing you can keep down, so you eat it 24/7) becomes associated with nausea—and actually starts to trigger it. If you're so sick of crackers that they're actually beginning to make you sick, switch off to another comforting carb (maybe it'll be Cheerios or watermelon next).

- If it makes you queasy, don't go there. Period. Don't force yourself to eat foods that don't appeal or, worse, make you sick. Instead, let your taste buds (and your cravings, and your aversions) be your guide. Choose only sweet foods if they're all you can tolerate (get your vitamin A and protein from peaches and yogurt at dinner instead of from broccoli and chicken). Or select only savories if they're your ticket to a less tumultuous tummy (have reheated pizza for breakfast instead of cereal).

- Smell (and see) no evil. Thanks to a much more sensitive sense of smell, pregnant women often find once appetizing aromas suddenly offensive—and offensive ones downright sickening. So stay away from smells that trigger nausea—whether it's the sausage and eggs your spouse likes to make on the weekends or the aftershave of his that used to make you head over heels (but now makes you head for the toilet). Steer clear, too, of foods that you can't stand the sight of (raw chicken is a common culprit).

- Supplement. Take a prenatal vitamin supplement to compensate for nutrients you may not be getting. Afraid you'll have trouble choking the pill down—or keeping it down? Actually, that one-a-day can decrease nausea symptoms (especially if you take a slow-releasing vitamin that's higher in quease-combating vitamin B_6). But take it at a time of day when you are least likely to chuck it back up, possibly with a substantial bedtime snack. If your symptoms are particularly rough, ask your practitioner about taking extra vitamin B_6, which can help relieve nausea in some women.

- Tread gingerly. It's true what the old wives (and midwives) have been saying for centuries: Ginger can be good for what ails a queasy pregnant woman. Use ginger in cooking (ginger-carrot soup, ginger muffins), steep it into tea, nibble on some ginger biscuits, nosh on some crystallized ginger, or suck on some ginger candy or lollipops. A drink made from real ginger (regular ginger ale isn't) may also be soothing. Even the smell of fresh ginger (cut open a knob and take a whiff) may quell the queasies. Or try another trick of the queasy trade: lemons. Many women find the smell—and taste—of lemons comforting (when life gives you morning sickness, make lemonade?). Sour sucking candies are the ticket to relief for others.

- Rest up. Get some extra sleep and relaxation. Both emotional and physical fatigue can exacerbate nausea.

- Go slow-mo. Don't jump out of bed and dash out the door—rushing tends to aggravate nausea. Instead, linger in bed for a few minutes, nibbling on that bedside snack, then rise slowly to a leisurely breakfast. This may seem impossible if you have other children, but try to wake up before they do so you can sneak in some quiet time, or let your spouse take the dawn shift.

- Minimize stress. Easing the stress can ease the quease. See page 141 for tips on dealing with stress during pregnancy.

- Treat your mouth well. Brush your teeth (with a toothpaste that doesn't increase queasiness) or rinse your mouth after each bout of vomiting, as well as after each meal. (Ask your dentist to recommend a good rinse.) Not only will this help keep your mouth fresh and reduce nausea, it will decrease the risk of damage to teeth or gums that can occur when bacteria feast on regurgitated residue in your mouth.

- Try Sea-Bands. These 1-inch-wide elastic bands, worn on both wrists, put pressure on acupressure points on the inner wrists and often relieve nausea. They cause no side effects and are widely available at drug and health food stores. Or your practitioner may recommend a more sophisticated form of acupressure: a battery-operated wristband—called the ReliefBand—that uses electronic stimulation.

- Go CAM crazy. There are a wide variety of complementary medical approaches, such as acupuncture, acupressure, biofeedback, or hypnosis, that can help minimize the symptoms of morning sickness—and they're all worth a try (see page 85). Meditation and visualization can also help.

Though there are medications that may help ease morning sickness (often a combo of doxylamine—an antihistamine found in Unisom Sleep Tabs—and vitamin B6), they'll usually only be recommended or prescribed when morning sickness is severe. Keep in mind, too, that the antihistamine part of the combo will make you drowsy—a good thing if you're going to sleep, but not such a good thing if you're driving to work. Don't take any medication (traditional or herbal) for morning sickness unless it is prescribed by your practitioner.

In fewer than 5 percent of pregnancies, nausea and vomiting become so severe that medical intervention may be needed. If this seems to be the case with you, see page 545.

Excess Saliva

"My mouth seems to fill up with saliva all the time—and swallowing it makes me queasy. What's going on?"

It may not be cool to drool (especially in public), but for many women in the first trimester, it's an icky fact of life. Overproduction of saliva is a common—and unpleasant—symptom of pregnancy, especially among morning sickness sufferers. And though all that extra saliva pooling in your mouth may add to your queasiness—and lead to a gaggy feeling when you eat—it's completely harmless, and thankfully short-lived, usually disappearing after the first few months.

Spitting mad about all that spit? Brushing your teeth frequently with a minty toothpaste, rinsing with a minty mouthwash, or chewing sugarless gum can help dry things up a bit.

Metallic Taste

"I have a metallic taste in my mouth all the time. Is this pregnancy related—or is it caused by something I ate?"

So your mouth tastes like loose change? Believe it or not, that metal mouth taste is a fairly common—though not often talked about—side effect of pregnancy, and one more you can chalk up to hormones. Your hormones always play a role in controlling your sense of taste. When they go wild (as they do when you have your period—and as they do with a vengeance when you're pregnant), so do your taste buds. Like morning sickness, that icky taste should ease up—or, if you're lucky, disappear altogether—in your second trimester when those hormones begin to settle down.

Until then, you can try fighting metal with acid. Focus on citrus juices, lemonade, sour sucking candy, and—assuming your tummy can handle them—foods marinated in vinegar (some pickles with that ice cream?). Not only will such assertive acidics have the power to break through that metallic taste, they'll also increase saliva production, which will help wash it away (though that could be a bad thing, if your mouth's already flooded with the stuff). Other tricks to try: Brush your tongue each time you brush your teeth, or rinse your mouth with a salt solution (a teaspoon of salt in 8 ounces of water) or a baking soda solution (¼ teaspoon baking soda in 8 ounces of water) a few times a day to neutralize pH levels in your mouth and keep away that flinty flavor. You might also ask your practitioner about changing your prenatal vitamin; some seem to lead to metal mouth more than others.

Frequent Urination

"I'm in the bathroom every half hour. Is it normal to be peeing this often?"

It may not be the best seat in the house, but for most pregnant women, it's the most frequented one. Let's face it, when you gotta go, you gotta go—and these days (and nights) you gotta go all the time. And while nonstop peeing might not always be convenient, it's absolutely normal.

What causes this frequent urination? First, hormones trigger not only an increase in blood flow but in urine flow, too. Second, during pregnancy the efficiency of the kidneys improves, helping your body rid itself of waste products more quickly (including baby's, which means you'll be peeing for two). Finally, your growing uterus is pressing on your bladder now, leaving less storage space in the holding tank for urine and triggering that "gotta go" feeling.

This pressure is often relieved once the uterus rises into the abdominal cavity during the second trimester and doesn't usually return until the third trimester or when the baby's head "drops" back down into the pelvis in the ninth month. But because the arrangement of internal organs varies slightly from woman to woman, the degree of urinary frequency in pregnancy may also vary. Some women barely notice it; others are bothered by it for most of the nine months.

Leaning forward when you urinate will help ensure that you empty your bladder completely, as can making it good to the last drop by double voiding (pee, then when you're done, squeeze out some more). Both tactics may reduce trips to the bathroom, though realistically, not by much.

Don't cut back on liquids thinking it'll keep you out of the bathroom. Your body and your baby need a steady supply of fluids—plus dehydration can lead to urinary tract infection (UTI). But do cut back on caffeine, which increases the need to pee. If you find that you go frequently during the night, try limiting fluids right before bedtime.

If you're always feeling the urge to urinate (even after you've just urinated), talk to your practitioner. He or she might want to run a test to see if you've got a UTI.

"How come I'm not urinating frequently?"

No noticeable increase in the frequency of urination may be perfectly normal for you, especially if you ordinarily pee often. But be sure you're getting enough fluids (at least eight 8-ounce glasses a day—more if you're losing some through vomiting). Not only can too little fluid intake cause infrequent urination, it can lead to dehydration and urinary tract infection.

Breast Changes

"I hardly recognize my breasts anymore—they're so huge. And they're tender, too. Will they stay that way, and will they sag after I give birth?"

Looks like you've discovered the first big thing in pregnancy: your breasts. While bellies don't usually do much growing until the second trimester, breasts often begin their expansion within weeks of conception, gradually working their way through the bra cup alphabet (you may ultimately end up three cups bigger than you started out). Fueling this growth are those surging hormones—the same ones that boost your bust premenstrually but at much greater levels. Fat is building up in your breasts, too, and blood flow to the area is increasing. And there's a swell reason for all this swelling—your breasts are gearing up to feed your baby when he or she arrives.

In addition to their expanding size, you will probably notice other changes to your breasts. The areola (the pigmented area around the nipple) will darken, spread, and may be spotted with even darker areas. This darkening may fade but not disappear entirely after birth. The little bumps you may notice on the areola are lubrication glands, which become more prominent during pregnancy and return to normal afterward. The complex road map of blue veins that traverses the breasts—often vivid on a fair-skinned woman and sometimes not even noticeable on darker women—represents a mother-to-baby delivery system for nutrients and fluids. After delivery—or, if you're breastfeeding, sometime after baby's weaned—the skin's appearance will return to normal.

Fortunately, that cup size gain won't continue to come with pain (or uncomfortable sensitivity). Though your breasts will probably keep growing throughout your nine months, they're not likely to stay tender to the touch past the third or fourth month. Some women find that the tenderness eases well before that. In the achy meantime, find relief in cool or warm compresses (whichever is more soothing).

As for whether or not your breasts will end up sagging, a lot of that's up to genetics (if your mom drooped, you may, too), but some of it's up to you. Sagging results not just from pregnancy itself but from a lack of support during pregnancy. No matter how firm your breasts are now, protect them for the future by wearing a supportive bra (though in that tender first trimester, you may want to avoid restrictive underwires). If your breasts are particularly large or have a tendency to sag, it's a good idea to wear a bra even at night. You'll probably find a cotton sports bra most comfortable for sleeping.

Not all women notice pronounced breast changes early in pregnancy, and some find the expansion takes place so gradually that it's not perceptible. As with all things pregnancy, what's normal is what's normal for your breasts. And don't worry: Though slower growth—or less substantial growth—means you won't have to replace bras so often, it won't have any impact on your ability to breastfeed.

"My breasts became very large in my first pregnancy, but they haven't seemed to change at all in my second. Is that normal?"

Last time your breasts were newbies—this time, they entered pregnancy with previous experience. As a result, they may not need as much preparation—or react as dramatically to those surging hormones—as they did in your first round of baby making. You may find that your breasts will enlarge gradually as your pregnancy progresses—or you may find that their expansion holds off until after delivery, when milk production begins. Either way, this slow growing is completely normal—and an early indication of how very different two pregnancies can be.

Lower Abdominal Pressure

"I've been having a nagging feeling of pressure in my lower abdomen. Should I be worried?"

It sounds like you're very tuned in to your body—which can be a good thing (as when it helps you recognize ovulation) or a not-so-good thing (when it makes you worry about the many innocuous aches and pains of pregnancy).

Don't worry. A feeling of pressure or even mild crampiness without bleeding is very common, especially in first pregnancies—and is usually a sign that everything's going right, not that something's going wrong. Chances are, that sensitive body radar of yours is just picking up some of the many dramatic changes that are taking place in your lower abdomen, where your uterus is currently located. What you're feeling may be the sensation of implantation, increased blood flow, the buildup of the uterine lining, or simply your uterus beginning to grow—in other words, your first growing pains (there will be many more to come). It could also be gas pains or bowel spasms that come with constipation (another common pregnancy side effect).

For further reassurance, ask your practitioner about the feeling (if you're still having it) at your next office visit.

Spotting

"I was using the toilet and noticed a small amount of blood when I wiped. Am I having a miscarriage?"

It's definitely scary to see blood down below when you're pregnant. But what's not definite is that bleeding is a sign that something's wrong with your pregnancy. Many women—about 1 in 5, in fact—experience some bleeding during pregnancy, and a very large majority go on to have a perfectly healthy pregnancy and baby. So if you're only noticing light spotting—similar to what you see at the beginning or end of your period—you can take a deep breath and read on for a probable (and probably reassuring) explanation. Such light spotting is usually caused by one of the following:

Implantation of the embryo into your uterine wall. Affecting 20 to 30 percent of women, such spotting (called "implantation bleeding" in the obstetrical business) will usually occur before (or in some cases around the time) you expected your period, around five to ten days after conception. Scantier than your monthly flow (and lasting anywhere from a few hours to a few days), implantation bleeding is usually light to medium pink or light brown in color and is spotty. It occurs when the little ball of cells you'll one day call your baby burrows its way into the uterine wall. Implantation bleeding is not a sign that something is wrong.

Intercourse or an internal pelvic exam or Pap smear. During pregnancy, your cervix becomes tender and engorged with blood vessels and can occasionally become irritated during intercourse or an internal exam, resulting in some light bleeding. This type of bleeding is common, can occur at any time during your pregnancy, and usually doesn't indicate

When to Call Your Practitioner

It's best to set up a protocol for emergencies with your practitioner before an emergency strikes. If you haven't, and you are experiencing a symptom that requires immediate medical attention, try the following: First call the practitioner's office. If he or she isn't available, leave a message detailing your symptoms. If you don't get a call back within a few minutes, call again or call the nearest emergency room and tell the triage nurse what's going on. If he or she tells you to come in, head to the ER and leave word with your practitioner. Call 911 if no one can take you to the ER.

When you report any of the following to your practitioner or to the triage nurse, be sure to mention any other symptoms you may be experiencing, no matter how unrelated they may seem to the immediate problem. Also be specific, mentioning when you first noticed each symptom, how frequently it recurs, what seems to relieve or exacerbate it, and how severe it is.

Call immediately if you experience:

- Heavy bleeding or bleeding with cramps or severe pain in the lower abdomen.

- Severe lower abdominal pain, in the center or on one or both sides, that doesn't subside, even if it isn't accompanied by bleeding.

- A sudden increase in thirst, accompanied by reduced urination, or no urination at all for an entire day.

- Painful or burning urination accompanied by chills and fever over 101.5°F and/or backache.

- Fever over 101.5°F.

- Very sudden and severe swelling or puffiness of hands, face, and eyes, accompanied by headache, vision difficulties, or sudden significant weight gain not related to overeating.

- Vision disturbances (blurring, dimming, double vision) that persist for more than a few minutes.

a problem, but do tell your practitioner about any post-intercourse or -exam spotting for extra reassurance.

Infection of the vagina or cervix. An inflamed or irritated cervix or vagina might cause some spotting (though the spotting should disappear once you're treated for the infection).

Subchorionic bleed. Subchorionic bleeding occurs when there is an accumulation of blood under the chorion (the outer fetal membrane, next to the placenta) or between the uterus and the placenta itself. It can cause light to heavy spotting but doesn't always (sometimes it is only

detected during a routine ultrasound). Most subchorionic bleeds resolve on their own and do not end up being a problem for the pregnancy (see page 545 for more).

Spotting is as variable in a normal pregnancy as it is common. Some women spot on and off for their entire pregnancies. Other women spot for just a day or two—and others for several weeks. Some women notice mucousy brown or pink spotting; others see small amounts of bright red blood. But happily, most women who experience any kind of spotting continue to have com-

- A severe headache or a headache that persists for more than two or three hours.

- Bloody diarrhea.

Call the same day (or the next morning, if it's the middle of the night) if you experience:

- Blood in your urine.

- Swelling or puffiness of your hands, face, eyes.

- Sudden excessive weight gain not related to overeating.

- Painful or burning urination.

- Fainting or dizziness.

- Chills and fever over 100°F in the absence of cold or flu symptoms (start bringing down any fever over 100°F promptly by taking acetaminophen, or Tylenol).

- Severe nausea and vomiting; vomiting more often than two or three times a day in the first trimester; vomiting later in pregnancy when you didn't earlier.

- Itching all over, with or without dark urine, pale stools, or jaundice (yellowing of skin and whites of the eye).

- Frequent (more than three times a day) diarrhea, especially if it's mucousy (if it's bloody, call right away).

Your practitioner may want you to call for different reasons or within different parameters, so be sure to ask him or her what protocol you should follow if you experience any of these symptoms.

Keep in mind, too, that there might be some times when you have none of the symptoms listed here, but you feel unusually exhausted, achy, not quite right. If a good night's sleep and some extra relaxation don't team up to make you feel better in a day or two, check with your practitioner. Chances are what you're feeling is normal—par for the pregnancy course. But it is also possible that you've become anemic or you're fighting an infection of some kind. Certain conditions—UTI, for example—can do their dirty work without causing any clear-cut symptoms. So when in doubt, check it out.

pletely normal and healthy pregnancies and end up delivering perfectly healthy babies. Which means that there's probably nothing for you to worry about (though, realistically, that doesn't mean you'll stop worrying).

For extra reassurance, put in a call to your practitioner (no need to call immediately or during non–office hours unless you're noticing spotting accompanied by cramping or bright red, soak-through-a-pad bleeding), who will likely order an ultrasound. If you're past the sixth week, you'll probably be able to see your baby's heartbeat during the ultrasound, which will reassure you that your pregnancy is progressing along just fine, even with the spotting.

What if the spotting progresses to heavier bleeding similar to a period? Though such a scenario is more cause for concern (especially if it's accompanied by cramps or pain in your lower abdomen) and does warrant an immediate call to your practitioner, it's not a sign that you're inevitably miscarrying. Some women bleed—even heavily— for unknown reasons throughout their pregnancies and still deliver healthy babies at term.

If it does end up that you're having a miscarriage, see page 536.

No Worries

Some expectant moms (and you know who you are) will always find something to worry about—especially in the first trimester and particularly in first pregnancies. Topping the list of most common concerns, understandably, is a fear of miscarriage.

Fortunately, most expectant worriers end up worrying unnecessarily. Most pregnancies continue uneventfully, and happily, to term. Just about every normal pregnancy includes some cramps, some abdominal aches, or some spotting—and many include all three. While any of these symptoms can be understandably unnerving (and when it comes to a stain on your underwear, downright scary), more often than not, they're completely innocuous—and not a sign that your pregnancy is in trouble. Though you should report them to your practitioner at your next visit (or sooner if you need some professional reassurance), the following are no cause for concern. So don't worry if you have:

- Mild cramps, achiness, or a pulling sensation in the lower abdomen or on one or both sides of the abdomen. This is probably caused by the stretching of ligaments that support the uterus. Unless cramping is severe, constant, or accompanied by significant bleeding, there's no need to worry.

- Slight spotting that isn't accompanied by cramps or lower abdominal

pain. There are plenty of reasons why pregnant women spot, and it often has nothing to do with a miscarriage. See page 137 for more on spotting.

Of course, it's not just symptoms that pregnant women worry about in early pregnancy—it's a lack of symptoms, too. In fact, not "feeling pregnant" is one of the most commonly reported first-trimester concerns. And that's not surprising. It's hard to feel pregnant this early on even if you're experiencing every early pregnancy symptom in the book—and it's far harder still to feel pregnant if you're relatively symptom-free. Without tangible proof yet of that baby-to-be growing inside you (a swelling belly, those first flutters of movement), it's pretty easy to start wondering whether the pregnancy is going well—or whether you're even still pregnant at all.

Once again, not to worry. A lack of symptoms—such as morning sickness or breast tenderness—is not a sign that something's wrong. Consider yourself lucky if you're spared these and other unpleasant early pregnancy symptoms—and also consider that you might be a late bloomer. After all, since every pregnant woman experiences pregnancy symptoms differently and at different times, these and other symptoms may be just around the corner for you.

HCG Levels

"My doctor gave me the results of my blood test and it says that my hCG level is at 412 mIU/L. What does that number mean?"

It means you're definitely pregnant! Human chorionic gonadotropin (hCG) is manufactured by the cells of the newly developing placenta within days after the fertilized egg implants in your uterine lining. HCG is found in your urine (you came face-to-stick with hCG the day that positive readout showed up on your home pregnancy test) and in your blood, which explains why your practitioner ran a blood test to find out your expectant status for sure. When you're very early in the pregnancy game (as you are), the level of hCG in your blood will be quite low (it's just starting to show up in your system, after all). But within days, it'll begin to soar, doubling every 48 hours (give or take). The rapid increase peaks somewhere between 7 and 12 weeks of pregnancy and then starts to decline.

But don't start swapping your numbers with those of your pregnant best friend. Just as no two women's pregnancies are alike, no two pregnant women's hCG levels are alike either. They vary enormously from day to day, person to person, even as early as the first missed day of a period and continuing throughout pregnancy.

What's more important and relevant to you is that your hCG level falls within the very wide normal range (see box, this page) and continues to increase over the coming weeks (in other words, look for a pattern of increasing levels instead of focusing on specific numbers). Even if your readings fall outside these ranges, don't worry. It's still quite likely that everything's fine (your due date might just be off—a very common cause of hCG number confusion—or you might be carrying more than one baby). As long as your pregnancy is progressing normally and your hCG levels are increasing during the first trimester, you don't have to obsess about these numbers or even try to find them out (plus, if your practitioner is happy with your numbers, then you can be, too). Ultrasound findings after five or six weeks of pregnancy are much more predictive of pregnancy outcome than are hCG levels. Of course, as always, if you are concerned, talk with your practitioner about your results.

HCG Levels

Really want to play the hCG numbers game? The following are ranges of "normal" hCG levels based on date. Keep in mind that anywhere in that wide range is normal—your baby doesn't have to be scoring off the charts for your pregnancy to be progressing perfectly—and that a slight miscalculation in your dates can throw the numbers off completely.

Weeks of Pregnancy	Amount of hCG in mIU/L
3 weeks	5 to 50
4 weeks	5 to 426
5 weeks	19 to 7,340
6 weeks	1,080 to 56,500
7 to 8 weeks	7,650 to 229,000
9 to 12 weeks	25,700 to 288,000

Stress

"My job is a high-stress one. I wasn't planning to have a baby now, but I got pregnant. Should I quit work?"

Depending on how you handle and respond to it, stress can be good for you (by sparking you to perform better, to function more effectively) or it can be bad for you (when it gets out of control, overwhelming and debilitating you). Research shows that pregnancy isn't affected by typical stress levels—and if you're able to cope well with your on-the-job stress (even if it's more than most people could take on), then your baby will be able to cope just fine, too. But if the stress makes you anxious,

Relaxation Made Easy

Is your growing bundle of joy making you a quivering bundle of nerves? Now's a great time to learn some soothing relaxation techniques—not just because they can help you cope with pregnancy concerns, but because they'll come in handy in your hectic life as a new mom. Yoga's a fabulous destresser, if you have time to take a prenatal class or practice with a DVD. If you don't, you can try this simple relaxation technique, which is easy to learn and to do anywhere, anytime. If you find it helpful, you can do it when anxiety strikes and/or regularly several times a day to try to ward it off.

Sit with your eyes closed and imagine a beautiful, peaceful scene (a sunset over your favorite beach, waves gently lapping the shore; a serene mountain vista, complete with babbling brook), or even your fantasized baby-to-be, wrapped in your arms on a sunny day in the park. Then, working your way up from your toes to your face, concentrate on relaxing every muscle. Breathe slowly, deeply, through your nose (unless it's stuffed up) and choose a simple word (such as "yes" or "one") to repeat aloud every time you exhale. Ten to 20 minutes should do the trick, though even a minute or two is better than nothing.

Since negative reactions to stress can take a toll, especially if they continue into the second and third trimesters—learning to handle the stress constructively, or cutting back on it, as needed, should become a priority now. The following should help:

Unload it. Allowing your anxieties to surface is the best way of ensuring that they don't get you down. Make sure you have somewhere to vent—and someone to vent to. Maintain open lines of communication with your spouse, spending some time at the end of each day (preferably not too close to bedtime, which should be as stress free as possible) sharing concerns and frustrations. Together you may be able to find some relief, some solutions—and ideally a good laugh or two. Is he too stressed to absorb enough of your stress? Find others who can lend an ear—a friend, another family member, coworkers (who will understand your workplace stress better?), or your practitioner (especially if you're concerned about the physical effects of your stress). Empathy helps, too, so try to find other expectant moms who can relate, either in a pregnancy group or online. If you need more than a friendly ear, consider counseling to help you develop strategies to better deal with your stress.

Do something about it. Identify sources of stress in your life and determine how they can be modified. If you're clearly trying to do too much, cut back in areas that are not high priority (this is something you're going to have to do big time anyway, once you have a bigger priority—a new baby—on the agenda). If you've taken on too many responsibilities at home or at work, decide which can be postponed or delegated. Learn to say no to new projects or activities before you're overloaded (another skill you're wise to cultivate pre-baby).

sleepless, or depressed, if it's causing you to experience physical symptoms (such as headache, backache, or loss of appetite), if it's causing you to turn to unhealthy behaviors (smoking, for instance), or if it is exhausting you, then it could eventually pose a problem.

Sometimes, sitting down with a pad or PDA and making lists of the hundreds of things you need to get done (at home or at work), and the order in which you're planning to do them, can help you feel more in control of the chaos in your life. Cross items off your list as they're taken care of for a satisfying sense of accomplishment.

Sleep it off. Sleep is the ticket to regeneration—for mind and body. Often, feelings of tension and anxiety are prompted by not getting enough shut-eye—and, of course, having too much tension and anxiety can also prevent you from getting enough shut-eye. If you're having trouble sleeping, see the tips on page 265.

Nourish it. Hectic lifestyles can lead to hectic eating styles. Inadequate nutrition during pregnancy can be a double whammy: It can hamper your ability to handle stress, and it can eventually affect your baby's well-being. So be sure to eat well and regularly (six mini meals will best keep you going when the going gets tough). Focus on complex carbs and protein, and steer clear of excesses of caffeine and sugar, two staples of the stressed life that can actually leave you less able to cope.

Wash it away. A warm bath is an excellent way to relieve tension. Try it after a hectic day; it will also help you to sleep better.

Run it off. Or swim it off. Or prenatal yoga it off. You might think that the last thing you need in your life is more activity, but exercise is one of the best stress relievers—and mood boosters. Build some into your busy day.

CAM it. Explore the many complementary and alternative therapies that can promise inner calm from CAM, among them biofeedback, acupuncture, hypnotherapy, massage (ask your spouse

Expect the Best

It's long been speculated that optimistic people live longer, healthier lives. Now it's been suggested that an expectant mother's optimistic outlook can actually improve the outlook for her unborn baby, too. Researchers have found that seeing the bright side reduces the chance of a high-risk woman delivering a preterm or low-birthweight baby.

A lower level of stress in optimistic women definitely plays a part in the lowered risk; high levels of stress, after all, have been implicated in a variety of health problems both in and out of pregnancy. But stress itself apparently doesn't tell the whole story. Women who are optimistic, not surprisingly, are more likely to take better care of themselves—eating well, exercising right, getting regular prenatal care, not smoking, drinking, or using drugs. And these positive behaviors—fueled by the power of positive thinking—can, of course, have a very positive effect on pregnancy and fetal well-being.

Researchers point out that it's never too late to start reaping the benefits of optimism, even if you're already pregnant. Learning how to expect the best—instead of the worst—can actually help make those expectations come true: a good reason to start seeing that glass of milk as half full instead of half empty.

for a back or shoulder rub, or splurge on a professional pregnancy massage). Meditation and visualization can also melt the stress away (just close your eyes and picture a bucolic scene, or keep them open and gaze at a soothing picture or photo placed strategically in your office). Practice relaxation techniques (see box, page 142), not just because they'll come in handy during childbirth, but because they can help drain the strain anytime. See page 85 for more on CAM techniques.

Get away from it. Combat stress with any activity you find relaxing. Lose it in reading; a good movie; listening to music (take your iPod to coffee breaks and lunch, or even use it while you work, if you can); knitting (you can relax while you get a head start on those booties); window-shopping for baby clothes; lunching with a fun friend; keeping a journal (another good way to vent your feelings); browsing baby sites online; scrapbooking. Or walk away

from it (even a quick stroll can be relaxing and rejuvenating).

Cut it back. Maybe what's causing the stress just isn't worth it. If it's your job that's got you too wired, consider taking early maternity leave or cutting back to part-time (if either of these options is financially feasible), or delegating at least part of your workload to reduce stress to a load that doesn't weigh you down. A change of jobs or careers might be impractical to pull off now that you're expecting, but it might be something to consider once your baby arrives.

Remember, your stress quotient is only going to increase once the baby is born; it makes sense to try to find ways of handling it better (or bringing it down to a manageable level) now.

Your Pampered Pregnancy

Talk about extreme makeovers. Pregnancy is a radical full-body transformation that may have you feeling your most beautiful (you glow, girl!), your least attractive (those zits! those chin hairs!), or both (in the same day). But it's also a time when your usual beauty regimen might need a makeover, too. Before you reach into your medicine cabinet for the acne cream you've been using since junior high or head to your favorite spa for a bikini wax and a facial, you'll need to know what's a beauty do—and what's a beauty don't—when you're expecting. Here's the lowdown from tip (highlights) to toes (pedicure) on how you can pamper your pregnant self beautifully—and safely.

Your Hair

When you're expecting, your hair can take a turn for the better (when lackluster hair suddenly sports a brilliant shine) or for the worse (when once-bouncy hair goes limp). One thing's for sure: Thanks to hormones, you'll have more of it than ever before (and sadly, not just on your head). Here's the heads-up on hair treatments:

Coloring. Here's the root of the problem when it comes to hiding your roots during pregnancy. Even though no evidence suggests the small amount of chemicals absorbed through the skin during hair coloring is harmful when you're expecting, some experts still advise waiting out the first trimester before heading back to the salon for retouching. Others maintain that it's safe to dye throughout pregnancy. Check with your practitioner—you'll likely get the green light on color. If you're uncomfortable with a full dye job, consider highlights instead of single-process color. This way the chemicals don't touch your scalp at all, plus highlights tend to last longer than all-over color, enabling you to revisit the salon fewer times during your pregnancy. You can also ask your colorist about less harsh processing (an ammonia-free base or an all-vegetable dye, for instance). Just keep in mind that hormonal changes can make your hair react strangely—so you might not get what you expect, even from your regular formula. Before you do your whole head, try a test strand so you don't wind up with punk purple instead of that ravishing red you were hoping for.

Straightening treatments or relaxers. Thinking about a straightening treatment to calm those curls? Though there's no evidence that hair relaxers are dangerous during pregnancy (the amount of chemicals that enter the body through the scalp is probably minimal), there's no proof they're completely safe, either. So check with your practitioner; you may hear that it's safest to let your hair do what comes naturally, especially during the first trimester. If you do decide to go straight, keep in mind that there's a possibility that your hormone-infused locks may respond oddly to the chemicals (you might end up with a helmet of frizz instead of ramrod-straight tresses). Plus, your hair will grow faster during pregnancy, making those curls reappear at your roots sooner than you'd like. Thermal reconditioning processes that involve different—and often gentler—chemicals to tame your frizz may be a safer option (again, ask first). Or

just buy a flat iron of your own, and coax your hair into smooth submission.

Permanents or body waves. So your hair's not as full as your figure's becoming? Ordinarily, a permanent or a body wave might be the answer for hair that's limping, but it probably isn't during pregnancy. Not because it isn't safe (it probably is, though check with your practitioner), but because hair responds unpredictably under the influence of pregnancy hormones. A permanent might not take at all—or might result in frizz instead of waves.

Hair removal and lightening treatments. If pregnancy has you looking like a resident of the Planet of the Apes, stay calm—this hairy situation is only temporary. Your armpits, bikini line, upper lip, even your belly may be fuzzier than usual due to all those raging hormones. But think twice and check with your practitioner before you turn to lasers, electrolysis, depilatories (and perhaps bleaching). No reliable studies have been done to determine for sure whether these popular hair-removal and lightening treatments are completely safe, but it's probably best to skip them until after you give birth (though some practitioners give the go-ahead after the first trimester). Don't worry about any electrolysis or laser treatments you've already had, because any risk is purely theoretical.

Shaving, plucking, and waxing. Unwanted hair can appear almost anywhere when you're expecting. That's the bad news. The good news is that you can pluck, shave, and wax it away safely when you're expecting. Even bikini waxing (including full-on Brazilian) is fine, but proceed with caution—pregnant skin can be extra-sensitive and easily irritated. If you're heading to the salon, let the esthetician know that you're expecting so she can be extra-gentle.

Your Face

Your pregnancy may not be showing in your belly yet, but it's almost certainly showing on your face. Here's the good, bad, and the ugly about face care when you're expecting.

Facials. Face facts: Not every mom-to-be is blessed with that expectant radiance you've always read about. If your glow decides not to show, a facial might be just the ticket, working wonders when it comes to clearing pores clogged by extra oil (thanks to extra hormones). Most facials are absolutely safe during pregnancy, though some abrasive treatments (like microdermabrasion or glycolic peels) may do more harm than good, as they might be especially irritating to skin made supersensitive by pregnancy hormones. Facials that use an electrical microcurrent are off limits during pregnancy. Discuss with the esthetician which preparations might be most soothing and least likely to provoke a reaction. If you're unsure about a particular treatment's safety, check with your practitioner before signing up.

Antiwrinkle treatments. A wrinkly baby is cute; a wrinkly mommy, not so much. But before you stop by your dermatologist's office to treat those fine lines (or fill those lips), consider this: The safety of injectable fillers (such as collagen, Restylane, or Juvederm) during pregnancy hasn't been established through studies yet. The same goes for Botox, which means you're better off staying unfilled (and uninjected) for now. As for antiwrinkle creams, it's best to read the fine print (and check with your practitioner). You'll likely be advised to bid a temporary farewell to products that contain vitamin A (in any of its many retinoid forms), vitamin K, or BHA (beta-hydroxy acid or salicylic acid). Check with your practitioner about other ingredients you're unsure about, too. Most practitioners will green-light products containing AHA (alpha-hydroxy acid) or fruit acids, but get the all-clear first. On the bright side, you may find that normal pregnancy fluid retention plumps up your face nicely, leaving your wrinkles less noticeable without the help of cosmetic procedures.

Acne treatments. Got more pimples than a high school marching band? You can blame pregnancy hormones for that. But before you march to the medicine cabinet for your usual zit zappers, check them out with your practitioner. Accutane (which causes serious birth defects) is definitely off-limits. So is Retin-A (ask your practitioner and dermatologist about over-the-counter products that contain retinol). Laser treatments and chemical peels for acne should also probably wait until after the baby is born. Two common topical acne medications, beta-hydroxy acid (BHA) and salicylic acid, have not been studied in pregnant women and may be absorbed through the skin. Ask your practitioner about the safety of products that contain these medications and those that contain benzoyl peroxide, another ingredient that's often not green-lighted. Glycolic acid and exfoliating scrubs, as well as azelaic and topical antibiotics like erythromycin, are probably safe to use (check first), though watch out for irritation. You can also try to tame eruptions naturally by drinking plenty of water, eating well, and keeping your face clean. And no popping or picking.

Your Teeth

You've got plenty to smile about now that you're expecting, but will your teeth be up to the task? Cosmetic dentistry's popular, but not always pregnancy approved.

Whitening products. Eager to flash your pearly whites? While there are no proven risks to tooth whitening during pregnancy, it's a procedure that probably falls into the better-safe-than-sorry category (so you'll be wise to wait a few months to debut that new million-dollar smile). Be sure to keep your teeth clean and well flossed, though. Your pregnancy-sensitive gums will thank you for the attention.

Veneers. Here's one more for the better-safe-than-sorry side, even though there are no proven risks to adding veneers to your teeth during pregnancy. There's another reason why you might consider waiting until you're postpartum before you veneer your teeth: Your gums might be extra-sensitive when you've got a baby on board, making any dental procedure—including veneers and whitening—more uncomfortable than usual.

Your Body

Your body definitely pays for the privilege of pregnancy—in ways you probably never imagined. So more than any body, it deserves some pampering. Here's how to give it what it needs—safely.

Massage. Aching for some relief from that nagging backache—or from that nagging anxiety that's keeping you up at night? There's nothing like a massage to rub away the aches and pains of pregnancy, as well as the stress and strain. But though a massage may be just what the feel-good doctor ordered, you'll need to follow some guidelines to ensure your pregnancy massages are not only relaxing but also safe:

■ Get rubbed by the right hands. Make sure your massage therapist is licensed and well versed in the do's and don'ts of prenatal massage.

■ Wait for your rub. Avoid massage during the first three months of pregnancy because it may trigger dizziness and add to morning sickness early on. But don't worry if you've already had a massage during your first trimester. There's no danger, just the potential for being uncomfortable.

■ Relax in the right position. It's best to avoid spending a lot of time on your back after the fourth month, so ask your massage therapist to use a table that's equipped with a cut-out for your belly, special pillows designed for pregnancy use, or a cushioned foam padding that conforms to your body, or to position you on your side.

■ Try some nonscents. Ask for an unscented lotion or oil, not only because your pregnancy-sharpened sniffer might be offended by strong fragrances, but also because some aromatherapy oils can stimulate contractions; see below.

■ Rub the right spots (and stay away from the wrong ones). Direct pressure on the area between the anklebone and heel can trigger contractions, so be sure your therapist stays away from there (another good reason to choose a massage therapist with prenatal training). He or she should also probably stay away from the abdomen area for comfort's sake. And if your therapist is working too deeply or if the massage is too intense, speak up. This is about you feeling good, after all.

Aromatherapy. When it comes to scents during pregnancy, it's good to use some common sense. Because the effects of many plant oils in pregnancy are unknown and some may be harmful, approach any kind of aromatherapy with caution. The following essential oils are considered safe for prenatal massage, though experts recommend that the oils be mixed at a concentration that's half the standard usage: rose, lavender, chamomile, jasmine, tangerine, neroli, and ylang-ylang. Pregnant women should particularly avoid the following oils because some of them can trigger uterine contractions: basil, juniper, rosemary, sage, peppermint, pennyroyal, oregano, and thyme. (Midwives often use these oils during labor precisely because they trigger contractions.) If you've had an aromatherapy massage with these oils (or used them in home baths or treatments), don't worry. The absorption of the oil is very low, especially because the skin on your back is pretty thick. Just steer clear of them in future treatments. Scented lotions or beauty products sold at bath and beauty shops (like peppermint foot lotion, for instance) are fine since the scents aren't concentrated.

Body treatments, scrubs, wraps, hydrotherapy. Body scrubs are generally safe, as long as they're gentle (some scrubs can be too vigorous for sensitive pregnant skin). Some herbal wraps can be safe, but most are off-limits because they might raise your body temperature excessively. A short warm bath (no hotter than 100°F) as part of hydrotherapy is safe and relaxing, but stay out of the sauna, steam room, and hot tub.

Tanning beds, sprays, lotions. Looking for a way to go beyond the pale (pale skin, that is) during your pregnancy? Sorry, but tanning beds are out. Not only are they bad for your skin, they up your chances of getting chloasma (the skin discoloration called the "mask of pregnancy"). Worse, tanning beds can raise your body temperature to a level that could be harmful to your developing baby. Still a fan of the tan? Before you fake it with sunless tanning lotions and sprays, talk to your practitioner. And

A Day at the Spa

Ahhhh, the spa. No one deserves —and needs—a day of pampering more than an expectant mother. And happily, more and more spas are offering treatments specifically catering to the pregnant set. But before you head off for your day of pampering, check out this chapter and ask your practitioner for any specific caveats for your situation. Then, when you call to make your appointment, tell the receptionist that you're expecting. Discuss any restrictions you may have so the spa can tailor treatments to fit your needs. Also be sure to inform any esthetician or therapist who will be working on you that you're pregnant.

even if you get the go-ahead, consider that your hormones can cause your skin to play games with the color (and take a turn for the terra-cotta). Plus, as your belly expands, applying a sunless tanner evenly might get tricky (especially once you can no longer see your legs, and even if you're getting a spray-on tan).

For information on the safety of tattoos, henna, and piercings during pregnancy, check out pages 160 and 180.

Your Hands and Feet

Yes, even your hands and feet will show the effects of pregnancy (though you won't be able to see the effects on your feet once you reach the third trimester). But even when you're feeling swell—as in fingers and ankles that are puffy with fluids—your hands and feet can still look their best.

Making Up for Pregnancy

Between breakouts, funky skin discolorations, and normal pregnancy swelling, your face will be facing some challenges over the next nine months. Luckily, you'll be able to make up for them with the right makeup:

- Go under cover. Corrective concealer and foundation can cover a multitude of pregnancy skin issues, including chloasma and other discolorations (see page 240). For those dark spots, look for brands that are designed to cover hyperpigmentation, but make sure all makeup is non-comedogenic and hypoallergenic. Match both to your skin tone, but select a concealer that's a shade lighter than your natural complexion. Apply the concealer only to the dark spots, stippling the edges to blend. Then lightly blend the foundation over the area. Less is definitely more when it comes to heavy coverage products, so use the least you can get away with—you can always top it off. Set with powder.

  Keep coverage lighter when it comes to pregnancy pimples to avoid calling attention to them (they'll likely call enough attention to themselves). Start with foundation, then apply a concealer—that matches your skin—directly to the zit, blending with your finger. If you're going to prespot before you cover up, use a pregnancy-approved topical that's clear.

- Play with shadows. Chip away at those chipmunk cheeks you'll likely be growing: After you've applied your all-over foundation, apply a highlighting shade (one shade lighter) to the center of your forehead, under your eyes, on the tops of your cheekbones, and on the tip of your chin. Then brush a contouring shade (one shade darker) down the sides of your face, starting at the temples. Blend, and presto—instant cheekbones!

- Stop the spread. Sure, you expect your belly to plump up, and maybe even your hips—but your nose? Don't worry—any widening is temporary, the result of pregnancy swelling. Slim a swollen sniffer by applying a highlighting shade (one shade lighter than your overall foundation) down the center of your nose; then contour the vertical edges of the sides of your nose with a darker shade. Make sure you blend well.

Manicure and pedicure. It's perfectly safe to polish while pregnant (and take advantage now because it's likely that your nails are growing faster and stronger than ever). If you get your nails done in a salon, make sure it's a well-ventilated one. Inhaling those strong chemical smells is never a good idea but especially not when you're breathing for two (and at the very least, the fumes might make you queasy). Do be sure the manicurist doesn't massage the area between your anklebone and heel when you're getting your pedicure (it could theoretically trigger contractions). As for acrylics, there's no proof that the chemicals are harmful, but you might want to err on the cautious side and forgo those tips until post-baby—not only because the application smell can be extremely strong, but because they can become a nail bed for infection, something you might be more prone to while you're pregnant. And remember, you may not need the extra length or strength of acrylics anyway because your nails will be growing at warp speed.

CHAPTER 7

The
Second
Month

Approximately 5 to 8 Weeks

E VEN IF YOU'RE NOT TELLING anyone you're expecting yet, and though no one around you could possibly know (unless you've already blabbed the big news), your baby's certainly spilling the beans to you. Not in so many words, but in so many symptoms. Like that nagging nausea that follows you wherever you go, or all that excess saliva pooling in your mouth (am I *drooling?*). Like the gotta-go feeling you're getting all day (and all night), and that 24/7 bloat you just can't seem to deflate.

Even with all this evidence you're pregnant, you're probably still getting used to the idea that a new life is developing inside you (after all, you've just found out for sure you've got a baby—and not a stomach bug—on board). You're also probably just getting used to the demands of pregnancy, from the physical (so that's why I'm tired!) to the logistical (the shortest route to the bathroom is . . .) to the dietary (make my Sea Breeze a virgin). It's a wild ride, and it's only just beginning. Hold on tight!

Your Baby This Month

Week 5 Your little embryo, which at this point resembles a tadpole more than a baby (complete with teeny tail), is growing fast and furious and is now about the size of an orange seed—still small, but a lot bigger than it's been. This week, the heart is starting to take shape. In fact, the circulatory system, along with the heart, is the first system to be operational. Your baby's heart (about the size of a poppy seed) is made up of two tiny channels called heart tubes—and though it's still far from fully functional, it's already beating—something you might be able to see on an early ultrasound. Also in the works is the neural tube, which will eventually become your baby's brain and spinal cord. Right now the neural tube is open, but it will close by next week.

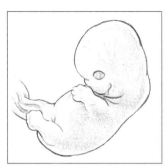

Your Baby, Month 2

Week 6 Crown (head) to rump (bottom) measurements are used for babies in utero because their tiny, newly forming legs are bent, making it difficult to measure the full length of the body. How's baby measuring up this week? That crown to rump measurement has reached somewhere between a fifth and a quarter of an inch (no bigger than a nail head). This week also sees the beginning of the development of your baby's jaws, cheeks, and chin. Little indentations on both sides of the head will form into ear canals. Small black dots on the face will form the eyes, and a small bump on the front of the head will turn into a button nose in a few weeks' time. Also taking shape this week: your baby's kidneys, liver, and lungs. Your baby's tiny heart is beating 80 times per minute and getting faster each day—a stat that's probably got your heart racing.

Week 7 Here's an amazing fact about your baby right now: He or she is 10,000 times bigger now than at conception—about the size of a blueberry. A lot of that growth is concentrated on the head (new brain cells are being generated at the rate of 100 cells per minute). Your baby's mouth and tongue are forming this week and so are his or her arm and leg buds, which are beginning to sprout into paddle-like appendages and to divide into hand, arm, and shoulder segments—and leg, knee, and foot segments. Also in place now are your baby's kidneys, and they're poised to begin their important work of waste management (i.e., urine production and excretion). At least you don't have to worry about dirty diapers yet!

Week 8 Your baby is growing up a storm, this week measuring about half an inch in length, or about the size of a large raspberry. And that sweet little raspberry of yours is looking less reptilian and more human (happily), as his or her lips, nose, eyelids, legs, and back continue to take shape. And though it's still too early to hear from the outside, your baby's heart is beating at the incredible rate of 150 times per minute (that's twice as fast as your heart beats). Something else new this week: Your baby is making spontaneous movements (twitches of the trunk and limb buds too tiny for you to feel).

What You May Be Feeling

As always, remember that every pregnancy and every woman is different. You may experience all of these symptoms at one time or another, or only one or two. Some may have continued from last month, others may be new. You may also have other, less common, symptoms. Don't be surprised, no matter what your symptoms (or lack thereof), if you don't "feel" pregnant yet. Here's what you might experience this month:

Physically

- Fatigue, lack of energy, sleepiness

- Frequent urination

- Nausea, with or without vomiting

- Excess saliva

- Constipation

- Heartburn, indigestion, flatulence, bloating

- Food aversions and cravings

- Breast changes: fullness, heaviness, tenderness, tingling; darkening of the areolas (the pigmented area around your nipples); lubrication glands in the areolas becoming prominent, like large goose bumps; a network of bluish lines that appear under your skin as the blood supply to your breasts increases

- Slight whitish vaginal discharge

- Occasional headaches

- Occasional faintness or dizziness

- A little rounding of your belly; your clothes feeling a little snugger

Emotionally

- Emotional ups and downs (like amped-up PMS), which may include

mood swings, irritability, irrationality, inexplicable weepiness

- Misgivings, fear, joy, elation—any or all of these

- A sense of unreality about the pregnancy ("Is there really a baby in there?")

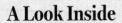

A Look Inside

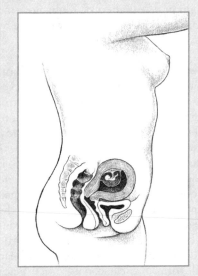

Even though you still won't look like you're pregnant to those around you, you might notice your clothes are getting a little tighter around the waist. You might also need a bigger bra now. By the end of this month, your uterus, usually the size of a fist, has grown to the size of a large grapefruit.

What You Can Expect at This Month's Checkup

If this is your first prenatal visit, see page 124. If this is your second exam, you'll find it will be a much shorter visit. And if those initial tests have already been taken care of, you probably won't be subjected to much poking and prodding this time. You can expect your practitioner to check the following, though there may be variations depending on your particular needs and your practitioner's style of practice.

- Weight and blood pressure

- Urine, for sugar and protein

- Hands and feet for swelling, and legs for varicose veins

- Symptoms you've been experiencing, especially unusual ones

- Questions or problems you want to discuss—have a list ready

What You May Be Wondering About

Heartburn and Indigestion

"I have indigestion and heartburn all the time. Why, and what can I do about it?"

No one does heartburn like a pregnant woman does heartburn. Not only that, but you're likely to keep doing it—and doing it at least as well—throughout your whole pregnancy (unlike many early pregnancy symptoms, this one's a keeper).

So why does it feel like you have a flamethrower stationed in your chest? Early in pregnancy, your body produces large amounts of the hormones progesterone and relaxin, which tend to relax smooth muscle tissue everywhere in the body, including the gastrointestinal (GI) tract. As a result, food sometimes moves more slowly through your system, resulting in indigestion (a feeling of fullness and bloating in the upper abdomen and chest; heartburn is a symptom of indigestion). This may be uncomfortable for you, but it's actually beneficial for your baby. The alimentary slowdown allows better absorption of nutrients into your bloodstream and subsequently through the placenta and into your baby.

Heartburn results when the ring of muscle that separates the esophagus from the stomach relaxes (like all the other smooth muscle in the GI tract), allowing food and harsh digestive juices to back up from the stomach to the esophagus. These stomach acids irritate the sensitive esophageal lining, causing a burning sensation right around where the heart is—thus the term heartburn—though the problem has nothing to do with your heart. During the last two trimesters, the problem can be compounded by your blossoming uterus as it presses up on your stomach.

It's nearly impossible to have an indigestion-free nine months; it's just one of the less pleasant realities of pregnancy. There are, however, some pretty effective ways of avoiding heartburn

Bringing up Reflux

If you have GERD (gastroesophageal reflux disease), heartburn's nothing new, but treating it during pregnancy might be. Now that you're expecting, ask your practitioner about whether the prescription meds you're used to taking are still okay to take. Some are not recommended for use during pregnancy, but most are safe. Many of the tips for fighting heartburn can also help with your reflux.

and indigestion most of the time, and of minimizing the discomfort when it strikes:

- Don't pull the triggers. If a food or drink brings on the burn (or other tummy troubles), take it off the menu for now. The most common offenders (and you're sure to know those that offend you) are spicy and highly seasoned foods, fried or fatty foods, processed meats, chocolate, coffee, carbonated beverages, and mint.

- Take it small. To avoid digestive system overload (and backup of gastric juices), opt for frequent mini meals over three large squares. The Six-Meal Solution is ideal for heartburn and indigestion sufferers (see page 91).

- Take it slow. When you eat too quickly, you tend to swallow air, which can form gas pockets in your belly. And rushing through meals means you're not chewing thoroughly, which makes your stomach work harder digesting your food—and makes heartburn more likely to happen. So even when you're starving or in a hurry, make an

Heartburn Today, Hair Tomorrow?

Feeling the burn bad? You may want to stock up on baby shampoo. New research has actually backed up what old wives have maintained for generations: The more heartburn you have during pregnancy, the more likely your baby will be born with a full head of hair. Implausible as it sounds, seems the hormones responsible for heartburn are the same ones that cause fetal hair to sprout. So pass the Tums, and the detangler.

effort to eat slowly, taking small bites and chewing well (your mother would be proud).

- Don't drink and eat. Too much fluid mixed with your food distends the stomach, aggravating indigestion. So try to take most of your fluids in between meals.

- Keep it up. It's harder for gastric juices to back up when you're vertical than when you're horizontal. To keep them where they belong (down in your stomach), avoid eating while lying down. Or lying down after eating—or eating a big meal before bed. Sleeping with your head and shoulders elevated about 6 inches can also fight the gastric backup with gravity. Another way: Bend at the knees, not at the waist. Anytime your head dips, you're more likely to experience burn.

- Keep it down. Your weight gain, that is. A gradual and moderate gain will minimize the amount of pressure on your digestive tract.

- Keep it loose. Don't wear clothing that's tight around your belly or waist. A constricted tummy can add to the pressure, and the burn.

- Pop some relief. Always keep a supply of Tums or Rolaids at popping distance (they'll also give you a healthy dose of calcium while they ease the burn), but avoid other heartburn medicines unless they've been cleared by your practitioner. Sick of antacids already? Try one of these burn-banishing folk remedies: a tablespoon of honey in warm milk, a handful of almonds, or some fresh or dried papaya.

- Chew on it. Chewing sugarless gum for a half hour after meals can reduce excess acid (increased saliva can neutralize the acid in your esophagus). Some people find that mint-flavored gum exacerbates heartburn; if so, choose a non-minty gum.

- Don't smoke (yet another reason to quit today, if you haven't already).

- Relax for relief. Stress compounds all gastric upset, especially heartburn, so learn to relax (see page 142). Also try some complementary and alternative medical (CAM) approaches, such as meditation, visualization, biofeedback, or hypnosis (see page 85).

Food Aversions and Cravings

"Certain foods that I've always loved taste strange now. Instead, I'm having cravings for foods that I never liked. What's going on?"

The pregnancy cliché of a harried husband running out in the middle of the night, raincoat over his pajamas, for a pint of ice cream and a jar of pickles to satisfy his wife's cravings has definitely played out more often in the heads of old-school sitcom writers than in real life. Not many pregnant women's cravings carry them—or their spouses—that far.

Still, most expectant moms find their tastes in food change somewhat in pregnancy. Most experience a craving for at least one food (most often ice cream, though usually without the pickles), and more than half will have at least one food aversion (poultry ranks right up there, along with vegetables of all varieties). To a certain extent, these suddenly eccentric (and sometimes borderline bizarre) eating habits can be blamed on hormonal havoc, which probably explains why they're most common in the first trimester of first pregnancies, when that havoc is at its height.

Hormones, however, may not tell the whole story. The long-held theory that cravings and aversions are sensible signals from our bodies—that when we develop a distaste for something, it's usually bad for us, and when we lust after something, it's usually something we need—often does seem to stand up. Like when you suddenly can't face the morning coffee you once couldn't face your morning without. Or when a glass of your favorite wine sips like vinegar. Or when you can't gobble down enough grapefruit. On the other hand, when you call "fowl" at the sight of chicken, or your beloved broccoli becomes bitter, or your cravings launch you into a full-fledged fudge frenzy—well, it's hard to credit your body with sending the smartest signals.

The problem is that body signals relating to food are always hard to read when hormones are involved—and may be especially tough to call now that humans have departed so far from the food chain (and now that so many food chains sell fast food). Before candy bars were invented, for instance, a craving for something sweet might have sent a pregnant woman foraging for berries. Now it's more likely to send her foraging for M&M's.

Do you have to ignore your cravings and aversions in the name of healthy pregnancy eating? Even if that were possible (hormone-induced food quirks are a powerful force), it wouldn't be fair. Still, it's possible to respond to them while also paying attention to your baby's nutritional needs. If you crave something healthy—cottage cheese by the crateful or peaches by the pile—don't feel like you have to hold back. Go for the nutritious gusto, even if it means your diet's a little unbalanced for a while (you'll make up for the variety later on in pregnancy when the cravings calm down).

If you crave something that you know you'd probably be better off without, then try to seek a substitute that satisfies the craving (at least somewhat) but also satisfies a nutritional requirement (and doesn't fill you up with too many empty calories): chocolate frozen yogurt instead of a frozen chocolate bar; a bag of trail mix instead of a bag of jelly beans; baked cheese puffs instead of the kind that turn your fingers orange. If substitutes don't fully satisfy, adding sublimation to the mix may be helpful. When MoonPies at the 7-Eleven howl your name, try doing something that takes your mind off them: taking a brisk walk, chatting with friends on a pregnancy message board, checking out maternity jeans online. And, of course, completely giving in to less nutritious cravings is fine (as is enjoying them, so leave that side of guilt off the menu when you indulge), as long as they don't include something risky (such as an alcoholic beverage) and as long as your indulgences don't take the place of nutritious foods in your diet on a regular basis.

Most cravings and aversions disappear or weaken by the fourth month. Cravings that hang in there longer may be triggered by emotional needs—the need for a little extra attention, for example. If both you and your spouse are aware of this need, it should be easy to satisfy. Instead of requesting a middle-of-the-night pint of Chunky Monkey (with or without the sour dills), you might settle for an oatmeal cookie or two and some quiet cuddling or a romantic bath.

Some women find themselves craving, even eating, such peculiar non-food substances as clay, ashes, and paper. Because this habit, known as pica, can be dangerous and may be a sign of nutritional deficiency, particularly of iron, report it to your practitioner. Craving ice may also mean you're iron deficient, so also report any compulsion to chew ice.

Visible Veins

"I have unsightly blue lines all over my breasts and belly. Is that normal?"

Not only are these veins (which can make your entire chest and belly look like a road map) normal and nothing to worry about, they are a sign that your body is doing what it should. They're part of the network of veins that has expanded to carry the increased blood supply of pregnancy, which will be nourishing your baby. They may show up earliest and be much more prominent in very slim or fair-skinned women. In some women, particularly those who are overweight or dark-skinned, the veins may be less visible or not noticeable at all, or they may not become obvious until later in pregnancy.

Spider Veins

"Since I became pregnant I've got awful-looking spidery purplish red lines on my thighs. Are they varicose veins?"

They aren't pretty, but they aren't varicose veins. They are probably spider nevi, commonly dubbed "spider veins," for obvious reasons. There are a few reasons why spider veins might choose to spin their web across your legs. First, the increased volume of blood you're carrying can create significant pressure on blood vessels, causing even tiny veins to swell and become visible. Second, pregnancy hormones can do a number on all your blood vessels, big and small. And third, genetics can predispose you to spider veins (thanks, Mom).

If you're destined to have spider veins, there's not much you can do to avoid them altogether, but there are ways to minimize their spread. Since your veins are as healthy as your diet is, try eating enough vitamin C foods (the body uses it to manufacture collagen and elastin, two important connective tissues that help repair and maintain blood vessels). Exercising regularly (to improve circulation and leg strength) and getting into the habit of not crossing your legs (which restricts blood flow) will also help keep spider veins at bay.

Prevention didn't do the trick? Some, though far from all, spider veins fade and disappear after delivery; if they don't, they can be treated by a dermatologist—either with the injection of saline (sclerotherapy) or glycerin, or with the use of a laser. These treatments destroy the blood vessels, causing them to collapse and eventually disappear—but they aren't recommended during pregnancy. In the meantime, you can try camouflaging your spider veins with flesh-toned concealers specifically designed for that purpose.

Varicose Veins

"My mother and grandmother both had varicose veins during pregnancy. Is there anything I can do to prevent them in my own pregnancy?"

Varicose veins run in families—and they definitely sound like they have legs in yours. But being genetically predisposed to varicose veins doesn't mean you have to be resigned to them, which is why you're wise to be thinking now about bucking your family tradition with prevention.

Varicose veins often surface for the first time during pregnancy, and they tend to worsen in subsequent pregnancies. That's because the extra volume of blood you produce during pregnancy puts extra pressure on your blood vessels, especially the veins in your legs, which have to work against gravity to push all that extra blood back up to your heart. Add to that the pressure your burgeoning uterus puts on your pelvic blood vessels and the vessel-relaxing effects of the extra hormones your body is producing, and you have the perfect recipe for varicose veins.

The symptoms of varicose veins aren't difficult to recognize, but they vary in severity. There may be a mild achiness or severe pain in the legs, or a sensation of heaviness, or swelling, or none of these. A faint outline of bluish veins may be visible, or serpentine veins may bulge from ankle to upper thigh. In severe cases, the skin overlying the veins becomes swollen, dry, and irritated (ask your practitioner about moisturizers that can help). Occasionally, superficial thrombophlebitis (inflammation of a surface vein due to a blood clot) may develop at the site of a varicosity, so always check with your practitioner about varicose vein symptoms.

To give your legs a leg up against varicose veins:

- Keep the blood flowing. Too much sitting or standing can compromise blood flow, so avoid long periods of either when you can—and when you can't, periodically flex your ankles. When sitting, avoid crossing your legs and elevate them if possible. When lying down, raise your legs by placing a pillow under your feet. When resting or sleeping, try to lie on your left side, the best one for optimum circulation (though either side will do).

- Watch your weight. Excess poundage increases the demands on your already overworked circulatory system, so keep your weight gain within the recommended guidelines.

- Avoid heavy lifting, which can make those veins bulge.

- Push gently during bowel movements. Straining can be a strain on those veins. Staying regular (see page 173) will help keep things moving.

- Wear support panty hose (light support hose seem to work well without being uncomfortable) or elastic stockings, putting them on before getting out of bed in the morning (before blood pools in your legs) and taking them off at night before getting into bed. While neither will contribute to your sexiest pregnancy moment, they help by counteracting the downward pressure of your belly and giving the veins in your legs a little extra upward push.

- Stay away from clothes that might restrict your circulation: tight belts or pants, panty hose and socks with elastic tops, and snug shoes. Also skip high heels, favoring flats or medium chunky heels instead.

- Get some exercise, such as a brisk 20- to 30-minute walk or swim every day. But if you're experiencing pain, avoid high-impact aerobics, jogging, cycling, and weight training.

- Be sure your diet includes plenty of foods rich in vitamin C, which helps keep blood vessels healthy and elastic.

Surgical removal of varicose veins isn't recommended during pregnancy, though it can certainly be considered a few months after delivery. In most cases, however, the problem will improve after delivery, usually by the time prepregnancy weight is reached.

An Achy, Swollen Pelvis

"My whole pelvic area feels achy and swollen, and really uncomfortable—and I think I felt an actual bulge in my vulva. What is that all about?"

Legs may have the market share of varicose veins, but they definitely don't have a monopoly. Varicose veins can also appear in the genital area (and in the rectum, where they're called hemorrhoids), for the same reason you might get them in your legs—and it sounds like they've made that appearance in you. Called pelvic congestion syndrome, or PCS, the symptoms (aside from bulging in the vulva) include chronic pelvic pain and/or abdominal pain, an achy, swollen, "full" feeling in the pelvic area and the genitals, and sometimes pain with intercourse. The tips for minimizing varicose veins in the legs will also help you (see previous question), but do be sure to check with your practitioner, both for the diagnosis and for possible treatment options (usually after delivery).

Breakouts

"My skin is breaking out the way it did when I was a teenager."

The glow of pregnancy that some women are lucky enough to radiate isn't just a result of joy, but of the stepped-up secretion of oils brought on by hormonal changes. And so, alas, are the less-than-glowing breakouts of pregnancy that some not-so-lucky expectant women experience (particularly those whose skin ordinarily breaks out like clockwork before their periods). Though such eruptions are hard to eliminate entirely, the following suggestions may help keep them at a minimum—and keep you from resembling your eighth-grade yearbook picture:

- Wash your face two or three times a day with a gentle cleanser. But don't get overaggressive with scrubs—not only because your skin is extra-sensitive during pregnancy, but because overstripped skin is actually more susceptible to breakouts.

- Get the all clear on any acne medications (topical or oral) before you use them. Some are considered safe to slather on; others aren't. Check with your practitioner, and see page 146.

- Use an oil-free moisturizer to keep skin hydrated. Sometimes skin that is overly dried by harsh acne soaps and other products is more pimple prone.

- Choose skin-care products and cosmetics that are oil free and labeled "non-comedogenic," which means they won't clog pores.

- Keep everything that touches your face clean, including those blush brushes at the bottom of your makeup bag.

- Pop (and pick) not. Just like your mother always told you, popping or picking at pimples won't make them go away—and can actually make them stick around longer by pushing bacteria back down into the zit. Plus, when you're pregnant, you're more prone to infections. Poked-at pimples can also leave scars.

- Eat well by following the Pregnancy Diet. It's good for your skin as well as for your baby.

- Don't pass a tap without filling your glass. Drinking water helps keep your skin moist and clear.

Dry Skin

"My skin is terribly dry. Is that pregnancy related, too?"

Feeling a tad reptilian these days? You can blame your hormones for your dry, often itchy, skin. Hormonal changes rob your skin of oil and elasticity, leaving you with that oh-so-sexy alligator look. To keep your skin as soft as your baby-to-be's bottom:

- Switch to a nonsoap cleanser such as Cetaphil or Aquanil, and use it no more than once a day (at night if you're taking off makeup). Wash with just water the rest of the time.

- Slather on moisturizer while your skin is still damp (after a bath or shower), and use the moisturizer as often as you can—and certainly before you turn in for the night.

- Cut down on bathing and keep your showers short (5 minutes instead of 15). Too much washing can dry out your skin. Make sure, too, that the water is lukewarm and not hot. Hot water removes natural oil from the skin, making it dry and itchy.

- Add unscented bath oils to your tub, but be careful with the slippery surface you've created. (Remember, as your belly grows, so will your klutz factor.)

- Drink plenty of fluids throughout the day to stay hydrated, and be sure to include good fats in your diet (those omega-3's that are so baby friendly are also skin friendly).

- Keep your rooms well humidified.

- Wear a sunscreen with an SPF of at least 15 (preferably 30) every day.

Eczema

"I've always been prone to eczema, but now that I'm pregnant, it's gotten much worse. What can I do?"

Unfortunately, pregnancy (or more accurately, its hormones) often exacerbates the symptoms of eczema, and for women who suffer from it, the itching and scaling can become practically unbearable. (Some lucky eczema sufferers find that pregnancy actually causes the eczema to go into remission.)

Belly Piercings

It's cool, it's stylish, it's sexy—and it's one of the cutest ways to show off a flat, toned tummy. But once your belly starts to bulge, will you have to give up on your belly piercing? Nope—not as long as your belly piercing is healed (read: your trip to the Piercing Pavilion wasn't last month) and healthy (in other words, not red, weeping, or inflamed). Remember, your belly button marks where you connected to your own mom in the womb, not where your baby connects to you—which means a piercing won't provide a path for pathogens to reach your baby. You also don't have to worry about a belly ring interfering with birth, or even a cesarean delivery.

Of course, as your pregnancy progresses and your tummy starts to jut out in earnest, you may find that your belly bar or belly ring becomes too uncomfortable to wear, thanks (or no thanks) to your taut, stretched-to-the-limit skin. The belly ring might also start to rub—and even get caught on—your clothing, especially when your belly button "pops" out later in pregnancy. And that rubbing can hurt, big time.

If you do decide to take out the jewelry entirely, just run your belly ring through the hole every few days to keep the piercing from closing up shop (unless you've had it for a number of years, in which case the likelihood that the hole will close is pretty slim). Or consider replacing your bar or ring with a flexible belly bar made of Teflon or PTFE (for polytetrafluoroethylene).

As far as getting your belly (or anywhere else on your body) pierced during pregnancy: better to hold off until after delivery. It's never a good idea to puncture the skin during pregnancy, because it ups the chances of infection.

Fortunately, low-dose hydrocortisone creams and ointments are safe to use during pregnancy in moderate amounts. Ask your practitioner or dermatologist which ones he or she recommends. Antihistamines may also be helpful in coping with the itchiness, but again, be sure to check with your practitioner first. Cyclosporine, long used on severe cases that don't respond to other treatment, is generally off limits during pregnancy. Some topical and systemic antibiotics may not be safe for use during pregnancy either, so check with your practitioner first. The newer nonsteroidals (Protopic and Elidel) aren't recommended because they haven't been studied in pregnancy and can't be ruled safe until more is known.

If you're an eczema sufferer, you know that prevention can go a long way in keeping the itch away. Try the following:

- Use a cold compress—not your fingernails—to curb the itch. Scratching makes the condition worse and can puncture the skin, allowing bacteria to enter and cause an infection. Keep nails short and rounded to decrease the likelihood that you will puncture the skin when you do inevitably scratch.

- Limit contact with potential irritants such as laundry detergents, household cleaners, soaps, bubble bath, perfumes, cosmetics, wool, pet dander, plants, jewelry, and juices from meats and fruits.

- Moisturize early and often (while skin is still damp, if you're just out of the water) to lock in the skin's own moisture and prevent dryness and cracking.

■ Don't spend too much time in the water (showers, baths, swimming pools), especially hot water.

■ Try not to get too hot or sweaty (two of the most common eczema triggers). Of course that's easier said than done when you're pregnant and already one hot, sweaty mama. Stay cool by wearing loose, cotton clothes and avoiding synthetic fabrics, wool, or any material that feels rough to the touch. Avoid overheating by favoring that layered look—and peeling off layers as you start to warm up.

■ Try to keep your cool, too, when it comes to stress—a common eczema trigger. When you feel anxiety creeping in, take some relaxation breaths (see page 230).

Something to keep in mind: Though eczema is hereditary (meaning that your baby has a chance of having it, too), research suggests that breastfeeding may prevent eczema from developing in a child. That's just one more good reason to nurse your baby if you can.

Come and Go Belly

"It's the strangest thing—one day it'll look like I'm showing, and the next day my belly will be completely flat again. What's up with that?"

What's up are your bowels, actually. Bowel distention (the result of constipation and excess gas, two of a newly pregnant woman's constant companions) can make a flat belly round in no time flat. And just as quickly as it appeared, your belly can disappear—once you've had a bowel movement, that is. A little unnerving, yes ("But I looked pregnant just yesterday!"), but completely normal.

Don't worry. Pretty soon you'll have a belly that doesn't come and go—and that's more baby than bowel. In the meantime, see page 173 for tips on fighting constipation.

Losing Your Shape

"Will I ever get my body back after I have a baby?"

Well, that kind of depends—mostly, on you. The 2 to 4 permanent pounds the average woman puts on with each pregnancy, and the flab that often goes with them, aren't inevitable. In fact, if you gain the right amount of weight, at the right rate, on the right foods, your chances of recovering your prepregnancy shape are really very good, particularly if you team your sensible eating efforts with pregnancy-approved exercise, and especially if you keep your regimen up after your baby arrives. Mind you, that recovery won't happen overnight (think three to six months, minimum).

So fear not your pregnancy weight gain. Remember, it's set to accumulate for the very best reason: the nourishment of your baby now, and, if you choose to breastfeed, later.

Measuring Small

"At my last prenatal visit, my midwife told me my uterus is measuring a little small. Does this mean the baby's not growing right?"

Parents rarely wait until their babies are born to begin worrying about their size. But—just as is usually the case after birth—there's rarely anything to worry about before. After all, trying to size up your uterus from the outside isn't an exact science anytime in pregnancy, and especially not this early in the game. Calculating what that size should be isn't easy either (unless you're certain about which day you conceived on), since the date of your pregnancy may be off by as much as several weeks on either side. Chances are your midwife is planning to schedule an ultrasound to pinpoint more precisely the size of your uterus and the date of your pregnancy and to see if there are any discrepancies, which there most likely aren't.

Measuring Big

"I was told my uterus is measuring ten weeks, but according to my dates I'm only eight weeks pregnant. Why is my uterus so large?"

There's a good chance that your uterus is bigger than it's supposed to be because you're further along than you think. It's likely that your dates are off, or that your size was miscalculated, both pretty common scenarios. To check this out, and because there are other, much less likely explanations (for example, that you might be carrying twins—though it's unlikely at this early stage that multiples would make a difference in uterine size), your practitioner will probably order an ultrasound.

Difficulty Urinating

"The last few days it's been really hard to urinate, even though my bladder seems very full."

It's possible that you might have a stubbornly tilted uterus (about 1 in 5 women has a uterus that tilts toward the back instead of the front) that has refused to right itself and is now pressing on your urethra, the tube leading from the bladder. The pressure of this increasingly heavy load can make urina-tion difficult. There may also be urinary leakage when the bladder becomes very overloaded.

In nearly all cases, the uterus shifts itself back into position by the end of the first trimester without any medical intervention. But if you're really uncomfortable now—or if you're finding it espcially difficult to urinate—put in a call to your practitioner. He or she might be able to manipulate your uterus by hand to move it off the urethra so you can pee easily again. Most of the time that works. In the unlikely event that it doesn't, catheterization (removing the urine through a tube) may become necessary.

One other possibility if you're having trouble urinating (and another good reason to put in that call to your practitioner): a urinary tract infection. See page 498 for more.

Mood Swings

"I know I should feel happy about my pregnancy—and sometimes I am. But other times, I feel so weepy and sad."

They're up—and they're down. The very normal mood swings of pregnancy can take your emotions places they've never gone before, both to exhilarating highs and depressing lows. Moods that can have you over-the-moon one moment, down-in-the-dumps the next—and weeping inexplicably over insurance commercials. Can you blame it on your hormones? You bet. These swings may be more pronounced in the first trimester (when hormonal havoc is at its peak) and, in general, in women who ordinarily suffer from marked emotional ups and downs before their periods (it's sort of like PMS pumped up). Feelings of ambivalence about the pregnancy once it's confirmed, which are common even when a pregnancy is planned, may exaggerate the swings still more. Not to mention all those changes you're experiencing (the physical ones, the emotional ones, the logistical ones, the relationship ones—all of which can overwhelm your moods).

Mood swings tend to moderate somewhat after the first trimester, once hormone levels calm down a little—and once you've adjusted to some of those pregnancy changes (you'll never adjust to all of them). In the meantime, though there's no sure way to hop off that emotional roller coaster, there are several ways to minimize the mood mayhem:

- Keep your blood sugar up. What does blood sugar have to do with moods? A lot. Dips in blood sugar—caused by long stretches between meals—can lead to mood crashes. Yet another compelling reason to ditch your usual three-meals-a-day (or fewer) eating routine and switch to the Six-Meal Solution (see page 91). Give complex carbs and protein starring roles in your mini meals for the longest lasting blood sugar—and mood—highs.

- Keep sugar and caffeine down. That candy bar, that doughnut, that Coke will give your blood sugar a quick spike—followed soon after by a downward spiral that can take your mood down with it. Caffeine can have the same effect, adding to mood instability. So limit both, for happier results.

- Eat well. In general, eating well will help you feel your best emotionally (as well as physically), so follow the Pregnancy Diet as best you can. Getting plenty of omega-3 fatty acids in your diet (through walnuts, fish, and enriched eggs, to name a few) may also help with mood moderating (and they're also super important for your baby's brain development).

- Get a move on. The more you move, the better your mood. That's because exercise releases feel-good endorphins, which can send your spirits soaring. With your practitioner's guidance, build exercise into your day—every day.

- Get a groove on. If you're in the mood for love (and if you're not too busy puking), making love can turn that frown upside down by releasing happy hormones. It can also bring you closer to your partner at a time when your relationship may be facing new challenges. If sex isn't in the cards, just taking the time for intimacy of any kind (cuddling, pillow talk, hand-holding on the sofa) can help boost your mood.

- Light up your life. Research has shown that sunlight can actually lighten your moods. When the sun's shining, try catching some daily rays (just don't forget to apply sunscreen first).

- Talk about it. Worried? Anxious? Feeling unsettled? Feeling unsure? Pregnancy is a time of many mixed emotions, which play themselves out in mood swings. Venting some of those feelings—to your spouse (who's probably feeling plenty of the same things), to friends who can relate, to other expectant moms on online pregnancy message boards (check out the ones on whattoexpect.com)—can help you feel better, or at least help you see that what you're feeling is normal.

- Rest up. Fatigue can exacerbate normal pregnancy mood swings, so make sure you're getting enough sleep (but not too much, since that can actually increase fatigue and emotional instability).

- Learn to relax. Stress can definitely take your moods down, so find ways of moderating it or coping with it better. See page 142 for tips.

If there's one person in your life who's more affected—and bewildered—by your mood swings than you are, it's your spouse. It'll help for him to understand why you're acting the way you are these days (that surges of pregnancy hormones are holding your emotions hostage), but it'll also help for him to know exactly how he can help you. So tell him what you need (more help around the house? a night out at your favorite restaurant?) and what you don't need (hearing that your rear's looking a little wide; his leaving a trail of socks and underwear down the hallway) right now, what makes you feel better and what makes you feel worse. And be specific: Even the most loving spouse isn't a mind reader. See Chapter 19 for more on coping strategies for fathers-to-be.

Depression

"I expected some mood swings with pregnancy, but I'm not just a little down— I'm depressed all the time."

Every pregnant woman has her ups and downs, and that's normal. But if your lows are consistent or frequent, you may be among the 10 to 15 percent of pregnant women who battle mild to moderate depression during pregnancy. Here are some of the factors that can put an expectant mom at risk for such depression:

- A personal or family history of mood disorder

- Financial or marital stress

- Lack of emotional support from and communication with the baby's father

- Hospitalization or bed rest because of pregnancy complications

- Anxiety about her own health, especially if she has a chronic medical condition or has previously experienced complications or illness during pregnancy

- Anxiety about her baby's health, especially if there is a personal or family history of miscarriage, birth defects, or other problems

The most common symptoms of true depression, in addition to feeling sad, empty, and emotionally lethargic, include sleep disturbances (you get too much or too little); changed eating habits (not eating at all or eating continually); prolonged or unusual fatigue and/or excessive agitation or restlessness; extended loss of interest in work, play, and other activities or pleasures; reduced ability to concentrate and focus; exaggerated mood swings; and even self-destructive thoughts. There may also be unexplained aches and pains. If that sounds like what you're experiencing, start by trying those tips for dealing with mood swings in the previous question.

If the symptoms continue for longer than two weeks, speak to your practitioner about your depression (he or she may want to test you for a thyroid condition since that can trigger depression) or ask for a referral to a therapist who can offer supportive psychotherapy. Getting the right help is important. Depression can keep you from taking optimum care of yourself and your baby, now and after delivery. In fact, depression during pregnancy can increase risks for complications—much as depression can adversely affect your health when you're not pregnant. Deciding whether antidepressant medication will be part of the treatment plan will require sitting down with your practitioner (and therapist) to weigh possible risks against possible benefits (see page 518 for a discussion of antidepressants during pregnancy).

Panic Attacks

Pregnancy can be a time of high anxiety, especially for those who are expecting for the first time (and consequently don't know what to expect). And a certain amount of worry is normal, and probably unavoidable. But what about when that worry turns to panic?

If you've had panic attacks in the past, you're probably all too aware of the symptoms (and most women who have panic attacks during pregnancy have had them before). They're characterized by intense fear or discomfort accompanied by an accelerated heart rate, sweating, trembling, shortness of breath, feeling of choking, chest pain, nausea or abdominal distress, dizziness, numbness or tingling, or chills or hot flashes that appear seemingly out of the blue. They can be incredibly unsettling, of course, particularly when they strike for the first time. But happily, though they definitely affect you, there is no reason to believe that panic attacks affect the development of your baby in any way.

Still, if you do experience such an attack, tell your practitioner. Therapy is always the first choice during pregnancy (and other times, too). But if medications are necessary to ensure your well-being (and your baby's—if anxiety is keeping you from eating or sleeping or otherwise taking care of your precious cargo), your practitioner, together with a qualified therapist, can work with you to decide which medication offers the most benefits for the fewest risks (and how low a dose you can take and still derive those benefits). If you've been on a medication for panic attacks, anxiety, or depression prepregnancy, a change or an adjustment of dose might be necessary, too.

While medication is one solution to extreme anxiety, it certainly isn't the only one. There are many nondrug alternatives that can be used instead of or in conjunction with traditional therapy. These include eating well and regularly (including plenty of omega-3 fatty acids in your diet may be especially helpful); avoiding sugar and caffeine (caffeine, in particular, can trigger anxiety); getting regular exercise; and learning meditation and other relaxation techniques (prenatal yoga can be incredibly calming). Talking your anxieties over with other expectant moms can also provide enormous relief.

Consult your practitioner, too, before turning to any alternative treatments. Over-the-counter supplements, such as SAM-e and St. John's wort, touted for their mood-elevating properties, have not been studied enough to consider them safe for use in pregnancy. But other CAM therapies (see page 85) might help, and bright light therapy (which increases levels of the mood-regulating hormone serotonin in the brain) cuts depressive symptoms during pregnancy in half. Eating foods rich in omega-3 fatty acids lowers the risk of depression during pregnancy and possibly during the postpartum period as well. You can also ask your practitioner about taking a pregnancy-safe omega-3 supplement.

Being depressed during pregnancy does put you at somewhat greater risk of postpartum depression. The good news is that getting the right treatment during pregnancy—and/or right after delivery—can help prevent postpartum depression. Ask your practitioner about this.

Weight Gain During Pregnancy

Put two pregnant women together anywhere—in a doctor's waiting room, on an elevator, at a business meeting—and the questions are certain to start flying. "When are you due?" "Have you felt the baby kicking yet?" "Have you been feeling sick?" And perhaps the most commonly posed of all: "How much weight have you gained?"

Everybody expects to gain weight while they're pregnant (and after spending half a lifetime dieting, lots of women actually look forward to it). And, in fact, gaining the right amount of weight is vital when you're growing a baby. But what is the right amount of weight? How much is too much? How much is too little? How fast should you gain it all? And will you be able to lose it all once your baby's delivered? (Answer: yes—if you gain the right amount of weight at the right rate on the right type of foods.)

How Much Should You Gain?

If there were ever a legitimate reason to pile on the pounds, pregnancy is it. After all, when you grow a baby, you've got to do some growing, too. But piling on too many pounds can spell problems for you, your baby, and your pregnancy. Ditto if you pile on too few pounds.

What's the perfect pregnancy weight gain formula? Actually, since every pregnant woman—and every pregnant body—is different, that formula can vary a lot. Just how many pounds you should aim on adding dur-

ing your 40 weeks of baby growing will depend on how many pounds you were packing before you became pregnant.

Your practitioner will recommend the weight gain target that's right for you and your pregnancy situation (and that's the guideline to follow, no matter what you read here). Generally, weight gain recommendations are based on your prepregnancy BMI (a measurement of body fat calculated by multiplying your weight in pounds by 703, then dividing by your height in inches squared; see *What to Expect: Eating Well When You're Expecting* for a chart). If your BMI is average (between 18.5 and 26), you'll probably be advised to gain between 25 and 35 pounds, the standard recommendation for the average-weight pregnant woman. If you start out pregnancy overweight (BMI between 26 and 29), your goal will be somewhat scaled back—to somewhere between 15 and 25 pounds. If you're obese (with a BMI greater than 29), you'll likely be told to tally a total of between 15 and 20 pounds, or perhaps even less than that. Super skinny (with a BMI of less than 18.5)? Chances are your target will be higher than average—upward of 28 to 40 pounds. For moms providing room and board for more than one, extra babies require extra pounds (see page 407).

It's one thing to set an ideal weight gain goal; it's another thing to get there. That's because ideals aren't always completely compatible with reality. Piling on the right number of pounds isn't just about piling the right amount of food on your plate. There are other factors at work, too. Your metabolism, your genes, your level of activity, your pregnancy symptoms (the heartburn and nausea that make eating too much like hard work; those cravings for high-calorie foods that make gaining too much too easy)—all play a role in helping you (or keeping you from) packing on the perfect pregnancy poundage. With that in mind, keep an eye on the scale to ensure that you're reaching your weight gain target.

At What Rate Should You Gain?

Slow and steady doesn't only win the race—it's a winner when it comes to pregnancy weight gain, too. A gradual weight gain is best for your body and your baby's body. In fact, the rate at which weight is gained is as important as the total number of pounds you gain. That's because your baby needs a steady supply of nutrients and calories during his or her stay in your womb—

deliveries that come in fits and spurts won't cut it once your little one starts doing some significant growing (as will happen during the second and third trimesters). A well-paced weight gain will also do your body good, allowing it to gradually adjust to the increased poundage (and the physical strains that come with it). Gradual gain also allows for gradual skin stretching (think fewer stretch marks). Need more convincing? Pounds put on at a slow and steady rate will come off more easily when the time comes (after you've delivered and you're anxious to get back to your prepregnancy shape).

Does steady mean spreading out those 30 pounds or so evenly over 40 weeks? No—even if that were a possible plan, it wouldn't be the best one. During the first trimester, your baby is only the size of a few poppy seeds, which means that eating for two doesn't require extra eating at all, and only a minimum of weight gain. A good goal for trimester 1 is between 2 and 4

Why More (or Less) Weight Gain Isn't More

What do you have to lose by gaining too much weight when you're expecting? Packing on too many pounds can present a variety of problems in your pregnancy. More padding can make assessing and measuring your baby more difficult, and added pounds can add to pregnancy discomforts (from backache and varicose veins to fatigue and heartburn). Gaining too much weight can also increase your risk of preterm labor, of developing gestational diabetes or hypertension, of ending up with an oversize baby that may be too large to deliver vaginally, of postcesarean complications, of a host of problems for your newborn, and of having

more trouble with breastfeeding. Not surprisingly, too, those extra pounds may be extra hard to shed postpartum—and, in fact, many women who gain too much weight during pregnancy end up never shedding them all.

Gaining too little weight can also be a losing proposition during pregnancy, and in some cases it can be more dangerous than gaining too much. Babies whose mothers gain under 20 pounds are more likely to be premature, small for their gestational age, and to suffer growth restriction in the uterus. (The exception: very overweight women, who can safely gain less than 20 pounds under close medical supervision.)

Breakdown of Your Weight Gain

(All weights are approximate)

Baby	7½ pounds
Placenta	1½ pounds
Amniotic fluid	2 pounds
Uterine enlargement	2 pounds
Maternal breast tissue	2 pounds
Maternal blood volume	4 pounds
Fluids in maternal tissue	4 pounds
Maternal fat stores	7 pounds

Total average	**30 pounds overall weight gain**

pounds—though many women don't end up gaining any at all or even losing a few (thanks to nausea and vomiting), and some gain somewhat more (often because their queasiness is comforted only by starchy, high-calorie foods), and that's fine, too. For those who start slowly, it should be easy to play weight gain catch-up during the next six months (especially once food starts tasting and smelling good again); for those who begin gangbusters, watching the scale a little more closely in the second and third trimester will keep their total close to target.

During the second trimester, your baby starts to grow in earnest—and so should you. Your weight gain should pick up to an average rate of about 1 to 1½ pounds per week during months 4 through 6 (totaling 12 to 14 pounds).

During your final trimester, baby's weight gain will pick up steam, but yours may start to taper off to about a pound a week (for a net gain of about 8 to 10 pounds). Some women find their weight holding steady—or even dropping a pound or two—during the ninth month when ever-tighter abdominal quarters can make finding room for food a struggle.

How closely will you be able to follow this rate of gain formula? Realistically, not that closely. There will be weeks when your appetite will rule and your self-control will waver, and it'll be a rocky road (by the half-gallon) to your weight gain total. And there will be weeks when eating will seem too much of an effort (especially when tummy troubles send whatever you eat right back up). Not to worry or stress over the scale. As long as your overall gain is on target and your rate averages out to that model formula (a half pound one week, 2 pounds the next, 1 the following, and so on), you're right on track.

So for best weight gain results, keep your eye on the scale, since what you don't know can throw your weight gain way off target. Weigh yourself (at the same time of day, wearing the same amount of clothes, on the same scale) once a week (more often and you'll drive yourself crazy with day-to-day fluid fluctuations). If once a week is too much (because you're scale-phobic),

Weight Gain Red Flags

If you gain more than 3 pounds in any one week in the second trimester, or if you gain more than 2 pounds in any week in the third trimester, especially if it doesn't seem to be related to overeating or excessive intake of sodium, check with your practitioner. Check, too, if you gain no weight for more than two weeks in a row during the fourth to eighth months.

twice a month should do the trick. Waiting until your monthly prenatal is fine, too—though keep in mind that a lot can happen in a month (as in 10 pounds) or not happen (as in no pounds), making it harder for you to stay on track.

If you find that your weight gain has strayed significantly from what you and your practitioner planned (for instance, you gained 14 pounds in the first trimester instead of 3 or 4, or you packed on 20 pounds in the second instead of 12), take action to see that the gain gets back on a sensible track, but don't try to stop it in its tracks. Dieting to lose weight is never appropriate when you're pregnant, and neither is using appetite-suppressing drinks or pills (these can actually be very dangerous). Instead, with your practitioner's help, readjust your goal to include the excess you've already gained and to accommodate the weight you still have to gain.

CHAPTER 8

The
Third
Month

Approximately 9 to 13 Weeks

As YOU ENTER THE LAST MONTH of your first trimester (great!), many of those early pregnancy symptoms are probably still going strong (not so great!). Which means it's probably hard to tell whether you're exhausted because of first-trimester fatigue—or because you woke up three times last night to go the bathroom (it's likely a little of both). But chin up, if you have the strength to lift it. There are better days ahead. If morning sickness has had you—and your appetite— down, there's a less queasy day soon to dawn. As energy levels pick up, you'll soon have more get-up-and-go—and as urinary urges ease, you may have to get up and go less often. Even better, you may hear the amazing sound of your baby's heartbeat at this month's checkup, which might make all those uncomfortable symptoms seem much more worthwhile.

Your Baby This Month

Week 9 Your baby (who has officially graduated now from embryo to fetus) has grown to approximately 1 inch in length, about the size of a medium green olive. His or her head is continuing to develop and take on more baby-like proportions. This week, tiny muscles are starting to form. This will allow your fetus to move his or her arms and legs, though it'll be at least another month before you'll be able to feel those little punches and kicks.

While it's way too early to feel anything, it's not too early to hear something (possibly). The glorious sound of your baby's heartbeat might be audible via a Doppler device at your practitioner's office. Take a listen—it's sure to make your heart beat a little faster.

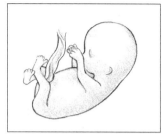

Your Baby, Month 3

istics by now, with hands and feet in the front of the body, ears nearly in their final shape (if not final location), open nasal passages on the tip of the nose, a tongue and palate in the mouth, and visible nipples.

Week 10 At nearly 1½ inches long (about the size of a prune), your baby is growing by leaps and bounds. And in gearing up for those first leaps and bounds (and baby steps), bones and cartilage are forming—and small indentations on the legs are developing into knees and ankles. Even more unbelievably for someone the size of a prune, the elbows on baby's arms are already working. Tiny buds of baby teeth are forming under the gums. Further down, the stomach is producing digestive juices, the kidneys are producing larger quantities of urine, and, if your baby's a boy, his testes are producing testosterone (boys will be boys—even this early on!).

Week 11 Your baby is just over 2 inches long now and weighs about a third of an ounce. His or her body is straightening out and the torso is lengthening. Hair follicles are forming, and fingernail and toenail beds are beginning to develop (nails will actually start to grow within the next few weeks). Those nails are forming on individual fingers and toes, having separated recently from the webbed hands and feet of just a few weeks ago. And though you can't tell baby's gender by looking yet (even with an ultrasound), ovaries are developing if it's a girl. What you would be able to see, if your womb had a view, is that your fetus has distinct human character-

Week 12 Your baby has more than doubled in size during the past three weeks, weighing in now at ½ ounce and measuring (crown to rump) about 2½ inches. About the size of a large fresh plum, your baby's body is hard at work in the development department. Though most of his or her systems are fully formed, there's still plenty of maturing to do. The digestive system is beginning to practice contraction movements (so your baby will be able to eat), the bone marrow is making white blood cells (so your baby will be able to fight off all those germs passed around the playgroup), and the pituitary gland at the base of the brain has started producing hormones (so your baby will one day be able to make babies of his or her own).

Week 13 As your first trimester comes to a close, your fetus (who seems to be working its way through the produce section) has reached the size of a peach, about 3 inches long. Your baby's head is now about half the size of his or her crown to rump length, but that cute little body is picking up steam and will continue growing overtime (at birth, your baby will be one-quarter head, three-quarters body). Meanwhile, your baby's intestines, which have been growing inside the umbilical cord, are now starting their trek to their permanent position in your baby's abdomen. Also developing this week: your baby's vocal cords (the better to cry with . . . soon!).

What You May Be Feeling

As always, remember that every pregnancy and every woman is different. You may experience all of these symptoms at one time or another, or only a few of them. Some may have continued from last month; others may be new. Still others may be hardly noticed because you've become so used to them. You may also have other, less common, symptoms. Here's what you might experience this month:

Physically

- Fatigue, lack of energy, sleepiness
- Frequent urination

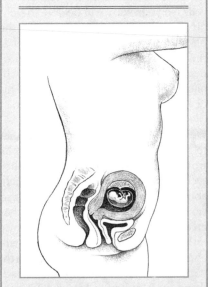

A Look Inside

This month, your uterus is a little bigger than a grapefruit and your waist may start to thicken. By the end of the month, your uterus can be felt right above your pubic bone in the lower abdomen.

- Nausea, with or without vomiting
- Excess saliva
- Constipation
- Heartburn, indigestion, flatulence, bloating
- Food aversions and cravings
- Increasing appetite, especially if morning sickness is easing
- Breast changes: fullness, heaviness, tenderness, tingling; darkening of the areolas (the pigmented area around your nipples); lubrication glands in the areolas becoming prominent, like large goose bumps; expanding network of bluish lines under your skin
- Visible veins on your abdomen, legs, and elsewhere, as your blood supply pumps up
- Slight increase in vaginal discharge
- Occasional headaches
- Occasional faintness or dizziness
- A little more rounding of your belly; your clothes feeling a little snugger

Emotionally

- Continued emotional ups and downs, which may include mood swings, irritability, irrationality, weepiness
- Misgivings, fear, joy, elation—any or all
- A new sense of calm
- Still, a sense of unreality about the pregnancy ("Is there really a baby in there?")

What You Can Expect at This Month's Checkup

This month, you can expect your practitioner to check the following, though there may be variations depending on your particular needs and your practitioner's style of practice:

- Weight and blood pressure

- Urine, for sugar and protein

- Fetal heartbeat

- Size of uterus, by external palpation (feeling from the outside), to see how it correlates to due date

- Height of fundus (the top of the uterus)

- Hands and feet for swelling, and legs for varicose veins

- Questions or problems you want to discuss—have a list ready

What You May Be Wondering About

Constipation

"I've been terribly constipated for the past few weeks. Is this common?"

Irregularity—that bloated, gassy, clogged-up feeling—is a very regular pregnancy complaint. And there are good reasons why. For one, the high levels of progesterone circulating in your expectant system cause the smooth muscles of the large bowel to relax, making them sluggish—and allowing food to hang around longer in the digestive tract. The upside: There's added time for nutrients to be absorbed into your bloodstream, allowing more of them to reach your baby. The downside: You end up with what amounts to a waste-product traffic jam, with nothing going anywhere anytime soon. Another reason for the clogged-up works: Your growing uterus puts pressure on the bowel, cramping its normal activity. So much for the process of elimination, at least as you once knew it.

But you don't have to accept constipation as inevitable just because you're pregnant. Try these measures to combat your colon congestion (and head off hemorrhoids, a common companion of constipation):

Fight back with fiber. You—and your colon—need about 25 to 35 grams of fiber daily. No need to actually keep count. Just focus on fiber-rich selections such as fresh fruit and vegetables (raw or lightly cooked, with skin left on when possible); whole-grain cereals and bread; legumes (beans and peas); and dried fruit. Going for the green can also help get things going—look for it not only in the form of green vegetables, but in the juicy, sweet kiwi, a tiny fruit that packs a potent laxative effect. If you've never been a big fiber fan, add these foods to your diet gradually or you may find your digestive tract protesting loudly. (But since flatulence is a common complaint of pregnancy as well as a frequent, but usually temporary, side effect of a newly fiber-infused diet, you may find your digestive tract protesting for a while anyway.)

Really plugged up? You can try adding some wheat bran or psyllium

Another Reason for Being Tired, Moody, and Constipated

Have you been tired, moody, and constipated lately? Welcome to the pregnancy club. Surging gestational hormones, of course, trigger those pesky symptoms in most pregnant women. However, a shortage of another hormone, thyroxine, can mimic these common pregnancy complaints, as well as many others—weight gain, skin problems of all kinds, muscle aches and cramps, a decrease in libido, memory loss, and swelling—especially of the hands and feet. (Another common symptom, an increased sensitivity to cold, is more clear-cut during pregnancy, since expectant moms tend to be warmer rather than chillier.) Consequently, hypothyroidism (a deficiency of the thyroid hormone due to an underactive thyroid gland) may be easy for physicians to miss in an expectant mom. Yet the condition, which affects 1 in 50 women, can have an adverse affect on pregnancy (also wreaking havoc in the postpartum period; see page 460), so proper diagnosis and treatment are vital.

Hyperthyroidism (when too much thyroid hormone is produced by an overactive gland) is seen less often in pregnancy, but it can also cause complications if left untreated. Symptoms of hyperthyroidism—many of which may also be hard to distinguish from pregnancy symptoms—include fatigue, insomnia, irritability, warm skin and sensitivity to heat, rapid heartbeat, and weight loss (or trouble gaining weight).

If you have ever been diagnosed with any thyroid problems in the past (even if they have since cleared up) or if you currently take medication for a thyroid condition, be sure to let your practitioner know. Because the body's need for thyroid hormone fluctuates during pregnancy, it's possible you may need medication again or need your dose adjusted (see page 531).

If you have never been diagnosed with a thyroid condition, but you're experiencing some or all of the symptoms of hypo- or hyperthyroidism (and especially if you have a family history of thyroid disease), check with your doctor. A simple blood test can determine whether you have a thyroid problem.

to your diet, starting with a sprinkle and working your way up, as needed. Don't overdo these fiber powerhouses, though; as they move speedily through your system, they can carry away important nutrients before they've had the chance to be absorbed.

Resist the refined. While high-fiber foods can keep things moving, refined foods can clog things up. So steer clear of the refiner things in life, such as white bread (and other baked goods) and white rice.

Drown your opponent. Constipation doesn't stand a chance against an ample fluid intake. Most fluids—particularly water and fruit and vegetable juices—are effective in softening stool and keeping food moving along the digestive tract. Another time-honored way to get things moving: Turn to warm liquids, including that spa staple, hot water and lemon. They'll help stimulate peristalsis, those intestinal contractions that help you go. Truly tough cases may benefit from that geriatric favorite, prune juice.

When you gotta go, go. Holding in bowel movements regularly can weaken muscles that control them and lead to constipation. Timing can help avoid this problem. For example, have your high-fiber breakfast a little earlier than usual, so it will have a chance to kick in before you leave the house—instead of when you're in the car stuck in traffic.

Don't max out at mealtime. Big meals can overtax your digestive tract, leading to more congestion. Opt for six mini meals a day over three large ones—you'll also experience less gas and bloating.

Check your supplements and medications. Ironically, many of the supplements that do a pregnant body good (prenatal vitamins, calcium, and iron supplements) can also contribute to constipation. Ditto every pregnant woman's best buddy, antacids. So talk to your practitioner about possible alternatives or adjustments in dosages or, in the case of supplements, switching to a slow-release formula. Also ask your practitioner about magnesium supplements that may help fight constipation.

Get some bacteria. Probiotics (aka "good bacteria") may stimulate the intestinal bacteria to break down food better, aiding the digestive tract in its efforts to keep things moving. Enjoy probiotics in yogurt and yogurt drinks that contain active cultures. You can also ask your practitioner to recommend a probiotic supplement—in powder form, it can be easily added to smoothies (and it has no taste of its own).

Get some exercise. An active body encourages active bowels, so fit a brisk walk of about half an hour into your daily routine (some people find even a 10-minute walk works); supplement it with any exercise you enjoy that is safe during pregnancy (see page 224).

If your efforts don't seem to be productive, consult with your practitioner. He or she may prescribe a bulk-forming stool softener for occasional use. Don't use any laxative (including herbal remedies or castor oil) unless your practitioner specifically recommends it.

Lack of Constipation

"All my pregnant friends seem to have problems with constipation. I don't—in fact, I've remained very regular. Is my system working right?"

From the sound of things, your system couldn't be working better. Chances are your digestive efficiency is attributable to your lifestyle—one you've been enjoying for a long while or one you've adopted since you learned you were expecting. Stepped-up consumption of fiber-rich foods and fluids, along with regular exercise, are bound to counteract the natural digestive slowdown of pregnancy and keep things moving smoothly. If this dietary style is new to you, the productivity of your digestive tract may decrease a little (and flatulence, which often temporarily accompanies such dietary changes, may ease up) as your system gets used to the rough stuff, but you will probably continue to be "regular."

Diarrhea

"I'm not at all constipated. In fact, for the last couple of weeks I've had loose stools—almost diarrhea. Is this normal?"

When it comes to pregnancy symptoms, normal is often what's normal for you. And in your case, more frequent, looser stools may be just that. Every body reacts differently to pregnancy hormones—yours may be reacting by stepping up, not slowing down, on production of bowel movements. It's also possible that this increased bowel activity is due to a positive change in your diet and exercise habits.

You can try cutting back on bowel-stimulating foods, such as dried fruits, and adding bulking foods (such as bananas) until your stool becomes more firm. To compensate for the fluids you're losing through loose stools, make sure you're drinking enough.

If your stools are very frequent (more than three a day) or watery, bloody, or mucousy, check with your practitioner; this kind of diarrhea could require prompt intervention during pregnancy.

Gas

"I'm very bloated and I'm passing gas all the time. Will it be like this the whole pregnancy?"

Are you passing gas like a college frat boy (make that *more* than a college frat boy)? Sorry, guys, but nobody does gas like a pregnant woman. Fortunately, while the same can't be said for those who work and live within hearing and sniffing distance of you, your baby is oblivious and impervious to your digestive distress. Snug and safe in a uterine cocoon that's protected on all sides by impact-absorbing amniotic fluid, he or she is probably soothed by the bubbling and gurgling of your gastric Muzak.

Baby won't be happy, though, if bloating—which often worsens late in the day and, yes, generally persists throughout pregnancy—prevents you from eating regularly and well. To cut down on the sounds and smells from down under and to make sure your nutritional intake doesn't suffer on account of your intestinal outtakes, take the following measures:

Stay regular. Constipation is a common cause of gas and bloating. See the tips on page 173.

Graze, don't gorge. Large meals just add to that bloated feeling. They also overload your digestive system, which isn't at its most efficient anyway in pregnancy. Instead of those two or three supersize squares, nibble on six mini meals.

Don't gulp. When you rush through meals or eat on the fly, you're bound to swallow as much air as food. This captured air forms painful pockets of gas in your gut, which will seek release the only way they know how.

Keep calm. Particularly during meals. Tension and anxiety can cause you to swallow air, which can give you a full tank of gas. Taking a few deep breaths before meals may help relax you.

Steer clear of gas producers. Your tummy will tell you what they are—they vary from person to person. Common offenders include onions, cabbage, fried foods, rich sauces, sugary sweets, carbonated beverages, and, of course, the notorious beans.

Don't be quick to pop. Ask your practitioner before popping your usual anti-gas medications (some are safe, others are not recommended) or any remedy, over-the-counter or herbal. Sipping a little chamomile tea, however, may safely soothe all kinds of pregnancy-induced indigestion. Ditto for hot water with lemon, which can cut through gas as well as any medication.

Headaches

"I find that I'm getting a lot more headaches than ever before. Can I take something for them?"

That women are more susceptible to headaches during the time they're

What's a Corpus Luteum Cyst?

If your practitioner has told you that you have a corpus luteum cyst, your first question will probably be—what is it? Well, here's all you need to know. Every month of your reproductive life, a small yellowish body of cells forms after you ovulate. Called a corpus luteum (literally "yellow body"), it occupies the space in the follicle formerly occupied by the egg. The corpus luteum produces progesterone and some estrogen, and it is programmed by nature to disintegrate in about 14 days. When it does, diminishing hormone levels trigger your period. When you become pregnant, the corpus luteum hangs around instead of disintegrating, continuing to grow and produce enough hormones to nourish and support your baby-to-be until the placenta takes over. In most pregnan-cies, the corpus luteum starts to shrink about six or seven weeks after the last menstrual period and stops functioning altogether at about 10 weeks, when its work of providing board for the baby is done. But in about 10 percent of pregnancies, the corpus luteum doesn't regress when it's supposed to. Instead, it develops into a corpus luteum cyst.

So now that you know what a corpus luteum cyst is, you're probably wondering—how will it affect my pregnancy? The answer: probably not at all. The cyst is usually nothing to worry about—or do anything about. Chances are it will go away by itself in the second trimester. But just to be sure, your practitioner will keep an eye on your cyst's size and condition regularly via ultrasound (which means you get extra peeks at your baby).

supposed to stay away from certain pain relievers is one of the ironies of pregnancy. It's an irony you'll have to live with, but it's not necessarily one you'll have to suffer with—at least, not too much. Prevention, teamed with the right remedies (medicinal and non), can offer relief from the normal recurrent headaches of pregnancy.

The best route to headache relief depends on the cause or causes. Pregnancy headaches are most commonly the result of hormonal changes (which are responsible for the increased frequency and severity of many types of headaches, including sinus headaches), fatigue, tension, hunger, physical or emotional stress, or any combination of these.

There are plenty of ways around a headache (and some surprisingly effective ones don't come in capsule form). In many cases you'll be able to fit the probable cause with the possible cure:

Relax. Pregnancy can be a time of high anxiety, with tension headaches a common result. Some women find relief through meditation and yoga (which also makes a fabulous pregnancy exercise). You can take a class, turn to a DVD or CD, read a book on these or other relaxation techniques, or try the one on page 142.

Of course, relaxation exercises don't work for everyone; some women find that they step up tension instead of easing it. If that sounds like you, lying down in a dark, quiet room or stretching out on the sofa or with your feet up on your desk for 10 or 15 minutes may be a better foil for tension and tension headaches.

Get enough rest. Pregnancy can also be a time of extreme fatigue, particularly in the first and last trimesters, and often for the full nine months for women who work long hours at a job and/or have other children to care for. Sleep can be elusive once the belly starts swelling ("How will I ever get comfortable?") and the mind starts racing ("How will I ever get everything done before the baby comes?"), which compounds fatigue. Making a conscious effort to get more rest, day and night, can help keep headaches at bay. But be careful not to sleep too much—excess sleep can also give you a headache, as can sleeping with the covers over your head.

Eat regularly. To avoid hunger headaches triggered by low blood sugar, be sure not to run on empty. Carry high-energy snacks (such as soy chips, granola bars, dried fruit and nuts) with you in your bag, stash them in the glove compartment of your car and in your office desk drawer, and always keep a supply on hand at home.

Seek some peace and quiet. Noise can give you a headache, especially if you're extra sound-sensitive. Make it a point to avoid noisy locales (the mall, loud parties, restaurants with bad acoustics). If your job is extra noisy, talk to your boss about taking steps to reduce the excess noise—or even ask for a transfer to a quieter area, if possible. At home, lower the volume on the telephone's ringer, the TV, and the radio.

Don't get stuffy. An overheated room or unventilated space can give anyone a headache—but especially an expectant mom, who's overheated to start with. So try not to get stuffy, but when you can't avoid it (it's two days before Christmas and you have to brave that jam-packed mall—or you work there), step out for a stroll and a breath of fresh air when

you can. Dress in layers when you know you're going somewhere stuffy, and keep comfortable (and hopefully, headache free) by removing layers as needed. Stuck inside? Try to crack a window, at least.

Switch lighting. Take the time to examine your surroundings, particularly the lighting around you, in a whole new . . . well, light. Some women find that a windowless work space lit by fluorescent bulbs can trigger headaches. Switching to incandescent lighting and/or a room with windows may help. If that's not practical, take outdoor breaks when you can.

Try alternatives. Some complementary and alternative medical approaches— including acupuncture, acupressure, biofeedback, and massage—can bring headache relief (see page 85).

Go hot and cold. For relief of sinus headaches, apply hot and cold compresses to the aching area, alternating 30 seconds of each for a total of 10 minutes, four times a day. For tension headaches, try ice applied to the back of the neck for 20 minutes while you close your eyes and relax. (Use an ordinary ice pack or a special neck pillow that holds a gel-based cold pack.)

Straighten up. Slouching or looking down to read or do other close work (knitting baby booties?) for long stretches of time can also trigger an aching head, so watch your posture.

Take two. Haven't got time for the pain? Acetaminophen (Tylenol) usually brings quick relief and is considered safe for pregnancy use (skip the ibuprofen and aspirin). Check with your practitioner for the right dosage and headache protocol. And don't take any pain medication (over-the-counter, prescription, or herbal) without your practitioner's okay.

If an unexplained headache persists for more than a few hours, returns very often, is the result of fever, or is accompanied by visual disturbances or puffiness of the hands and face, notify your practitioner.

"I suffer from migraine headaches. I heard they're more common in pregnancy. Is this true?"

Some women find their migraines strike more frequently during pregnancy; luckier ones find they are less frequent. It isn't known why this should be true, or even why some people have recurrent migraines and others never have a single one.

If you've had migraines in the past, discuss with your physician which migraine medications are safe to take during pregnancy so you'll be prepared for dealing with these killer headaches should they strike while you're expecting. Think prevention, too. If you know what brings on an attack, you can try to avoid the culprit. Stress is a common one, as are chocolate, cheese, and coffee. Try to determine what, if anything, can stave off a full-blown attack once the warning signs appear. You may be helped by one or more of the following: splashing your face with cold water or applying a cold cloth or ice pack; avoiding noise, light, and odors by lying down in a darkened room for two or three hours, eyes covered (napping, meditating, or listening to music, but not reading or watching TV); or trying CAM techniques such as biofeedback or acupuncture (see page 85).

Stretch Marks

"I'm afraid I'm going to get stretch marks. Can they be prevented?"

Nobody likes stretch marks, especially come skin-baring season. Still, they're not easy to escape when you're expecting. The majority of pregnant women develop these pink or reddish (sometimes purplish), slightly indented, sometimes itchy streaks on their breasts, hips, and/or abdomen sometime during pregnancy.

As their name implies, stretch marks are caused by tiny tears in the supporting layers of tissue under your skin as it becomes stretched to its limit. Expectant mothers who have good elastic skin tone (because they inherited it and/or earned it through years of excellent nutrition and exercise) may slip through several pregnancies without a single telltale mark. And actually, your mother may be your best crystal ball when it comes to predicting whether you'll end up with stretch marks or not; if she sailed through her pregnancies with smooth skin intact, odds are you will, too. If stretch marks struck her, they'll likely strike you, too.

You might be able to minimize, if not prevent, stretch marks by keeping weight gain steady, gradual, and moderate (the faster skin stretches, the more likely the stretching is to leave its mark). Promoting elasticity in your skin by nourishing it with a good diet (especially those vitamin C foods) may also help. And though no topical preparation has been proven to prevent stretch marks from zigzagging their way across your skin, there's no harm in applying moisturizers, such as cocoa butter. Even without the scientific proof to back them up, some women swear they work—and if nothing else, they'll prevent the dryness and itching associated with pregnancy-stretched skin. An added plus: It may be fun for your spouse to rub them on your tummy (and baby will enjoy the massage, too).

If you do develop stretch marks (frequently referred to as the red badge of motherhood), you can console yourself

Body Art for Two?

Heading off to The House of Ink for a "hot mama" tattoo? Think before you ink. While the ink itself won't enter your bloodstream, there is a risk of infection any time you get stuck with a needle, and why take that risk when you've got a baby on board?

Something else to ponder before getting a tattoo for two. What looks symmetrical on your pregnant skin might become lopsided or distorted after you regain your prepregnancy shape. So keep your skin free of any new marks for now, and wait until after you've weaned your baby to express yourself through body art.

If you already have a tattoo, no problem—just sit back and watch it stretch. And don't worry about that lower back tattoo and how it might affect the epidural you were hoping for come labor day. As long as the tattoo ink is fully dried and the wound healed, sticking that epidural needle through it won't be risky.

What about using henna to decorate your body during pregnancy? Since henna is plant based—and temporary—it's probably safe to use during pregnancy. Still, it's wise to follow certain caveats: Make sure the henna artist uses natural henna (it stains the skin reddish brown), not the kind that contains the potentially irritating chemical paraphenylendiamine (which stains black), and check the artist's references (read: no fair doing it at a street fair). To be extra-cautious (always the best way to be), ask your practitioner before using henna.

Keep in mind, too, that pregnant skin is often extra-sensitive skin, so there's a chance you'll have an allergic reaction to the henna, even if you've had it applied before without incident. To test your reaction to it, place a small amount of henna on a patch of skin and wait 24 hours to make sure no irritation appears.

---

with the knowledge that they will gradually fade to a silvery sheen some months after delivery. You can also discuss with a dermatologist the possibility of reducing their visibility postpartum with laser therapy or Retin-A. In the meantime, wear them with pride.

First-Trimester Weight Gain

"I'm nearing the end of the first trimester and I'm surprised that I didn't gain any weight yet."

Many women have trouble putting on an ounce in the early weeks—some even lose a few pounds, usually courtesy of morning sickness,

and others, because they started out overweight, don't need to gain any this early on. Fortunately, nature has your baby's back, offering protection even if you're too queasy or food-averse to eat. Tiny fetuses have tiny nutritional needs, which means that your lack of weight gain now won't have any effect on your baby. Not so, however, once you enter the second trimester. As your baby gets bigger and your baby-making factory picks up steam, calories and nutrients will be more and more in demand— and you'll need to begin playing weight gain catch-up, piling the pounds on at a steady pace.

So definitely don't worry, but do start eating (hopefully any morning sickness will ease up soon). And from the fourth month on, start watching your weight to make sure it begins to move upward at the appropriate rate (see page 167). If you continue to have trouble gaining weight, try packing more of a nutritional wallop with the calories you take in, through efficient eating (see page 91). Try, too, to eat a little more food each day, by not skipping meals and by adding more frequent snacks. If you can't eat a lot at one sitting (which isn't so good for pregnancy digestion anyway), graze on six small meals daily instead of three big squares. Save salads and soups and fill-you-up beverages for after your main course to avoid putting a damper on your appetite. Enjoy foods high in good fats (nuts, seeds, avocados, olive oil). But don't try to add pounds by adding lots of junk food to your diet. That kind of weight gain is more likely to round out your hips and thighs than your baby.

"I'm 12 weeks pregnant and I was shocked to find out that I'd already gained 13 pounds. What should I do now?"

First of all, don't panic. Lots of women have that "oops" moment—when they step on the scale at the end of their first trimester and discover they've gained 8, 10, a dozen pounds, or more in three short months. Sometimes it's because they've taken "eating for two" just a tad too literally (you are eating for two, but one of you is really, really small), relishing sweet release from a lifetime of dieting. Sometimes it's because they've found that comfort from queasiness can come in high-calorie packages (ice cream, pasta, burgers, or just bread by the loaf).

Either way, all is not lost if you've gained a little too much in the first trimester. True, you can't turn back the scales—or apply the first three months' gain neatly to the next six. Your baby needs a steady supply of nutrients (espe-cially in the second and third trimester, when he or she will be growing over-time), so cutting way back on calories now isn't a smart plan. But you can aim to keep your gain on target for the rest of your pregnancy—to slow it down, without putting the brakes on it alto-gether—by watching the scale (and what you eat) more carefully.

Check with your practitioner and work out a safe and sensible weight gain goal for the next two trimesters. Even if you stay in the pound-a-week club through month 8 (most women find their weight gain slows or stops in the ninth month), you won't end up more than a couple of pounds over 35 pounds, the outside limit for recommended weight gain. Check out the Pregnancy Diet (Chapter 5) to find out how to eat healthily for two without ending up looking like two (of you). Gaining effi-ciently, on the highest-quality foods pos-sible, will not only accomplish that goal but make the weight you do gain easier to shed in the postpartum period.

Boys Will Be Boys

Hungry, Mom? As you close in on your second trimes-ter, you'll likely notice that your appetite (which you may have lost somewhere around week 6 or so) is starting to make a comeback. But if you're bellying up to the refrigera-tor with the regularity of a teenage boy, you may be expecting one (or, at least, a male fetus on his way to becoming a teenage boy). Research shows that moms-to-be carrying boys tend to eat more than moms expecting girls—which could explain why boys tend to be heavier at birth than girls. Food (and more food) for thought!

Showing Early

"Why am I already showing if I'm only in my first trimester?"

Have lots more to show for your first trimester than you expected? Because every belly's different, some stay flat far into the second trimester while others seem to pop before the home pregnancy test is dry. An early bump can be disconcerting ("If I'm this big *now,* what will I look like in a few months?"), but it can also be welcome, tangible proof that there's actually a baby in there.

Several possibilities might explain why you're showing so early:

- **Small build.** If you're slender to begin with, your growing uterus may have nowhere to hide, causing a bulge even when it's still relatively little.

- **Less muscle tone.** A pregnant woman with loose abdominal muscles is more likely to produce a pronounced pooch faster than a mom-to-be with a taut and toned torso. That's why second timers tend to show earlier—their abdominal muscles have already been stretched.

- **Overeating.** If you've been eating for two (but forgetting that one of those two is only prune-sized right now), your belly might be sporting more fat than baby. If you've gained more than 4 or 5 pounds by this point, that could explain your prematurely protruding tummy.

- **Wrong dates.** A sooner-than-expected show time could be the result of a miscalculated conception date.

- **Bloating.** Excess gas and bloating could be behind that supersize stomach of yours. So could bowel distention if you've been going long stretches between movements.

- **More than one on board.** Some women who sport an impressive bump in their first trimester later discover they're having twins. But before you start doubling up the layette, keep in mind that most women whose bellies balloon early turn out to be carrying just one baby. A relatively round belly in the first trimester is not generally considered a reliable sign that an expectant mother is carrying multiples (see next question).

Carrying Multiples?

"How will my doctor know if I'm carrying twins or not?"

Have a hunch that there's more than one baby on board? There are plenty of clues you can look for when trying to determine whether or not you're toting twins:

A large-for-date uterus. The size of the uterus, not of the abdomen, is what counts in the diagnosis of multiples. If your uterus seems to be growing more rapidly than expected for your due date, a multiple pregnancy might be suspected. A big belly alone doesn't count.

Exaggerated pregnancy symptoms. When carrying twins, the typical troubles of pregnancy (morning sickness, indigestion, and so on) can be doubled, or at least seem that way. But all of these can also be exaggerated in a one-fetus pregnancy.

Predisposition. Several factors make a woman more likely to have nonidentical, or fraternal, twins. These include nonidentical twins in the mother's family, advanced age (women over 35 more frequently release more than one egg at a time), the use of fertility drugs to stimulate ovulation, and in vitro fertilization. Some evidence indicates that identical twins might also be genetically influenced (something in your egg or your spouse's sperm could cause a fertilized egg to split).

As for your practitioner, he or she might try to listen for two (or more) distinctly separate heartbeats, but it's not an exact science (the heartbeat of a single fetus may be heard at several locations), so twins aren't often diagnosed this way. The best diagnostic tool for detecting multiples is an early ultrasound. In virtually every case (except in the rare instance where one camera-shy fetus remains stubbornly hidden behind the other), this technique accurately diagnoses a multiple pregnancy. If you are carrying twins (or more), see Chapter 16.

Baby's Heartbeat

"My friend heard her baby's heartbeat at 10 weeks. I'm a week ahead of her, and my doctor hasn't picked up my baby's yet."

Hearing the first lub-dub of your baby's heartbeat is definitely music to every mom-to-be's (and dad-to-be's) ears. Even if you've already seen your little one's steady drumbeat on an early ultrasound, there's nothing like hearing it through the Doppler (a handheld ultrasound device that amplifies the sound with the help of a special jelly on the belly) in your practitioner's office.

Even though a heartbeat can be heard as early as the 10th or 12th week with a Doppler, not all expectant moms get to feast their ears on this fetal symphony that early. Your baby's position may be the cause of the inaudible heartbeat, or maybe the location of the placenta (or extra fat padding your belly) is muffling the sound. A slightly miscalculated due date may also explain why you're not hearing your baby's beat yet. By your 14th week, the miraculous sound of your baby's heartbeat is certain to be available for your listening pleasure. If it isn't, or if you are very anxious, your practitioner will likely do

At-Home Dopplers

Tempted to buy one of those inexpensive prenatal "heart listeners" so you can stay tuned in to your baby's heartbeat between practitioner visits? Being able to monitor your baby's heart rate can be loads of fun and may even help you have a better night's sleep if you're a stresser by nature. But listen to this: Though these devices are considered safe to use, they're not as sophisticated as the one your practitioner uses—and most aren't nearly sensitive enough to pick up fetal heart tones until after the fifth month of pregnancy. Use one before then, and you'll likely be met with silence instead of a steady beat, which can increase worry unnecessarily

instead of putting it to rest. Even later on in pregnancy, at-home Dopplers can't always pick up what you're looking for (baby's position or a bad angle on the device can easily throw off an at-home Doppler). The readings might not be accurate, either—or might be different enough from the ones you're used to getting at your checkups to prompt undue concern. So do try this at home, if you like (though you should get your practitioner's okay before placing your order, especially because the FDA requires a prescription for them). Just keep in mind that you get what you pay for, and you might get somewhat less than you bargained for.

The Heart of the Matter

Is it a boy or a girl, and can your baby's heart rate give you a clue? While old wives—and some practitioners—have been telling tales for ages (a heart rate of above 140 promises a girl, one under 140 delivers a boy), studies show no correlation between fetal heart rate and gender. It may be fun to make predictions based on your baby's heart rate (you'll be right 50 percent of the time, after all), but you might not want to make nursery color choices based on it.

an ultrasound, which will see a heartbeat that, for some reason, was difficult to hear with the Doppler.

When you do get to hear the heartbeat, listen carefully. Your normal heart rate is usually under 100 beats per minute, but your baby's will be around 110 to 160 beats per minute during early pregnancy and average between 120 and 160 beats per minute by midpregnancy. Don't compare fetal heartbeats with your pregnant friends, though—every baby beats to his or her own drummer, and normal fetal heart rates vary a lot.

Starting at about 18 to 20 weeks, the heartbeat can be heard without Doppler amplification, using a regular stethoscope.

Sexual Desire

"All of my pregnant friends say that they had an increased sex drive early in pregnancy. How come I feel so unsexy?"

Pregnancy is a time of change in many aspects of your life, not the least of

them sexual. Hormones, which, as you've undoubtedly noticed, play a role in every physical and emotional high and low, also play an important role in sexuality. But those hormones hit every woman differently, turning up the heat for some and throwing ice water on others. Some women who have never had either an orgasm or much of a taste for sex suddenly experience both for the first time when they're expecting. Other women, accustomed to having a voracious appetite for sex and to being easily orgasmic, suddenly find that they're completely lacking in desire and are difficult to arouse. And even if your hormones have pushed your passion turn-on button, pregnancy symptoms (that nausea, that fatigue, those painfully tender breasts) can stand between you and a good time. These changes in sexuality can be disconcerting, guilt-provoking, wonderful, or a confusing combination of all three. And they are all perfectly normal.

Most important is recognizing that your sexual feelings during pregnancy—and your partner's as well—may be more erratic than erotic; you may feel sexy one day and not the next. Mutual understanding and open communication will see you through, as will a sense of humor. And remember (and remind your partner) that many women who've lost that loving feeling in the first trimester get it back in the second, in spades, so don't be surprised if a very warm front moves into your bedroom soon. Until then, you might want to try the tips on the next page to help heat things up.

"Ever since I became pregnant, I'm turned on all the time and I can't get enough of sex. Is this normal?"

Feeling a little hot under the collar (and under those very snug jeans)? Is your turn-on switch always on? Lucky you. While some women find their sex lives coming to a screeching halt in the first trimester (what with all those early pregnancy symptoms kicking their libidos out the bedroom door), others—like you—find they just can't get enough of a good thing. You can thank those extra hormones surging through your body these days, as well as the increase in blood flow to your pelvic region (which can make your genitals feel wonderfully engorged and ever-tingly), for turning up the sexual thermostat. On top (so to speak) of that are the new curves you're sprouting and the bigger-than-life breasts you're likely sporting, all of which can make you feel like one sexy mama. Plus, it might be the first time in your sexual life that you're able to make love when the mood moves you—without having to spoil the moment while you run to the bathroom for your diaphragm or calculate your fertility with an ovulation predictor. This happy state of sensual affairs may be most pronounced during the first trimester, when hormonal havoc is at its height, or it can continue right up until delivery day.

Since your increased sexual appetite is perfectly normal (as is a lack of sexual desire), don't worry or feel guilty about it. And don't be surprised or concerned if your orgasms are more frequent or more intense than ever (and if you're having orgasms for the first time, that's even more reason to celebrate). As long as your practitioner has green-lighted lovemaking in all its forms (and that's usually the case), seize the moment and your partner. Explore different positions before that belly of yours makes many of them a physical impossibility. And most of all, enjoy that cozy twosome while you can (and before that libido of yours takes its very likely postpartum nosedive).

"I'm interested in sex all the time, but my husband's never in the mood these days. I'm starting to take it personally."

What's putting your man off his favorite feed now that there's a bun in the oven? There are several possible explanations. One could be fear—of hurting you or hurting the baby (even though he can't). Another could be the weirdness factor of making love "in front of" the baby—or the nagging thought that the baby can see or feel his penis when it's inside you (which, by the way, is giving himself way too much credit). Maybe he's having a tricky time getting used to the changes in your body or adjusting to the idea that you're about to become somebody's mother. Or maybe he's just so focused on becoming a father that being a lover has taken a back seat. There might even be a physical trigger: Expectant and new fathers often experience a drop in testosterone and a surge in female hormones that can give their libidos a cold shower.

No matter what's causing your husband to run for cover every time he spies you with "that look," don't take it personally. But also don't resign yourself to a nine-month dry spell. Instead, initiate some frank pillow talk. Tell him how you're feeling (all revved up and no place to go), and find out what's going on in his head (which can explain what's not going on below his belt). Have him read the section on sex starting on page 255, as well as Chapter 19, which will reassure him that sex is perfectly safe in a normal pregnancy and that babies are completely oblivious to parental goings-on and gettings-it-on (and completely out of reach, even for the particularly gifted dad). Be understanding and patient if he has baggage he needs to unpack before you hit the sack again. Honest, open communication will allow the two of you to come to a meeting of the minds—and hopefully, a meeting of the bodies.

And don't just passively wait for love (and him) to land in your lap. Turn up his heat with some naughty lingerie that accentuates all your new (and dangerous) curves, add some mood lighting and music, and offer up a massage (complete with scented oils). If that just makes him feel more uncomfortable (and more pressured to perform), take the opposite tack. Cozy up on the sofa for some cuddling instead. Perhaps when the pressure's off, he might feel inspired to jump on the jumping-you bandwagon.

Cramp After Orgasm

"I get a cramp in my abdomen after orgasm. Is that normal, or does it mean something's wrong?"

Not to worry—and not to stop enjoying sex, either. Cramping (sometimes accompanied by lower backache)—both during and after orgasm—is common and harmless during a low-risk pregnancy. Its cause can be physical: a combination of the normal increased blood flow to the pelvic area during pregnancy, the equally normal congestion of the sexual organs during arousal and orgasm, and the normal contractions of the uterus following orgasm. Or it can be psychological: a result of the common, but unfounded, fear of hurting the baby during sex. Or it can be a combination of physical and psychological factors, since the mind-body connection is so strong when it comes to sex.

In other words, that cramping isn't a sign that you're hurting your baby while you're enjoying yourself. In fact, unless your practitioner has advised you otherwise, it's perfectly safe to mix the pleasure of sex and the business of making a baby. If the cramps bother you, ask your partner for a gentle low back rub. It may relieve not only the cramps but any tension that might be triggering them. Some women also experience leg cramps after they have sex; see page 271 for tips on relieving those.

Pregnant on the Job

If you're pregnant, you've already got your work cut out for you. Add a full-time job to the full-time job of baby making, and your workload doubles. Juggling it all—practitioner visits with client meetings, trips to the bathroom with trips to the mailroom, morning sickness with business lunches, telling your best friend in accounting (who'll be excited for you) with telling your boss (who might not be), staying healthy and comfortable with staying motivated and successful, preparing for baby's arrival with preparing for maternity leave—can be a 9-to-5 challenge that keeps you working overtime. Here's some help for the pregnant and employed.

When to Tell the Boss

Wondering when to belly up to your boss's desk to spill the pregnancy beans? There's no universally perfect time (though it's a sure bet you should do it before that bump gets noticeably big). A lot will depend on how family friendly (or unfriendly) your workplace is. Still more will depend on your feelings (the physical and emotional). Here are some factors to consider:

The Pregnant Worker's Rights

There is much room for improvement in the U.S. workplace when it comes to families and their needs. Though individual policies vary from company to company, here's what federal law recognizes:

■ The Pregnancy Discrimination Act of 1978. This act prohibits discrimination based on pregnancy, childbirth, or related medical conditions. Under this law, employers must treat you as they would treat any employee with a medical disability. However, it does not protect you if you end up not being able to do the job you were hired to do.

It is considered discriminatory—and illegal—to pass up a woman for a promotion or a job or fire her solely on the basis of her pregnancy. But this kind of discrimination, like all kinds of discrimination, can be difficult to prove. Complaints of pregnancy discrimination can be reported to the U.S. Equal Employment Opportunity Commission (EEOC), (800) 669-4000; eeoc.gov.

■ The Family and Medical Leave Act (FMLA) of 1993. All public agencies and private-sector companies that employ at least 50 workers within a 75-mile radius of each other are subject to regulation under this act. If you have worked for such a company for at least a year (and at least 1,250 hours during the year),

you are entitled to take up to 12 weeks of unpaid leave during your pregnancy and for a child's (or other member of your family's) illness each year that you are employed. Barring unforeseen complications or early delivery, you must notify your employer of your leave 30 days in advance. During your leave, you must continue to collect all benefits (including health insurance), and when you return, you must be restored to an equivalent position with equal pay and benefits. Keep in mind, too, that you can use FMLA for weeks during your pregnancy if you're not feeling well. (In some cases, companies may be able to exclude from FMLA women who are considered key employees—those the company can't do without for 12 weeks and who are in the top 10 percent compensation bracket.) The Wage and Hour Division of the U.S. Department of Labor can offer information on FMLA. For more help, contact them at (800) 827-5335; or go online to dol.gov.

■ State and local laws. Some state and local laws offer additional protection against pregnancy discrimination. A very small handful of states and some larger companies also offer "temporary disability insurance," which allows for partial wages during time off for medical disabilities, including pregnancy.

How you're feeling and whether you're showing. If morning sickness has you spending more time hovering over the toilet than sitting at your desk; if first-trimester fatigue has you barely able to lift your head off your pillow in the morning; or if you're already packing a paunch that's too big to blame on your breakfast, you probably won't be able to keep your secret long. In that case, telling sooner makes more sense than waiting until your boss (and everyone else in the office) has come to his or her own conclusions. If, on the other hand, you're feeling fine and still zipping your pants up with ease, you may be able to hold off on the announcement until later.

What kind of work you do. If you work under conditions or with substances that could be harmful to your pregnancy or your baby, you'll need to make your announcement—and ask for a transfer or change of duties, if at all feasible—as soon as possible.

How work is going. A woman announcing her pregnancy at work may unfortunately—and unfairly—raise many red flags, including, "Will she still have the stamina to produce while pregnant?" and "Will her mind be on work or on her baby?" and "Will she leave us in the lurch?" You may head off some of those concerns by making your announcement just after finishing a report, scoring a deal, ringing up record sales, coming up with a great idea, or otherwise proving that you can be both pregnant and productive.

Whether reviews are coming up. If you're afraid your announcement might influence the results of an upcoming performance or salary review, wait until the results are in before sharing your news. Keep in mind that proving you've been passed up for a promotion or raise based solely on the fact that you're expecting (and that you'll soon be a worker and a mother, not necessarily in that order) may be difficult.

Whether you work in a gossip mill. If gossip is one of your company's chief products, be especially wary. Should word of mouth of your pregnancy reach your boss's ears before your announcement does, you'll have trust issues to deal with in addition to the pregnancy-related ones. Make sure that your boss is the first

to know—or, at least, that those you tell first can be trusted not to squeal.

What the family-friendliness quotient is. Try to gauge your employer's attitude toward pregnancy and family if you're not sure what it is. Ask other women who have walked in your soon-to-be-swollen footsteps before, if there are any (but keep inquiries discreet). Check the policies on maternity leave in your copy of the employee handbook that's been gathering dust on your desk. Or set up a confidential meeting with someone in human resources or the person in charge of benefits. If the company has had a history of being supportive of mothers and mothers-to-be, you may be inclined to make the announcement sooner. Either way, you'll have a better sense of what you'll be facing.

Making the Announcement

Once you've decided when to make your announcement, you can take some steps to ensure that it's well received:

Prepare yourself. Before you break the news, do your research. Learn everything you need to know about your employer's maternity-leave policies. Some companies offer paid leave, others unpaid. Still others allow you to use sick days or vacation days as part of your leave.

Know your rights. Pregnant women—and parents in general—have fewer rights in the United States than in most every other industrialized country. Still, some baby steps have been made on behalf of expectant workers on the federal level through the Pregnancy Discrimination Act and the Family and Medical Leave Act (see box, page 187) and on the state level (many states have

The Juggling Act

Even if you don't have any kids at home yet, staying on the job while you're expecting will require that you practice the fine art of juggling work and family (or, at least, a family-to-be). Especially during the first trimester and the last, when the symptoms of pregnancy may be dragging you down and the distractions of pregnancy may be competing for your attention, this juggling act may be exhausting, and sometimes overwhelming—in other words, good preparation for the years of working and parenting you may have ahead of you. These tips won't make working simultaneously at those two jobs easier, but they may help make your working life work more smoothly with your making-a-baby life:

- **Schedule smart.** Make appointments for checkups, ultrasounds, blood tests, glucose tolerance tests, and other procedures before your workday begins (you may be too tired afterward) or during your lunch break. If you need to leave work in the middle of the day, explain to your boss that you have a doctor's appointment, and keep a log of these visits (just in case anyone accuses you of slacking off). If necessary, request a note from your practitioner verifying your appointment, and give this to your employer or someone in your human resources department.

- **Remember not to forget.** If your brain cells seem to be dropping like flies, you can blame your hormones—and start taking precautions so your pregnancy-impaired memory doesn't get you into workplace hot water. To ensure that you don't forget that meeting, that lunch date, those calls that had to be made by noon: Make lists, write yourself reminders (Post-its are a pregnant worker's best friend), and keep your PDA handy (if you can remember where you put it).

- **Know your limits and stop before you reach them.** This isn't the time to volunteer to take on extra projects or extra hours unless it's absolutely necessary. Focus on what needs to be done—and realistically can be done—without wearing yourself out. To avoid feeling overwhelmed, complete one task at a time.

- **Just say "yes."** If colleagues offer to help out when you're not feeling well, don't hesitate to take them up on their kindness (maybe you can return the favor someday). And attention all expectant micromanagers: If there was ever a time to learn how to delegate, this would be it.

- **Recharge as needed.** When you find yourself emotionally overwhelmed, and you will (a stuck stapler can start the tears flowing when you're pregnant), take a brief walk, a bathroom break, or some relaxation breaths to clear your head. Or indulge in a private moment of mom-to-be madness—you deserve it.

- **Speak up.** Not only are you only human, but you're human and pregnant. Which means you can't do it all and do it all well—especially if you feel crappy, as you will sometimes feel. If you can barely lift your head off your pillow (or leave the bathroom for more than five minutes) and you've got a pile of stuff on your desk or a major deadline looming, don't panic. Tell your boss you need extra time or extra help. And don't beat yourself up—or let anyone else beat you up. You're not lazy or incompetent, you're pregnant.

equal employment opportunity laws that protect against pregnancy discrimination). Many other big steps have been taken voluntarily by forward-thinking, family-friendly companies. Become familiar with what the law says you're entitled to, so you'll know what you can and probably can't ask for.

Put together a plan. Efficiency is always appreciated on the job, and being prepared invariably impresses people. So before you go in to make your announcement, prepare a detailed plan that includes how long you plan to stay on the job (barring any unforeseen medical problems), how long your maternity leave will be, how you plan to finish up business before you leave, and how you propose that any unfinished business be handled by others. If you would like to return part-time at first, propose that now. Writing up your plan will ensure you won't forget the details, plus it'll score you extra efficiency points.

Set aside the time. Don't try to tell your boss the news when you're in a taxi on the way to a meeting or when he or she's got one foot out the door Friday night. Make an appointment to meet, so no one will be rushed or distracted. Try to make it on a day and at a time that is usually less stressful at your office. Postpone the meeting if things suddenly take a turn for the tense.

Accentuate the positive. Don't start your announcement with apologies or misgivings. Instead, let your boss know that you are not only happy about your pregnancy but confident in your ability and committed in your plan to mix work and family.

Be flexible (but not spineless). Have your plan in place, and open it up to discussion. Then be ready to compromise (make sure there is room for negotiation built into your plan) but not to back down completely. Come up with a realistic bottom line and stick with it.

Set it in writing. Once you've worked out the details of your pregnancy protocol and your maternity leave, confirm it in writing so there won't be any confusion or misunderstanding later (as in "I never said that . . .").

Never underestimate the power of parents. If your company is not as family friendly as you'd like, consider joining forces to petition for better parental perks. Realize, however, that you and other parents may be met with hostility by childless employees; as family policies become more generous, resentment tends to build among those who can't take advantage of them. Making sure that similar allowances are made for employees who must take time off to care for sick spouses or parents may help unite, rather than divide, the company.

Staying Comfortable on the Job

Between nausea and fatigue, backaches and headaches, puffy ankles and a leaky bladder, it's hard for any expectant mom to have a completely comfortable day. Put her at a desk or on her swollen feet or at a job that requires bending or lifting and you've got a recipe for even more pregnancy discomfort. To stay as comfortable as possible on the job when you're expecting, try these tips:

- Dress for success and comfort. Avoid tight, restrictive clothing, socks or knee-highs that cut off circulation, as well as heels that are too high or too flat (wide 2-inch heels are best). Wearing support hose designed for pregnancy will help ward off or minimize a variety of symptoms, from

Carpal Tunnel Syndrome

If you spend your day (and maybe your nights, too) tap-tap-tapping on a keyboard, you may already be familiar with the symptoms of carpal tunnel syndrome (CTS). A well-known worker's malady, CTS causes pain, tingling, and numbness in the hands and most often strikes those who spend a lot of time doing repetitive tasks (typing, punching numbers, working a PDA). What you might not know, however, is that CTS affects the majority of pregnant women. Even moms-to-be who never touch a computer keyboard are prone to it, thanks to swollen tissue in the body that presses on nerves. The good news is that carpal tunnel syndrome is not dangerous—just uncomfortable, especially on the job. Even better, you can try a number of remedies until you see the light at the end of the carpal tunnel:

- Raise your office chair so your wrists are straight and your hands are lower than your elbows as you type.

- Switch to a wrist-friendly ergonomic keyboard (one that has a wrist rest) as well as a mouse that offers wrist support.

- Wear a wrist brace while typing.

- Take frequent breaks from the computer.

- Use a speakerphone or headset if you're on the phone a lot.

- In the evenings, soak your hands in cool water to reduce any swelling.

- Ask your practitioner about other possible remedies, including vitamin B_6 supplements, acupuncture, or pain relievers.

swelling to varicose veins, and may be especially important if you're spending a lot of the day on your feet.

- Watch the weather—inside you. No matter the climate in your city (or your office), when you're pregnant, the forecast is for wildly swinging body temperatures. Sweating one minute and chilly the next, you'll want to favor the layered look—and have a layer ready for every possible condition. Thinking of bundling up in a wool turtleneck to brave a 12°F day? Don't do it unless you've got a lightweight layer underneath that you can strip down to when a hormone-driven heat wave starts burning inside. And even if you're usually toasty in just a tee, stash a sweater in your drawer or locker. Your body temp goes both ways fast these days.

- Stay off your feet—at least as much as possible. If your job demands that you stand for long stretches, take sitting or walking breaks. If possible, keep one foot on a low stool, knee bent, while you stand, to take some of the pressure off your back. Switch feet regularly. Flex them periodically, too.

- Put your feet up. Find a box, a wastebasket, or another sturdy object on which to discreetly rest your weary feet under your desk.

- Take a break. Often. Stand up and walk around if you've been sitting; sit down with your feet up if you've been standing. If there's a spare sofa and a slot in your schedule, lie down for a few minutes. Do some stretching exercises, especially for your back, legs, and neck. At least once (or even twice) every hour, do this 30-second stretch:

Raise your arms above your head, clasp your fingers, palms up, and reach up. Next, place your hands on a desk or table, step back a bit, and stretch out your back. Sit down and rotate your feet in both directions. If you can bend over and touch your toes—even from a seated position—go for it to release the tension in your neck and shoulders.

- Adjust your chair. Back hurt? Slip on a lumbar cushion for extra support. Bottom sore? Slide a soft pillow onto your seat. If your chair reclines, consider setting it back a few notches to create more (and more!) space between your belly and your desk.

- Hang out by the water cooler. Not for the latest gossip (though that certainly can be a perk) but for frequent refills of your cup. Or keep a refillable water bottle at your desk. Drinking at least 64 ounces of water a day can keep many troublesome pregnancy symptoms at bay, including excessive swelling, and may help prevent a UTI.

- Don't hold it in. Emptying your bladder as needed (but at least every two hours) also helps prevent UTIs. A good strategy: Plan to pee every hour or so, whether you need to or not. You'll feel better overall if you avoid getting to the bursting point. (Now's not the time to have to sprint to the bathroom.)

- Take time for your tummy. Every expectant mom's job description includes feeding her baby regularly, no matter what else is on her workday agenda. So plan accordingly—making room in even your busiest days for three meals, plus at least two snacks (or five to six mini meals). Scheduling meetings as working meals (and trying to have some say about what's served) may help. So will keeping a supply of nutritious snacks in your desk and your purse, as well as in the office fridge, if there is one. Rediscover brown bags—they're not particularly glam, but they can keep you and baby fed when time's not on your side.

- Keep an eye on the scale. Make sure job stress—or erratic eating—isn't keeping you from gaining enough or is contributing to excess weight gain (as it can for stress eaters, especially if they work near a vending machine or another easy junk food outlet).

- Pack a toothbrush. If you're suffering from morning sickness, brushing your teeth can protect them between bouts of vomiting—plus it helps freshen up your breath when it most needs freshening. Mouthwash will also be a welcome addition to the breath-freshening team, and it can help dry out a mouth that's full of excess saliva (which is common in the first trimester and can be extra embarrassing at work).

- Lift with care. Do any necessary lifting properly, to avoid strain on the back (see page 237).

- Watch what you breathe. Stay out of smoke-filled areas; not only is smoke bad for you and your baby, it can also increase fatigue.

- Take an occasional chill pill. Too much stress isn't good for you or your baby. So try to use breaks to relax as fully as you can: Bring an iPod so you can listen to music; close your eyes and meditate or indulge in some daydreaming; do some soothing stretches; take a five-minute stroll around the building.

- Listen to your body. Slow down your pace if you're feeling tired; go home early if you're exhausted (and can leave).

Staying Safe on the Job

Most jobs are completely compatible with the job of feeding and caring for an unborn baby, which is very good news to the millions of expectant mothers who must manage to work full time at both occupations. Still, some jobs are obviously safer and better suited to pregnant women than others. Most on-the-job problems can be avoided with the right precautions or a modification of duties (check with your practitioner for other workplace recommendations in your case):

Office work. Anyone with a desk job knows the pain of stiff necks, aching backs, and headaches, all of which can make a pregnant woman feel more uncomfortable than she already is. No harm done to baby—but a lot of wear and tear on your achy expectant body. If you spend a lot of time sitting, be sure to stand up, stretch, and walk away from your desk frequently. Stretch your arms,

---

Quiet, Please

By about 24 weeks, your baby's outer, middle, and inner ear are well developed. By 27 to 30 weeks, your baby's ear is mature enough to start to respond to the sounds that filter through to him or her. The sounds, of course, are muffled—and not just by the physical barrier of amniotic fluid and your own body. In his or her fluid-filled home, a baby's eardrum and middle ear can't do their normal job of amplifying sounds. So even sounds that are quite loud to you won't be for the baby.

Still, since noise is one of the most prevalent of all occupational hazards and has long been known to cause hearing loss in those (adults) exposed to it regularly, you might want to play it safe when it comes to excessive noise during pregnancy. That's because studies suggest that *prolonged* and *repeated* exposure to very loud noise raises the odds of a baby suffering some hearing loss, especially at lower frequencies. Such prolonged noise exposure—say, an eight-hour-a-day shift in an industrial workplace, where the sound level is more than 90 or 100 decibels (about the same as standing next to a loud lawn mower or a chain saw)—can also increase the risk of premature delivery and low-birthweight babies. Extremely intense sound, 150 or 155 decibels (ever stand right next to a screaming jet engine?), can cause similar problems for the baby. Generally, it's safest to avoid more than eight hours of continuous exposure to noises louder than 85 or 90 decibels (such as a lawn mower or truck traffic) and more than two hours a day of exposure to noise louder than 100 decibels (such as that from a chain saw, pneumatic drill, or snowmobile).

More research needs to be done, but in the meantime, expectant mothers who work in an extremely noisy environment—such as a club where loud music is played, in a subway, or in a factory where protective hearing devices are required (you can't put these devices on your fetus)—or who are exposed to heavy vibrations on the job should play it safe and seek a temporary transfer or a new job. And try to avoid prolonged exposure to very loud noises in your everyday life: Listen to the concert from the middle of the amphitheater, or better yet, head back to the lawn seats; turn down the volume in your car; and wear headphones instead of blasting the music while you're vacuuming.

neck, and shoulders while sitting in your chair, put your feet up to reduce swelling (your boss may not appreciate your tootsies on the desk, so rest your feet on a low stool or box instead), and support your back with a cushion.

What about computer safety? Luckily, computer monitors are not a hazard to pregnant women, and neither are laptops. More worrisome is the multitude of physical discomforts, including wrist and arm strain, dizziness, and headaches, that can result from too much time spent in front of the computer. For fewer aches and pains, use a height-adjustable chair with a backrest that supports your lower back. Adjust the monitor to a comfortable height; the top should be level with your eyes and about an arm's length away from you. Use an ergonomic keyboard, designed to reduce the risk of carpal tunnel syndrome (see box, page 191), if possible, and/or a wrist rest. When you put your hands on the keyboard, they should be lower than your elbows and your forearms should be parallel to the floor.

Health care work. Staying healthy is every health care professional's top on-the-job priority, but it ranks even higher when you're staying healthy for two. Among the potential risks you'll need to protect yourself and your baby from are exposure to chemicals (such as ethylene oxide and formaldehyde) used for sterilization of equipment; to some anticancer drugs; to infections, such as hepatitis B and AIDS; and to ionizing radiation (such as that used in diagnosis or treatment of disease). Most technicians working with low-dose diagnostic X-rays are not exposed to dangerous levels of radiation. It is recommended, however, that women of childbearing age working with higher-dose radiation wear a special device that keeps track of daily exposure, to ensure that cumulative annual exposure does not exceed safe levels.

Depending on the particular risk you are exposed to, you might want to either take safety precautions as recommended by NIOSH (see box) or switch to safer work for now.

Manufacturing work. If you have a factory or manufacturing job that has you operating heavy or dangerous machinery, talk to your boss about a change of duties while you're pregnant. You can also contact the machinery's manufacturer (ask for the corporate medical director) for more information about the product's safety. How safe conditions are in a factory depends on what's being

---

Getting All the Facts

By law, you have the right to know what chemicals you are exposed to on the job; your employer is obliged to tell you. The Occupational Safety and Health Administration (OSHA) is the regulatory body that monitors those laws. Contact them for more information on your rights regarding workplace safety: (800) 321-OSHA—(800) 321-6742; osha.gov. Further information on workplace hazards can also be obtained by contacting the National Institute for Occupational Safety and Health (NIOSH), Clearinghouse for Occupational Safety and Health Information, (800) CDC-INFO—(800) 232-4636; cdc.gov/niosh/topics/repro.

If your job does expose you to hazards, either ask to be transferred temporarily to a safer post or, finances and company policy permitting, begin your maternity leave early.

made in it and, to a certain extent, on how responsible and responsive the people who run it are. OSHA lists a number of substances that a pregnant woman should avoid on the job. Where proper safety protocols are implemented, exposure to such toxins can be avoided. Your union or other labor organization may be able to help you determine if you are properly protected. You can also get useful information from NIOSH or OSHA (see box, facing page).

Physically strenuous work. Work that involves heavy lifting, physical exertion, long hours, rotating shifts, or continuous standing may somewhat increase a woman's risk for preterm delivery. If you have such a job, you should request a transfer, by 20 to 28 weeks, to a less strenuous position until after delivery and postpartum recovery. (See page 196 for recommendations on how long it is safe for you to stay at various strenuous jobs during your pregnancy.)

Emotionally stressful work. The extreme stress in some workplaces seems to take its toll on workers in general and on pregnant women in particular. So it makes sense to cut down on the stress in your life as much as possible, especially now. One obvious way to do that is to switch to a job that is less stressful or take early maternity leave. But these approaches aren't feasible for everyone; if the job is critical financially or professionally, you may find yourself even more stressed if you leave it.

You might, instead, consider ways of reducing stress, including meditation and deep breathing, regular exercise (to release those feel-good endorphins), and having more fun (seeing a movie instead of working until 10 P.M.). Talking to your employer, explaining that overtime, overwork, and general stress could affect your pregnancy, may help, too. Explain that being allowed to set your own pace at work may make your pregnancy more comfortable (this kind of stress seems to increase the risk of backaches and other painful pregnancy side effects) and help you do a better job. If you're self-employed, cutting back may be even tougher (you're probably your own most demanding boss), but it's something you'd be wise to consider.

Other work. Teachers and social workers who deal with young children may come into contact with infections that can potentially affect pregnancy, such as chicken pox, fifth disease, and CMV. Animal handlers, meat cutters, and meat inspectors may be exposed to toxoplasmosis (but some may well have developed immunity already, in which case their babies would not be at risk). If you work where infection is a risk, be sure you're immunized as needed and take appropriate precautions, such as washing hands frequently and thoroughly, wearing protective gloves, a mask, and so on.

Flight attendants or pilots may be at a slightly higher risk for miscarriage or preterm labor (though studies are inconclusive) due to exposure to radiation from the sun during high-altitude flights, and they might want to consider switching to shorter routes (they're usually flown at lower altitudes and require less standing time) or to ground work during pregnancy.

Artists, photographers, chemists, cosmeticians, dry cleaners, those in the leather industry, agricultural and horticultural workers, and others may be exposed to a variety of possibly hazardous chemicals in the course of work, so be sure to wear gloves and other protective gear. If you work with any suspect substances, take appropriate precautions, which in some cases may mean avoiding the part of the job that involves the use of chemicals.

Staying on the Job

Planning to work until that first contraction hits? Many women successfully mix business with baby making right through the ninth month, without compromising the well-being of either occupation. Still, some jobs are better suited to pregnant women during the long haul (so to speak) than other jobs. And chances are, the decision of whether you'll continue to work until delivery will have at least something to do with the kind of work you're involved in. If you have a desk job, you can probably plan to go straight from the office to the birthing room. A sedentary job that isn't particularly stressful may actually be less of a strain on both you and baby than staying at home with a vacuum cleaner and mop, trying to tidy up the nest for your new arrival. And some walking—an hour or two daily, on the job or off—is not only harmless but beneficial (assuming you aren't carrying heavy loads as you go).

Jobs that are strenuous, very stressful, and/or involve a great deal of standing, however, may be another, somewhat controversial, matter. One study found that women who were on their feet 65 hours a week didn't seem to have any more pregnancy complications than women who worked many fewer and usually less stressful hours. Other studies, however, suggest that steady strenuous or stressful activity or long hours of standing after the 28th week—particularly if the expectant mother also has other children to care for at home—may increase the risk of certain complications, including premature labor, high blood pressure, and a low-birthweight baby.

Should women who stand on the job—salespeople, chefs and other restaurant workers, police officers, doctors, nurses, and so on—work past the 28th week? Most practitioners give the green light to work longer if a woman feels fine and her pregnancy is progressing normally. Standing on the job all the way to term, however, may not be a good idea, less because of the theoretical risk to the pregnancy than the real risk that such pregnancy discomforts as backache, varicose veins, and hemorrhoids will be aggravated.

It's probably a good idea to take early leave, if possible, from a job that requires frequent shift changes (which can upset appetite and sleep routines, and worsen fatigue); one that seems to exacerbate any pregnancy problems, such as headache, backache, or fatigue; or one that increases the risk of falls or other accidental injuries. But the bottom line: Every pregnancy, every woman, and every job is different. Together with your practitioner, you can make the decision that's right for your situation.

Changing Jobs

With all the changes going on in your life (like your growing belly and the ever-expanding responsibilities that come with it), it may seem counterintuitive to want to add another to your list. But there are dozens of valid reasons why an expectant mom might consider a job change. Maybe your employer isn't family friendly and you're concerned about balancing career and motherhood when you return from maternity leave. Maybe the commute is too long, the hours inflexible, or the grind all-consuming. It could be that you're bored or not fulfilled (and, hey—change is in the air anyway, so why not make the most of it?). Or perhaps you're worried that your current workplace might be hazardous to you and your developing baby. Whatever your reason, here are some things to consider before you make a job move:

▪ Looking for work takes time, energy, and focus, three things you may be lacking these days as you concentrate on having a healthy pregnancy. Typically, you'll be asked to come in for several interviews and meetings before an offer is made (and if you're already suffering from pregnancy forgetfulness, forming the kind of sentences that make a good impression may be challenging). Starting a new job also demands a great deal of concentration (all eyes are on you, so you have to be extra careful not to make mistakes), and you should be certain you have the stamina and commitment to take these steps.

- Before you jump ship, you'll need to be sure the new job you're seeking out is really all it's cracked up to be (in your mind, at least). Does the company you're smitten with offer twice as much vacation time but charge double for health insurance? Do they allow people to work from home yet expect them to be on call morning, noon, and night? Are the salaries far higher and, likewise, the travel demands? Keep in mind that what looks like a great job now may not be so great when you're juggling it with new-baby care (your home life will be a lot more complicated, so you might not want your workplace life to be). Also bear in mind that companies often offer fewer paid short-term disability days or pay a lower percentage of your salary during leave if you have been employed for less than one year.

- By law, your potential employer has no right to ask whether you're pregnant (if it isn't already obvious), nor can he or she deny you an offer in light of the news. Still, some companies simply can't bring you on and let you leave so quickly. And not all employers appreciate what they consider to be a bait-and-switch strategy (you tell them you want to work there, then after you begin, you tell them you'll be

Unfair Treatment at Work

Think you're being treated unfairly on the job because of your pregnancy? Don't just sit there, do something. Let someone you trust—your supervisor, someone in human resources—know how you feel. If that doesn't fix the problem, see if there is a procedure for employees to follow in the case of pregnancy discrimination (you can probably find it in your employee handbook, if there is one). If that still doesn't work, contact the U.S. Equal Employment Opportunity Commission (eeoc.gov) to find your local office. They'll be able to help you determine if you have a legitimate complaint.

Remember to keep records of everything that'll bolster your claim (copies of e-mails, letters, a diary of events). This paper trail will also be helpful in case you ever need to contact an attorney.

out on maternity leave). So though it may be smart in the short run to keep your pregnancy a secret as you interview, it may damage your relationship with the company in the end. On the other hand, sometimes it's better to secure the offer first and then discuss the future once you know the company wants to hire you—but before you accept the position.

What if you started a new job before you found out you were pregnant? Be up front about what happened, and then get down to the business of doing your job to the best of your expectant ability. Just make sure you know your rights about job security should the situation take a negative turn.

CHAPTER 9

The
Fourth
Month

Approximately 14 to 17 Weeks

F INALLY, THE BEGINNING OF THE second trimester—which, for many pregnant women, is the most comfortable of the three. And with the arrival of this momentous milestone (one down, two to go!) come some welcome changes. For one, most of the more pesky early pregnancy symptoms may be gradually easing up or even disappearing. That queasy cloud may be lifting (which means that food may actually smell and taste good for the first time in a long time). Your energy level should be picking up (which means you'll finally be able pick yourself up off the sofa), and your visits to the bathroom should be dropping off. And though your breasts will likely still be super-size, they're less likely to be super-tender. Another change for the better: By the end of this month, the bulge in your lower abdomen may be looking less like the remains of a large lunch and more like the beginnings of a pregnant belly.

Your Baby This Month

Week 14 Beginning in the second trimester, fetuses (like the children they'll eventually become) start growing at different paces, some faster than others, some more slowly. Despite the differences in growth rates, all babies in utero follow the same developmental path. This week, that path is leading your baby—who is about the size of your clenched fist—toward a straighter position as the neck is getting longer and the head more erect. And on top of that cute little head, your baby might actually be sprouting some hair.

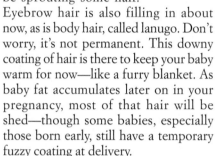

Your Baby, Month 4

Eyebrow hair is also filling in about now, as is body hair, called lanugo. Don't worry, it's not permanent. This downy coating of hair is there to keep your baby warm for now—like a furry blanket. As baby fat accumulates later on in your pregnancy, most of that hair will be shed—though some babies, especially those born early, still have a temporary fuzzy coating at delivery.

Week 15 Your baby, who measures 4½ inches this week and weighs around 2 to 3 ounces, is about the size of a navel orange. Looking more and more like the baby you're picturing in your dreams, his or her ears are positioned properly on the sides of the head (they used to be in the neck), and the eyes are moving from the side of the head to the front of the face. By now your baby has the coordination, strength, and smarts to wiggle his or her fingers and toes and even suck a thumb. But that's not all your baby can do now. He or she can also breathe (or at least make breathing movements), suck, and swallow—all in preparation for the big debut and life outside the womb. And though it's unlikely that you'll be feeling any movements from your little one this week, your baby is certainly getting a workout—kicking, flexing, and moving those arms and legs.

Week 16 With a whopping weight of anywhere from 3 to 5 ounces and a length (crown to rump) of 4 to 5 inches, your baby is growing up fast. Muscles are getting stronger (you'll start to feel

movement in a few weeks), especially the back muscles, enabling your little one to straighten out even more. Your baby-to-be is looking more and more adorable, with a face that has eyes (complete with eyebrows and eyelashes) and ears in the right spots. What's more, those eyes are finally working! Yes, it's true: Your baby's eyes are making small side-to-side movements and can even perceive some light, though the eyelids are still sealed. Your baby is also becoming more sensitive to touch. In fact, he or she will even squirm if you poke your belly (though you probably won't be able to feel those squirms just yet).

Week 17 Take a look at your hand. Your baby is about palm-size now, with a crown-to-rump length of 5 inches and an approximate weight of 5 (or more) ounces. Body fat is beginning to form (baby's fat, that is, though yours is probably forming pretty quickly these days, too), but your little one is still quite skinny, with skin that is practically translucent. This week, your baby is all about practice, practice, practice in preparation for birth. One important skill your baby is sharpening now: sucking and swallowing—to get ready for that first (and second . . . and third) suckle at breast or bottle. Your baby's heart rate is regulated by the brain (no more spontaneous beats) and clocks in at 140 to 150 beats per minute (roughly twice your own heart rate).

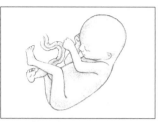

More Baby

For week-by-week pics of your baby's amazing development, go to whattoexpect.com.

What You May Be Feeling

As always, remember that every woman and every pregnancy is different. You may experience all of these symptoms at one time or another, or only a few of them. Some may have continued from last month; others may be new. Still others may be hardly noticed because you've become so used to them. You may also have other, less common, symptoms. Here's what you might experience this month:

Physically

- Fatigue

- Decreasing urinary frequency

- An end to, or a decrease in, nausea and vomiting (for a few women, morning sickness will continue; for a very few, it is just beginning)

- Constipation

- Heartburn, indigestion, flatulence, bloating

- Continued breast enlargement, but usually decreased tenderness

- Occasional headaches

- Occasional faintness or dizziness, particularly with sudden change of position

- Nasal congestion and occasional nosebleeds; ear stuffiness

- Sensitive gums that may bleed when you brush

- Increased appetite

- Mild swelling of ankles and feet, and occasionally of hands and face

- Varicose veins of legs and/or hemorrhoids

- Slight increase in vaginal discharge

- Fetal movement near the end of the month (but usually not this early, unless this is your second or subsequent pregnancy)

Emotionally

- Mood swings, which may include irritability, irrationality, inexplicable weepiness

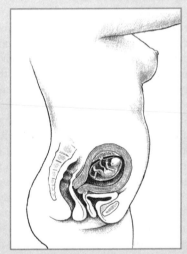

A Look Inside

Your uterus, now about the size of a small melon, has grown large enough to rise out of the pelvic cavity and by the end of the month, you'll be able to feel the top of it around 2 inches below your belly button (if you don't know what you're feeling for, ask your practitioner for some pointers at your next visit). If you haven't done so already, you'll probably begin to outgrow your regular clothes.

- Excitement and/or apprehension—if you have started to feel and look pregnant at last

- Frustration at being "in between"—your regular wardrobe doesn't fit anymore, but you're not looking

pregnant enough for maternity clothes

- A feeling you're not quite together—you're scattered, forgetful, drop things, have trouble concentrating

What You Can Expect at This Month's Checkup

This month, you can expect your practitioner to check the following, though there may be variations depending on your particular needs and on your practitioner's style of practice:

- Weight and blood pressure

- Urine, for sugar and protein

- Fetal heartbeat

- Size of uterus, by external palpation (feeling from the outside)

- Height of fundus (top of the uterus)

- Hands and feet for swelling, and legs for varicose veins

- Symptoms you've been experiencing, especially unusual ones

- Questions or problems you want to discuss—have a list ready

What You May Be Wondering About

Dental Problems

"My mouth has suddenly become a disaster area. My gums bleed every time I brush, and I think I have a cavity. Is it safe to have dental work done?"

Smile—you're pregnant! But with so much of your attention centered on your belly during pregnancy, it's easy to overlook your mouth—until it starts screaming for equal time, as frequently happens during pregnancy. For starters, pregnancy hormones aren't kind to your gums—which, like your other mucous membranes, become swollen, inflamed, and tend to bleed easily. Those same hormones also make the gums more sus-

ceptible to plaque and bacteria, which can soon make matters worse in some women, possibly leading to gingivitis (inflammation of the gums) and even tooth decay.

To keep your mouth happy—and your smile safe—while you're growing a baby:

- Floss and brush regularly, and use toothpaste with fluoride for cavity protection. Brushing your tongue while you're at it will also help combat bacteria while keeping your breath fresher.

- Ask your dentist to recommend a rinse to reduce bacteria and plaque, protecting your gums and your teeth.

A Gum Alert

If it's not one thing in pregnancy, it's another. If you notice a nodule on the side of your gum that bleeds when you brush, get it checked out. It's most likely a canker sore or something called a pyogenic granuloma (also known by the ominous-sounding term "pregnancy tumor," despite the fact that it's perfectly harmless). More of a nuisance than anything else, such nodules usually regress on their own after delivery, but if it becomes very annoying before that, it can be removed by a doctor or dentist.

- When you can't brush after eating, chew a stick of sugarless gum (the action of chewing increases the amount of saliva, which rinses the teeth—and if the gum's sweetened with xylitol, chewing can actually help prevent decay). Or nibble on a chunk of hard cheese (it decreases the acidity in your mouth, and it's the acid that causes tooth decay).

- Watch what you eat, particularly between meals. Save sweets (particularly sticky ones) for times when you can brush soon after. Consume plenty of foods high in vitamin C, which strengthens gums, reducing the possibility of bleeding. Also be sure to fill your calcium requirements daily.

Pearly White Wisdom

Wondering if you can use teeth-whitening products while you're pregnant? Check out page 147 for the latest facts.

Calcium is needed throughout life to keep teeth strong and healthy.

- Whether or not you're experiencing dental discomfort, be sure to make an appointment with your dentist at least once during the nine months for a checkup and cleaning, preferably earlier than later. The cleaning is important to remove plaque, which can not only increase the risk of cavities but also make your gum problems worse. If you've had gum problems in the past, also see your periodontist during your pregnancy.

If you suspect a cavity or other tooth or gum trouble, make an appointment with your dentist or periodontist right away. Untreated gingivitis can develop into a more serious gum condition, periodontitis, which has actually been associated with a variety of pregnancy complications. Decay that isn't cleaned up or other tooth issues that aren't tended to can also become a source of infection (and infection isn't good for you or your baby).

What happens if major dental work becomes necessary during pregnancy? Luckily, in most dental procedures, a local anesthetic will suffice, and that's safe. A low dose of nitrous oxide (laughing gas) is also safe to use after the first trimester, but more serious sedation should be avoided during pregnancy. In some cases, it may be necessary to take an antibiotic before or after major dental work; check with your practitioner.

Breathlessness

"Sometimes I feel a little breathless. Is this normal?"

Take a deep breath (if you can!) and relax. Mild breathlessness is normal, and many pregnant women experience it beginning in the second trimester.

Expecting X-Rays?

Routine dental X-rays (and other routine X-rays or CT scans) are usually postponed until after delivery, just to be on the extra-safe side. But if putting off dental (or other) X-rays during pregnancy just isn't a good idea (the risk of having one is outweighed by the risk of not having one), most practitioners will green-light the procedure. That's because the risks of X-rays during pregnancy are really very low and can be easily made even lower. Dental X-rays are targeted to your mouth, of course, which means the rays are directed far away from your uterus. What's more, a typical diagnostic X-ray of any kind rarely delivers more radiation than you'd get from spending a few days in the sun at the beach. Harm to a fetus, however, only occurs at very high doses, doses you're extremely unlikely to ever be exposed to. Still, if you do need an X-ray during pregnancy, keep the following guidelines in mind:

- Always inform the doctor ordering the X-ray and the technician performing it that you're pregnant, even if you're pretty sure they know.

- Have any necessary X-ray done in a licensed facility with well-trained technicians.

- The X-ray equipment should, when possible, be directed so that only the minimum area necessary is exposed to radiation. A lead apron should be used to shield your uterus and a thyroid collar should protect your neck.

- Follow the technician's directions precisely, being especially careful not to move while he or she is taking the picture, so retakes won't be needed.

Most important, if you had an X-ray before you found out you were pregnant, don't worry.

And, once again, you can blame your pregnancy hormones. Here's why: Those hormones stimulate the respiratory center to increase the frequency and depth of your breaths, giving you that out-of-breath feeling after nothing more strenuous than a trip to the bathroom. They also swell the capillaries in the body—including those of the respiratory tract—and relax the muscles of the lungs and bronchial tubes, making those breaths seem even harder to catch. Your uterus will also likely contribute to your breathlessness as pregnancy progresses, pushing up against your diaphragm as it grows, crowding your lungs and making it more difficult for them to expand fully.

Fortunately, though the mild breathlessness you're experiencing may make you feel uncomfortable, it doesn't affect your baby—who's kept well stocked with oxygen through the placenta. But if you're having a very hard time breathing, if your lips or fingertips seem to be turning bluish, or if you have chest pain and a rapid pulse, call your practitioner right away.

Nasal Stuffiness and Nosebleeds

"My nose has been stuffed up a lot, and sometimes it bleeds for no apparent reason. Is it pregnancy related?"

Your belly's not the only thing that's starting to swell these days. Thanks to the high levels of estrogen and progesterone circulating in your body, which bring with them increased blood flow, the mucous membranes of your nose start to swell, too, and soften (much as the cervix does in preparation for childbirth). Those membranes also produce more mucus than ever, with the intention of keeping infections and germs at bay. What's not so swell is the result—which your nose undoubtedly already knows: congestion, and possibly even nosebleeds. Also not so swell: The stuffiness may only get worse as your pregnancy progresses. You may develop postnasal drip, too, which in turn can occasionally cause coughing or gagging at night (as if you didn't have enough other things keeping you up—or enough gagging going on).

You can safely try saline sprays or nasal strips, especially if the congestion takes a turn for the truly uncomfortable. A humidifier in your room may also help overcome the dryness associated with any congestion. Medications or antihistamine nasal sprays are usually not prescribed during pregnancy, but do ask your practitioner what he or she recommends (some practitioners okay decongestants or steroid nasal sprays after the first trimester).

Taking an extra 250 mg of vitamin C (with your practitioner's okay), plus eating plenty of vitamin C–rich foods, may help strengthen your capillaries and reduce the chance of bleeding. Sometimes a nosebleed will follow overly energetic nose blowing, so easy does it.

To stem a nosebleed, sit or stand leaning slightly forward, rather than lying down or leaning backward. Using your thumb and forefinger, pinch the area just above your nostrils and below the bridge of your nose, and hold for five minutes; repeat if the bleeding contin-

ues. If the bleeding isn't controlled after three tries, or if the bleeding is frequent and heavy, call your practitioner.

Snoring

"My husband tells me that I've been snoring lately. Why is this happening?"

Snoring can disrupt a good night's sleep, for both the snorer and her bedmate, but it's usually not something to lose sleep over when you're expecting. Your nocturnal nasal symphony may simply be triggered by normal pregnancy stuffiness, in which case sleeping with a humidifier (or a nasal strip) on and with your head well elevated may help. Extra weight can also contribute to snoring, so make sure you aren't gaining too much.

Rarely, snoring can be a sign of sleep apnea, a condition in which breathing stops briefly during sleep. Since you're breathing for two, it's probably a good idea to mention your snoring to your practitioner at your next visit.

Snooze or Lose?

Are pregnancy hormones—or that growing belly—getting between you and a good night's sleep? Sleep problems are common in pregnancy, and while insomnia may be good preparation for the sleepless nights that lie ahead once your baby arrives, you're likely eager to catch some expectant z's. Before turning to over-the-counter (or prescribed) sleep aids, however, talk to your practitioner. He or she may have other suggestions to help summon the sandman. You can also read the tips on page 265 to help with your insomnia.

Allergies

"My allergies seem to have gotten worse since my pregnancy began. My nose is runny all the time."

Expectant noses are stuffy noses, so it's possible that you're mistaking the normal (though uncomfortable) congestion of pregnancy for allergies. But it's also possible that pregnancy has aggravated your allergies. Though some lucky expectant allergy sufferers (about a third) find a temporary respite from their symptoms during pregnancy, the less lucky (also about a third) find their symptoms get worse, and the rest (that final third) find their symptoms stay about the same. Since it sounds like you're among the less lucky, you're probably itching (and tearing and sneezing) for relief. But before you join the rest of the other allergy sufferers in the antihistamine aisle at the drugstore, check with your practitioner to see what you can safely pull off the shelf or have filled at the pharmacy. Some antihistamines and other medications are safe for use in pregnancy; others, which may or may not include your usual over-the-counter or prescription medication, may not be (though don't worry about any that you took before you knew you were pregnant).

Allergy shots are considered safe for pregnant women who have been on the receiving end of them for a while before they conceived. Most allergists say it's not a good idea to start allergy shots during pregnancy because they may cause unexpected reactions.

In general, however, the best approach to dealing with allergies in pregnancy is prevention—which can be worth a pound of tissues this season. Steering clear of what causes your allergies may also reduce the risk that your baby will develop allergies to those triggers.

No Peanuts for Your Little Peanut?

It's as American as the sandwich bread it's spread on—plus it makes a convenient and wholesome snack—but is peanut butter safe for the little peanut you're feeding in utero? It's long been known that moms (and much less so, dads) who have or have had allergies may pass allergic tendencies—though not necessarily the specific allergies—to their unborn child. Some research suggests that *allergic* mothers who eat highly allergenic foods (such as peanuts and dairy products) while they're nursing may be more likely to pass on allergies to those foods in their offspring. The good news for expectant peanut butter lovers (and those who like to wash their PB&J down with a glass of milk) is that the research on this connection during pregnancy has been inconclusive thus far. Still, if you have ever suffered from allergies, speak to your practitioner and an allergist about whether you should think about restricting your diet while you're pregnant and/or breastfeeding. If not, there's no need to skip the Skippy.

To ease the sneeze, try these tips:

- If pollens or other outdoor allergens trouble you, stay indoors in an air-conditioned and air-filtered environment as much as you can during your susceptible season. When you come indoors, wash your hands and face and change clothes to remove pollen. Outdoors, wear large curved sunglasses to keep pollens from floating into your eyes.

- If dust is a culprit, make sure someone else does the dusting and sweeping (how's that for a good excuse to get out of housecleaning?). A vacuum cleaner (especially one with a HEPA filter), a damp mop, or a damp cloth-covered broom kicks up less dust than an ordinary broom, and a microfiber cloth will do better than a traditional feather duster. Stay away from musty places like attics and libraries full of old books.

- If you're allergic to certain foods, stay away from them, even if they're good foods for pregnancy. Check out the Pregnancy Diet (Chapter 5) for substitutes.

- If animals bring on allergy attacks, let friends know of the problem in advance so that they can rid a room of both pets and their dander before you visit. And of course, if your own pet is suddenly triggering an allergic response, try to keep one or more areas in your home (particularly your bedroom) pet free.

- Tobacco smoke allergy is easier to control these days, since there are fewer smokers around, and fewer places where they can smoke. To ease your allergy, as well as for the benefit of your baby, avoid exposure to cigarette, pipe, and cigar smoke.

Vaginal Discharge

"I've noticed a slight vaginal discharge that's thin and whitish. Does this mean I have an infection?"

A thin, milky, mild-smelling discharge (known in the obstetrics business as leukorrhea) is normal throughout pregnancy. Its purpose is noble: to protect the birth canal from infection and maintain a healthy balance of bacteria in the

vagina. Unfortunately, in achieving its noble purpose, leukorrhea can make a mess of your underwear. Because it increases until term and may become quite heavy, some women are more comfortable wearing panty liners during the last months of pregnancy. Don't use tampons, which could introduce unwanted germs into the vagina.

Though it might offend your esthetic sensibilities (and possibly your partner's, during oral sex), and make you feel a little icky and sticky on occasion, this discharge is nothing to worry about. Keeping yourself clean, fresh, and dry will help, of course, but do not douche. Douching upsets the normal balance of microorganisms in the vagina and can lead to bacterial vaginosis (BV; see page 500). For information on vaginal infection and its symptoms, see page 499.

Elevated Blood Pressure

"My blood pressure was up a little bit at my last visit. Should I be worried?"

R elax. Worrying about your blood pressure will only send the readings higher. Besides, a slight increase at one visit is probably nothing to worry about. Maybe you were stressed because you were caught in traffic on the way to your appointment or because you had a pile of papers to finish back at work. Maybe you were just nervous—you were afraid you'd gained too much weight or not enough, or you had some strange symptoms to report, or you were anxious to hear the baby's heartbeat. Or maybe medical settings just make you edgy, giving you what is known as "white coat hypertension." An hour later, when you were relaxed, your pressure might very well have been perfectly normal. To make sure anxiety doesn't do a number on those numbers again, try to do some relaxation exercises (see page 142) while you're waiting for your next appointment—and, especially, while your blood pressure's being taken (think happy baby thoughts).

Even if your blood pressure remains slightly elevated at your next reading, such transient high blood pressure (which about 1 to 2 percent of women develop during pregnancy) is perfectly harmless and disappears after delivery (so you can still relax).

Most expectant mothers will see a slight drop in blood pressure readings during the second trimester as blood volume increases and the body starts working long hours to get that baby-making factory up to speed. But when you hit the third trimester, it usually begins to rise a bit. If it rises too much (if systolic pressure—the upper number—is 140 or more or the diastolic pressure—the lower number—is over 90) and stays up for at least two readings, your practitioner will monitor you more closely. That's because if such mildly elevated blood pressure is also accompanied by protein in the urine, swelling of the hands, ankles, and face, and/or sudden weight gain, it may turn out to be preeclampsia; see page 548.

Sugar in the Urine

"At my last office visit, the doctor said that there was sugar in my urine, but that it wasn't anything to worry about. Isn't it a sign of diabetes?"

Take your doctor's advice—don't stress. Your body is probably doing just what it's supposed to do: making sure that fetus of yours, which depends on you for its fuel supply, is getting enough glucose (sugar).

The hormone insulin regulates the level of glucose in your blood and

Get Your Flu Shots

The Centers for Disease Control and Prevention recommends that every woman who will be pregnant during flu season (generally October through April) be given the flu shot. The shot will not affect your baby and is unlikely to cause you any side effects. (The worst that can happen is you'll develop a mild fever and feel more tired than usual for a few days.) Ask if you can get the thimerosal-free (or reduced) vaccine, if available. Pregnant women should not get FluMist, the nasal spray flu vaccine. FluMist, unlike the flu shot, is made from live flu virus and could actually give you a mild case of the flu.

ensures that enough is taken in by your body cells for nourishment. Pregnancy triggers anti-insulin mechanisms to make sure enough sugar remains circulating in your bloodstream to nourish your fetus. It's a perfect idea that doesn't always work perfectly. Sometimes the anti-insulin effect is so strong that it leaves more than enough sugar in the blood to meet the needs of both mother and child—more than can be handled by the kidneys. The excess is "spilled" into the urine. Thus "sugar in the urine" is not uncommon in pregnancy, especially in the second trimester, when the anti-insulin effect increases. In fact, roughly half of all pregnant women show some sugar in the urine at some point in their pregnancies.

In most women, the body responds to an increase in blood sugar with an increased production of insulin, which usually eliminates the excess sugar by the next office visit. This may well be the case with you. But some women, especially those who are diabetic or have tendencies toward diabetes (because of a family history or because of their age or weight), may be unable to produce enough insulin at one time to handle the increase in blood sugar, or they may be unable to use the insulin they do produce efficiently. Either way, these women continue to show high levels of sugar in both blood and urine. In those who were not previously diabetic, this is known as gestational diabetes (see page 546).

You—like every pregnant woman—will be given a glucose screening test around the 28th week to check for gestational diabetes (those at higher risk may be screened earlier). Until then, don't give the sugar in your urine another thought.

Anemia

"A friend of mine became anemic during pregnancy—is that common?"

Iron-deficiency anemia is common during pregnancy—but it's also incredibly easy to prevent. And when it comes to prevention, your practitioner has your back. You were already tested for anemia at your first prenatal visit, though it's unlikely you were low on iron then. That's because iron stores are quickly replenished once those monthly periods stop.

As your pregnancy progresses and you hit the halfway mark (around 20 weeks, coming right up), your blood volume expands significantly and the amount of iron needed for producing red blood cells dramatically increases, depleting those stores once again. Fortunately, filling those stores up again—and effectively preventing anemia—is as easy as taking a daily iron

supplement (in addition to your prenatal vitamin), which your practitioner may prescribe starting midway through pregnancy. You should also pump up your diet by eating foods loaded with iron (though dietary sources, such as the ones listed on page 100, may not do the job alone, they provide a great backup for your supplement). For extra absorption, chase your iron down with vitamin C–rich foods (your morning OJ instead of your morning java, which will actually reduce the amount of iron absorbed).

Symptoms of Anemia

Pregnant women with mild iron deficiency rarely have symptoms. But as oxygen-carrying red blood cells are further depleted, an anemic mother-to-be becomes pale, extremely weak, easily tired or breathless, and might even experience fainting spells. This may be one of the few instances where fetal nutritional needs are met before Mom's, since babies are rarely iron deficient at birth.

Though all pregnant women are susceptible to iron-deficiency anemia, certain groups are at particularly high risk: those who have had several babies in quick succession, those who have been vomiting a lot or eating little because of morning sickness, and those who came to pregnancy undernourished (possibly because of an eating disorder) and/or have been eating poorly since they conceived. Daily iron supplementation, as prescribed by your practitioner, should prevent (or relieve) anemia.

Fetal Movement

"I haven't felt the baby moving yet; could something be wrong? Or could I just not be recognizing the kicking?"

Forget that positive pregnancy test, the early ultrasound, that expanding belly, or even the lub-dub of a baby's heartbeat. Nothing says you're pregnant like fetal movement.

That is, when you finally feel it. And you're sure you felt it. However, few expectant moms, particularly first timers, feel the first kick—or even the first flutter—in the fourth month. Though the embryo begins to make spontaneous movements by the seventh week, these movements, made by very tiny arms and legs, don't become apparent to mom until much later. That first momentous sensation of life, or "quickening," can occur anywhere between the 14th and 26th weeks, but generally closer to the average of the 18th to 22nd week. Variations on that average are common. A woman who's had a baby before is likely to recognize movement earlier (both because she knows what to expect and because her uterine and abdominal muscles are more lax, making it easier to feel a kick) than one who is expecting her first child. A very slender woman may notice very early, weak movements, whereas a woman who's sporting lots of padding on her belly may not be aware of movements until much later, when they've become more vigorous. The position of the placenta can also play a role: If it's facing front (an anterior placenta), it can muffle the movements and make the wait for those kicks weeks longer.

Sometimes, fetal movements aren't noticed when expected because of a miscalculated due date. Other times, mom doesn't recognize the movement when she feels it—or mistakes it for gas or other digestive gurgles.

So what do early movements feel like? They're almost as hard to describe as they are to recognize. Maybe it'll feel like a flutter (sort of like the "butterflies" you can get when you're nervous). Or a twitch. Or a nudge. Or even like the growling of hunger pangs. Maybe it'll feel like a bubble bursting—or that upside-down, inside-out sensation you get on a roller coaster. No matter what it feels like, it's bound to put a smile on your face—at least once you figure out for sure what it is.

Body Image

"I've always watched my weight—and now when I look in the mirror or step on a scale, I get so depressed. I look so fat."

When you've watched your weight your whole life, watching the numbers on the scale creep up can be unnerving—and maybe a little depressing, too. But it shouldn't be. If there's one place where thin is never in, it's in pregnancy. You're supposed to gain weight when you're pregnant. And there's an important difference between pounds added for self-indulgent reasons (just too many midnight dates with Ben and Jerry) and pounds gained for the best and most beautiful of reasons: your child and its support system growing inside you.

In the eyes of many beholders, a pregnant woman isn't just beautiful inside but outside as well. Many women and most spouses (and others who ogle) consider the rounded pregnant silhouette the most lovely—and sensuous—of feminine shapes. So instead of longing for the thin old days (you'll have them back soon enough), try getting on board with your expectant body. Embrace those new curves (which will become even more fun to embrace as they grow). Celebrate your new shape. Relish being rounder. Enjoy the pounds

A Pregnant Pose

If you've been dodging the camera lately ("no need to put yet another 10 pounds on me!"), consider striking a pregnant pose. Even if you may prefer to forget what you look like pregnant, your child-to-be will definitely relish seeing his or her first "baby" pictures one day—and so will you, eventually. To preserve your pregnant progress for posterity, have someone take a photo of your profile each month. Dress in something form-fitting (or belly-baring) for more dramatic documentation of your silhouette, and compile your photos in a pregnancy album or post them in an online photo gallery for easy sharing with family and friends, alongside the ultrasound shot, if you have one.

you pack on, instead of dreading them. As long as you're eating well and not exceeding the recommended guidelines for pregnancy weight gain, there's no reason to feel "fat"—just pregnant. The added inches you're seeing are all legitimate by-products of pregnancy and will disappear soon enough after the baby is born.

If you are exceeding the guidelines, feeling depressed about it won't keep you from getting fatter (and, if you're a typical estrogen producer, will only send you to the freezer for that vat of mint chocolate chip more often), but taking a good look at your eating habits might. Remember, the idea isn't to stop the weight gain (that's unsafe during pregnancy)—only to slow it down to the right rate if it's adding up a little too quickly. Instead of cutting back on the Pregnancy Diet requirements, just become more efficient in filling them

(a smoothie made with yogurt to fill a Calcium serving instead of a pint of ice cream).

Watching your weight gain isn't the only way to give your appearance an edge. Exercise will definitely help, too, by ensuring that the weight you do gain ends up in all the right places (more belly, less hips and thighs). Another workout plus: It'll give you a mood lift (it's hard to feel depressed when you've got an exercise-induced endorphin high going).

Being maternity fashion-forward can also help you make friends with your mirror. Instead of trying to squeeze into your civilian wardrobe (nothing flattering about the muffin-top look, especially when buttons keep popping), choose from the vast selection of creative maternity styles that accentuate the pregnant shape, rather than trying to hide it. You'll like your mirror image better, too, if you get a hairstyle that's slimming, pamper your complexion, and experiment with new makeup routines (the right techniques can take pounds off your pregnancy-rounded face; see page 149).

Maternity Clothes

"I can't squeeze into my jeans anymore, but I dread buying maternity clothes."

There's never been a more styling time to be pregnant. Gone are the days when pregnancy wardrobes were limited to tentlike muumuus intended to hide the expectant shape under yards and yards of polyester. Not only are today's maternity clothes a lot more fashion-forward and practical to wear, but they're designed to hug (and highlight) your beautiful baby-filled belly. Visit a nearby maternity store (or shop one online) and you'll likely be filled with excitement, instead of dread.

Looking Slim When You're Bulking Up

Big is beautiful when you're expecting, but that doesn't mean you can't try some tricks of the trim. With the right fashion choices, you can highlight your belly while slimming your overall silhouette. Here's how to show in all the right places:

Think black. And navy blue, chocolate brown, or charcoal. Dark colors are slimming, minimizing body bulk and giving you an overall trimmer appearance, even if you're wearing a T-shirt and yoga pants.

Think monotone. One color fits all—or at least looks slimmer. Sticking to a single hue (or to one color with slight variations) from top to bottom will make you look longer and leaner. A two-tone look, however, will create a break in your figure, causing the eye to stop right at the color change (and possibly right where your hips start spreading).

Think vertical. It's the oldest trick in the fashion book, but for good reason—it works. As you widen, choose clothes with vertical lines (which create height and give you a leaner look) instead of horizontal lines (which widen you even further). Look for clothes with vertical stripes, vertical zippers, vertical stitching, and vertical rows of buttons.

Focus on the pluses. Like those probably plus-size breasts of yours (there's never been a better time to spotlight your cleavage). And minimize attention to the spots that you might be less inclined to want to show off, such as those swollen ankles (keep them under pants or comfortable boots, or wear slimming black tights).

Stay fit. With your clothes, that is. While you'll definitely want clothes that have room to grow in the bust and the belly, look for tops—shirts, sweaters, jackets, and dresses—that fit you well in the shoulders (probably the only part of your body that won't be widening). Hanging shoulders will give you a sloppy (and bulky) look. And though clinging can be slimming, watch out for clothes that are so clingy they appear too tight, like you've outgrown them (which you probably have). The overstuffed sausage look is never in style, after all.

Here are some tips to consider when making your purchases:

- You still have a long way to grow. So don't set off on a whirlwind spending spree on the first day you can't button your jeans. Maternity clothes can be costly, especially when you consider the relatively short period of time they can be worn. So buy as you grow, and then buy only as much as you need (once you've checked what you can use that's already in your closet, you may end up needing a lot less than you'd figured). Though the pregnancy pillows available in try-on rooms in maternity stores can give a good indication of how things will fit later, they can't predict how you will carry (high, low, big, small) and which outfits will end up being the most comfortable when you crave comfort most.

- You're not limited to maternity clothes. If it fits, wear it, even if it isn't from the maternity department. Buying non-maternity clothing for maternity use (or using items you already own) is, of course, the best way of avoiding throwing away a fortune on clothes you'll only wear briefly. And depending on what the stores are showing in a particular season, anywhere from a few to many of the fashions on the regular racks may be suitable for pregnant shapes (though you may need to size up). Still, be wary of spending a lot on such purchases. Though you may love the clothes now, you may love them considerably less after you've worn them throughout your pregnancy. Plus, if you've bought them on the big side, they may not fit once you've shed your baby fat.

■ You've got it, so flaunt it. Bellies are out of the closet—and out from under those polyester pup tents. Many maternity fashions celebrate the pregnant belly, with clingy fabrics and styles. And that's something to celebrate, since belly-accentuating maternity wear actually slims your silhouette down, rather than bulking you up. Another great option: low-cut jeans and pants that can be worn under your belly. A low cut's also elongating (and what expectant mom couldn't use a little elongating?).

■ Don't overlook those accessories the public never sees. A well-fitting, supportive bra should be your bosom buddy during pregnancy, especially as that bosom expands . . . and expands. Skip the sale racks and put yourself in the hands of an experienced fitter at a well-stocked lingerie department or shop. With any luck, she will be able to tell you approximately how much extra room and support you need and which kind of bra will provide it. But don't stock up. Buy just a couple (one to wear and one to wash), and then go back for another fitting when you start growing out of them.

Special maternity underwear isn't usually necessary, but if you do decide to go that route, you'll probably be relieved to find that it's a lot sexier than it used to be (good-bye granny panties, hello thongs and bikinis). You can also opt for regular bikini panties—bought in a larger-than-usual size if you need the room—worn under your belly. Buy them in favorite colors and/or sexy fabrics to give your spirits a lift (but make sure the crotches are cotton).

■ Dip into your partner's drawers. It's all there for the taking (though it's probably a good idea to ask first): oversize T-shirts and regular shirts that look great over pants or leggings, sweatpants that accommodate more inches than yours do, running shorts that will keep up with your waistline for at least a couple more months, belts with the few extra notches you need. Keep in mind, though, that by the sixth month (possibly a lot sooner), no matter how big your man is, you're likely to outgrow him and his clothes.

■ Both a borrower and a lender be. Accept all offers of used maternity clothes, as long as they fit. In a pinch, any extra dress, skirt, or pair of jeans may do—you can make any borrowed item more "yours" with accessories (a fabulous scarf or a flashy pair of sneakers, for example). When your term is over, offer to lend those maternity outfits you bought and can't or don't want to wear postpartum to newly pregnant friends; between you and your friends, you'll be getting your money's worth from your maternity clothes.

■ Cool is hot. Hot stuff (fabrics that don't breathe, such as nylon and other synthetics) isn't so hot when you're pregnant. Because your metabolic rate is higher than usual, making you warmer, you'll feel more comfortable in cottons. You'll also be less likely to get heat rash (a common complaint among the pregnant set). Knee-highs or thigh-highs will also be more comfortable than pantyhose, but avoid those that have a narrow constrictive band at the top. Light colors, mesh weaves, and looser fits will also help you keep your cool in warm weather. When the weather turns cold, dressing in layers is ideal, since you can selectively peel off as you heat up or when you go indoors.

Pre-Baby Jitters

"Now that my abdomen is swelling, the fact that I'm really pregnant has finally sunk in. Even though we planned this pregnancy, we suddenly feel scared."

Sounds like you've got a little case of the pre-baby jitters—which, you'll be relieved to hear, many parents-to-be come down with at some point in their pregnancies. Even the most eager of expectant couples may find themselves with second thoughts once pregnancy starts to become a reality—and that isn't so surprising when you think about it. After all, a little person you haven't even met yet is already turning your lives upside down, making unexpected demands on you, both physically and emotionally. Every aspect of your lifestyle—from how you spend your evenings and your money to what you eat and drink to how often (and how) you make love—may already be changing, with plenty more changes on the postpartum horizon.

Not only is the prenatal ambivalence you're confronting completely understandable and extremely common, it's really pretty healthy. Facing it now gives you a chance to work out these feelings—and adjust to these major life changes—before baby arrives. The best way to do this is to talk it all out, both with each other and with friends who've already made the transition to parenthood (and will be able to offer you a reassuring perspective).

Without a doubt, becoming a parent is a life-changing experience—in other words, your life will never be the same. But as any parent will tell you—and as you'll soon find out for yourselves—it's a life-changing experience that's likely to bring a change for the better. Or even more likely, the best.

Unwanted Advice

"Now that it's obvious I'm expecting, everyone—from my mother-in-law to strangers on the elevator—has advice for me. It drives me crazy."

There's just something about a bulging belly that brings out the so-called expert in everyone, and that brings down social barriers that usually keep strangers minding their own business. Take your morning jog around the park and someone is sure to chide, "You shouldn't be running in your condition!" Lug home two bags of groceries from the supermarket and you're bound to hear, "Do you think you ought to be carrying that?" Double dip at the ice cream parlor, and expect the fingers to start wagging: "That baby fat's not going to be easy to lose, honey."

Between the pregnancy police, the gratuitous advice-givers, and all those inevitable predictions about the sex of the baby, what's an expectant mother to do? First of all, keep in mind that most of what you hear is probably nonsense. Old wives' tales that do have foundation in fact have been scientifically substantiated and have become part of standard medical practice. Those that do not might still be tightly woven into pregnancy mythology but can be confidently dismissed. Those recommendations that leave you with a nagging doubt ("What if they're right?") are best checked out with your doctor, midwife, or childbirth educator.

Whether it's possibly plausible or obviously ridiculous, however, don't let unwanted advice get you going—who needs the added stress anyway? Instead, keep your sense of humor handy and take one of two approaches: Politely inform the well-meaning stranger, friend, or relative that you have a trusted practitioner who counsels you on your pregnancy and that, even though you appreciate the thought, you can't accept advice from anyone else. Or, just as politely, smile, say thank you, and go on your way, letting their comments go in one ear and out the other—without making any stops in between.

But no matter how you choose to handle unwanted advice, you might also want to get used to it. If there's anyone who attracts a crowd of advice-givers faster than a woman with a belly, it's a woman with a new baby.

Unwanted Belly Touching

"Now that my pregnant belly is showing, friends, colleagues, even strangers come up to me and touch it—without even asking. I'm uncomfortable with that."

They're round, they're cute, and they're filled with something even cuter. Let's face it, pregnant bellies just scream out to be touched. Still, touching a pregnant belly may be an irresistible impulse, but it's also an inappropriate one—particularly without the owner's permission.

Some women don't mind being the center of so much touching attention; others actually enjoy it. But if all this uninvited rubbing is rubbing you the wrong way, don't hesitate to say so. You can do this bluntly (though politely): "I know you find my belly tempting to touch, but I'd really rather you didn't."

Or a playful "No touching, please—the baby's sleeping!" can discourage those uninvited advances. Or you can try a little belly turning, rubbing the rubber right back (patting someone's potbelly might make him or her think twice next time before reaching out and touching another pregnant belly without permission). Or make your statement without saying a word: Cross your arms protectively over your belly, or take the rubber's hand off your midsection and place it somewhere else (like on his or her own belly).

Forgetfulness

"Last week I left the house without my wallet; this morning I completely forgot an important business meeting. I can't focus on anything, and I'm beginning to think I'm losing my mind."

You're in good (forgetful) company. Many pregnant women begin to feel that as they're gaining pounds, they're losing brain cells. Even women who pride themselves on their organizational skills, their capacity to cope with complicated issues, and their ability to maintain their composure suddenly find themselves forgetting appointments, having trouble concentrating, and losing their cool (along with their wallets and cell phones). And it's not in their heads—it's in their brains. Researchers have found that a woman's brain-cell volume actually decreases during pregnancy (which could explain why you won't remember what you just read about in that last paragraph). And—for reasons unknown—women pregnant with girls are more forgetful, on average, than those carrying boys (who would have guessed?). Fortunately, the pregnancy brain fog (similar to what many women experience premenstrually, only thicker) is only temporary. Your brain will plump back up a few months after delivery.

Like numerous other symptoms, forgetfulness is caused by the hormonal changes of pregnancy. Sleep deprivation can also play a role (the less you sleep, the less you remember), as can the fact that you're constantly zapped of energy—energy your brain needs to stay focused. Also contributing to your scatterbrained self: the mother-to-be mind overload that's keeping all brain circuits busy contemplating nursery colors and negotiating baby names.

Feeling stressed about this intellectual fogginess will only make it worse (stress also compounds forgetfulness). Recognizing that it is normal (and not imagined), even accepting it with a sense of humor, may help to ease it—or, at least, make you feel better about it. Realistically, it might just not be possible to be as efficient as you were before you took on the added job of baby making. Keeping written checklists at home and at work can help contain the mental chaos. So can setting reminders (to show up for that meeting, to call your dad on his birthday) on your phone and computer, and recording important information on a PDA, if you have one (and can remember where you put it). Strategically placed Post-its (one on the front door to remind you to take your keys so you don't lock yourself out, for instance) can also help keep you on track.

Although ginkgo biloba has been touted for its memory-boosting properties, it is not considered safe for use during pregnancy, so you'll have to forget about using this and any other herbal preparation in your battle against pregnancy-induced forgetfulness.

And you might as well get used to working at a little below peak efficiency. The fog may well continue after your baby's arrival (due to fatigue, not hormones) and perhaps may not lift completely until baby (and you) start sleeping through the night.

Exercise During Pregnancy

You're aching and you can't sleep and your back is killing you and your ankles are swelling and you're constipated and bloated and you're passing more gas than a busload of high school football players. In other words, you're pregnant. Now if only there were something you could do that might minimize the aches and pains and unpleasant side effects of pregnancy.

Actually, there is, and it'll take just minutes (make that 30 minutes) a day: exercise. Thought pregnancy was a time to take it easy? Not anymore. Lucky for you (or unlucky, if you're a member of the couch potato club), the official advice of ACOG reads like a personal trainer's pep talk: Women with normal pregnancies should get 30 minutes or more a day of moderate exercise on most (if not all) days.

More women than ever are taking that advice, making fitness a part of their daily—or almost daily—routine. And barring any red light from your practitioner, you can, too. It doesn't matter whether you started out as an iron woman in peak physical condition or a sofa slacker who hasn't laced up sneakers since your last high school gym class (except as a fashion statement). There are plenty of health perks to exercising for two.

The Benefits of Exercise

So what's in it for you? Regular exercise can help:

- Your stamina. It seems paradoxical, but sometimes getting too much rest can actually make you feel more tired. A little exercise can go a long way when it comes to giving your energy level the boost it needs.

- Your sleep. Many pregnant women have a hard time falling asleep (not to mention staying asleep), but those who exercise consistently often sleep better and wake up feeling more rested.

- Your health. Exercise may prevent gestational diabetes, a growing problem among pregnant women.

- Your mood. Exercise causes your brain to release endorphins, those feel-good chemicals that give you a

Working in Workouts

Your mission when it comes to exercise during pregnancy, should you choose to accept it (and there are lots of reasons why you should), is to work your way up to 30 minutes of some sort of activity a day. And if that sounds daunting, keep in mind that three 10-minute walks sprinkled throughout the day are just as beneficial as 30 minutes on the treadmill. And even non-exercise activity—like 15 minutes of vacuuming and 15 minutes of light yard work—counts toward your daily goal. (See, it's not as hard as it sounds.)

Still not convinced that you have the time? To make your mission possible, try thinking of exercise as part of your day—like brushing your teeth and going to work—and build it into your routine (that's how it becomes routine, after all).

If there's no place in your schedule to block out gym time, just incorporate exercise into your daily activities: Get off the bus two stops from the office, and walk the rest of the way. Park your car in a faraway spot at the mall instead of cruising for the closest (and while you're at the mall, take a few extra laps around—those count, too). Take a brisk walk to the deli instead of ordering in your sandwich. Use the stairs instead of the elevator. Walk up the escalator instead of going along for the ride. Visit the ladies' room at the far end of your office instead of the one across the hall.

Have the time but lack the motivation? Find it in a pregnancy exercise class (the camaraderie will help cheer you on) or by exercising with a friend (form a lunchtime walking club or hit the hiking trails with your buds on Saturdays before your weekly brunch). Just plain bored with your workouts? Switch it up—try pregnancy yoga if you're tired (literally) of running, or swimming (or water aerobics) if the stationary cycle is getting you nowhere. Find your exercise excitement in a pregnancy DVD workout.

Sure, there'll be days (especially in those fatigue-prone first and third trimesters), when you're too pooped to lift your legs off the coffee table, never mind actually do leg lifts. But there's never been a better time, or better reasons, to get yourself moving.

natural high—improving your mood, diminishing stress and anxiety.

- **Your back.** A strong set of abs is the best defense against back pain, which plagues many pregnant women. But even exercise that's not directly targeting the tummy can also relieve back pain and pressure.

- **Your (tense) muscles.** Stretching does your body good—especially a pregnant body, which is more prone to muscle cramps in the legs (and elsewhere). Stretching can help you uncover little pockets of tension, warding off sore muscles. Plus you can do it anywhere, anytime—even if you spend most of your day sitting down—and you don't even have to break a sweat.

- **Your bowels.** An active body encourages active bowels. Even a 10-minute stroll helps get things going.

- **Your labor.** Though exercise during pregnancy can't guarantee that you'll race through childbirth, moms who exercise tend to have shorter labors and are less likely to need labor and delivery interventions (including C-sections).

- **Your postpartum recovery.** The more fit you stay during pregnancy, the faster you'll recover physically after childbirth (and the sooner you'll be zipping up those prepregnancy jeans again).

What's in it for baby? Plenty. Researchers theorize that changes in heart rate and oxygen levels in exercising moms-to-be stimulate their babies. Babies are also stimulated by the sounds and vibrations they experience in the womb during workouts. Exercise regularly during pregnancy, and your baby might end up being:

Can You Kegel?

If you do only one exercise during your pregnancy, make it this one. Kegels help strengthen your pelvic floor (the muscle group that controls the flow of urine and the contraction of the vagina and anal sphincter). One of the many benefits of doing your Kegels is that they prevent urinary incontinence, a pretty common complaint late in pregnancy and during postpartum—as well as fecal incontinence, which, though less common, can be even more uncomfortable and embarrassing. They can also tone your pelvic floor in preparation for labor and delivery—and possibly help you avoid an episiotomy or a tear. Finally, flexing your pelvic muscles through Kegels can improve sexual satisfaction postpartum, when those muscles will need some tightening up. For more about Kegels and instructions on how to flex those amazing muscles, see page 295.

- **More fit.** Babies of moms who exercise during pregnancy are born at healthier weights, are better able to weather labor and delivery (they're less stressed by it), and recover from the stresses of birth more quickly.

- **Smarter.** Believe it or not, research shows that babies of moms who exercise throughout pregnancy score higher, on average, on general intelligence tests by age 5 (meaning that your workout may boost both your muscle power and baby's brain power!).

- **Easier.** Babies of pregnant exercisers tend to sleep through the night sooner, are less prone to colic, and are better able to soothe themselves.

Exercise Smarts

Exercising with a baby on board? Remember to use your exercise smarts:

- Drink before you exercise. To avoid becoming dehydrated, have a drink before your workout—even if you're not thirsty (waiting until you're thirsty means you've waited too long). End your workout with a drink, also, to replenish the fluids you lost through sweat.

- Bring on the snacks. A light but sustaining before-workout snack will help keep your energy up. Follow up with a light snack, too, especially if you've burned a lot of calories.

- Stay cool. Any exercise or environment that raises a pregnant woman's temperature more than 1.5 degrees should be avoided (it causes blood to be shunted away from the uterus to the skin as the body attempts to cool off). So stay out of saunas, steam rooms, or hot tubs, and don't exercise outdoors in very hot or humid weather or indoors in a stuffy, overheated room (no Bikram yoga). If you generally walk outdoors, try an air-conditioned mall instead when the temperature soars.

- Dress for exercise success. Play it cool by wearing loose, breathable, stretchable clothes. Choose a bra that provides plenty of support for your larger-than-life breasts but that doesn't pinch once you get moving (a sports bra can be a great addition to your maternity wardrobe).

- Put your feet first. If your sneakers are showing their age, replace them now to minimize your chances of injury or falls. And make sure you choose workout shoes that are designed for the sport you're pursuing.

- Select the right surface. Indoors, a wood floor or a tightly carpeted sur-

Exercising the Right Way When You're Expecting

Not only does your pregnant body not fit into your regular workout clothes anymore, it also may not fit into your regular workout routine. Now that you're exercising for two, you'll need to make doubly sure you're exercising the right way. Here are some pointers, whether you're a gym junkie or a Sunday stroller:

The starting line is the practitioner's office. Before you lace up your sneaks and hit the aerobics class, make a pit stop at your practitioner's office for the green light. It's highly likely you'll get it—most women do. But if you have any medical or pregnancy complications, your practitioner may limit your exercise program, nix it entirely, or—if you have gestational diabetes—even encourage you to be a little more active. Be sure you're clear about what exercise programs are appropriate for you and whether your normal fitness routine (if you have one) is safe to continue when you're expecting. If you're in good health, your practitioner will likely encourage you to stick with your regular routine as long as you feel up to it, with certain modifications (especially if your regular routine includes pregnancy-taboo sports, like ice hockey).

face is better than tile or concrete for your workouts. (If the surface is slippery, don't exercise in socks or footed tights.) Outdoors, soft running tracks and grassy or dirt trails are better than hard-surfaced roads or sidewalks; level surfaces are better than uneven ones.

■ **Stay off the slopes.** Because your growing abdomen will affect your sense of balance, ACOG suggests women in the latter part of pregnancy avoid sports that come with a higher risk of falling or abdominal injury. These include gymnastics, downhill skiing, ice-skating, vigorous racquet sports (play doubles instead of singles), and horseback riding, as well as cycling and contact sports such as ice hockey, soccer, or basketball (see page 224 for more).

■ **Stay on the level.** Unless you're living at high altitudes, avoid any activity that takes you up more than 6,000 feet. On the flip(per) side, scuba diving, which poses a risk of decompression sickness for your baby, is also off-limits, so you'll have to wait until you're no longer carrying a passenger to take your next dive.

■ **Stay off your back.** After the fourth month, don't exercise flat on your back. The weight of your enlarging uterus could compress major blood vessels, restricting circulation.

■ **Avoid risky moves.** Pointing, or extending, your toes—at any time in pregnancy—could lead to cramping in your calves. Flex your feet instead, turning them up toward your face. Full sit-ups or double leg lifts pull on the abdomen, so they're probably not a good idea when you've got a baby on board. Also avoid any activity that requires "bridging" (bending over backward) or other contortions, or that involves deep flexion or extension of joints (such as deep knee bends), jumping, bouncing, sudden changes in direction, or jerky motions.

Respect your body as it changes. Expect your routines to change as your body does. You'll need to modify your workouts as your sense of balance shifts, and you'll probably also have to slow down to avoid taking a spill (especially once you can no longer see your feet). Also expect workouts to seem different, even if you've been doing a particular routine for years. If you're a walker, for example, you'll feel more pressure on your hips and knees as your pregnancy progresses and as your joints and ligaments loosen. You'll also have to accommodate your pregnant body by avoiding any exercise that requires you to lie flat on your back or stand without moving (like some yoga and tai chi poses do) after the first trimester. Both can restrict your blood flow.

Start slow. If you're new at this, start slowly. It's tempting to start off with a bang, running 3 miles the first morning or working out twice the first afternoon. But such enthusiastic beginnings usually lead not to fitness but to sore muscles, sagging resolve—and abrupt endings. Start the first day with 10 minutes of warm-ups followed by 5 minutes of a more strenuous workout (but stop sooner if you begin to tire) and a 5-minute cool-down. After a few days, if your body has adjusted well, increase the period of strenuous activity by about 5 minutes until you are

Thirty Minutes Plus?

Is more (exercise) more—or less? That depends. If you're really ambitious (or just really fit), and you've been green-lighted by your practitioner (based on your fitness level), it's safe to work out for up to an hour or even more, as long as you listen to your body. Moms-to-be tend to fatigue sooner than they used to, and tired bodies are more apt to injure themselves. Plus, overexertion could lead to other problems (dehydration, for one, if you don't take in enough fluids; for another, lack of oxygen to the baby if you're short of breath for long periods). Burning more calories during your marathon sessions also means you'll need to take in more, so be sure to compensate appropriately (the best part of a workout, wouldn't you say?).

up to 30 minutes or more, if you feel comfortable.

Of course, if you're already a gym rat, remember that while pregnancy is a great time to maintain your fitness level, it's not a time to increase it (you can set new personal bests after baby is on the scene).

Get off to a slow start every time you start. Warm-ups can be tedious when you're eager to get your workout started—and over with. But as every athlete knows, they're an essential part of any exercise program. They ensure that the heart and circulation aren't taxed suddenly and reduce the chances of injury to muscles and joints, which are more vulnerable when cold—and particularly during pregnancy. So walk before you run; swim slowly or jog in place in the pool before you start your laps.

Finish as slowly as you start. Collapse may seem like the logical conclusion to a workout, but it isn't physiologically sound. Stopping abruptly traps blood in the muscles, reducing blood supply to other parts of your body and to your baby. Dizziness, faintness, extra heartbeats, or nausea may result. So finish your exercise with exercise: about 5 minutes of walking after running, easy paddling after a vigorous swim, light stretching exercises after almost any activity. Top off your cool-down with a few minutes of relaxation. You can help avoid dizziness (and a possible fall) if you get up slowly when you've been exercising on the floor.

Watch the clock. Too little exercise won't be effective; too much can be debilitating. A full workout, from warm-up to cool-down, can take anywhere from 30 minutes to an hour. But keep the level of exertion mild to moderate.

Divide and conquer your workout. Can't find time in your day for a 30-minute workout? Divide your exercise schedule into two, three, or even four shorter ones. Not only will any combo that adds up to 30 minutes do the trick, this can tone muscles more effectively.

Keep it up. Exercising erratically (four times one week and none the next) won't get you in shape. Exercising regularly (three or four times a week, every week) will. If you're too tired for a strenuous workout, don't push yourself, but do try to do the warm-ups so that your muscles will stay limber and your discipline won't dissolve. Many women find they feel better if they do some exercise—if not necessarily their full workout—every day.

Compensate for the calories you burn. Perhaps the most fun part of a pregnancy exercise program is the extra eating you'll have to do. You'll have to

Shoulder and Leg Stretches

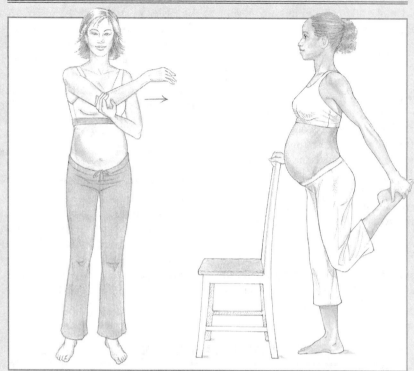

▲ **Shoulder stretch.** To ease tension in your shoulders (especially good if you spend a lot of time at the computer), try this simple move: Stand with your feet shoulder-width apart and knees slightly bent. Bring your left arm out in front of you at chest height and bend it slightly. Take your right hand, place it on your left elbow, and then gently pull your left elbow toward your right shoulder as you exhale. Hold the stretch for 5 to 10 seconds, then switch sides.

▲ **Standing leg stretch.** Give your legs a much-needed break with this easy stretch: Stand and hold on to a countertop, the back of a heavy chair, or another sturdy object for support. Bend your right knee and bring your right foot back and up toward your buttocks. Grasp your foot with your right hand and bring your heel toward your buttocks while extending your thigh backward from the hip joint. Keep your back straight and hold the stretch for 10 to 30 seconds. Repeat with the left leg.

consume about 150 to 200 additional calories for every half hour of moderate exercising. If you believe you're consuming enough calories but you still are not gaining weight, you may be exercising too much.

Replace the fluids you use up. For every half hour of moderate activity, you will need at least a full glass of extra liquid to compensate for fluids lost through perspiration. You will need more in warm weather, or whenever you're sweating a lot: Drink before, during, and after exercising—but no more than 16 ounces at a time. It's a good idea to start your fluid intake 30 to 45 minutes before your planned workout.

Choose the right group. If you prefer a group approach to exercise, take an exercise class that is specifically designed for pregnant women (ask for the instructor's credentials before enrolling). For some women, classes are better than solo exercising (particularly when self-discipline is lacking) and provide support and feedback. The best programs maintain moderate intensity, meet at least three times weekly, individualize to each woman's capabilities, and have a network of medical and exercise specialists available for questions.

Make it fun. Any workout, group or otherwise, should be an experience you look forward to rather than dread, one you think of as fun, not as torture. If you choose something you like doing, it'll be easier to stick with—particularly on days when you have no energy, feel the size of an SUV, or both. Some women find it helpful to pick a workout with a social component, from a prenatal yoga class to a romantic after-dinner walk. Exercising with a mate or a pal, incidentally, increases the odds of sticking with a program. So instead of meeting a friend for a coffee and scone, meet for a walk.

Do everything in moderation. Never exercise to the point of exhaustion, especially when you're pregnant. (Even if you're a trained athlete, don't exercise to your fullest capacity, whether it exhausts you or not.) There are several ways of checking to see whether you're overdoing it. First, if it feels good, it's probably

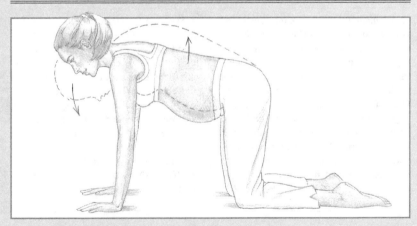

Dromedary Droop

A great way to relieve back pressure (your constant companion these days) is to get down on your hands and knees and relax your back, keeping your head straight and making sure your neck is lined up with your spine. Then arch your back—you'll feel your abs and buttocks tighten. Let your head gently droop down. Slowly return to your original position. Repeat several times—and do several times a day if you can, especially if you're standing or sitting a lot on the job.

Neck Relaxer

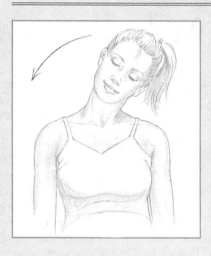

This exercise will ease tension in your neck. Sit up straight in a supportive chair. Close your eyes and breathe deeply, then gently tilt your head to one side and let it slowly drop toward your shoulder. Don't raise your shoulder to meet your head, and don't force your head down. Hold for 3 to 6 seconds, then switch sides. Repeat three or four times. Gently bring your head forward, letting your chin relax into your chest. Roll your cheek to the right toward your shoulder (again, don't force the motion, and don't move your shoulder toward your head) and hold for 3 to 6 seconds. Switch sides and repeat. Do three or four sets per day.

okay. If there's any pain or strain, it's not. A little perspiration is fine; a drenching sweat is a sign to slow down. So is being unable to carry on a conversation as you go. Work hard enough so you feel yourself breathing more heavily, but never be so out of breath that you aren't able to talk, sing, or whistle while you work(out). Needing a nap after completing a workout means you've worked too hard. You should feel exhilarated, not drained, after exercising.

Know when to stop. Your body will signal when it's time by saying, "Hey, I'm tired." Take the hint right away, and throw in the towel. More serious signals suggest a call to your practitioner: pain anywhere (hip, back, pelvis, chest, head, and so on); a cramp or stitch that doesn't go away when you stop exercising; uterine contractions and chest pain; lightheadedness or dizziness; very rapid heartbeat; severe breathlessness; difficulty walking or loss of muscle control; sudden headache; increased swelling of your hands, feet, ankles, or face; amniotic fluid leakage or vaginal bleeding; or, after the 28th week, a slowing down or total absence of fetal movement. In the second and third trimesters, you may notice a gradual decrease in your performance and efficiency. This is normal and another signal to take it easier.

Taper off in the last trimester. Most women find that they need to slack off somewhat in the third trimester, particularly during the ninth month, when stretching routines and brisk walking or water workouts will probably provide enough exercise. If you feel up to sticking with a more vigorous program (and you're in excellent athletic shape), your practitioner may green-light your usual exercise agenda right up until delivery, but definitely ask first.

Even when you're not working out . . . don't just sit there. Sitting for an extended period without a break causes blood to pool in your leg veins, can cause your feet to swell, and could lead to other problems. If your work entails a lot of sitting, or if you watch TV for hours at a time or travel long distances frequently, be sure to break up every hour or so of sitting with 5 or 10 minutes of walking. And while at your seat, periodically do some exercises that enhance circulation, such as taking a few deep breaths, extending your lower legs, flexing your feet, and wiggling your toes. Also try contracting the muscles in your abdomen and buttocks (a sort of sitting pelvic tilt). If your hands tend to swell, periodically stretch your arms above your head, opening and closing your fists several times as you do.

Choosing the Right Pregnancy Exercise

While it's true that pregnancy isn't the time to learn to water-ski or enter a horse-jumping competition, you will still be able to enjoy most fitness activities—and use many of the machines at the gym (with a few caveats). You can select, too, from the growing number of exercise programs specifically designed for expecting moms (pregnancy water aerobics and prenatal yoga classes, for example). But be sure to ask your practitioner about what's okay and what's not when it comes to choosing an exercise program or sport. You'll probably find that most of the activities that are off-limits when you're expecting are ones you'd probably have a hard time doing well anyway once you have a basketball-size belly (like competitive basketball . . . or football or scuba diving or downhill racing or mountain biking). Here are the do's and don'ts of pregnancy workouts:

Walking. Just about anyone can do it— and do it just about anywhere, anytime.

Pelvic Tilt

This simple routine can help improve your posture, strengthen your abs, reduce back pain, and help prepare you for labor. To do a pelvic tilt, stand with your back against a wall and relax your spine. As you inhale, press the small of your back against the wall. Exhale; then repeat several times. For a variation that also helps reduce the pain of sciatica, try rocking your pelvis back and forth—keeping your back straight—while either kneeling on all fours or standing up. Do pelvic tilts regularly (take a 5-minute pelvic-tilt break several times during your workday).

Biceps Curl

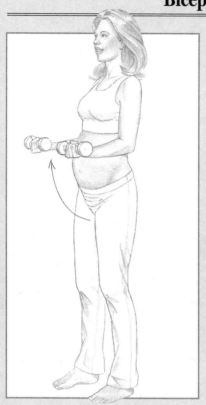

Start by selecting light weights (3- or 5-pound weights if you're a beginner, and never lift more than 12-pound weights). Stand with your legs shoulder-width apart, making sure not to lock your knees. Keep your elbows in and your chest up. Slowly raise both weights toward your shoulders by bending your elbows and keeping your arms in front of you (remember to breathe), stopping when your forearms are perpendicular to the floor and the weights are facing the ceiling. Lower slowly and repeat. Try to do 8 to 10 repetitions, but take breaks if needed and don't overdo it. You'll feel a burn in your muscles, but never strain or start holding your breath.

There's no easier exercise to fit into your busy schedule than walking (don't forget, all the walking you do counts, even if it's walking two blocks to the market or 10 minutes while the dog does its business). And you can continue to fit it in right up until delivery day (and even on delivery day if you're anxious to get those contractions moving along). Best of all, there's no equipment necessary—and no gym membership or classes to pay for, either. All you need is a supportive pair of sneakers and comfortable, breathable clothes. If you're just beginning a walking routine, go slowly at first (start out at a stroll before you move on to a brisk pace). Need some time for yourself? Walking alone can give you that quiet moment you crave. But if you'd rather have company along for the walk, stroll with your partner, friends, or colleagues. You can even start a walking club (in the morning with neighbors or at lunchtime with coworkers). Weather's not cooperative? Do the mall walk.

Jogging. Experienced runners can stay on track during pregnancy—but you may want to limit your distances and stick to level terrain or use a treadmill (if you weren't a runner prepregnancy, stick to walking for now). Keep in mind that loosening ligaments and joints during pregnancy can make running harder

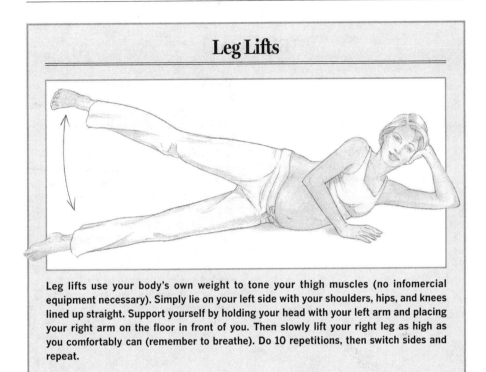

Leg Lifts

Leg lifts use your body's own weight to tone your thigh muscles (no infomercial equipment necessary). Simply lie on your left side with your shoulders, hips, and knees lined up straight. Support yourself by holding your head with your left arm and placing your right arm on the floor in front of you. Then slowly lift your right leg as high as you comfortably can (remember to breathe). Do 10 repetitions, then switch sides and repeat.

on your knees and also make you more prone to injury—yet another reason not to overdo it.

Exercise machines. Treadmills, ellipticals, and stair-climbers are all fine during pregnancy. Adjust the machines' speed, incline, and tension to a level that's comfortable for you (starting out slowly if you're a novice). During your last trimester, though, you may find a machine workout too strenuous. You may also have to be more conscious of avoiding stumbles on the machine when you're no longer able to see your feet.

Aerobics. Experienced athletes in good shape can continue dance and aerobic workouts during pregnancy. Tone down the intensity level, and never exert yourself to the point of exhaustion. If you're a beginner, choose low-impact aerobics or consider the water version, which is uniquely suited to the pregnant set.

Step routines. As long as you're already in good shape and have experience doing step routines, it's usually fine to continue them during much of your pregnancy. Just remember that your joints are more prone to injury when you're pregnant, so stretch out well beforehand and don't overexert yourself. And, of course, don't step on something too high off the ground. As your abdomen expands, avoid any activities that require careful balance.

Kickboxing. Kickboxing takes a great deal of grace and speed—two things pregnant women don't typically possess. Many pregnant kickboxers find they can't kick as high or move as quickly, but if you're still comfortable getting your exercise from getting your kicks, and you have plenty of experience (no novices now), it's okay to continue while you're expecting. Just be sure to avoid any movements that you have difficulty with or cause you to strain. Make sure you keep a safe distance from other kickboxers (you don't want to be kicked in the belly by accident) by leaving two leg lengths of space between you and those around you. Be sure, too, that everyone in the class knows you're pregnant, or look for pregnancy-specific classes (where everyone around you is pregnant—and far away).

Swimming and water workouts. You might not feel like slipping into a teeny bikini right now, but consider this: In the water, you weigh just a tenth of what you do on land (how often do you have the chance to be close to weightless these days?), making water workouts the perfect choice for a pregnant woman. Working out in the water boosts your strength and flexibility but is gentle on your joints—plus there's much less risk of overheating (unless the pool is overheated). What's more, many pregnant women report that water workouts help ease swelling in their legs and feet and relieve sciatic pain. Most gyms with a pool offer water aerobics, and many have classes specifically designed for expectant moms. Just be careful when walking on slippery poolsides, and don't dive. And stick to workouts in chlorinated pools.

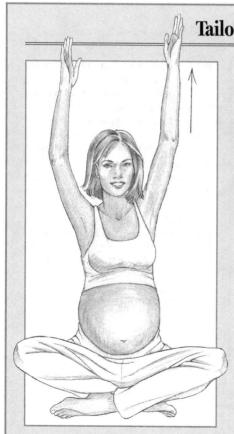

Tailor Stretch

Sitting cross-legged and stretching will help you relax and get in touch with your body (the more familiar you are with your body as you move into labor and delivery, the better). Experiment with different arm stretches while sitting—try placing your hands on your shoulders, then try reaching them over your head and stretching toward the ceiling. You can also alternate stretching one arm higher than the other or leaning to one side. (Do not bounce when stretching.)

Outdoor sports (hiking, skating, bicycling, skiing). Pregnancy isn't the time to take up a new sport—especially one that challenges your balance—but experienced athletes should be able to continue these activities (with their practitioner's approval and some precautions). When hiking, be sure to avoid uneven terrain (especially later on in pregnancy when it won't be easy to see that rock in your path), high altitudes, and slippery conditions (and of course, rock climbing is out). When biking, be extra careful—wear a helmet; don't ride on wet pavement, winding paths, or bumpy surfaces (falling is never a good idea but especially not when you're pregnant);

and don't lean forward into racing posture (it can tax your lower back, plus this isn't the time for racing; slow and steady should win all your races now). As for ice-skating, you can give it a whirl (and a figure eight) early in pregnancy if you're experienced and careful—later on, you'll probably face balance issues, so stop as soon as you get more bulky than graceful. Ditto for in-line skating and horseback riding. Avoid downhill skiing or snowboarding altogether, even if you've got years of double black diamonds under your belt; the risk of a serious fall is too great (after all, even pros take the occasional tumble). Cross-country skiing and snowshoeing are okay

Hip Flexors

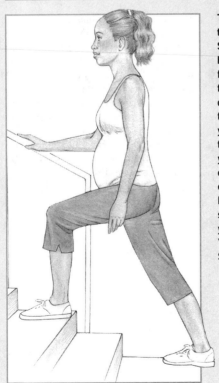

The hip flexor muscles are what allow you to lift your knees and bend at the waist. Stretching these muscles periodically will help keep you limber and make it easier for you to spread your legs when it's time for the baby to exit (not to mention during sex). To flex your flexors, stand at the bottom of a flight of stairs as though you were about to climb them. (Hang on to the railing with one hand for support if you need to.) Place one foot on the first or second stair up (whatever you can comfortably reach) and bend your knee. Keep your other leg behind you, knee straight, foot flat on the floor. Lean into your bent leg, keeping your back straight. You'll feel the stretch in your straight leg. Switch legs and repeat.

Squats

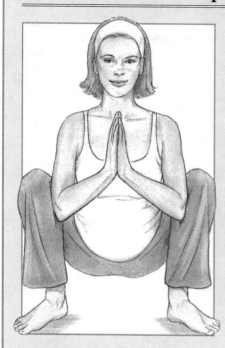

This exercise strengthens and tones your thighs and is particularly useful for women who plan to deliver in the squatting position. To begin, stand with your feet shoulder-width apart. Keeping your back straight, bend at the knees and slowly lower yourself as close to the ground as you comfortably can, keeping your feet flat on the floor. If you can't, try moving your feet farther apart. Hold the squat for 10 to 30 seconds, then slowly come back to a standing position. Repeat five times. (Note: Squats are fine, but avoid lunges and deep knee bends because your joints will be more prone to injury.)

for the experienced during pregnancy, but you'll have to be extra careful to avoid falling. And, of course, no matter what activity's taking you outdoors (or to the indoor rink), make sure you don't work out to the point of exhaustion.

Weight training. Using weights can increase your muscle tone, but it's important to avoid heavy weights or those that require grunting or breath holding, which may compromise blood flow to the uterus. Use light weights with multiple repetitions instead.

Yoga. Yoga encourages relaxation, focus, and paying attention to your breathing—so it's just about perfect for pregnancy (and great preparation for childbirth, as well as for parenting). It also increases oxygenation (bringing more oxygen to the baby) and increases flexibility, mak-

ing pregnancy—and delivery—easier. Select a class that's specifically tailored to expectant women or ask your instructor how to modify poses so that they're safe for you. For instance, you won't be able to exercise on your back after the fourth month, and your center of gravity changes with pregnancy, so you'll have to adjust your favorite poses accordingly. One important caveat: Avoid Bikram yoga. It's done in a hot room (one that's generally 90°F to 100°F), and you need to pass on any exercises that heat you up too much.

Pilates. Pilates is similar to yoga in that it's a low- to no-impact discipline that improves your flexibility, strength, and muscle tone. The focus is on strengthening your core, which will improve your posture and ease backaches. Look for

Waist Twists

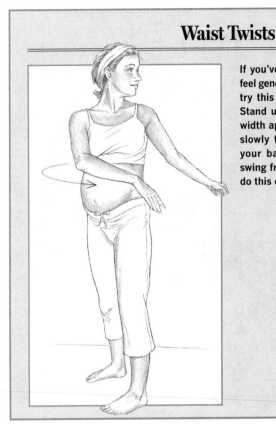

If you've been sitting for a while or just feel generally tensed up or uncomfortable, try this easy circulation-boosting move. Stand up and place your feet shoulder-width apart. Twist gently from the waist, slowly turning from side to side. Keep your back straight and let your arms swing freely. Can't get up? You can even do this exercise while you're sitting.

a class specifically tailored to pregnant women, or let your instructor know that you're expecting so you can avoid pregnancy-inappropriate moves (including those that overstretch).

Tai chi. An ancient form of meditative exercises, tai chi's basic slow movements allow even the stiffest person the opportunity to relax and strengthen the body without the risk of injury. If you're comfortable with it and have plenty of experience, it's fine to continue tai chi when you're expecting. Look for pregnancy-specific classes, or only do moves that you can easily complete—take care with the balancing poses.

Breathing. Believe it or not, you even get exercise credit for breathing—at least, if you do it right. Deep breathing is relaxing, improves body awareness, and allows for better oxygen intake than the shallow chest breaths most people take. Here's how to do it: Sit up straight and place your hands on your belly. Feel it rise and fall as you inhale (through your nose, unless it's too stuffy) and exhale (out your mouth). Concentrate on your

Exercise in Bed

Have you been sent to bed (rest)? Not only will continuing to flex your muscles (in a modified way) be possible, it'll be extra important. See page 571 for more.

breathing by counting: As you inhale, count to 4; as you exhale, count to 6. Try taking a few minutes each day to focus on breathing deeply.

If You Don't Exercise

Exercising during pregnancy can certainly do the average pregnant body good. But sitting it out (whether by choice or on practitioner's orders) and getting most of your exercise from opening and closing your car door won't hurt, either. In fact, if you're abstaining from exercise on practitioner's orders, you're helping your baby and yourself. Your practitioner will almost certainly restrict exercise if you have a history of miscarriages or of premature labor, or if you

have an incompetent cervix, bleeding or persistent spotting in the second or third trimester, heart disease, or a diagnosis of placenta previa or preeclampsia. Your activity may also be limited if you're expecting multiples; have high blood pressure, thyroid disease, anemia or other blood disorders, or a fetus that isn't thriving; are seriously over- or underweight; or have had an extremely sedentary lifestyle up until now. A history of precipitous (very brief) labor or of a fetus that didn't thrive in a previous pregnancy might also be a reason for a red light (or at least a yellow one) on exercise. In some cases, arm-only exercises or water workouts designed for pregnancy may be okayed when other exercises are taboo. Check with your practitioner for your pregnancy exercise protocol.

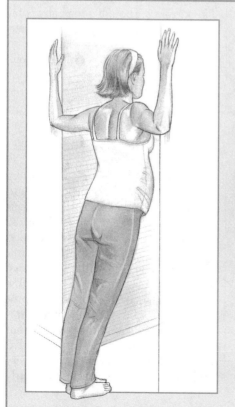

Chest Stretches

Pregnancy changes your posture and center of gravity, and it causes you to make a number of new and strange bodily adjustments—many of which can lead to aches and pains. Gently stretching your chest muscles will help you feel more comfortable while improving your circulation. Here's how: With your arms bent and at shoulder level, grasp both sides of a doorway. Lean forward, feeling the stretch in your chest. Hold this position for 10 to 20 seconds and release; do five reps.

The
Fifth
Month

Approximately 18 to 22 Weeks

WHAT WAS ONCE COMPLETELY abstract is fast becoming palpable, literally. Chances are that sometime this month or the beginning of the next, you will feel your baby's movements for the first time. That miraculous sensation, along with the serious rounding of your belly, will finally make the pregnancy feel more like a reality. Though your baby is far from ready to make a personal appearance in the nursery, it's really nice to know for sure there's actually someone in there.

Your Baby This Month

Week 18 At 5½ inches long and about 5 ounces in weight (as much as that chicken breast you're having for dinner, but a lot cuter), your baby is filling out nicely and getting large enough that you might even be feeling those twists, rolls, kicks, and punches he or she is perfecting. Another set of skills your baby is mastering now is yawning and hiccupping (you might even begin to feel those hiccups soon!). And your one-of-a-kind baby is truly one of a kind now, complete with unique fingerprints on his or her fingertips and toes.

Week 19 This week your baby is hitting the growth charts at 6 inches long and a full half pound in weight. What fruit is it this week? Your baby's about the size of a large mango. A mango dipped in greasy cheese, actually. Vernix caseosa—a greasy white protective substance (it resembles cheese)—now covers your baby's sensitive skin, protecting it from the surrounding amniotic fluid. Without that protection, your baby would look very wrinkled at birth. The coating sheds as delivery approaches, but some babies born early are still covered with vernix at delivery.

Week 20 You've got a baby the size of a small cantaloupe in your melon-size belly this week, about 10 ounces and 6½ inches (crown to rump). Your

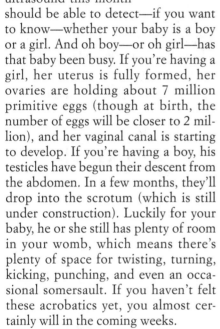

Your Baby, Month 5

ultrasound this month should be able to detect—if you want to know—whether your baby is a boy or a girl. And oh boy—or oh girl—has that baby been busy. If you're having a girl, her uterus is fully formed, her ovaries are holding about 7 million primitive eggs (though at birth, the number of eggs will be closer to 2 million), and her vaginal canal is starting to develop. If you're having a boy, his testicles have begun their descent from the abdomen. In a few months, they'll drop into the scrotum (which is still under construction). Luckily for your baby, he or she still has plenty of room in your womb, which means there's plenty of space for twisting, turning, kicking, punching, and even an occasional somersault. If you haven't felt these acrobatics yet, you almost certainly will in the coming weeks.

Week 21 How big is baby this week? About 7 inches in length (think large banana) and almost 11 ounces in weight. And talking about bananas, you might want to eat some this week if you'd like your baby to have a taste for them. Some carrots, too. That's because amniotic fluid differs from day to day depending on what you've eaten (hot chili one day, sweet banana another), and now that your baby is swallowing amniotic fluid each day (for hydration, nutrition, and also to get practice swal-

lowing and digesting), he or she will be getting a taste of—and a taste for—whatever's on your menu. Here's another baby update: Arms and legs are finally in proportion, neurons are now connected between the brain and muscles, and cartilage throughout the body is turning to bone. Which means that when your baby makes his or her moves (which you're probably feeling by now), they're much more coordinated—no more jerky twitches.

Week 22 Forget about ounces, baby. This week, we're talking a whopping weight of 1 pound and a length of nearly 8 inches, about the size of a small doll. But your doll is a living one—with developing senses, including touch, sight, hearing, and taste. What's your baby touching? He or she may grab onto the umbilical cord (there's not much else to hang onto in there) and practice the strong grip that will soon be clutching your fingers (and pulling on your hair). What's your baby seeing? Though it's dark in the uterine cocoon—and even with fused eyelids—fetuses this age can perceive light and dark. If you shine a flashlight over your belly, you might feel your baby react, perhaps trying to turn away from the "bright" light. What's your baby hearing? The sound of your voice and that of your partner, your heart beating, the whoosh-whoosh of your blood circulating through your body, those gastric gurgles produced by your stomach and intestines, the dog barking, sirens, a loud TV. And what's your baby tasting? Pretty much everything you're tasting (so pass the salad).

What You May Be Feeling

As always, remember that every pregnancy and every woman is different. You may experience all of these symptoms at one time or another, or only a few of them. Some may have continued from last month; others may be new. Still others may be hardly noticed because you've become so used to them. You may also have other, less common, symptoms. Here's what you might experience this month:

Physically

- More energy
- Fetal movement (probably by the end of the month)
- Increasing vaginal discharge
- Achiness in the lower abdomen and along the sides (from stretching of the ligaments supporting the uterus)
- Constipation
- Heartburn, indigestion, flatulence, bloating
- Occasional headaches, faintness, or dizziness
- Backache
- Nasal congestion and occasional nosebleeds; ear stuffiness
- Sensitive gums that may bleed when you brush
- Hearty appetite
- Leg cramps
- Mild swelling of ankles and feet, and occasionally of hands and face
- Varicose veins of legs and/or hemorrhoids
- Skin color changes on abdomen and/or face

- A protruding navel
- Faster pulse (heart rate)
- Easier—or more difficult—orgasm

Emotionally

- A growing sense of reality about the pregnancy
- Fewer mood swings, though you'll likely still be weepy and irritable occasionally
- Continued absentmindedness

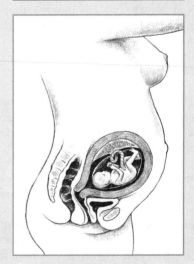

A Look Inside

You're halfway through your pregnancy now—and the top of your uterus will hit your belly button sometime around the 20th week. By the end of this month, your uterus will be about an inch above your belly button. By this point, there is no hiding the fact that you're pregnant.

What You Can Expect at This Month's Checkup

Yet another checkup, and by this time you probably know the drill. This month, you can expect your practitioner to check the following, though there may be variations depending on your particular needs and your practitioner's style of practice:

- Weight and blood pressure

- Urine, for sugar and protein

- Fetal heartbeat

- Size and shape of uterus, by external palpation (feeling from the outside)

- Height of fundus (top of uterus)

- Feet and hands for swelling, and legs for varicose veins

- Symptoms you have been experiencing, especially unusual ones

- Questions or problems you want to discuss—have a list ready

What You May Be Wondering About

Heating Up

"I feel hot and sweaty all the time these days, even when everybody else is cool. What's that about?"

Feeling like hot stuff these days? You can thank your hormones (as always), increased blood flow to the skin, and a hopped-up pregnancy metabolism for that perpetually damp feeling. Throw in a particularly warm climate or the hottest summer on record (or even just an over-heated office in the middle of winter), and the heat is on—big time. Luckily, there are plenty of ways to stay comfort-able when the temperature—outdoors, indoors, or inside of you—is soaring. To stay cool while you're heating for two:

- Wear loose, light clothing in breath-able fabrics, such as cotton, and dress in layers so you can peel them off as you heat up.

- Avoid exercising outside in the heat of the day; take your power walks before breakfast or after dinner instead, or attend exercise classes in an air-conditioned fitness center. Always quit before you feel overheated.

- Stay out of the sun as much as pos-sible, particularly on very hot days.

- Take a tepid bath or shower to cool off. Or go for a swim, if that's practi-cal—it's the one exercise that's almost sure not to overheat you.

- Seek out AC. Fans alone won't help you keep your cool when the tempera-ture is over 90°F, so if you have no air-conditioning at home, spend time at the movies, a museum, a pal's house, or a mall.

- Be a thermostat hog. Commandeer the temperature control at home so you're always comfortable. Let your partner add a sweater or a blanket if he's chilly.

- Drink, drink, drink. Staying hydrated will help keep you from feeling weak and dizzy when you heat up. Down at least eight 8-ounce glasses of water a day, more if you're exercising and/or perspiring a lot.

■ A sprinkle of powder can help absorb some moisture (plus help to prevent heat rash).

On the plus side, while you'll be sweating more—you'll be smelling less. That's because the production of apocrine perspiration (the stinkier kind produced by glands under the arms and breasts and in the genital area) actually slows down when you're expecting.

Dizziness

"I feel dizzy when I get up from a sitting or lying-down position. And yesterday I nearly fainted while I was shopping. Am I okay?"

Feeling a little dizzy can definitely be disconcerting when you're pregnant (especially because you might already be having a hard enough time staying on your feet), but it isn't dangerous. In fact, it's a pretty common—and almost always a normal—symptom of pregnancy. Here's why:

■ In the first trimester, dizziness may occur because there's not yet an adequate blood supply to fill your rapidly expanding circulatory system; in the second trimester, it may be caused by the pressure of your expanding uterus on your blood vessels.

■ Throughout your pregnancy, high levels of your old friend progesterone cause your blood vessels to relax and widen, increasing the flow of blood to your baby (good for baby) but slowing the return of blood to you (not so good for mom). Less blood flow to you means lower blood pressure and reduced blood flow to your brain, which can contribute to that light-headed, dizzy feeling.

■ Getting up too quickly, which results in a sudden blood pressure drop, can trigger an especially light-headed moment. The cure for that kind of dizziness is simple: Just get up very gradually. Jumping up in a hurry to answer the phone is likely to land you right back on the sofa.

■ You might also feel dizzy when your blood sugar is low—something expectant moms are particularly prone to. To avoid those blood sugar dips, get some protein and complex carbs at every meal (the combo helps maintain even blood sugar levels) and eat more frequently (choosing the minimeal approach or snacking in between meals). Carry a bag of trail mix, a piece of fruit, a granola bar, or some soy chips in your bag for quick blood sugar lifts.

When Too Much Is Too Much

Feel breathless or exhausted when you're jogging? What about when you're doing heavy cleaning—does the vacuum suddenly feel as if it weighs a ton? Stop before you drop. Exerting yourself to the point of exhaustion is never a good idea. During pregnancy it's a particularly bad one, because overwork takes its toll not only on you but on your baby as well. Instead of marathon activity sessions, pace yourself. Work or exercise a bit, rest a bit. Ultimately, the work, or the workout, gets done, and you won't feel drained afterward. If occasionally something doesn't get done, consider it good training for the days when the demands of parenthood will often keep you from finishing what you started.

- Dizziness can be a sign of dehydration, so be sure you're getting your full quota of fluids—at least 8 cups a day, more if you've been sweating.

- A dizzy spell can also be triggered by indoor stuffiness—in an overheated or crowded store (which might explain why you felt faint while you were shopping), office, or bus—especially if you're overdressed. In that case, getting some fresh air by stepping outside or opening a window may bring relief. Taking off your coat and loosening your clothes—especially around the neck and waist—should help, too.

If you feel dizzy or faint, lie down on your left side—with your legs elevated, if you can—or sit with your head lowered between your knees. Take deep breaths, and loosen any tight clothing (like that button on your jeans you struggled to close in the first place). As soon as you feel a little better, get something to eat and drink.

Tell your practitioner about the dizzy spells at your next visit. Actual fainting is rare, but if you do faint, there is no need for concern—it won't affect your baby. But do call right away (once you come to, of course).

Backache

"I'm having a lot of back pain. I'm afraid I won't be able to stand up at all by the ninth month."

The aches and discomforts of pregnancy aren't designed to make you miserable, though that's often the upshot. They're the side effects of the preparations your body is making for that momentous moment when your baby is born. Backache is no exception. During pregnancy, the usually stable joints of the pelvis begin to loosen up to allow easier (hopefully) passage for the baby at delivery. This, along with your oversize abdomen, throws your body off balance. To compensate, you tend to bring your shoulders back and arch your neck. Standing with your belly thrust forward—to be sure that no one who passes fails to notice you're pregnant—compounds the problem. The result: a deeply curved lower back, strained back muscles, and pain.

Even pain with a purpose hurts. But without defeating the purpose, you can conquer (or at least subdue) the pain. The following should help:

- Sit smart. Sitting puts more stress on your spine than almost any other activity, so it pays to do it right. At home and at work, make sure the chairs you use most provide good support, preferably with a straight back, arms, and a firm cushion. A chair back that reclines slightly can also help take the pressure off. Use a footrest to elevate your feet slightly (see illustration on page 239), and don't cross your legs, which can cause your pelvis to tilt forward, exacerbating those strained back muscles.

- Sitting for long periods can be as bad for your back as sitting the wrong way. Try not to sit for more than an hour without taking a walking and stretching break; setting a half-hour limit would be even better.

- Try not to stand too long, either. If you work on your feet, keep one foot on a low stool to take some pressure off your lower back. When you're standing on a hard-surfaced floor—in the kitchen while cooking or washing dishes, for example—put a small skid-proof rug underfoot to ease the pressure.

- Avoid lifting heavy loads, but if you must, do it slowly. Stabilize yourself by assuming a wide stance; bend at the knees, not at the waist; and lift with your arms and legs, not your back (see illustration below.) If you have to carry a heavy load of groceries, divide them between two shopping bags and carry one in each arm rather than carrying it all in front of you.

- Try to keep weight gain within the recommended parameters (see page 166). Excess pounds will only add to the load your back is struggling under.

- Wear the right shoes. Extremely high heels are a pain for your back—as are very flat ones. Experts recommend a chunky 2-inch heel to keep your body in proper alignment. You might also consider orthotics, orthopedic shoe inserts designed for muscle support.

- A comfortable sleeping position aided by a body pillow (one that's at least 5 feet long) will help minimize aches

and pains when you're awake. When getting out of bed in the morning, swing your legs over the side of the bed to the floor rather than twisting to get up.

- Consider a crisscross support sling designed specifically for a pregnant figure, which will help take the burden of your belly's weight off your lower back.

- No reaching for the stars—or the crackers on the top shelf. Use a low, stable step stool to get items from high places and you'll avoid additional strain.

- Alternate cold and heat to temporarily relieve sore back muscles. Use an ice pack for 15 minutes, followed by a heating pad for 15 minutes. Wrap both cold pack and heating pad in a towel or cloth.

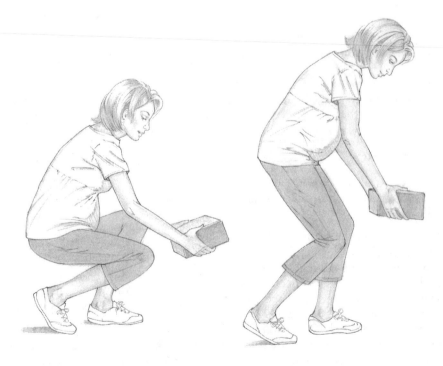

Bend at the knees when you lift

- Take a warm (but not hot) bath. Or turn the shower head to pulsating and enjoy the back massage.

- Rub your back the right way. Treat yourself to a therapeutic massage (with a massage therapist who knows you're pregnant and is trained in the art of prenatal massage).

- Learn to relax. Many back problems are aggravated by stress. If you think yours might be, try some relaxation exercises when pain strikes. Also follow the suggestions beginning on page 141 for dealing with stress in your life.

- Do simple exercises that strengthen your abdominal muscles, such as the Dromedary Droop (page 222) and the Pelvic Tilt (page 224). Or sit on an exercise ball and rock back and forth (or lie back on it to ease back—and hip—discomfort). Join a pregnancy yoga or water gymnastics class, or consider water therapy if you can find a medically (and pregnancy) savvy water therapist.

- If pain is significant, ask your practitioner about physical therapists or alternative medicine specialists (such as acupuncturists or those who specialize in biofeedback), who might be able to help.

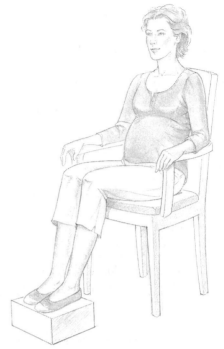

Sit comfortably

Abdominal Aches

"What are those aches and pains I've been getting on the lower sides of my abdomen?"

What you're probably feeling is the pregnancy equivalent of growing pains: the stretching of muscles and ligaments supporting your enlarging uterus. Technically, it's known as round ligament pain (though when it's tugging at your sides, do you really care what the pros call it?), and most expectant moms experience it. But there's a wide variety of ways to experience it. The pain may be crampy, sharp and stabbing, or achy, and it may be more noticeable when you're getting up from bed or from a chair, or when you cough. It can be brief, or it may last for several hours. And it's completely normal. As long as it is occasional and fleeting, and there are no other symptoms accompanying it (such as fever, chills, bleeding, or light-headedness), this kind of pain is absolutely nothing to be concerned about.

Kicking up your feet (though not literally) and resting in a comfortable position should bring some relief. Of course, mention the pain—like all pains—to your practitioner at your next visit so you can be reassured that this is just another normal, if annoying, part of pregnancy.

The New Skin You're In

If you haven't already noticed, pregnancy impacts just about every inch of your body—from head (that forgetfulness!) to toes (those expanding feet!) and everything in between (breasts, belly!). So it's not surprising that your skin is also showing the effects of pregnancy. Here are some changes you may expect when it comes to your expectant skin:

Linea nigra. Sporting a zipper down the center of your burgeoning belly? Just as those pregnancy hormones caused the hyperpigmentation, or darkening, of the areolas, they are now responsible for the darkening of the linea alba, the white line you probably never noticed that runs between your belly button and your pubic area. During pregnancy, it's renamed the linea nigra, or black line, and may be more noticeable in dark-skinned women than in those who are fair-skinned. It usually starts to appear during the second trimester and most often will begin to fade a few months after delivery (though it may never go away entirely). Interested in a round of "guess-the-sex-of-my-baby"? According to an old wives' tale, if the linea nigra runs only up to the belly button, you're having a girl. If it runs past the navel up to the xiphoid process (near your ribs), it's a boy.

Mask of pregnancy (chloasma). Around 50 to 75 percent of expectant mothers, particularly those with darker complexions, develop discolorations—in a masklike configuration or a confetti-like appearance—on foreheads, noses, and cheeks. The patches are dark in light-skinned women and light in dark-skinned women. Not a fan of the blotchy look? Never fear. Chloasma will fade within a few months after delivery; if it doesn't (or if you'd like to speed up its postpartum retreat), a dermatologist can prescribe a bleaching cream (if you aren't nursing) or recommend another treatment (such as a laser or a peel). Because those treatments are no-no's for now, bring on the concealer and foundation in the meantime (see page 149).

Other skin hyperpigmentation. Many women also find that freckles and moles become darker and more noticeable and that darkening of the skin occurs in high-friction areas, such as between the thighs. All this hyperpigmentation should fade after delivery. Sun can intensify the discoloration, so use a sunscreen with an SPF of 15 or more on all exposed skin and avoid spending long hours in the sun (even with sunscreen on). A hat that completely shades your face and long sleeves to protect your arms (if you can take the heat) can also help.

Red palms and soles. It's your hormones at work again (plus an increase

Foot Growth

"My shoes are all beginning to feel uncomfortably tight. Could my feet be growing, too?"

The belly isn't the only part of the pregnant body that's prone to expansion. If you're like many expectant women, you'll discover that your feet are growing, too. Good news if you're looking to revamp your entire shoe collection; not so good if you've just indulged in a pricey pair or two.

What causes your feet to go through a growth spurt? While some expansion in blood flow), and this time they're causing red, itchy palms (and sometimes soles of the feet) in more than two thirds of white and one third of nonwhite pregnant women. There's no specific treatment, but some women find relief by soaking their hands and/or feet in cold water or applying an ice bag for a few minutes a couple of times a day. Steer clear of anything that heats up your hands and feet (such as taking hot baths, washing dishes, wearing wool gloves), because that can make the condition worse. Also, stay away from potential irritants, such as harsh soaps or scented lotions. The dishpan look will disappear soon after delivery.

Bluish, blotchy legs. Due to stepped-up estrogen production, many expectant women experience this kind of transitory, mottled discoloration on their legs (and sometimes their arms) when they're chilly. It's harmless and will disappear postpartum.

Skin tags. A skin tag, which is essentially a tiny piece of excess skin, is another benign skin problem common in pregnant women and often found in high-friction areas, such as under the arms. Skin tags frequently develop in the second and third trimesters and may regress after delivery. If they don't, your physician can easily remove them.

Heat rash. Though heat rashes are usually associated with babies, pregnant women get them, too. Caused by the combination of an already overheated pregnant body, dampness from excessive perspiration, and the friction of skin rubbing against itself or against clothing (as it tends to do when there's more skin to rub), heat rash can be irritating. It is most common in the crease between and beneath the breasts, in the crease where the bulge of the lower abdomen rubs against the top of the pubic area, and on the inner thighs. (The pregnancy beauty bonuses just keep on coming, don't they?) A cool, damp compress can take some of the heat out of your heat rash. Patting on some powder after your shower and trying to keep as cool as possible will help minimize discomfort and recurrence. A dab of calamine lotion can also be soothing and is safe to use, but before you apply any medicated lotions, check with your practitioner. If any rash or irritation lasts longer than a couple of days, ask your practitioner about next steps.

Irritated skin rashes. Often, rashes are triggered by pregnancy-sensitive skin reacting to a product you've used prepregnancy without a reaction. Switching to a gentler product often relieves these contact rashes, but still do let your practitioner know about any persistent rash.

But wait, there's more. Believe it or not, there are a host of other skin changes you might experience. For information on stretch marks, see page 179; itchy pimples, see page 288; dry or oily skins, see pages 158–59; spider veins, see page 156.

can be attributed to the normal fluid retention and swelling of pregnancy (or to new fat in your feet if your weight gain has been substantial or quick), there's another reason, too. Relaxin, the pregnancy hormone that loosens the ligaments and joints around your pelvis so your baby can fit through, doesn't discriminate between the ligaments you'd want loosened up (like those pelvic ones) and those you'd rather it just leave alone (like those in your feet). The result: When the ligaments in the feet are loosened, the bones under them tend to spread slightly, resulting, for many women, in a half or whole shoe-size increase. Though the joints will tighten back up again after delivery, it's possible that your feet will be permanently larger.

In the meantime, try the tips for reducing excessive swelling (see page 286) if that seems to be your problem, and get a couple of pairs of shoes that fit you comfortably now and will meet your "growing" needs (so you won't end up barefoot and pregnant). When shoe shopping, put comfort before style— even if it's just this once. Look for shoes with heels that are no more than 2 inches high and have both nonskid soles and plenty of space for your feet to spread out (shop for them at the end of the day when your feet are the most swollen). The shoes should be made from a material that will allow your swollen, sweaty dogs to breathe (nothing synthetic).

Are your feet and legs achy, especially at the end of the day? Shoes and orthotic inserts specially designed to correct the distorted center of pregnancy gravity not only can make your feet more comfortable but can reduce back and leg pain as well. Getting off your feet periodically during the day can (obviously) help with swelling and pain, as can elevating (and periodically flexing) your feet when you get the chance. You can also try slipping on elasticized slippers while you're at home; wearing them for several hours a day may not make a great fashion statement, but it can ease fatigue and achiness.

Fast-Growing Hair and Nails

"It seems to me that my hair and nails have never grown so fast before."

Though it may seem as if pregnancy hormones only team up to make you miserable during your nine months (constipation, heartburn, and nausea come to mind), those same hormones are actually responsible for a substantial pregnancy perk: nails that grow faster than you can manicure them and hair that grows before you can secure appointments with your stylist (and if you're really lucky, hair that is thicker and more lustrous). Those pregnancy hormones trigger a surge in circulation and a boost in metabolism that nourish hair and nail cells, making them healthier than ever before.

Of course, every perk has its price. That extra nourishment can, unfortunately, have less than happy effects, too: It can cause hair to grow in places you would rather it didn't (and probably didn't know it could, at least on a woman). Facial areas (lips, chin, and cheeks) are most commonly plagued with this pregnancy-induced hairiness, but arms, legs, chest, back, and belly can be affected, too. (To read about which hair removal treatments are safe during pregnancy, see page 145). And though your nails might be long, they can also turn dry and brittle.

Do keep in mind that these hair and nail changes are only temporary. Your good-hair-day run ends with delivery— when the normal daily hair loss that's suppressed during pregnancy (thus the thicker hair) resumes with a vengeance. And your nails will likely go back to their slower growth schedule postpartum, too (probably not such a bad thing—you'll want to keep your nails short anyway with a new baby around).

Vision

"My eyesight seems to be getting worse since I got pregnant. And my contact lenses don't seem to fit anymore. Am I imagining it?"

Nope, you're not seeing things— that is, you're not seeing things as well as you were prepregnancy. The eyes are just another of the seemingly unrelated body parts that can fall prey to pregnancy hormones. Not only can your vision seem less sharp, but your contact lenses, if you wear them, may suddenly no longer feel comfortable. Eye dryness, which is caused by a hormone-induced decrease in tear production, may be at least partially to blame for irritation and discomfort. If that's not enough, fluid increases that change the eye lenses' shape can actually cause some pregnant women to become more near- or farsighted. Your vision should clear up and your eyes return to normal after delivery (so don't bother to get a new prescription unless the change is so pronounced that you really can't see well anymore).

Now isn't the time to consider corrective laser eye surgery. Though the procedure wouldn't harm the baby, it could overcorrect your vision and take longer to heal, possibly requiring a second corrective surgery later on (plus the eyedrops used aren't recommended for pregnant women). Ophthalmologists recommend avoiding the surgery during pregnancy, in the six months preconception, and for at least six months postpartum (and if you're nursing, six months postweaning).

Though a slight deterioration in visual acuity is not unusual in pregnancy, other symptoms do warrant a call to your practitioner. If you experience blurring or dimming vision or often see spots or floaters, or have double vision that persists for more than two or three hours, don't wait to see if it passes; call your practitioner at once. Briefly seeing spots after you have been standing for a while or when you get up suddenly from a sitting position is fairly common and nothing to worry about, though you should report it at your next visit.

Fetal Movement Patterns

"I felt little movements every day last week, but I haven't felt anything at all today. What's wrong?"

Feeling your baby twist, wriggle, punch, kick, and hiccup is simply one of pregnancy's biggest thrills (it sure beats heartburn and puffy feet). There may be no better proof that a brand-new—and impressively energetic—life is developing within you. But fetal movements can also drive a mom-to-be to distraction with questions and doubts: Is my baby moving enough? Too much? Moving at all? One minute you're sure those were kicks you were feeling, the next you're second-guessing yourself (maybe it was just gas?). One day you feel your baby's twists and turns nonstop. The next day your little athlete seems to have been benched, and you barely feel a thing.

Not to worry. At this stage of pregnancy, concerns about your baby's movements—while understandable—are usually unnecessary. The frequency of noticeable movements at this point varies a great deal, and patterns of movement are erratic at best. Though your baby is almost certainly on the move much of the time, you probably won't be feeling it consistently until he or she is packing a more powerful punch. Some of those dance moves may be missed because of the fetal position (facing and kicking inward, for instance, instead of outward). Or because of your own activity—when you're walking or moving about a lot, your fetus may be rocked to sleep; or it may be awake, but you may be too busy to notice its movements. It's also possible that you're sleeping right through your baby's most active period; for many babies that's in the middle of the night. (Even at this stage, babies are most likely to act up when their moms are lying down.)

One way to prompt fetal movement if you haven't noticed any all day is to lie down for an hour or two in the evening, preferably after a glass of milk, orange juice, or other snack. The combination of your inactivity and the jolt of food energy may be able to get your fetus going. If that doesn't work, try again in a few hours, but don't worry. Many moms-to-be find they don't notice movement for a day or two at a time, or even three or four days, this early on. If you're still worried, call your practitioner for reassurance.

After the 28th week, fetal movements become more consistent, and it's a good idea to get into the habit of checking on your baby's activity daily (see page 289).

Second-Trimester Ultrasound

"I'm having a perfectly normal pregnancy, with no problems at all. But my practitioner is still recommending that I have an ultrasound this month. Is it really necessary?"

These days, it's pretty much routine for women in their second trimester to be scheduled for a level 2 ultrasound, no matter how normally their pregnancies seem to be proceeding. That's because practitioners have found that it's a great way to see how a baby is developing and to offer reassurance that everything is going exactly the way it should be. On the plus side for parents, it's fun to get a sneak peek at your baby—and to take home a souvenir photo to start the album with and to start bonding with. It can also give you the 4-1-1 on baby's sex (on a want-to-know basis, of course; see next question).

Even if you had a first-trimester (level 1) sonogram to confirm or date your pregnancy, or as part of a first-trimester screening test, the more detailed level 2 sonogram (also called an anatomy scan), typically performed between 18 and 22 weeks, gives your practitioner additional valuable information about what's going on in that belly of yours. For example, it can measure the size of your baby and check out all the major organs. It can determine the amount of amniotic fluid to make sure there's just the right amount, and evaluate the location of your placenta. In short, this second-trimester ultrasound—besides being fun to watch—will give you and your practitioner a clear picture (literally) of the overall health of your baby and your pregnancy.

If you're concerned about the upcoming picture show (and what those grainy images reveal), talk to your practitioner about what he or she is looking for. Chances are you'll come away enlightened (and relieved).

A Picture That Lasts a Lifetime

Now that you've got your baby's first portrait, courtesy of your second-trimester ultrasound exam, you'll want to preserve it forever—right? To make sure that precious picture doesn't get damaged (or fade), scan it into your computer and save it on your hard drive or onto a CD. Or scan it into a photo website and have it printed out on acid-free paper with real photo ink. That way your memories won't fade with, well, your memory.

Baby's First Mall Portrait

Want a womb with a view? Ultrasound is a window into the wonderful world of your womb, and to get a sneak peek into that world, you often don't have to go farther than your local mall. But is it safe to take that peek inside your tummy on the way to Sears?

The FDA hasn't yet established rules for these storefront prenatal photography studios, but it does warn against having ultrasounds for fun (instead of for medical reasons), since the three-dimensional imaging machines they use are much higher powered than the typical ultrasound machines at your doctor's office. What's more, many medical professionals fear that nervous moms-to-be will come away wrongly convinced there's something wrong with their babies, or, worse, that the less-trained wand wavers will miss real problems that a pro would detect.

If you're still intrigued by the idea, check with your practitioner before you leap (or in this case heave yourself) onto the exam table at the mall. If you decide to go ahead with this kind of elective sonography, do so wisely: Limit your visits to one or two, with each ultrasound no more than 15 minutes in length. And bring your wallet. The image may be priceless, but some studios charge a hefty price for that suitable-for-framing photo, CD, and DVD of your baby-to-be.

"I'm going for my 20-week ultrasound, and we're not sure whether to find out the baby's sex or not."

This is one pregnancy decision only a mom and dad can make—and there's no right or wrong when it comes to making it. Some parents opt to know for practical reasons: It makes layette shopping, nursery painting, and name selection (only one to pick!) a lot simpler. Others opt to know because they simply can't stand the suspense. But many parents still prefer the guessing game, and they decide to find out the old-fashioned way—when baby's lower half finally makes its way out into the world. The choice is yours.

If you do decide to find out now, keep in mind that determining the sex of a baby through ultrasound is not an exact science (unlike amniocentesis, which determines the sex of the baby through chromosomal analysis). Very occasionally, parents are told by the sonographer that they're expecting a girl only to hear at delivery, "It's a boy!" (or vice versa). So if you do choose to find out your baby's gender when you go for your ultrasound, remember that it's only a guess, however educated it may be.

Placenta Position

"The doctor said my ultrasound showed that the placenta was down near the cervix. She said that it was too early to worry about it, but of course I started worrying."

Think your baby is the only thing moving around in your uterus? Think again. Like a fetus, a placenta can move around during pregnancy. It doesn't actually pick up and relocate, but it does appear to migrate upward as the lower segment of the uterus stretches and grows. Though an estimated 10 percent of placentas are in the lower segment in the second trimester (and an even larger percentage before 14 weeks), the vast majority move into the upper segment by the time delivery nears. If this doesn't happen and the placenta remains low in the uterus, partially or completely covering the cervix (the mouth of the uterus), a diagnosis of "placenta previa" is made. This complication occurs in very few full-term pregnancies (about 1 in 200). In other words, your doctor is right. It's too early to worry—and statistically speaking, the chances are slim that you'll ever have to worry.

"During my ultrasound, the technician told me I have an anterior placenta. What does that mean?"

It means your baby is taking a backseat to the placenta. Usually, a fertilized egg situates itself in the posterior uterus—the part closest to your spine, which is where the placenta eventually develops. Sometimes, though, the egg implants on the opposite side of the uterus, closest to your belly button. When the placenta develops, it grows on the front (or anterior) side of your uterus, with the baby behind it. And that, apparently, is what happened in your case.

Happily, your baby doesn't care which side of the uterus he or she is lying on, and where the placenta is located certainly makes no difference to his or her development. The downside for you is that you might be less able to feel (and later see) your baby's early kicks and punches because the placenta will serve as a cushion between your baby and your tummy (which could lead to unnecessary worrying). For the same reason, your doctor or midwife may find it a bit harder to hear fetal heart sounds (and it could make amniocentesis a little more challenging). But despite those slight inconveniencies—which are nothing to be concerned about—an anterior pla-

centa is inconsequential. What's more, it's very likely that the placenta will move into a more posterior position later on (as anterior placentas commonly do).

Sleeping Position

"I've always slept on my stomach. Now I'm afraid to. And I just can't seem to get comfortable any other way."

Unfortunately, two common favorite sleeping positions—on the belly and on the back—are not the best (and certainly not the most comfortable) choices during pregnancy. The belly position, for obvious reasons: As your stomach grows, it's like sleeping on a watermelon. The back position, though more comfortable, rests the entire weight of your pregnant uterus on your back, your intestines, and major blood vessels. This pressure can aggravate backaches and hemorrhoids, make digestion less efficient, interfere with optimum circulation, and possibly cause hypotension, or low blood pressure, which can make you dizzy.

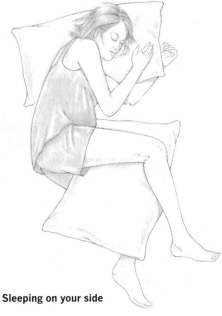

Sleeping on your side

Carrying Baby, Fifth Month

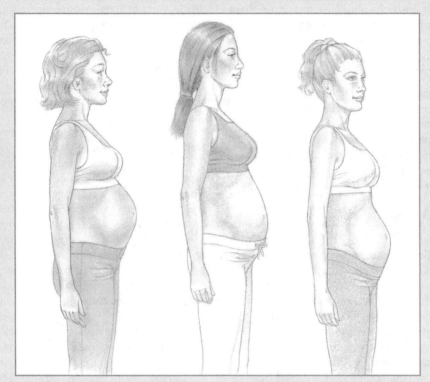

Here are just three of the very different ways that a woman may carry near the end of her fifth month. The variations on these are endless. Depending on your size, your shape, the amount of weight you've gained, and the position of your uterus, you may be carrying higher, lower, bigger, smaller, wider, or more compactly.

This doesn't mean you have to sleep standing up. Curling up or stretching out on your side—preferably the left side, though either side is fine—with one leg crossed over the other and with a pillow between them (see illustration, facing page), is ideal for both you and your fetus. It not only allows maximum flow of blood and nutrients to the placenta but also enhances efficient kidney function, which means better elimination of waste products and fluids and less swelling (edema) of ankles, feet, and hands.

Very few people, however, manage to stay in one position through the night. Don't worry (repeat: do not worry) if you wake up and find yourself on your back or abdomen. No harm done (repeat: no harm done); just turn back to your side. You may feel uncomfortable for a few nights, but your body will soon adjust to the new position. A body pillow that's at least 5 feet long or a wedge-shaped pillow can offer support, making side sleeping much more comfortable and staying on your side much easier.

If you don't have either of these, you can improvise with any extra pillows, placing them against your body in different positions until you find that perfect combination for catching z's.

Class Womb?

"I have a friend who insists that taking her unborn baby to concerts will make him a music lover, and another one whose husband reads to her tummy every night to give their baby a love of literature. Should I be trying to stimulate my baby, too?"

All parents want only the best for their children—or in this case, for their children-to-be. But it's important to keep some perspective before switching on the Beethoven and reciting the Shakespeare.

While it's true the fetus's ability to hear is well developed by the end of the second trimester, there is no proof that an in utero concerto or a lesson in the great classics gives the baby a head start in education (or on a musical or literary career). Promoting an educational or cultural agenda this early can also come with a potential downside—especially if it signals the start of extremely premature parental pushiness, and begins placing too much emphasis on achievement at a too-tender age (and before birth is definitely too tender an age). Fetuses (like the babies and children they'll become before you know it) develop—and later, learn—best at their own pace, no prodding necessary. There's also the theoretical risk that when parents attempt to turn the womb into a classroom, they may unwittingly disrupt the natural sleep patterns of their baby-to-be, actually hampering development instead of nurturing it (just as waking up a newborn for a game of name-this-letter might).

That said, there's nothing wrong—and a lot right—with providing a uterine environment that's rich in language and music, and much more important, about finding ways to get close to your little one long before you even have that first cuddle. Talking, reading, or singing to your baby while in the womb (no amplification necessary) won't guarantee a scholarship to Yale, but it will guarantee that your baby will know your voice at birth—and will give you both a head start on bonding.

Playing classical music now may increase the likelihood that your newborn will appreciate, and even be soothed by, these sounds later on (though it's been shown that exposure to music and literature has a much more significant effect once your baby is actually born than it does prenatally—so keep the sonatas handy once baby's arrived). And don't underestimate the power of touch. Since this sense also begins to develop in utero, stroking your belly now may also help strengthen the bond between you and your baby later.

So turn on the Mozart, bring on the Bach, pull out those dusty Shakespeare sonnets and read away to your belly if you like (and if you can do it without cracking up). Just make sure you're doing it all to get closer to your baby—not to get your baby closer to an Ivy League degree.

Of course, if you feel silly performing for your bloated belly, there's no reason to worry that your baby will miss out on getting to know you. He or she is getting used to the sound of your voice—and Dad's, too—every time you speak to each other or someone else. So enjoy making baby contact now, but definitely don't worry about early learning this early. As you'll discover, kids grow up all too soon anyway. There's no need to rush the process, particularly before birth.

Carrying Older Children

"I have a three-year-old who always wants to be carried. Is it okay to keep doing it at this point in pregnancy? It's definitely killing my back."

Carrying moderately heavy loads (even some 35 or 40 pounds of preschooler) is safe throughout pregnancy unless your practitioner has told you otherwise. What giving in to those choruses of "carry me" can end up doing to your back is another story—a probably painful one. Breaking her of the being-carried habit would definitely be a better strategy than continuing to break your back—so try making walking fun for her. Challenge her to mini races, or climb the stairs to a song. Don't forget to applaud her efforts when she does agree to walk on her own two feet instead of hailing the mommy taxi—and try to blame your back (not her sibling-to-be) for the slowdown in pick ups. Compensate, too, with plenty of holding and hugging from a sitting position. And because there will be times when she definitely won't take "walk" for an answer, save your back some strain by learning the proper way to lift her (see page 237).

Approaching Parenthood

"I keep wondering if I will be happy with this whole parenthood thing. I have no clue what it'll really be like."

Most people approach any major change in their lives—and there's no more major change than an upcoming birth—wondering whether it will be a change they'll be happy with. And it's always much more likely to be a happy change if you keep your expectations realistic.

So, if you have images of bringing a cooing, smiling, picture-perfect baby home from the hospital, you may want to read up on what newborns are really like. Not only won't your newborn be smiling or cooing for many weeks, he or she may hardly communicate with you at all, except to cry—and this will almost invariably be when you're sitting down to dinner or starting to get busy in bed, have to go to the bathroom, or are so tired you can't move.

And if your visions of parenthood consist of nothing but leisurely morning walks through the park, sunny days at the zoo, and hours coordinating a wardrobe of miniature, picture-perfect clothes, another reality check is probably in order. You'll have your share of walks in the park, but there will also be many mornings that turn into evenings before you and your baby have the chance to see the light of day; many sunny days that will be spent largely in the laundry room; very few tiny outfits that will escape unstained by spit-up, pureed bananas, and baby vitamins.

What you can expect realistically, however, are some of the most wondrous, miraculous experiences of your life. The fulfillment you will feel when cuddling a warm, sleeping bundle of baby (even if that cherub was howling moments before) is incomparable. That—along with that first toothless smile meant just for you—will be well worth all the sleepless nights, delayed dinners, mountains of laundry, and frustrated romance.

Happy? Just you wait, Mom.

Wearing a Seat Belt

"Is it safe to buckle my seat belt in the car? And is the air bag an issue when you're pregnant?"

There's no safer way for an expectant mother—and her unborn baby—to travel than buckled up. Plus, it's the law in most places. For maximum safety and minimum discomfort, fasten the belt below your belly, across your pelvis and upper thighs. Wear the shoulder harness over your shoulder (not under your arm), diagonally between your breasts and to the side of your belly. And don't worry that the pressure of an abrupt stop will hurt your baby; he or she is well cushioned by amniotic fluid and uterine muscle, among the world's best shock-absorbing materials.

As for air bags, it's safest to keep your distance. So if you're sitting in the passenger seat, set the seat as far back as you can (your legs will appreciate the stretching room, too). If you're driving, tilt the wheel up toward your chest, away from your tummy, and sit at least 10 inches from the steering wheel, if possible.

Travel

"Is it safe for me to go ahead and take the vacation we had planned for this month?"

Never again will it be so easy to vacation with your baby. Fast-forward to next year when you'll be lugging a car seat, diapers, toys, and child-proofing kits wherever you go, and you'll see why. And there's no better time for pregnant travel than the second trimester. After all, the fatigue, queasiness, and emotional extremes of the first trimester are behind you—but you're not yet at the point where your belly has a life of its own, making it hard enough to drag yourself around, never mind the luggage.

So don't have reservations about those reservations you've made. But before you pack your suitcase, do get the go-ahead from your practitioner. Chances are your vacation plans will be green-lighted, since travel is rarely restricted during pregnancy unless there's an obstetrical or medical complication.

Once you've been cleared for takeoff, you'll only need to do a little planning to ensure a safe and pleasant expectant voyage, whether it's a quick business trip or a leisurely babymoon:

Time it right. When you're planning a pregnancy vacation, timing is everything. For long-distance travel, the second trimester is the clear winner. Far-flung travel during the first trimester, even in a low-risk pregnancy, can be pretty uncomfortable, especially if morning sickness, fatigue, and other early symptoms have hit hard. Likewise, roaming far from home isn't recommended in the last part of the last trimester for obvious reasons: Should you go into labor early, you'd be stranded far from your practitioner.

Choose a suitable destination. A hot, humid climate may be hard for you to handle because of your hopped-up metabolism; if you do choose such a locale, make sure that your hotel and transportation are air-conditioned

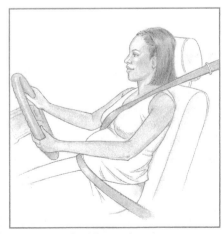

Buckling up for two

Jettisoning Jet Lag

Add jet lag to the normal fatigue of pregnancy and you're likely to want to end your trip before it begins. So it makes sense to try to minimize—if you can't completely eliminate—the physically draining effects of travel across time zones. Here's how:

Start switching time zones before you leave. Ease yourself into the time zone you're headed for by setting your watch—and your schedule—gradually back or forward. If you're heading east, start getting up a little earlier and going to bed a little earlier a few days before your departure. If you're heading west, go to bed a little later and get up a little later (if you can). On your plane ride, try to sleep if it's an appropriate sleeping time at your destination, or stay awake if it's not.

Live on local time. Once you arrive at your destination, start living on local time full-time. If you arrive at your Paris hotel room at 7 A.M., exhausted from an overnight flight, resist the urge to nap until noon. Instead, try to get a second wind going with a shower and a hearty breakfast, and then step out for a slow-paced day. Don't push yourself—take frequent breaks to sit down with your feet up—but do try hard to stay vertical. Lie down and you're sure to surrender to sleep. Dine, too, according to the local clock and not your internal one (snack if you're hungry, but hold off on a full meal until the clock strikes "eat"), and strive to stay awake until as close to your usual bedtime (local time) as possible. This should help you sleep through the local night. Avoid sleeping in, too, which could make going to bed at a normal time the next night more difficult. Ask for a wake-up call, even if you think you won't need it.

Seek out sun. Getting some sunlight will help you reset your biological clock, so be sure to spend some time outdoors on your first day at your new destination. If there's no sun to be found, at least spend some time outdoors. If you've gone west to east, the best sun to seek is morning sun; if you've gone east to west, get your daylight in the late afternoon.

Eat, drink, and be less jet-lagged. Anyone who travels frequently knows how dehydrating air travel can be. And dehydration can make jet lag symptoms more severe (not to mention put you at risk for pregnancy complications). So drink plenty of water on the plane, and continue drinking once you have arrived. Take time to eat regularly, too. Concentrate on foods that are high in long-term energy boosters, such as protein and complex carbohydrates, preferably eaten in combo. Getting some exercise (nothing strenuous; a walk in a park or a few laps in the hotel pool are just right) will also help you feel less fatigued.

Don't look for a miracle. Don't use any over-the-counter, prescription, or herbal preparation for jet lag (or any purpose) without your practitioner's approval.

Give it time. You should start to feel less tired and more in sync with the local schedule within a couple of days.

You may find sleep problems—and the fatigue that inevitably accompanies them—continue to plague you during the entire trip. But let's face it, that may have less to do with jet lag and more to do with the fact that you're carrying around a lot of extra baggage—the kind you can't ask a skycap or bellman to help you with.

Pregnant at a High Altitude

Women who are accustomed to breathing thinner air because they live at a high altitude are far less likely to encounter an altitude-induced problem in their pregnancies (hypertension, water retention, a somewhat smaller-than-average baby) than those who just moved there after a lifetime at sea level. For that reason, many practitioners suggest postponing a contemplated move or visit from low altitude to high until after delivery. And scaling Mount Rainier is definitely out for now.

If you must make a trip to a destination at a high altitude, try to ascend gradually, if possible (if you're driving, for example, try to go up 2,000 feet a day, rather than going up 8,000 feet all at once). To minimize the risk of developing acute mountain sickness (AMS), also plan on limiting exertion for a few days after your arrival, drink lots of fluids, eat frequent small meals instead of three large ones, avoid rich and heavy food, and seek sleeping accommodations, if feasible, at a somewhat lower altitude.

and that you stay hydrated and out of the sun. Travel to areas at high altitude (more than 7,000 feet above sea level) may be unsafe, because adjusting to the decrease in oxygen may be too taxing for both you and your baby. Other inappropriate destinations are developing regions of the world for which vaccinations would be necessary, since some vaccines may be hazardous during pregnancy (check with your practitioner). Not insignificantly, these same locales may be hotbeds of certain potentially dangerous infections for which there are no vaccines—another reason to avoid them when you're expecting. Not to mention the risk of food- and water-borne illnesses common in those parts.

Plan a trip that's relaxing. A single destination trumps a whirlwind tour that takes you to six cities in six days. A vacation for which you set the pace is a lot better than one where a group tour guide sets it for you. A few hours of sightseeing or shopping (or meetings) should be alternated with time spent with your feet up. You'll need to listen

to your pregnant body, which may have to set the agenda.

Insure yourself. Sign up for reliable travel insurance, in case a pregnancy complication should require you to change your plans and stick close to home. Consider medical evacuation insurance as well if you're traveling overseas, in case you need to return home quickly and under medical supervision. Medical travel insurance may also be useful if your regular insurance plan does not include foreign medical care. Check your policy ahead of time.

Pack a pregnancy survival kit. Make sure you take enough prenatal vitamins to last the trip; some healthy snacks; Sea-Bands if you're susceptible to motion sickness and a medication for traveler's stomach that's been recommended by your practitioner; comfortable shoes roomy enough to accommodate feet swelled by long hours of sightseeing or work; and sunscreen.

If you're traveling overseas, have the name of a local obstetrician handy, just in case. Contact the International

Association for Medical Assistance to Travelers (IAMAT) at (716) 754-4883 or at iamat.org, which can provide you with a directory of English-speaking physicians throughout the world. Some major hotel chains can also provide you with this kind of information. When you're overseas, if for any reason you find yourself in need of a doctor in a hurry and your hotel can't provide you with one, you can call the American embassy, an American military base, or the nearest teaching hospital. Or you can head for the hospital's emergency room. If you have medical travel insurance, you should have a number to call for help.

Take healthy eating habits with you. You may be on vacation, but your baby is working as hard as ever at growing and developing and has the same nutritional requirements as always. Order thoughtfully and you will be able to savor the local cuisine while also fulfilling your baby's requirements. Most important: Eat regularly and snack as needed. Don't skip breakfast or lunch to save up for a six-course dinner.

Eat selectively. In some regions, it may not be safe to eat raw unpeeled fruits or vegetables or salads. (Peel fruit yourself, washing the fruit first and your hands after peeling to avoid transferring germs to the fruit; bananas and oranges tend to be safer than other fruits because of their thick skins.) No matter where you roam, avoid cooked foods that are lukewarm or at room temperature, raw or undercooked meat, fish, and poultry, as well as unpasteurized or unrefrigerated dairy products and juice and food sold by street vendors, even if it's hot. For complete information on such restrictions, on other foreign health hazards, and on immunizations for travel, contact the Centers for Disease Control and Prevention's Traveler's Hotline at (877) FYI-TRIP (394-8747) or at wwwn

.cdc.gov/travel. Travel warnings are also available from the State Department at (202) 647-5225 or at travel.state.gov.

Don't drink the water (or even brush your teeth with it) unless you're certain it's safe. If the purity of the water is questionable at your destination, plan to use bottled water for drinking and brushing (and always make sure the seal on the bottle cap is intact when you open it). Avoid ice, too, unless you are certain it was made from bottled or boiled water.

Don't swim in the water, either. In some areas, lakes and oceans may be polluted.

Pregnant Women Are Delicious

If mosquitoes seem to love snacking on you more than ever now that you're pregnant, it's not just your imagination. Scientists have found that pregnant women attract twice as many mosquitoes as non-pregnant women do, possibly because those pesky bugs are fond of carbon dioxide and pregnant women tend to take more frequent breaths, thereby releasing more of this mosquito-friendly gas. Another reason why mosquitoes make a bee-line for expectant mothers: They're heat-seeking, and expectant mothers generally have higher body temperatures, what with all that baby making going on. So if you live in or travel to an area where mosquitoes are a problem (especially if they pose a health risk), take proper precautions. You can avoid their bites by staying indoors in heavily mosquito-infested areas, by using tight-fitting screens on windows, and by using a non-DEET-based insect repellent.

Check with the CDC about the waters at your destination to be sure of safety before taking a dip. Any pool you swim in should be properly chlorinated (a whiff will usually clue you in).

Head off traveler's irregularity. Changes in schedule and diet can compound constipation problems. So make sure you get plenty of the three most effective constipation combaters: fiber, fluids, and exercise. It may also help to eat breakfast (or at least a morning snack) a little early so you'll have time to use the bathroom before you set out for the day.

When you've gotta go, go. Don't encourage a UTI or constipation by postponing trips to the bathroom. Go as soon as you feel the urge (and can find a rest room).

Get the support you need. Support hose, that is, particularly if you already suffer from varicose veins. But even if you only suspect you may be predisposed to them, consider wearing support hose when you'll be doing a lot of sitting (in cars, planes, or trains, for example) and when you'll be doing a lot of standing (in museums, in airport lines). They'll also help minimize swelling in your feet and ankles.

Don't be stationary while on the move. Sitting for long periods can restrict the circulation in your legs, so be sure to shift in your seat frequently, and stretch, flex, wiggle, and massage your legs often—and avoid crossing your legs. If possible, take your shoes off and elevate your feet a bit. Get up at least every hour or two to walk the aisles when you are on a plane or train. When traveling by car, don't go for more than two hours without stopping for a stretch and a stroll.

If you're traveling by plane. Check with the airline in advance to see if it has spe-cial regulations concerning pregnant women (many airlines do). Arrange ahead of time for a seat in the bulkhead (preferably on the aisle, so you can get up and stretch or use the rest room as needed), or if seating is not reserved, ask for preboarding.

When booking your flight, ask whether any meal will be served or available for purchase. More and more often, the so-called friendly skies are also the go-hungry skies. If the pickings will be slim (half an ounce of snack mix) at best, bring along a meal of your own (a sandwich or salad, for instance). Even if you will be scoring a meal, keep in mind that it may be (a) tiny (b) inedible (c) a long time in coming due to flight delays, or (d) all of the above. Pack snacks accordingly: cheese sticks or wedges, raw vegetables, fresh fruit, trail mix, dry cereal, some healthy chips. And don't forget to drink plenty of bottled water (don't drink airplane tap water or water that you suspect might have originated in the airplane tap), milk, and juice to counter the dehydration caused by air travel. This tactic will also encourage trips to the bathroom, which will ensure your legs get stretched periodically.

Wear your seat belt comfortably fastened below your belly. If you're traveling to a different time zone, take jet lag (see box, page 251) into account. Rest up in advance, and plan on taking it easy for a few days once you arrive.

If you're traveling by car. Keep a bagful of nutritious snacks and a thermos of juice or milk handy for when hunger strikes. For long trips, be sure the seat you will occupy is comfortable; if it isn't, consider buying or borrowing a special cushion for back support, available in auto supply or speciality stores or online. A pillow for neck support may also add to your comfort. For car safety tips, see page 250.

If you're traveling by train. Check to be sure there's a dining car with a full menu. If not, bring adequate meals and snacks along. If you're traveling overnight, book a sleeper car, if you can. You don't want to start your trip exhausted.

Sex and the Pregnant Woman

Religious and medical miracles aside, every pregnancy starts with sex. So why does what probably got you here in the first place become so complicated now that you're here? Whether you're having it more often or you're having it less often, whether you're enjoying it more or enjoying it less—or whether you're not doing it or enjoying it at all—chances are that making a baby has changed the way you make love. From sorting out what is and isn't safe in bed (or on the living room rug or on the kitchen counter) to figuring out which positions best accommodate your ever-bigger belly; from mismatched moods (you're turned on, he's turned off; he's turned on, you're turned off) to hormones gone wild (leaving your breasts more enticing than ever, yet too tender to touch), pregnancy sex is full of challenges on both sides of the bed. But not to worry. A little creativity, a good sense of humor, plenty of patience (and practice), and lots of love will conquer all when it comes to pregnancy lovemaking.

Sex Through the Trimesters

Down-up-down. While that might sound like a new sex position, it's actually a good description of the roller-coaster pattern most couples can expect their sex lives to follow during their nine months of pregnancy. In the first trimester, many women find that their libidos take a nosedive, plummeting promptly as soon as pregnancy hormones kick in. And that slowdown in sexual interest should come as no shocker. After all, fatigue, nausea, vomiting, and painfully tender nipples don't make great sex partners. But as with all things pregnancy, no two women are alike, which means no two libidos are alike, either. If you're lucky, you might actually find that the first trimester makes you hotter than ever, thanks to the happy side of hormonal changes: genitals that are ultrasensitive and evertingly, and breasts that are extra big and extra fun to touch (or have touched).

Interest often—though not always—picks up during the second trimester, when early pregnancy symptoms have subsided and there's more energy to put into lovemaking (and when less time in the bathroom leaves more time in the bedroom). Never had multiple orgasms before (or any orgasms)? This may be your lucky break—and your chance to get lucky again and again. That's because extra blood flow to the labia, clitoris, and vagina can make it easier to climax than ever before—and to have orgasms that are stronger and longer lasting, too. But again, nothing's a given during pregnancy. Some women actually lose that loving feeling in the second trimester—or never end up finding it at all during their nine months, and that's normal, too.

As delivery nears, libido usually wanes again, sometimes even more drastically than in the first trimester, for obvious reasons: First, your watermelon-size abdomen makes the target more difficult for your partner to reach, even with creative positioning; second, the aches and discomforts of advancing pregnancy can cool even the hottest passion; and third, late in the trimester it's hard to concentrate on anything but that eagerly and anxiously awaited event. Still, some couples manage to overcome those late-pregnancy obstacles and keep up the action until that first contraction.

What's Turning You On (or Off)?

With all the many physical changes you're undergoing during your nine months of pregnancy, it's no wonder desire and sexual pleasure are being affected, both positively and negatively. You'll have to learn to accommodate some of the negative effects so their interference in your sex life is minimal.

Nausea and vomiting. Morning sickness can certainly come between you and a good time. After all, it's hard to purr with pleasure when you're busy gagging up dinner. So use your time wisely. If your morning sickness rises with the sun, put after-dark hours to good use. If your evenings are queasy, hop on the morning love train. If morning sickness stays with you day and night, you and your spouse may just have to wait out its symptoms, which typically taper off by the end of the first trimester. Whatever you do, don't pressure yourself to feel sexy when you're feeling lousy; the result won't be satisfying for anyone.

Fatigue. It's hard to get busy when you barely have the energy to get undressed. Happily, the worst of pregnancy fatigue should pass by the fourth month (though exhaustion will probably return in the last trimester). Until then, make love while the sun shines (when the opportunity presents itself) instead of trying to force yourself to stay up for after-dinner romance. Cap off a weekend afternoon of lovemaking with a nap or the other way around. Have the kind of breakfast in bed that doesn't leave crumbs.

Your changing shape. Making love can be both awkward and uncomfortable when your bulging belly seems to loom as large and forbidding as a Himalayan mountain. As pregnancy progresses, the gymnastics required to scale that growing abdomen may not seem, to some couples, worth the effort. (But there are ways to manage that mountain; read on for more.) What's more, your fuller-than-ever figure may make you feel less sexy (though some women—and most partners—find that pregnant shape the most sensual of all female forms). If your body is a turnoff to you, try dressing it up in lacy lingerie or lighting your love nest with the flattering glow of candles. Also try to shed those negative body images by thinking: Big (in pregnancy) is beautiful.

Your engorged genitals. Increased blood flow to the pelvic area, caused by hormonal changes of pregnancy, can make some women more sexually responsive than ever. But it can also make sex less satisfying (especially later in pregnancy) if a residual fullness persists after orgasm, leaving you feeling as though you didn't quite make it. For your partner, too, the engorgement of your genitalia may increase pleasure (if he feels pleasantly and snugly caressed) or decrease it (if the fit is so tight he loses his erection).

Leakage of colostrum. Late in pregnancy, some women begin producing the pre-

The Ins and Outs of Sex During Pregnancy

Wondering what's safe and what's not when it comes to making love during pregnancy? Here's the lowdown:

Oral sex. Cunnilingus (oral stimulation of the female genitals) is as safe as it is potentially pleasurable throughout pregnancy, so don't hesitate to go for it (just make sure your partner doesn't forcefully blow air into your vagina). Fellatio (oral stimulation of the penis) is always safe during pregnancy (as is swallowing semen), and for some couples is a very satisfactory substitute when intercourse isn't permitted. It's wise to avoid oral sex if your partner has an STD.

Anal sex. Anal sex is probably safe during pregnancy, but proceed to the back door with caution. First, it probably won't be comfortable if you have hemorrhoids, an occupational hazard of pregnancy—and it can make them bleed (which can really spoil

the moment). Second, you'll need to remember the same safety rule of anal sex whether you're pregnant or not, but be especially fastidious about following it now: Never go from anal to vaginal sex without cleaning up first. Doing so may introduce harmful bacteria into your vaginal canal, setting you up for infection and risk to the baby.

Masturbation. Unless orgasm is off-limits because of a high-risk pregnancy or premature labor, masturbating during pregnancy is perfectly safe—and a great way to release all that tension you're feeling.

Vibrators or dildos. As long as your practitioner has okayed vaginal penetration, dildos and vibrators are safe to use during pregnancy; after all, they're just mechanical versions of the real thing. But be sure anything you introduce into the vagina is clean before you use it, and be careful not to penetrate the vagina too deeply with it.

milk called colostrum, which can leak from the breasts during sexual stimulation and can be a little disconcerting (and messy) in the middle of foreplay. It's nothing to worry about, of course, but if it bothers you or your partner, concentrate on other parts of the body (like that possibly trigger-happy clitoris of yours!).

Breast tenderness. For some couples, pregnant breasts (full, firm, and possibly larger than life) are favorite toys that can't get enough play time. But for many, that early pregnancy swelling comes with a high price—painful tenderness—and along with it, a look-but-don't-touch policy. If your breasts are bringing you more pain than pleasure, make sure your

partner gets the memo—and remind him that the tenderness will ease up by the end of the first trimester, at which point he'll be able to enjoy a hands-on approach.

Changes in vaginal secretions. Wet isn't always wild when you're expecting. Normal vaginal secretions increase during pregnancy and also change in consistency, odor, and taste. If you've always been on the dry or narrow side, that extra lubrication may make sex more enjoyable. But sometimes, too much of a good thing can make the vaginal canal so wet and slippery that it actually decreases sensation for both of you—and even makes it more difficult for your partner to keep his erection or reach orgasm. (A little extra foreplay for him may help him out in that department.) The heavier scent and taste of the secretions may also make oral sex off-putting. Massaging scented oils into the pubic area or the inner thighs (but not the vagina) may help.

Some expectant moms experience vaginal dryness during sex, even with all those extra secretions. Unscented water-based lubricants, such as K-Y or Astroglide, are safe to use as needed when you're having a dry spell.

Bleeding caused by the sensitivity of the cervix. The mouth of the uterus also becomes engorged during pregnancy—crisscrossed with many additional blood vessels to accommodate increased blood flow—and is much softer than before pregnancy. This means that deep penetration can occasionally cause spotting, particularly late in pregnancy when the cervix begins to ripen for delivery (but also at any time during pregnancy). This type of bleeding is usually nothing to be concerned about, though do mention it to your practitioner for extra reassurance.

There are also plenty of psychological hang-ups that can get between you, your partner, and full sexual enjoyment during pregnancy. These, too, can often be minimized.

Fear of hurting the fetus or causing a miscarriage. Stop worrying and start enjoying. In normal pregnancies, sex isn't harmful. Your baby is well cushioned and protected inside the amniotic sac and uterus, and your uterus is securely sealed off from the outside world by a mucous plug in the mouth of your cervix. Your practitioner will let you know if there's a reason why you shouldn't have sex during your pregnancy. Otherwise, go for it.

Fear that having an orgasm will stimulate miscarriage or early labor. Although the uterus does contract following orgasm—and these contractions can be quite powerful in some women, lasting as long as half an hour after intercourse—such contractions are not a sign of labor and aren't harmful in a normal pregnancy. Again, if there's a reason why you should avoid orgasm while you're expecting (because you're at high risk for miscarriage or preterm labor, or have a placenta problem, for instance), your practitioner will let you know.

Fear that the fetus is "watching" or "aware." Not possible. Though your baby may enjoy the gentle rocking of uterine contractions during orgasm, he or she can't see what you're doing, has no clue what's happening, and will certainly have no memory of it. Fetal reactions (slowed movement during sex, then furious kicking and squirming and a speeded-up heartbeat after orgasm) are solely responses to uterine activity.

Fear of "hitting" the baby on the head. Though your partner may not want to admit it, no penis is big enough to hurt a fetus—or big enough to get close to it. Once again, the baby is well sealed off in a cozy uterine home. Even if your baby's head is engaged in your pelvis, deep penetration can't do any harm (though if it's uncomfortable, avoid it).

Fear that sex will cause infection. As long as your partner doesn't have a sexually transmittable disease and your cervix is not open, there is no danger of infection to either mother or fetus through intercourse. In the amniotic sac, the baby is safely sealed off from both semen and infectious organisms.

Anxiety over the coming attraction. Sure, you're both preoccupied and maybe a little (or a lot) stressed out. You might be experiencing mixed feelings, too, over your baby's imminent arrival. And it's

Sexercise

There's no better way to mix business with pleasure than performing Kegels during sex. These exercises tone the perineal area in preparation for childbirth, reducing the likelihood that you'll need an episiotomy, as well as minimizing the risk of a tear. Doing Kegels often will also speed postpartum recovery in the area. And though you can perform Kegels anywhere, anytime (see page 295 for how), doing them during intercourse can double the pleasure for you both. Exercise was never this much fun!

---

sometimes hard to have sexy thoughts when your mind's cluttered with worries about all those upcoming responsibilities and lifestyle changes, not to mention the financial and emotional cost of bringing up baby. Your best move? Talk about these feelings openly and often—and don't bring them to bed.

The changing relationship. Maybe you're having trouble adjusting to those impending changes in your family dynamic—the idea that you'll no longer be just lovers, or partners, but mother and father as well. Or you may be discovering that the new dimension in your relationship brings a new intimacy to lovemaking—and with it, a new excitement.

Resentment. Feelings of resentment—of your partner toward you, perhaps because he is jealous that you and the pregnancy have become the center of attention, or of you toward him because you feel you're doing all the heavy lifting for the baby you both want and will both

enjoy—can keep things chilly under the sheets. Such feelings are important to talk out, but again, do your chatting before you hit the sack.

Belief that sex later in pregnancy will cause labor to begin. It is true that the uterine contractions triggered by orgasm become stronger as pregnancy proceeds. But unless the cervix is ripe and ready, these contractions do not appear to bring on labor—as many hopeful and eager overdue couples can attest. In fact, studies show that couples who are sexually active during late pregnancy are more likely to carry to term.

Of course, psychological factors can also add to pregnancy sex pleasure (good news!). For one, some couples who worked hard at becoming pregnant may be happy to switch from procreational to recreational sex. Instead of being slaves to ovulation predictor kits, charts, calendars, and monthly anxiety, they can enjoy spontaneous sex for pleasure's sake. For another, many couples find that creating a baby brings them closer together than ever before, and they find the belly a symbol of that closeness—instead of an awkward obstacle.

When Sex May Be Limited

Since lovemaking has so much to offer you and your partner when you're expecting, it would be wonderful if every couple could take advantage of those perks throughout pregnancy. Alas, for some this isn't possible. In high-risk pregnancies, intercourse may be restricted at certain times or even for the full nine months. Or intercourse may be permitted without orgasm for the woman. Or foreplay may be allowed as long as penetration is avoided. Or penetration is permitted but only if a condom is used. Knowing precisely what is safe and when it's safe is essential, so ask for details if your practitioner instructs you to abstain. Find out why sex is off the table and whether that refers to intercourse, orgasm, or both, and whether the restrictions are temporary or apply for the entire pregnancy.

Sex will probably be restricted under the following, and possibly other, circumstances:

- If you are experiencing signs of preterm labor or, possibly, if you have a history of preterm labor

- If you've been diagnosed with incompetent cervix or placenta previa

- Possibly, if you are experiencing bleeding or if you have a history of miscarriages

If penetration is off-limits, but orgasm's allowed, consider mutual masturbation. If orgasm's taboo for you,

you might get pleasure out of pleasuring your partner this way (he certainly won't object). If intercourse has been okayed—but orgasm's prohibited—you could try making love without your reaching climax. Though this definitely won't be completely satisfying for you (and may be impossible if you climax easily), you'll still get some of the intimacy you're both craving while providing pleasure for your partner. If all lovemaking activities have been banned for the duration, try not to let that come between you as a couple. Focus on other ways of getting close—the romantic, G-rated kinds you might not have tapped into since early on in your relationship (like hand-holding, cuddling, and old-fashioned making out).

Enjoying It More, Even If You're Doing It Less

Good, lasting sexual relationships are rarely built in a day (or even a really hot night). They grow with practice, patience, understanding, and love. This is true, too, of an already established sexual relationship that undergoes the emotional and physical changes of pregnancy. Here are a few ways to "stay on top":

- Enjoy your sex life instead of analyzing it. Seize the moment as you seize each other. Don't focus on how frequently or infrequently you're having sex (quality is always more important than quantity, but especially when you're expecting) or compare prepregnancy sex with your sex life now (they're two different animals and, for that matter, so are both of you).

- Accentuate all the positives. Think of making love as good physical preparation for labor and delivery—especially true if you remember to do your Kegels during intercourse. (Not many

---

Getting Comfortable

When you're making love at this point in your pregnancy (and later on, too), position matters. Side-lying positions (front-to-front or front-to-back) are often most comfortable because they keep you off your back. Ditto woman on top (which allows you more control over penetration). Rear entry can work well, too. Man on top is fine for quickies (as long as he keeps his weight off you by supporting himself with his arms), but after the fourth month, it's not a good idea to spend too much time flat on your back.

athletes have this much fun in training.) Think of sex as relaxing—and relaxation is good for all involved (including baby). Think of the roundness of your pregnant body as sensual and sexy. Think of every embrace as a chance to get closer as a couple, not just a chance to get closer to closing the deal.

- Get adventurous. The old positions don't fit anymore? Look at this as an opportunity to try something new (or a lot of somethings new). But give yourselves time to adjust to each position you try. You might even consider a "dry run"—trying out a new position fully clothed first, so that it'll be more familiar (and you'll be more successful) when you try it for real. See the box on the facing page for ideas.

- Keep your expectations within reality's reach. Pregnant sex presents plenty of challenges, so cut yourself some slack in the sack. Though some women achieve orgasm for the first time during pregnancy, other women find the big "O" more elusive than ever. Your goal doesn't always have to be mutual

fireworks. Remind yourself that getting close is sometimes the best, and most satisfying, part of getting it on.

- Don't forget the other kind of intercourse (talking, that is). Communication is the foundation of every relationship, particularly one that's going through life-changing adjustments. Discuss any problems you're facing as a couple openly instead of trying to sweep them under the bed (and instead of taking them to bed). If any problems seem too big to handle by yourselves, seek professional help. There was never a better time to work on your twosome than now that it's about to become a threesome.

Good, bad, or indifferent, remember, too, that every couple feels differently about sex during pregnancy, both physically and emotionally. The bottom line (whether you're on top, on bottom, side to side, or not doing it at all): What's normal, as is almost always the case when you're expecting, is what's normal for you and your partner. Embrace that, embrace each other—and try not to sweat the rest.

The
Sixth
Month

Approximately 23 to 27 Weeks

NO DOUBT ABOUT THOSE TUMMY moves these days: They're all baby, not gas (though you're probably still having plenty of that, too). And as those little arms and legs start to pack more of a punch, these baby calisthenics—and sometimes bouts of baby hiccups—will become visible from the outside and may even entertain those around you. This month marks the last of the second trimester, which means you're almost two thirds of the way there. Still, you've got a ways to go, and a ways to grow—as does baby, who's a relatively light load compared to what you'll be carrying around in a month or two. Take advantage—and while you can still see your feet (if not touch your toes), kick up your 2-inch heels a little.

Your Baby This Month

Week 23 A window into your womb would reveal that your baby's skin is a bit saggy, hanging loosely from his or her little body. That's because skin grows faster than fat develops, and there's not much fat to fill that skin out yet. But don't worry—the fat is about to start catching up. Beginning this week, your baby (who is around 8 inches long and just over a pound in weight) begins to pack on the pounds (which means you will, too!). In fact, by month's end, your baby will be double the weight he or she is now (fortunately, you won't be).

Once those fat deposits are made, your baby will be less transparent, too. Right now, the organs and bones can still be seen through the skin, which has a red hue thanks to the developing blood veins and arteries just underneath. But by month 8, no more see-through baby!

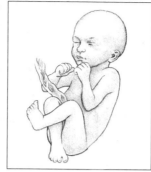

Your Baby, Month 6

Week 24 At a weight of 1½ pounds and a length of about 8½ inches, your baby has outgrown the fruit references and is now the size of a standard letter (but would take a lot more than a standard stamp to mail). Baby's weekly weight gain is now about 6 ounces—not quite as much as you're putting on, but getting a lot closer. Much of that weight is coming from accumulating baby fat, as well as from growing organs, bones, and muscle. By now, your baby's tiny face is almost fully formed, and achingly adorable—complete with a full set of eyelashes and eyebrows and a good sprinkling of hair on that head. Is your baby a brunette, a blond, or a redhead? Actually, right now, he or she's snow white, since there's no pigment in that hair just yet.

Week 25 Baby's growing by leaps and bounds (and inches and ounces), this week reaching 9 inches in length and more than 1½ pounds in weight. And there are exciting developments on the horizon, too. Capillaries are forming under the skin and filling with blood. By week's end, air sacs lined with capillaries will also develop in your baby's lungs, getting them ready for that first breath of fresh air. Mind you, those lungs aren't ready for prime-time breathing yet—and they have a lot of maturing left to do before they will be. Though they're already beginning to develop surfactant,

a substance that will help them expand after birth, your baby's lungs are still too undeveloped to sufficiently send oxygen to the bloodstream and release carbon dioxide from the blood (aka breathe). And talking about breathing, your baby's nostrils, which have been plugged up until now, are starting to open up this week. This enables your baby to begin taking practice "breaths." Your baby's vocal cords are functioning now, leading to occasional hiccups (which you'll certainly be feeling).

Week 26 Next time you're browsing through the meat department, pick up a 2-pound chuck roast. No, not for dinner—just so you can get a sense of how big your baby is this week. That's right—your baby now weighs a full 2 pounds and measures in at 9-plus inches long. Another momentous development this week: Your baby's eyes are beginning to open. The eyelids have been fused for the past few months (so the retina, the part of the eye that allows images to come into focus, could develop). The colored part of the eye (the iris) still doesn't have much pigmentation, so it's too early to start guessing your baby's eye color. Still, your baby is now able to see—though there's not much to see in the dark confines of his or her uterine home. But with the heightened sense of sight and hearing that your baby now possesses, you may notice an increase in activity when your baby sees a bright light or hears a loud noise. In fact, if a loud vibrating noise is brought close to your belly, your baby will respond by blinking and startling.

Week 27 Your baby graduates onto a new growth chart this week. No longer will he or she be measured crown to rump, but rather from head to toe. And this week that head-to-toe length is a full 15 inches (more than a foot long)! Your baby's weight is creeping up the charts as well, coming in at just over 2 pounds this week. And here's an interesting fetal factoid: Your baby has more taste buds now than he or she will have at birth (and beyond). Which means that not only is your baby able to taste the difference in the amniotic fluid when you eat different foods, he or she might even react to it. For instance, some babies respond to spicy foods by hiccupping. Or by kicking when they get that spicy kick.

What You May Be Feeling

As always, remember that every pregnancy and every woman is different. You may experience all of these symptoms at one time or another, or only a few of them. Some may have continued from last month; others may be new. Still others may be hardly noticed because you've become so used to them. You may also have other, less common, symptoms. Here's what you might experience this month:

Physically

- More definite fetal activity

- Continued vaginal discharge

- Achiness in the lower abdomen and along the sides (from stretching of ligaments supporting the uterus)

- Constipation

- Heartburn, indigestion, flatulence, bloating

- Occasional headaches, faintness, or dizziness

- Nasal congestion and occasional nosebleeds; ear stuffiness

- Sensitive gums that may bleed when you brush

- Hearty appetite

- Leg cramps

- Mild swelling of ankles and feet, and occasionally of hands and face

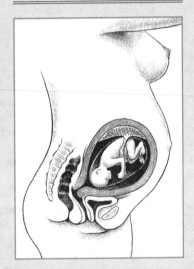

A Look Inside

At the beginning of this month, your uterus is around 1½ inches above your belly button. By the end of the month, your uterus has grown an inch higher and can be felt approximately 2½ inches above your belly button. Your uterus is the size of a basketball now, and you might even look like that's what you're carrying around in your belly.

- Varicose veins of the legs and/or hemorrhoids
- Itchy abdomen
- A protruding navel
- Backache
- Skin pigmentation changes on abdomen and/or face
- Stretch marks
- Enlarged breasts

Emotionally

- Fewer mood swings
- Continued absentmindedness
- Some boredom with the pregnancy ("Can't anyone think about anything else?")
- Some anxiety about the future
- Plenty of excitement about the future

What You Can Expect at This Month's Checkup

It will probably be business pretty much as usual at this month's checkup. As you end your second trimester, you can expect your practitioner to check the following, though there may be variations, depending on your particular needs and on your practitioner's style of practice:

- Weight and blood pressure
- Urine, for sugar and protein
- Fetal heartbeat

- Height of fundus (top of uterus)
- Size of uterus and position of fetus, by external palpation (feeling from the outside)
- Feet and hands for swelling, and legs for varicose veins
- Symptoms you may have been experiencing, especially unusual ones
- Questions and problems you want to discuss—have a list ready

What You May Be Wondering About

Trouble Sleeping

"I've never had a sleep problem in my life—until now. I can't seem to settle down at night."

Between midnight bathroom runs, a racing mind, cramping legs, heartburn that's keeping you upright, a hopped-up metabolism that's keeping the heat on even when it's off, and

the impossibility of getting comfortable when you're sporting a basketball in your midsection, it's no wonder that you can't settle in for a good night's sleep. While this insomnia is definitely good preparation for the sleepless nights you'll encounter as a new parent, that doesn't mean you have to take it lying down. Try the following tips for summoning the sandman:

- Move your body during the day. A body that gets a workout by day will be sleepier at night. But don't exercise too close to bedtime, since the postexercise high could keep you from crashing when your head hits the pillow.

- Clear your mind. If you've been losing sleep over problems at work or at home, unload them on your spouse or a friend during the early evening so they don't weigh you down at bedtime. If no one's around to talk them over with, write your concerns down. Putting them on paper can be therapeutic, plus it may help you figure out some solutions. As bedtime approaches, put those worries aside, empty your head, and try thinking happy thoughts only.

- Take your (dinner)time. Instead of wolfing your dinner down (as hungry as you are by the time it's in front of you), serve up a leisurely approach to your evening meal. Eating slowly and calmly will take a bite out of nighttime heartburn and ideally keep you from tossing and turning when you turn out the light. And don't go straight from dinner to bed, because a full tummy can leave you too energized—and too uncomfortable—to sleep.

- Top off before you turn in. Too much food right before bed can interfere with sleep, but so can too little. To keep the midnight munchies from waking you, have a light snack as part of your bedtime routine. That old sleepy-time standard, a glass of warm milk, may be especially effective, probably because it reminds you of being tucked in with your teddy bear. You'll get a similar soporific effect by combining any light protein with some complex carbs, so nibble on fruit and cheese or yogurt and raisins, or dunk a muffin or some oatmeal cookies in your milk.

- Slow the flow. If frequent trips to the bathroom are standing between you and a good night's sleep, limit fluids after 6 P.M. (just make sure you get your daily quota of fluids before then). Drink if you're thirsty, but don't guzzle a 16-ounce bottle of water right before bedtime.

- Don't get buzzed. Avoid caffeine in all its forms in the afternoon and evening (its effects can keep you buzzing for up to six hours). Ditto for sugar (especially combined with caffeine, as in chocolate), which will give you an energy boost when you least want one and then leave your blood sugar levels wobbly during the night.

- Give yourself a bedtime routine. It's not just for kids. The relaxing repetition of the right bedtime rituals can help adults settle down for a good night's sleep, too. Easy does it, so focus on activities that slow you down after dinner, preferably practiced in a predictable order. Good options to consider adding to your routine: light reading (but nothing you can't put down) or television (though steer clear of anything that's violent or emotionally wrenching), soothing music, some stretching, serene yoga poses or relaxation exercises, a warm bath, a backrub, some lovemaking.

- Get comfy. There is no such thing as too many pillows when you're pregnant. Use them to prop you up, support you where you need it, or just cozy up to. The sooner in pregnancy you learn to sleep comfortably on your side, the easier it will be for you to do it later on. Be sure, too, that your mattress is comfortable and your bedroom isn't too hot or too cold.

- Get some air. It's hard to get sleepy when you're stuffy, especially when you're heating for two. So open a window in all but the coldest or hottest weather (when a fan or air-conditioning can help circulate the air). And don't sleep with the covers over your head. This will decrease the oxygen and increase the carbon dioxide you breathe in, which can cause headaches.

- Ask before you pop. While there are sleep aids that are safe for occasional pregnancy use, don't take any sleep aid (prescription, over-the-counter, or herbal) unless it's been prescribed by your practitioner. If your practitioner has recommended that you take a magnesium supplement (or a calcium-magnesium supplement) to combat constipation or leg cramps, it makes sense to take it before bed because magnesium has natural relaxing powers.

- Smell your way to sleep. A lavender-scented pillow that you tuck into bed with you or a dried lavender sachet slipped between the pillowcase and pillow can help relax you and bring on sleep faster.

- Save your bed for sleep (and sex). Don't invite activities you associate with being wide awake and possibly stressed (answering office e-mails on your laptop, paying bills) into your bed. Take care of business in other parts of your home, and reserve your bedroom for its more traditional purposes.

- Go to bed when you're tired. Climbing into bed before you're sleepy is a recipe for a restless night. Putting off your bedtime may, paradoxically, help you sleep better. But don't wait until you're overtired and less able to settle down.

- Avoid clock-watching. Judge whether you're getting enough sleep by how you feel, not by how many hours you stay in bed. Keep in mind that many people who believe they have sleep problems actually get more sleep than

they think—and as much as they need. You're getting enough rest if you're not chronically tired (beyond the normal fatigue of pregnancy). And speaking of clocks, if the sight of that glowing dial (and the hours ticking by) stresses you out, turn it so you can't see it.

- Don't just lie there. When sleep's eluding you—and you've run out of sheep to count—get up and do something relaxing (read, watch TV) until you feel sleepy.

- Don't lose sleep over losing sleep. Stressing about your lack of shut-eye will only make it harder to grab any. In fact, sometimes just letting go of that "will I ever fall asleep?" worry is all it takes to drop off into dreamland.

Save Time (in a Capsule)

Time flies when you're having babies—and raising them. Before it has a chance to fly away, preserve your pregnancy for posterity by making a time capsule. Years from now, your baby (who won't be a baby anymore) will get a kick out of seeing the way things were back in the day, before he or she arrived on the scene. Just take a box (or a capsule) and put in pictures of you (pregnant, of course), your spouse, any pets, and your house and car. Add ultrasound pictures, a menu from the restaurant that always delivers your cravings to the door, a current magazine and newspaper—and any other souvenirs of this expectant era you'd like to hold on to. No need to bury it—just seal it and put it away (don't forget where next time you move) until your baby's old enough to appreciate it.

Protruding Navel

"My belly button used to be a perfect 'innie.' Now it's sticking all the way out. Will it stay that way even after I deliver?"

Has your innie been outed? Is it poking straight through your clothes these days? Taking on a life of its own? Don't worry: There's nothing novel about navels that pop during pregnancy. Just about every belly button does at some point. As the swelling uterus pushes forward, even the deepest "innie" is sure to pop like a timer on a turkey (except, on most women, the navel "pops" well before baby's "done"). Your belly button should revert back to its regular position a few months after delivery, though it may bear the mommy mark: that stretched-out, lived-in look. Until then, you can look at the bright side of your protruding navel: It gives you a chance to clean out all the lint that's accumulated there since you were a kid. If you find that the outie look doesn't quite work with the clingy fashion statement you're trying to make, consider taping it down (you can use a Band-Aid, as long as it doesn't irritate, or specially designed belly button tape). But in the meantime, remember, it's just one more pregnancy badge of honor to wear proudly.

Baby Kicking

"Some days the baby is kicking all the time; other days he seems very quiet. Is this normal?"

Fetuses are only human. Just like us, they have "up" days, when they feel like kicking up their heels (and elbows and knees), and "down" days, when they'd rather lie back and take it easy. Most often, their activity is related to what you've been doing. Like babies out of the womb, fetuses are lulled by rocking. So when you're on the go all day, your baby is likely to be pacified by the rhythm of your routine, and you're likely not to notice much kicking—partly because baby's slowed down, partly because you're so busy. As soon as you slow down or relax, he or she is bound to start acting up (a pattern babies, unfortunately, tend to continue even after they're born). That's why you're more apt to feel fetal movement in bed at night or when you're resting during the day. Activity may also increase after you've had a meal or snack, perhaps in reaction to the surge of sugar in your blood. You may also notice increased fetal activity when you're excited or nervous—about to give a presentation, for example—possibly because the baby is stimulated by your adrenaline response.

Babies are actually most active between weeks 24 and 28, when they're small enough to belly dance, somersault, kickbox, and do a full aerobic step class in their roomy uterine home. But their movements are erratic and usually brief, so they aren't always felt by a busy mother-to-be, even though they are visible on ultrasound. Fetal activity usually becomes more organized and consistent, with more clearly defined periods of rest and activity, between weeks 28 and 32. It's definitely felt later and less emphatically when there's an anterior placenta getting in the way (see page 246).

Don't be tempted to compare baby movement notes with other pregnant women. Each fetus, like each newborn, has an individual pattern of activity and development. Some seem always active; others mostly quiet. The activity of some fetuses is so regular their moms could set their watches by it; in others there's no discernible activity pattern at all. As long as there is no radical slowdown or cessation of activity, all variations are normal.

Keeping track of your baby's kicks isn't necessary until week 28 (see page 289).

"Sometimes the baby kicks so hard it hurts."

As your baby matures in the uterus, he or she becomes stronger and stronger, and those once butterfly-like fetal movements pack more and more punch. Which is why you shouldn't be surprised if you get kicked in the ribs or poked in the abdomen or cervix with such force it hurts. When you seem to be under a particularly fierce attack, try changing your position. It may knock your little linebacker off balance and temporarily stem the assault.

"The baby seems to be kicking all over. Could I be carrying twins?"

At some point in her pregnancy, just about every woman begins to think that she's carrying either twins or a human octopus. That's because until a fetus grows out of room to move (usually at about 34 weeks), it's able to perform numerous acrobatics. So, while it may sometimes feel as if you're being pummeled by a dozen fists (or a litter), it's more likely to be two fists that really get around—along with tiny knees, elbows, and feet. (And if you did have a second passenger on board, you would have likely made that discovery during one of your ultrasounds.)

Itchy Belly

"My belly itches constantly. It's driving me crazy."

Join the club. Pregnant bellies are itchy bellies, and they can become progressively itchier as the months pass. That's because as your belly grows, the skin stretches rapidly, becoming increasingly moisture-deprived—leaving it itchy and uncomfortable. Try not to scratch, which will only make you itchier and could cause irritation. Moisturizer can temporarily curb the itching; apply a gentle one frequently and liberally. An anti-itching lotion (such as calamine) may provide more relief, as can an oatmeal bath. If you have an all-over itch that's not related to dry or sensitive skin, however, or develop a rash on your abdomen, check with your practitioner.

Clumsiness

"Lately I've been dropping everything I pick up. Why am I suddenly so clumsy?"

Like the extra inches on your belly, the extra thumbs on your hands and those two left feet you suddenly feel you're sporting are part of the pregnancy package. This real (and, unfortunately, plain for everyone to see) pregnancy-induced clumsiness is caused by the loosening of joints and ligaments and the retention of water, both of which can make your grasp on objects less firm and sure. Other factors include a lack of concentration as a result of pregnancy forgetfulness (see page 214) or a lack of dexterity as a result of carpal tunnel syndrome (see next question). And it certainly doesn't help matters that your growing belly has shifted your center of gravity, throwing your balance off-kilter. This uneasiness in balance—whether conscious or not—is most apparent when you're climbing a flight of stairs, walking on a slippery surface (something you really shouldn't be doing anyway), or carrying something heavy (ditto). Not being able to see past your belly to your feet (which, if it hasn't happened yet, definitely will) can also make tripping—over curbs, on steps, on the sneakers your spouse left in front of the bathroom door—a lot easier to do. Finally, pregnancy fatigue can keep you off your game (or knock you off your feet), making it easier to both trip and drop.

Most pregnancy clumsiness is just annoying. Repeatedly retrieving the car keys from the floor, for instance, is merely an ongoing pain in the neck (as well as a pain in the back if you don't remember to bend from the knees). Falls, however, can be a more serious matter, which is why "caution" should be your middle name when you're expecting.

If you're feeling like a bull in a china shop these days, you'll have to make some modifications to your daily activities. Definitely stay out of china shops (and keep your clumsy paws off the good china at home). Leave your favorite crystal on the shelf for the duration and let someone else load and unload the dishwasher, especially when the good stuff's involved. It'll also help to slow down, walk more deliberately and carefully (especially when there's ice or snow underfoot), use extra caution in the tub or shower, keep hallways and stairs clear of objects that might trip you up, refrain from standing on any chairs (no matter what you need to reach), and avoid pushing yourself (the more tired you are, the more clumsy you'll be). Most important, recognize your current limitations and your lack of coordination, and try to have a sense of humor about it.

Numbness in the Hands

"I keep waking up in the middle of the night because some of the fingers on my right hand are numb. Is that related to pregnancy?"

Feeling all atingle these days? Chances are it isn't romance or even excitement about the baby—it's the normal numbness and tingling in the fingers and toes that many women experience during pregnancy, probably the result of swelling tissues pressing on nerves. If the numbness and pain are confined to your thumb, index finger, middle finger, and half of your ring finger, you probably have carpal tunnel syndrome (CTS). Though this condition is most common in people who regularly perform tasks that require repetitive motions of the hand (such as piano playing or typing), it is also extremely common in pregnant women—even in those who don't do repetitive hand motions. That's because the carpal tunnel in the wrist, through which the nerve to the affected fingers runs, becomes swollen during pregnancy (as do so many other tissues in the body), with the resultant pressure causing numbness, tingling, burning, and pain. The symptoms can also affect the hand and wrist, and they can radiate up the arm.

Though the pain of CTS can strike at any time of day, you might feel yourself wrestling with wrist pain more at night. That's because fluids that accumulate in your lower extremities during the day are redistributed to the rest of your body (including your hands) when you're lying down. Sleeping on your hands can make the problem worse, so try elevating them on a separate pillow at bedtime. When numbness occurs, shaking your hands may relieve it. If that doesn't do the trick, and the numbness is interfering with your sleep, discuss the problem with your practitioner. Often wearing a wrist splint is helpful. Acupuncture can also bring relief.

The nonsteroidal anti-inflammatory drugs and steroids usually prescribed for CTS may not be recommended during pregnancy. Check with your practitioner. Luckily, when the regular swelling of pregnancy resolves once you've delivered, the carpal tunnel symptoms will diminish, too.

If you think the CTS is related to your work habits (or at-home computer use) as well as your pregnancy, see page 191.

Leg Cramps

"I have leg cramps at night that keep me awake."

Between your overloaded mind and your bulging belly, you probably have enough trouble catching those z's without leg cramps cramping your sleeping style. Unfortunately, these painful spasms that radiate up and down your calves and occur most often at night are very common among the expectant set in the second and third trimesters.

No one's quite sure what causes leg cramps. Various theories blame fatigue from carrying pregnancy weight, compression of the blood vessels in the legs, and possibly diet (an excess of phosphorus and a shortage of calcium or magnesium). You might as well blame hormones, too, since they seem to cause so many pregnancy aches and pains.

Whatever the cause, there are ways of both preventing and alleviating them:

- When a leg cramp strikes, be sure to straighten your leg and flex your ankle and toes slowly up toward your nose (don't point your toes). This should soon lessen the pain. Doing this several times with each leg before turning in at night may even help ward off the cramps.

- Stretching exercises can also help stop cramps before they strike. Before you head to bed, stand about 2 feet away from a wall and put your palms flat against it. Lean forward, keeping your heels on the floor. Hold the stretch for 10 seconds, then relax for 5. Try this three times. (See the illustration.)

- To ease the daily load on your legs, put your feet up as often as you can, alternate periods of activity with periods of rest, and wear support hose during the day. Flex your feet periodically.

- Try standing on a cold surface, which can sometimes stop a spasm.

- You can add massage or local heat for added relief, but don't massage or add heat if neither flexing nor cold helps the situation.

- Make sure you're drinking enough fluids—at least eight glasses a day.

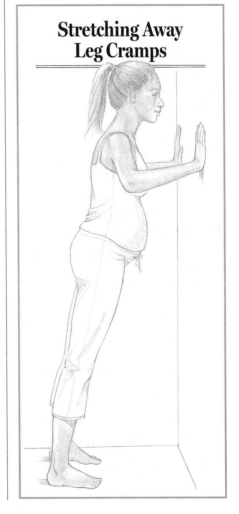

Stretching Away Leg Cramps

When Something Just Doesn't Feel Right

Maybe it's a twinge of abdominal pain that feels too much like a cramp to ignore, a sudden change in your vaginal discharge, an aching in your lower back or in your pelvic floor— or maybe it's something so vague you can't even put your finger on it. Chances are it's just par for the pregnancy course, but to play it safe, check page 138 to see if a call to your practitioner is in order.

If you can't find your symptoms on the list, it's probably a good idea to call anyway. Reporting odd symptoms could help identify early signs of premature labor or other pregnancy complications, which could make a big difference in your pregnancy. Remember, you know your body better than anyone. Listen up when it's trying to tell you something.

- Eat a well-balanced diet that includes plenty of calcium and magnesium.

Really bad cramps (like a charley horse) can cause muscle soreness that lasts a few days. That's nothing to worry about. But if the pain is severe and persists, contact your practitioner because there's a slight possibility that a blood clot may have developed in a vein, making medical treatment necessary (see page 563).

Hemorrhoids

"I'm dreading getting hemorrhoids—I've heard they're common during pregnancy. Is there anything I can do to prevent them?"

It's a big pain in the butt, but more than half of all pregnant women experience hemorrhoids. Just as the veins of the legs are more susceptible to varicosities at this time, so, too, are the veins of the rectum. Pressure from your enlarging uterus, plus increased blood flow to the pelvic area, can cause the veins in your rectal wall to swell, bulge, and itch (how's that for a pleasant thought?).

Constipation can aggravate, or even cause, hemorrhoids (also called piles because of the resemblance these swollen veins sometimes bear to a pile of grapes or marbles), so your best prevention is to avoid constipation in the first place (see page 173). Doing your Kegels (see page 295) can also ward off hemorrhoids by improving circulation to the area, as can taking the pressure off by sleeping on your side, not your back; avoiding long hours of standing or sitting; and not lingering on the toilet (keep this book and other reading material out of the bathroom so you aren't tempted to just sit and read). Sitting with your feet on a step stool may make that other stool easier to pass.

To soothe the sting of hemorrhoids, try witch hazel pads or ice packs. A warm bath might reduce discomfort, too. If sitting is a pain, use a doughnut-shaped pillow to ease pressure. Ask your practitioner before using any medication, topical or otherwise. But forget about your grandma's cure—downing a spoonful of mineral oil—which can carry valuable nutrients right out the back door.

Hemorrhoids can sometimes bleed, especially when you're bearing down during a bowel movement, though anal fissures (painful cracks in the skin of the anus caused by straining from constipation) can also be the cause of rectal bleeding. Rectal bleeding should always be evaluated by your physician, but hemorrhoids or fissures are probably the culprits. Hemorrhoids aren't dangerous (just uncomfortable) and usually go away after delivery—though they can also develop postpartum as a result of pushing during delivery.

Breast Lump

"I'm worried about a small tender lump on the side of my breast. What could it be?"

Though you're still months away from being able to nurse your baby, it sounds like your breasts are already gearing up. The result: a clogged milk duct. These red, tender-to-the-touch, hard lumps in the breast are very common even this early in pregnancy, especially in second and subsequent pregnancies. Warm compresses (or letting warm water run on it in the shower) and gentle massage will probably clear the duct up in a few days, just as it will during lactation. Some experts suggest that avoiding underwire bras also helps, but make sure you get ample support from the bra you do wear.

Keep in mind that monthly self-exams of your breasts shouldn't stop when you're pregnant. Though checking for lumps is trickier when you're expecting because of the changes in your breasts, it's still important to try. Show any lump to your practitioner at your next visit.

Childbirth Pain

"I'm eager to become a mother, but not so eager to experience childbirth. Mostly, I worry about the pain."

Almost every expectant mother eagerly awaits the birth of her child,

---

Bleeding in Mid- or Late Pregnancy

It's always unsettling to see pink or red on your underwear when you're expecting, but light or spotty bleeding in the second or third trimester is generally not a cause for concern. It's often the result of bruising to the increasingly sensitive cervix during an internal exam or sexual intercourse, or it is sometimes simply triggered by causes unknown and innocuous.

Still, let your practitioner know about any bleeding or spotting in case it's a sign something more serious is going on. If you're bleeding heavily or if the spotting is accompanied by pain or discomfort, give your practitioner a call right away. An ultrasound exam can often determine whether or not there's a problem.

---

but few look forward to labor and delivery—and far fewer still to the pain of labor and delivery. And many, like you, spend much of the months leading up to this momentous event obsessing about the pain. That's not surprising. For those who've never experienced significant discomfort (except maybe a toothache here, a pulled muscle there), the fear of labor pain—which is, after all, an unknown quantity of pain—is very real and very normal.

But it's important to keep in mind the following: Childbirth is a normal life process, which women have been experiencing as long as there have been women. Sure it comes with pain, but it's a pain with a positive purpose (though it won't necessarily feel positive when you're in it): to thin and open your cervix, and bring your baby into your arms. And it's also a pain with a built-in time limit. You might not believe it (especially somewhere around the 5-cm mark), but labor won't last forever. Not only that, but the pain of childbirth is a pain you don't even have to put up with at all. Pain medication is always just a request

away, should you end up wanting it or needing it—or both.

So there's no point in dreading the pain (especially because you have the option of avoiding it, or at least, avoiding most of it), but there's a lot to be said for being prepared for it—and for preparing realistically and rationally, with eyes wide open to every option and every eventuality. Preparing now (both your body and mind—since both are involved in how you experience pain) should help reduce the anxiety you're feeling now and the amount of discomfort you'll feel once those contractions kick in.

Get educated. One reason earlier generations of women found labor so frightening was that they didn't understand what was happening to their bodies or why. They only knew that it hurt. Today, a good childbirth education class can reduce fear (and ultimately pain) by increasing knowledge, preparing women and their coaches, stage by stage and phase by phase, for labor and delivery. If you can't take a class or if you just don't want to, read up as much as you can on the subject of labor and delivery. What you don't know can worry you more than it has to. Taking classes makes sense, by the way, even if you're planning on having an epidural—or even if you have a cesarean delivery scheduled.

Get moving. You wouldn't consider running a marathon without the proper physical training. Neither should you consider signing up for labor (which is no less challenging an event) untrained. Work out with all the breathing, stretching, and toning-up exercises your practitioner and/or childbirth educator recommends, plus plenty of Kegels.

Team up. Whether you have your partner there to comfort you and feed you ice chips, a doula (see page 298) to mas-

---

Diagnosing Preeclampsia

Chances are you've heard of (or know) someone who developed preeclampsia (or pregnancy-induced hypertension) during pregnancy. But the reality is that it isn't that common, occurring in only 3 to 7 percent of pregnancies, even in its mildest form. And luckily, in women who are receiving regular prenatal care, preeclampsia can be diagnosed and treated early, preventing needless complications. Though routine office visits sometimes seem a waste of time in a healthy pregnancy ("I have to pee in a cup again?"), the earliest signs of preeclampsia can be picked up at such visits.

Early symptoms of preeclampsia include sudden weight gain apparently unrelated to overeating, severe swelling of the hands and face, unexplained headaches, pain in the stomach or the esophagus, all-over itching, and/or vision disturbances. If you experience any of these, call your practitioner. Otherwise, assuming you are getting regular medical care, there's no reason to worry about preeclampsia. See pages 524 and 548 for more information on and tips for dealing with high blood pressure and preeclampsia.

sage your back, or a friend to wipe your brow—or if you really like company, all three—a little support can go a long way in easing your fears. Even if you end up feeling more tense than chatty during labor, it will be comforting to know that you're not going it alone. And make sure your team is trained, too. Have your coach attend childbirth classes with you, or if that's not possible, suggest that he read the section on labor and delivery beginning on page 380, so that he'll know what to expect—and how best to help.

Have a plan—and a backup plan. Maybe you've already decided that an epidural has your name on it. Maybe you're hoping to breathe your way through those contractions—or use hypnosis or another CAM approach to pain management. Maybe you're waiting to make that decision until you see how much pain you're facing. Either way, think ahead, and then keep your mind open (because labor has a way of not always following plans). In the end, you'll need to do what's best for you and your baby (even if that's accepting pain relief when you were hoping to tough it out). Remember, you don't have to be a martyr to be a mother. This is one time when you can have the gain without the pain. In fact, sometimes pain relief's absolutely necessary to keep a laboring mom at her most effective. See page 301 for more on pain relief during labor and delivery.

Labor Inhibitions

"I'm afraid I'll do something embarrassing during labor."

That's because you're not in labor yet. Sure, the idea of screaming, cursing, or involuntarily emptying your bladder or bowel might seem embarrassing now—but during labor, embarrassment will be the furthest thing from your mind. Besides, nothing you can do or say during labor will shock your birth attendants, who've seen and heard it all before—and then some. So check your inhibitions when you check into the hospital or birthing center and feel free to do what comes naturally, as well as what makes you most comfortable. If you are ordinarily a vocal, emotive person, don't try to hold in your moans or hold back your grunts and groans—or even your ear-shattering screams. But if you're normally very soft-spoken or stoic and would prefer to whimper quietly into your pillow, don't feel obligated to out yell the woman next door.

Calling the Labor Shots

"I have pretty definite ideas of what I'd like to happen during labor and delivery. I don't like the idea of losing control of the situation."

If you're a take-charge kind of person, the thought of handing control of your labor and delivery over to the medical team can be a little unnerving. Of course you want the doctors, nurses, and midwives to take the best possible care of you and your baby. But you'd still like to call as many shots as possible (including whether or not you get those shots). And chances are you'll be able to, especially if you prepare thoroughly for labor and delivery at your childbirth preparation exercises, become familiar with the birth process, and develop an open and productive rapport with your practitioner, if you haven't already. Setting up a birth plan (see page 294), specifying what you would like to happen and not happen during a normal labor and delivery, also increases your control.

But with that said and done and written down, it's important to understand that you won't necessarily be able to call all the shots during labor, no matter how well prepared you are and no matter what type of practitioner you are laboring with. The best-laid plans of obstetrical patients and their practitioners can give way to a variety of unforeseeable circumstances, and it makes sense to prepare for that possibility, too. For instance, you'd planned to go through labor completely unmedicated, but an extremely long and trying active phase has sapped you of your strength. Or you'd hoped for an epidural, but your labor's going extremely quickly and the anesthesiologist doesn't arrive in time. Learning when it's necessary to relinquish the reins—and be flexible—is also in the best interest of you and your baby, and it is an important part of your childbirth education.

Hospital Tours

"I've always associated hospitals with sick people. How can I get more comfortable with the idea of giving birth in one?"

The labor and delivery floor is by far the happiest in the hospital. Still, if you don't know what to expect, you can arrive not only with contractions, but with apprehension. That's why the vast majority of hospitals and birthing centers encourage expectant couples to take advance tours of maternity facilities. Ask about such tours when you preregister, and look online, too. Some hospitals and birthing centers have websites that offer virtual tours. You can also stop in for an informal peek during visiting hours; even if the actual labor and delivery area is off-limits then, you'll be able to view postpartum rooms and take a good look at the nursery. Besides making you feel more comfortable about the surroundings where you'll be giving birth, this will give you the opportunity to check out what real newborns look like before you hold your own in your arms.

Chances are you'll be happily surprised by what you see when you pay your visit. Facilities vary from hospital to hospital and from birthing center to birthing center, but as competition for obstetrical patients increases, the range of amenities and services offered in many areas has become more and more impressive—less hospital, more hotel. Comfy birthing rooms are the rule, rather than the exception, in more and more hospitals (they've always been common at birthing centers staffed by midwives).

Childbirth Education

The countdown is on—and baby's just around the corner (give or take a few months). Of course you're eagerly awaiting the arrival of your little one. But are you just as eager for the arrival of labor and delivery? Could that be trepidation (make that panic) mixed in with that excited anticipation?

Relax. It's normal to be a little nervous about childbirth—or even a lot, especially if you're a first timer. Just about every parent-to-be is. But fortunately, there's a great way to ease jitters, to calm worries, and to feel less anxious and more confident when that first contraction strikes: by getting educated.

A little knowledge and a lot of preparation can go a long way in helping you feel more comfortable when you enter the birthing room. Reading all about childbirth can definitely give you an idea of what to expect (and you can start doing that on page 380), but a good childbirth education class can fill in even more blanks. So it's back to school, Mama (and Papa).

Benefits of Taking a Childbirth Class

What's in a childbirth education class for you and your coach? That depends, of course, on the course you take, the instructor who teaches it, and on your attitudes (as was true back in your school days, the more you put in, the more you tend to get out of a childbirth education class). No matter what, there's something in it for every soon-to-be-laboring team. Some potential benefits include:

- A chance to spend time with other expectant couples who are at the same stage of pregnancy as you are—to share experiences and tips; compare progress; trade tales of woes, worries, aches, and pains; and swap notes on baby gear, nursery gear, pediatricians, and child care. In other words, lots of expectant camaraderie and empathy. It's also a chance to make friends with other couples who, like you, will soon be parents (a definite plus if your current crowd of friends hasn't taken the baby plunge yet). Keep in touch with these classmates after delivery and you've got yourself a ready-to-go parent's group—and playgroup for the kids. Many classes hold "reunions" once everyone has delivered.

- A chance for dad to join in. So much of pregnancy revolves around mom, which can sometimes leave an expectant father feeling like he's on the outside looking in. Childbirth education classes are aimed at both parents and help to get dad feeling like the valued member of the baby team he is—particularly important if he hasn't been able to attend all the prenatal visits. Classes will also get dad up to speed on labor and delivery so that he can be a more effective coach when those contractions start coming. Best of all, perhaps, he'll be able to hang out with other guys who can relate—among other things, to those maternal mood swings he's been on the receiving end of and to nagging feelings of daddy self-doubt. Some courses include a special session for fathers only, which gives them the chance to open up about concerns they might otherwise not feel comfortable expressing.

- A chance to ask questions that come up between prenatal visits or that you don't feel comfortable asking your practitioner (or that you never seem to have the time to ask in the context of a hurried visit).

- A chance to learn all about it—labor and delivery, that is. Through lecture, discussion, models, and video, you'll get an inside peek at what childbirth's all about—from prelabor symptoms to crowning to cutting the cord. The more you know, the more comfortable you'll feel when it's actually happening to you.

- A chance to learn all about your pain relief options, from Demerol to an epidural to a spinal—even to CAM approaches.

- A chance to get hands-on instruction in breathing, relaxation, and other alternative approaches to pain relief and to get feedback from an expert as you learn. Mastering these coping strategies—and coaching techniques—may help you be more relaxed during labor and delivery, while somewhat decreasing your perception of pain. They'll also come in handy if you're planning on signing up for an epidural or other pain meds.

- A chance to become familiar with the medical interventions sometimes used during childbirth, including fetal monitoring, IVs, vacuum extraction, and C-sections. You may not encounter any of the available interventions during your labor—or only one or two—but knowing about them ahead of time will make labor a little less intimidating.

- A chance to have a relatively more enjoyable labor—and a relatively less stressful one—thanks to all of the above. Couples who've had childbirth preparation generally rate their childbirth experiences as more satisfying overall than those who haven't.

- A chance to become empowered. Knowledge is always power, but it can be especially powerful when you're in labor. By eliminating the fear of the unknown (what you don't know, in this case, can definitely hurt your confidence), a childbirth education class can leave you feeling more in control, more empowered—ready to handle just about any labor scenario that nature throws your way.

Choosing a Childbirth Class

So you've decided to take a childbirth class. But where do you begin looking for one? And how do you choose?

In some communities, where childbirth class options are limited, the choice of which class to take is a rela-tively simple one. In others, the variety of offerings can be overwhelming and confusing. Courses are run by hospitals, by private instructors, by practitioners through their offices. There are "early bird" prenatal classes, taken in the first or second trimester, which cover such pregnancy topics as nutrition, exercise, fetal development, and sex; and there are down-to-the-wire 6- to 10-week childbirth preparation classes, usually begun in the seventh or eighth month, which concentrate on labor, delivery, and postpartum mother and baby care. There are even weekend getaway classes.

If the pickings are slim, any childbirth class is probably better than none at all. If there is a selection of courses where you live, it may help to con-

Back To School

Besides studying up on childbirth techniques these days, there's another class you should consider signing up for now: infant CPR and first aid. Even though you don't actually have the baby yet, there's no better time to learn how to keep that little bundle you're about to deliver safe and sound. First, because you won't have to line up a babysitter to attend class now. And second—and more important—because you'll be able to bring baby home, secure in the knowledge that you have all the necessary know-how at your fingertips in case of an emergency. You can find a course by contacting the American Red Cross (redcross.org) or the American Heart Association (americanheart.org/cpr), or check with your local hospital.

sider the following when making your decision:

Who sponsors the class? A class that is run by, under the auspices of, or recommended by your practitioner often works out best. Also useful could be a class provided by the hospital or birthing center where you'll be delivering. If the laboring and delivering philosophy of your childbirth education teacher varies a lot from that of the person or staff who will be assisting you during labor and delivery, you're bound to run into contradictions and conflicts. If differences of opinion do arise, make sure you address them with your practitioner well before your delivery date.

What's the size of the class? Small is best. Five or six couples to a class is ideal; more than 10 or 12 may be too large. Not only can a teacher give more time and individual attention to couples in an intimate group—particularly important during the breathing and relaxation technique practice sessions—but the camaraderie in a small group tends to be stronger.

What's the curriculum like? To find out, ask for a course outline. A good course includes a discussion of cesarean delivery (recognizing that more than a quarter of the students may end up having one) and of medication (recognizing, too, that many will need or want it). It deals with the psychological and emotional as well as the technical aspects of childbirth.

How is the class taught? Are films of actual childbirths shown? Will you hear from mothers and fathers who've recently delivered? Will there be ample opportunity for parents-to-be to ask questions? Is enough time allowed during class for practicing the various techniques that are taught?

For Information on Pregnancy/Childbirth Classes

Ask your practitioner about classes in your area, or call the hospital where you plan to deliver. The following organizations can also give you referrals to local classes:

Lamaze International:
(800) 368-4404; lamaze.org

Bradley: The Bradley Method:
(800) 4-A-BIRTH (422-4784);
bradleybirth.com

International Childbirth Education Association:
(952) 854-8660; icea.org

Association of Labor Assistants and Childbirth Educators:
(617) 441-2500; alace.org

New Way Childbirth:
(864) 268-1402;
newwaychildbirth.com

The American Society of Clinical Hypnosis:
(630) 980-4740; asch.net

Society for Clinical and Experimental Hypnosis:
(617) 469-1981; sceh.us

Childbirth Education Options

Childbirth education classes in your area may be taught by nurses, nurse-midwives, or other certified professionals. Approaches may vary from class to class, even among those trained in the same programs. The most common classes include:

Lamaze. The Lamaze approach to childbirth education, pioneered by Dr. Fernand Lamaze in the 1950s, is probably the most widely used in the United States. Its foundation is the use of relaxation and breathing techniques by the laboring woman, along with continuous support from a spouse (or other coach) and trained nurse to allow the laboring woman to experience a more "natural" childbirth (remember, back in the 1950s, most delivering moms were put to sleep). According to the Lamaze philosophy, birth is normal, natural, and healthy, and a woman's confidence and ability to give birth naturally can be either enhanced or diminished by the level of support she receives from her care provider, as well as by the comfort of the birthing environment (which could be a birthing center or home as well as a hospital).

The goal of Lamaze training is active concentration based on relaxation and rhythmic breathing patterns. To help with concentration, women are encouraged to direct their attention to a focal point. Courses also cover comfortable labor and birthing positions; breathing, distraction, and massage techniques; communication skills; and other comfort measures, as well as information on the early postpartum period and breastfeeding. Though the Lamaze philosophy states that women have a right to give birth free from routine medical interventions, classes generally cover most common interventions (including pain relief) to prepare couples for any birthing scenario. A traditional Lamaze course consists of six 2- to 2½-hour sessions.

Bradley. This approach emphasizes deep abdominal breathing rather than panting. Bradley recommends that the laboring woman concentrate within herself and tune in to her own body to control the pain of the contractions, rather than relying on distractions. In Bradley classes, women learn to mimic their nighttime sleeping positions and breathing (which is deep and slow) for use during labor and to use relaxation techniques to make labor more comfortable.

According to the Bradley technique, during labor a woman needs darkness, quiet, physical comfort aided by pillows, and closed eyes. Bradley teachers acknowledge that labor hurts, and they stress acceptance of pain. Medication is reserved for complications and C-sections (which are discussed so parents can be prepared for any eventuality), and about 87 percent of Bradley graduates who have vaginal births go without it. The typical Bradley course runs 12 weeks, beginning in the fifth month, and most are taught by married couples. "Early bird" Bradley classes, which focus on matters prenatal, are available.

International Childbirth Education Association (ICEA) classes. These classes tend to be broader in scope, covering more of the many options available today to expectant parents in family-centered maternity care and newborn care. They also recognize the importance of freedom of choice, and so classes focus on a wide range of possibilities rather than on a single approach to childbirth. Teachers are certified through ICEA.

Hypnobirthing. Classes for individuals or groups that teach how to use hypnosis to reduce discomfort and pain (and in some highly suggestible women, to eliminate it entirely), achieve a deep state of relaxation, as well as improve mood and attitude during labor and childbirth, are becoming more available. Check with your practitioner or a national clinical hypnosis organization for names of licensed health professionals who teach hypnobirthing. (For more on hypnobirthing, see page 306.)

Other childbirth classes. The range is wide. Association of Labor Assistants and Childbirth Educators (ALACE) champions a woman's right to a natural or unmedicated birth when at all possible. Rather than try to teach expectant parents how to avoid labor and childbirth pain, classes provide coping tools to work with the discomfort. Childbirth Education Preparation (CEP) certifies nurses and practical nurses as childbirth educators who are trained to run classes that explain and teach the many options, including Lamaze and Bradley, available to expectant parents during labor. In addition, there are childbirth education classes designed to prepare parents to deliver in a particular hospital, and classes sponsored by medical groups, health maintenance organizations (HMOs), or other health care provider groups. In some areas, prenatal classes, which cover all aspects of pregnancy as well as childbirth, are also offered, usually beginning in the first trimester.

Home study. If you are on bed rest, live in a remote area, or for some other reason can't or don't want to attend a group class, you can look into the Lamaze program on video or DVD available from Lamaze International.

Weekend classes at resorts. These offer the same curriculum as typical classes, packed into a single weekend instead of spaced out over a series of weeks, and they are a nice choice for those who can—and would like to—get away. In addition to promoting camaraderie

Classes for Second Timers

Been there, done that? Pregnant with your second baby? Even seasoned pros stand to benefit from taking a childbirth education class. First of all, every labor and delivery is different, so what you experienced last time may not be what you can expect this time. Second, things change quickly in the delivery business, and they may have changed quite a bit, even if it's only been a couple of years since you were last on a birthing bed. There may be different childbirth options available than there were last time: Certain procedures that were routine may now be uncommon; certain procedures that were uncommon may now be routine. Taking another course may be especially useful if you'll be using a different hospital or birthing center. Chances are, however, that you won't have to sit in with the rookies. "Refresher" courses are available in most areas.

among expectant parents (especially rewarding if you don't have other pregnant friends to talk to at home), these weekends can promote romance, too—a nice plus for twosomes who are about to become threesomes. Plus, they're a great opportunity for some pre-baby pampering.

CHAPTER 12

The
Seventh
Month

Approximately 28 to 31 Weeks

WELCOME TO YOUR THIRD—and final!—trimester. Believe it or not, you're two thirds of the way to the finish line, and just three months away from holding (and kissing, and cuddling) your prize. In this last stretch of pregnancy (definitely the biggest stretch, at least as far as your belly is concerned), you'll probably find the excitement and anticipation mounting—along with your pregnancy aches and pains, which tend to multiply as the load you're lugging gets heavier and heavier. Drawing near to the end of pregnancy also means you're closing in on labor and delivery, an event you'll begin planning for, preparing for, and getting educated about. Time to think about signing up for those classes, if you haven't already.

Your Baby This Month

Week 28 This week, your amazing baby has reached 2½ pounds and may be almost 16 inches long. Baby's skill of the week: blinking. Yes, along with the other tricks in a growing repertoire that already includes coughing, sucking, hiccupping, and taking practice breaths, your baby can now blink those sweet little eyes. Dreaming about your baby? Baby may be dreaming about you, too, courtesy of the REM (rapid eye movement) sleep he or she has started getting. But this little dreamer isn't ready for birth day just yet. Though his or her lungs are nearly fully mature by now (making it easier for your baby—and you—to breathe a little easier if he or she were born now), your baby still has a lot of growing to do.

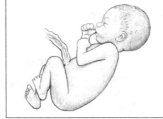

Your Baby, Month 7

Week 29 Your baby can be as tall as 17 inches now and can weigh nearly 3 pounds. Though already coming pretty close (within 3 inches or so) of his or her ultimate birth length, baby still has lots to gain. In fact, over the next 11 weeks, your baby more than doubles—and may even come close to tripling—his or her weight. Much of that weight will come from the fat accumulating under his or her skin right now. And as your baby plumps up, the room in your womb will start to feel a little cramped, making it less likely that you'll feel hard kicks from your little one, and more likely that you'll be feeling jabs and pokes from elbows and knees.

Week 30 What's 17 inches long, just over 3 pounds in weight, and cute all over? It's your baby—and he or she is getting bigger by the day (in case you couldn't tell from the size of your belly). Also getting bigger daily is baby's brain, which is preparing for life outside the womb—and for a lifetime of learning. Starting this week, your baby's brain is starting to look like one, taking on those characteristic grooves and indentations. These wrinkles allow for future expansion of brain tissue that is crucial as your baby goes from helpless newborn to responsive infant to verbal toddler to curious preschooler and beyond. Your baby's bigger and better brain is also starting to take on tasks previously delegated to other parts of the body, like temperature regulation. Now that the brain is capable of turn-ing up the heat (with the help of that growing supply of baby fat), your baby will start shedding lanugo, the downy, soft body hair that has been keeping him or her warm up to this point. Which means that by the time your baby is born, he or she probably won't be fuzzy wuzzy anymore.

Week 31 Though your baby still has 3 to 5 pounds more to gain before delivery, he or she is weighing in at an impressive 3-plus pounds this week. And at 18 inches long (give or take a couple because fetuses this age come in all sizes), your baby is quickly approaching his or her birth length. Also developing at an impressive clip these days: your baby's brain connections (baby has to make trillions of them). And he or she is able to put that complex web of brain connections to good use, too—already processing information, tracking light, and perceiving signals from all five senses. Your brainy baby is also a sleepy one, putting in longer stretches of snooze time, specifically in REM sleep—which is why you're probably noticing more defined patterns of awake (and kicking) and sleeping (quiet) times from your little one.

Baby Brain Food

Have you been feeding your baby's brain? Getting enough of those fabulous fats, the omega-3's, is more important than ever in the third trimester when your baby's brain development is being fast-tracked. See page 101 for all the good-fat facts.

What You May Be Feeling

As always, remember that every pregnancy and every woman is different. You may experience all of these symptoms at one time or another, or only a few of them. Some may have continued from last month, others may be new. Still others may hardly be noticed because you've become so used to them. You may also have other, less common, symptoms. Here's what you might experience this month:

A Look Inside

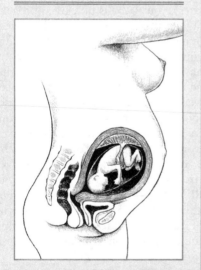

At the beginning of this month, your uterus is approximately 11 inches from the top of your pubic bone. By the end of the month, your baby's home has grown another inch in height and can be felt around 4½ inches above your belly button. You may think that there's no more room for your womb to grow (it seems to have already filled up your abdomen), but you still have 8 to 10 more weeks of expansion ahead of you!

Physically

- Stronger and more frequent fetal activity

- Increasing vaginal discharge

- Achiness in the lower abdomen or along the sides

- Constipation

- Heartburn, indigestion, flatulence, bloating

- Occasional headaches, faintness, or dizziness

- Nasal congestion and occasional nosebleeds; ear stuffiness

- Sensitive gums that may bleed when you brush

- Leg cramps

- Backache

- Mild swelling of ankles and feet, and occasionally of hands and face

- Varicose veins of the legs

- Hemorrhoids

- Itchy abdomen

- Protruding navel

- Stretch marks

- Shortness of breath

- Difficulty sleeping

- Scattered Braxton Hicks contractions, usually painless (the uterus hardens for a minute, then returns to normal)

- Clumsiness

- Enlarged breasts

- Colostrum, leaking from nipples (though this premilk substance may not appear until after delivery)

Emotionally

- Increasing excitement (the baby's coming soon!)

- Increasing apprehension (the baby's coming soon!)

- Continued absentmindedness

- Strange and vivid dreams

- Increased boredom and weariness with pregnancy or a sense of contentment and well-being, particularly if you're feeling great physically

What You Can Expect at This Month's Checkup

A couple of new items are on the agenda at this month's checkup, along with the old standards. As you enter your last trimester, you can expect your practitioner to check the following, though there may be variations depending on your particular needs and on your practitioner's style of practice:

- Weight and blood pressure

- Urine, for sugar and protein

- Fetal heartbeat

- Height of fundus (top of uterus)

- Size and position of fetus, by external palpation (feeling from the outside)

- Feet and hands for swelling, and legs for protruding varicose veins

- Glucose screening test

- Blood test for anemia

- Symptoms you have been experiencing, especially unusual ones

- Questions and problems you want to discuss—have a list ready

What You May Be Wondering About

Fatigue Revisited

"I was feeling really energetic for the last few months, and now I'm starting to drag again. Is this what I have to look forward to in the third trimester?"

Pregnancy is full of ups and downs—not only when it comes to moods (and libidos) but when it comes to energy levels. That trademark first-trimester fatigue is often followed by a second-trimester energy high, making those typically comfortable middle months the ideal time to pursue just about any activity (Exercise! Sex! Travel! All three in one weekend!). But by the third trimester, many moms-to-be find themselves once again dragging—and eyeing the sofa longingly.

And that's not surprising. Though some women continue to sprint as they close in on the pregnancy finish line (remember, every pregnancy is different, even when it comes to energy levels), there are lots more good reasons why you might be lagging behind. The best reason can be found around your midsection. After all, you're carrying much more weight there (and other places) than you were earlier on—and carting those extra pounds can be exhausting. Another reason: These days, that extra bulk may be lying (literally) between you and a good night's sleep, leaving you less rested each morning. Your baby-overloaded mind (jam-packed with shopping lists, to-do lists, baby-name lists, questions-to-ask-the-doctor lists) may also be costing you z's—and energy. Add other, unrelated life responsibilities to the mix—a job, the care and feeding of other children, and so on—and the fatigue factors multiply exponentially.

But just because fatigue often comes with the third-trimester territory doesn't mean you have to resign yourself to three months of exhaustion—or relocate yourself to the sofa for the duration. As always, fatigue is a signal from your body, so pay attention. If you've been living life in the fast lane (too much baby prep, not enough rest), slow down the pace a bit. Cut back on any nonessential essentials (no fair calling them all essential), and start building some R&R into your daily schedule. Get some exercise, but make sure it's the right kind (a 30-minute walk may leave you energized, an hour run will have you running for the sofa), at the right time (not too close to bedtime, so it'll induce sleep, not prevent it). And since running on empty can bench you in a hurry, don't forget to fuel your energy levels. Keeping your blood sugar levels up with frequent healthy snacks (cheese and crackers, trail mix, a yogurt smoothie) will give those levels a longer lasting boost than caffeine or sugar. Most of all, remember that third-trimester fatigue is nature's way of telling mothers-to-be to conserve their energy. You'll need every bit of strength you can save up now for labor, delivery, and, more important, what follows. For more energy-saving tips, revisit the ones on page 128.

If you do get the extra rest your body is calling for but you still feel consistently run-down, talk to your practitioner. Sometimes, extreme fatigue that doesn't ease up is triggered by third-trimester anemia (see page 208), which is why most practitioners repeat a routine blood test for it in the seventh month.

Swelling

"My ankles and feet seem to be swollen, especially at the end of the day. What's going on?"

Your belly's not the only thing that's swelling these days. That puff mama look often extends to the extremities, too. And although all that swelling's not so swell—especially as your shoes and watch get uncomfortably tight and your rings become harder and harder to pry off your fingers—mild swelling (aka edema) of the ankles, feet, and hands is completely normal, related to the necessary increase in body fluids in pregnancy. In fact, 75 percent of women develop such swelling at some point in their pregnancies, usually around this point (the other 25 percent never notice any at all, which is normal, too). As you've probably already noticed, the puffiness is likely to be more pronounced late in the day, in warm weather, or after spending too much time sitting or standing. In fact, you may find that much of the swelling disappears overnight or after several hours spent lying down (another good reason to get that rest).

Generally, this type of swelling means nothing more than a little discomfort—and a few fashion compromises if you can no longer squeeze your ankles into stylish shoes. Still, you'll want to find ways to deflate, if you can. To spell swell relief, keep these tips in mind:

- Stay off your feet and off your butt. If long periods of standing or sitting are part of your job description—at home or at the office—take periodic breaks. Have a seat if you've been standing, and get up if you've been sitting. Or for best results, take a brisk 5-minute walk to rev up your circulation (which should get those pooled fluids flowing).

- Put 'em up—your legs, that is. Elevate them when you're sitting. If anyone deserves to put her feet up, it's you.

- Get some rest on your side. If you're not already in the side-lying habit, time to try it now. Lying on your side helps keep your kidneys working at peak efficiency, enhancing waste elimination and reducing swelling.

- Choose comfort. Now's the time to make a comfort statement, not a fashion statement. Favor shoes that are accommodating (those slinky sling-backs don't fit now, anyway), and once home, switch to soft slippers.

- Move it. Keeping up your exercise routine (if your practitioner has green-lighted one) will actually keep down the swelling. Walking (you'll probably soon call it waddling) is swell for swollen feet since it'll keep the blood flowing instead of pooling. Swimming or water aerobics are even better because the water pressure pushes tissue fluid back into your veins; from there it goes into your kidneys, after which you'll be able to pee it out.

- Wash away that water weight. Though it sounds counterintuitive, it's true: The more water you drink, the less you'll retain. Drinking at least eight to ten 8-ounce glasses of liquid a day will help your system flush out waste products. Restricting fluid intake, on the other (puffy) hand, will *not* decrease swelling.

- Use salt to taste. It used to be believed that salt restriction would help keep the swelling down, but it is now known that limiting salt increases swelling. So salt to taste, but as with most everything, moderation is key.

- Get the support you need. Support hose may not be sexy, but they're very effective in relieving swelling. Several types are available for pregnancy wear, including full panty hose (with roomy tummy space) and knee- or thigh-highs (which are at least cooler to wear), though avoid those with tight elastic tops.

The good news about edema, besides that it's normal, is that it's temporary. You can look forward to your ankles deflating and your fingers depuffing soon after you give birth (though

Take Them Off, While You Can

Have your rings been getting snugger and snugger? Before they get too tight for comfort (and much too tight to remove), you might want to consider taking them off and putting them away for safekeeping until your fingers have slimmed down again. Having trouble prying them off already? Try taking them off in the morning and after cooling your hands down (the hotter they are, the puffier they'll be). Some liquid soap can make the rings slippery and easier to slide off, too.

some moms find it takes at least a few weeks, sometimes a month or more, for swelling to disappear completely). In the meantime, look on the bright side: Pretty soon your belly will be so big, you won't even be able to see how swollen your feet are.

If your swelling seems to be more than mild, talk to your practitioner. Excessive swelling can be one sign of preeclampsia, but when it is, it's accompanied by a variety of other symptoms (such as sudden excessive and unexplained weight gain, elevated blood pressure, and protein in the urine). If your blood pressure and urine are normal (they're checked at each prenatal visit), there's nothing to be concerned about. If, along with your swelling, you've suddenly and inexplicably gained a lot of weight in a short time, or if you're experiencing severe headaches or vision disturbances, call your practitioner and describe what's going on.

Strange Skin Bumps

"As if it's not bad enough that I have stretch marks, now I seem to have some kind of itchy bumps breaking out in them."

Cheer up. You have less than three months left until delivery, when you'll be able to bid a grateful good-bye to most of the unpleasant side effects of pregnancy—among them, these new eruptions. Until then, it may help to know that although they may be uncomfortable (and slightly unsightly), the bumps aren't dangerous to you or your baby. Known medically—and unpronounceably—as pruritic urticarial papules and plaques of pregnancy (try saying that fast three times), aka PUPPP, or PEP (polymorphic eruption of pregnancy), the condition generally disappears after delivery and doesn't recur in subsequent pregnancies. Though PUPPP most often

develops in abdominal stretch marks, it sometimes also appears on the thighs, buttocks, or arms of expectant moms. Show your rash to your practitioner, who may prescribe topical medication, an antihistamine, or a shot to ease any discomfort.

A variety of other skin conditions and rashes can develop during pregnancy (lucky you!), making you less than happy with the skin you're in. Though you should always show any rash that crops up to your practitioner, keep in mind that they're rarely cause for concern. See page 240 for more.

Lower Back and Leg Pain (Sciatica)

"I've been having pain on the side of my lower back, running right down my hip and leg. What's that about?"

Sounds like your baby's getting on your nerves—your sciatic nerve, that is. Toward the middle to end of your pregnancy, your baby begins to settle into the proper position for birth (a big positive). In doing that, however, his or her head—and the weight of your ever-enlarging uterus—may settle on the sciatic nerve in the lower part of your spine (a big negative). Such so-called sciatica can result in sharp, shooting pain, tingling, or numbness that starts in your buttocks or lower back and radiates down the back of either of your legs. Sciatica can be quite intense at times, and though it may pass if your baby shifts positions, it can also linger until you've delivered—and sometimes linger for a little while postpartum.

How can you get baby off your nerves and relieve the pain of sciatica? Try these tips:

- Take a seat. Getting off your feet can ease some of the leg and lower back pain associated with sciatica. Lying down can also relieve pressure—as long as you find the position that feels best.

- **Warm it up.** A warm heating pad applied on the spot where you feel the pain can help ease it, as can a long soak in a warm bath.

- **Work it out.** Pelvic tilts or just some stretches can take off some of the pressure.

- **Get in the swim of things.** Since swimming and water exercises aren't weight bearing, they are particularly good choices when you've got sciatic pain. Swimming stretches and strengthens the muscles in your back, providing relief for that searing pain.

- **Seek an alternative.** CAM therapies, such as acupuncture, chiropractic medicine, or therapeutic massage (always with a trained and licensed practitioner), might help relieve your sciatica.

If your pain is particularly bad, ask your practitioner if pain medications would be helpful in your case.

Restless Leg Syndrome

"As tired as I am at night, I can't seem to settle down because my legs feel so restless. I've tried all the tips for leg cramps, but they don't work. What else can I do?"

With so many other things coming between you and a good night's sleep in your last trimester, it hardly seems fair that your legs are, too. But for the 15 percent or so of pregnant women who experience restless leg syndrome (RLS)—yes, it's got a name— that's exactly what happens. The name captures it all—that restless, creeping, crawling, tingling feeling inside the foot

---

Count Your Kicks

From the 28th week on, it may be a good idea to test for fetal movements twice a day—once in the morning, when activity tends to be sparser, and once in the more active evening hours. Your practitioner may recommend a test, or you can use this one: Check the clock and start counting. Count movements of any kind (kicks, flutters, swishes, rolls). Stop counting when you reach 10, and note the time (if you like, you can use the fetal movement tracker in the *What to Expect Pregnancy Journal and Organizer*). Often, you will feel 10 movements within 10 minutes or so—sometimes it will take longer.

If you haven't counted 10 movements by the end of an hour, have some juice or a snack, walk a bit, even jiggle your belly a little; then lie down, relax, and continue counting. If two hours go by without 10 movements, call your practitioner. Though such an absence of activity doesn't necessarily mean something's wrong, it can occasionally be a red flag that needs quick evaluation.

The closer you are to your due date, the more important regular checking of fetal movements becomes.

---

and/or leg that keeps the rest of your body from settling down. It's most common at night, but it can also strike in the late afternoon or pretty much any time you're lying or sitting down.

Experts aren't certain what causes RLS in some pregnant women (though there does seem to be a genetic component to it), and they're even less sure of how to treat it. None of the tricks of the leg cramp trade—including rubbing or flexing—seem to bring relief.

Medications may not be a good option, either, because many of those currently used to treat RLS aren't safe for use during pregnancy (check with your practitioner).

It's possible that diet, stress, and other environmental factors may contribute to the problem, so it may help to keep track of what you eat, what you do, and how you feel each day so you can see what lifestyle habits, if any, bring on symptoms. Some women, for instance, find that eating carbohydrates late in the day can worsen RLS. It's also possible that iron-deficiency anemia may cause RLS, so it's worth asking your practitioner about testing to rule that out, as well as asking him or her for any other suggested treatments. Acupuncture may help some women, as can yoga, meditation, or other relaxation techniques. And, of course, it couldn't hurt to try the sleep tips on page 266. Unfortunately, however, some women continue to find relief—and sleep—elusive. If you are one of them, RLS is something you may just have to put up with until delivery. If you came into pregnancy with the condition, you may have to wait until after delivery (and possibly after weaning, if you're nursing) to resume any drug treatment you were using.

Fetal Hiccups

"I sometimes feel regular little spasms in my abdomen. Is this kicking, or a twitch, or what?"

Believe it or not, your baby's probably got hiccups, a phenomenon not uncommon among fetuses during the last half of pregnancy. Some get hiccups several times a day, every day. Others never get them at all. The same pattern may continue after birth.

But before you start holding your breath or trying other hiccup tricks, you should know that hiccups don't cause the same discomfort in babies—in or out of the uterus—as they do in adults, even when they last 20 minutes or more. So just relax and enjoy this little entertainment from within.

Accidental Falls

"I missed the curb today when I was out walking and fell belly first on the pavement. Could the fall have hurt the baby?"

Is pregnancy tripping you up? That's not surprising—after all, once you enter the third trimester, there are plenty of factors that can combine to literally put you head over heels. For one, your impaired sense of balance, which has been thrown off-kilter as your center of gravity keeps shifting forward, along with your belly. For another, your looser, less stable joints, which add to awkwardness and make you prone to minor falls, especially those belly flops. Also contributing to clumsiness are your tendency to tire easily, your predisposition to preoccupation and daydreaming, and the difficulty you may be having seeing past your belly to your feet—all of which makes those curbs and other stumbling blocks easy to miss.

But while a curbside spill may leave you with multiple scrapes and bruises (particularly on your ego, if it was a public flop), it's extremely rare for a fetus to suffer the consequences of its mother's clumsiness. Your baby is protected by one of the world's most sophisticated shock absorption systems, comprised of amniotic fluid, tough membranes, the elastic, muscular uterus, and the sturdy abdominal cavity, which is girded with muscles and bones. For it to be penetrated, and for your baby to be hurt, you'd have to sustain very serious injuries, the kind that would very likely land you in the hospital.

If you're concerned, however, do call your practitioner for extra reassurance.

Orgasm and Baby's Kicking

"After I have an orgasm, my baby usually stops kicking for about half an hour. Does that mean that sex isn't safe at this point in pregnancy?"

No matter what you do these days, your baby's along for the ride. And when it comes to lovemaking, the ride can make baby very sleepy. The rocking motion of sex and the rhythmic uterine contractions that follow orgasm often lull fetuses to dreamland. Some babies, on the other hand (because every baby's an individual), become more lively after their parents make love. Either reaction is normal and healthy, and it is in no way a sign that sex isn't safe. Nor, in case you're wondering, is it a sign that baby's in the know about what's going on between those sheets (baby's completely in the dark, literally).

In fact, unless your practitioner has prescribed otherwise, you can continue enjoying lovemaking—and orgasms—until delivery. And you might as well get that sex in while you can. Let's face it—it may be a while before it's this convenient to make love with your baby in the house again.

Dreams and Fantasies

"I've been having so many vivid dreams—day and night—about the baby that I'm beginning to think I'm losing my mind."

Been catching some pretty strange late shows along with your z's? Dreams—and daydreams and fantasies—from the horrifying (like the one about leaving the baby on the bus) to the heartwarming (snuggling chubby cheeks, pushing strollers through a sunny park), to the bizarre (giving birth to an alien baby with a tail or to a litter of puppies) are healthy, normal, and very, very common during pregnancy. And though they may make you feel as though you're losing your mind (was that really a giant salami that chased you around the parking lot of Babies "R" Us last night?), they're actually helping you stay sane. They're just one way that your subconscious works through your mind's overload of pre-baby anxieties, fears, hopes, and insecurities and comes to terms with the impending upheaval in your life—an outlet for the 1,001 conflicting emotions (from ambivalence to trepidation to overwhelming excitement and joy) you're feeling but may be uneasy expressing any other way. Think of it as therapy you can sleep through.

Hormones contribute, also, to your heavier-than-usual dream schedule (what don't they contribute to?). Plus, they can make your dreams much more vivid. The lighter sleep you've been getting also plays a part in your ability to recall your dreams—and recall them in high definition. Because you're waking up more often than you used to, whether to use the bathroom, kick off some blankets, or just toss, turn, and try to get comfortable, you have more opportunities to wake up in the middle of a REM dream cycle. With the dreams so fresh in your mind each time you awaken, you're able to remember them in greater—and sometimes unnerving—detail.

Here are some of the most commonly reported dream and fantasy themes during pregnancy. Some probably sound familiar.

■ Oops! dreams. Dreaming about losing or misplacing things (from your car

Preparing Fido and Whiskers

Already a parent—to the kind of baby that has four legs, fur, and a tail? Concerned that your pet, who's used to ruling the roost (and curling up on your bed and your lap), will suffer from a bad (and possibly dangerous) case of sibling rivalry when you show up with a new baby? Taking steps now to prepare your dog or cat for when baby makes three (people, that is) is crucial. See *What to Expect the First Year* for tips and recommendations on preparing the family pet for baby's arrival.

keys to your baby); forgetting to feed the baby; missing a doctor's appointment; going out to shop and leaving baby home alone; being unprepared for the baby when he or she arrives can reveal the common fear that you're not up to being a mother.

- Ouch! dreams. Being attacked or hurt—by intruders, burglars, animals; or falling down the stairs after a push or a slip—may represent a sense of vulnerability.

- Help! dreams. Dreams of being enclosed or unable to escape—trapped in a tunnel, a car, a small room; drowning in a pool, a lake of snowy slush, a car wash—can signify the fear of being tied down by the expected new family member, of losing your once carefree life to a demanding newborn.

- Oh no! dreams. Dreams of gaining no weight or gaining a lot of weight overnight; overeating; eating or drinking the wrong things (a tray of sushi washed down with a pitcher of marti-

nis)—are common among those trying to stick to a dietary regimen.

- Ugh! dreams. Dreaming about becoming unattractive or repulsive to your spouse or about your spouse taking up with someone else—expresses the common fear that pregnancy will destroy your looks forever and make you unappealing to your partner.

- Sexual dreams. Dreams about sexual encounters—either positive or negative, pleasure or guilt provoking—may reflect the sexual confusion and ambivalence often experienced during pregnancy.

- Memory dreams. Dreaming of death and resurrection—lost parents or other relatives reappearing—may be the subconscious mind's way of linking old and new generations.

- Life with baby dreams. Dreaming about getting ready for the baby and loving and playing with the baby in a dream is practice parenting, a way that your subconscious bonds you with your baby before delivery.

- Imagining baby dreams. Dreaming about what your baby will be like can reveal a wide variety of concerns. Dreams about the baby being deformed, sick, or too large or too small express anxiety about its health. Fantasies about the infant having unusual skills (like talking or walking at birth) may indicate concern about the baby's intelligence and ambition for his or her future. Premonitions that the baby will be a boy or a girl could mean your heart's set on one or the other. So could dreams about the baby's hair or eye color or resemblance to one parent or the other. Nightmares of the baby being born fully grown could signify your fear of having to handle a tiny infant.

■ **Labor dreams.** Dreaming about labor pain—or lack of it—or about not being able to push the baby out may reflect your anxieties about labor.

Bottom line about your dreams and fantasies—don't lose any sleep over them. They're completely normal and as common among expectant moms as heartburn and stretch marks (just ask around and you'll get an interesting earful). Keep in mind, too, that you may not be the only one in your bed who's dreaming up a sometimes unsettling storm. Expectant dads may also have strange dreams and fantasies as they attempt to work out their conscious and subconscious anxieties about impending fatherhood (and it's not as easy for them to blame it on the hormones). Swapping dreams in the morning can be fun (can you top this one?) as well as therapeutic, making that transition into real-life parenthood easier—plus it can help bring you closer together. So dream on!

Handling It All

"I'm beginning to worry that I won't be able to manage my job, my house, my marriage—and the baby, too."

Here's the first thing you should know about doing it all: You can't do it all, do it all well, do it all well at the same time, and do it all well all the time. Every mom's super, but even the best among us are only human. Many new mothers have tried to don the cape—handling a full workload on the job; keeping the house spotless, the laundry basket empty, the refrigerator stocked, and home-cooked meals on the table; being a doting (read: sexy) partner and an exemplary parent; and leaping the occasional building at a single bound—but most have realized somewhere in midflight that something's gotta give.

Just how well you'll manage your new life will probably depend on how quickly you come to that realization. And there's no better time than now—before your latest (and cutest) life challenge arrives—to start.

First, you'll need to give some thought to what your priorities are so you can begin arranging them in order of importance (and not everything can make that top spot). If baby, spouse, and job are priorities, perhaps keeping the house clean will have to take a (messy) backseat. Maybe home-cooked will give way to home-delivered, at least some of the time, or the laundry basket will become someone else's responsibility. If you're thinking that full-time motherhood might have your name on it, and you can afford to stay home for a while, maybe you can put your career on hold temporarily. Or you might consider working part-time or job sharing with another mom, if you can swing it, or working from home, if possible.

Once you've settled on your priorities, you'll need to let go of your unrealistic expectations (you know, the ones your daydreams are filled with). Check in with experienced moms, and you'll get a reality check fast. As every mother finds out sooner or later—and you'll save yourself a lot of stress if you find out sooner—nobody's perfect. As much as you'll want to do everything right, you won't be able to—and there will be those days when it seems like you can't do anything right. Despite your best efforts, beds may go unmade and laundry unfolded, takeout may take over your dinner table, and getting "sexy" may mean finally getting around to washing your hair. Set your standards too high—even if you were able to meet them in your preparenting days—and you'll set yourself up for a whole lot of unnecessary disappointment.

However you decide to rearrange your life, it will be easier if you don't have to go it alone. Beside most successful moms is a dad who not only shares equally in household chores but also is a full partner in parenting, in every department from diapering to bathing to cuddling. If dad's not available as much as you'd like (or isn't in the picture at all), then you are going to need to consider other sources of assistance: baby's grandparents or other relatives, child care or household help, baby-sitting co-ops, or child-care centers.

A Birth Plan

"A friend who recently delivered said she worked out a birth plan with her doctor before delivery. Should I?"

Decisions, decisions. Childbirth involves more decisions than ever

Some Cookies with That Birth Plan?

Once you've passed your approved birth plan on to your practitioner, it should become part of your chart and find its way to your delivery. But just in case it doesn't make it in time, you might want to print up several copies of the plan to bring along to the hospital or birthing center, just so there's no confusion about your preferences. Your coach or doula can make sure that each new shift (with any luck, you won't have to labor through too many of these) has a copy for reference. Some expectant parents have found that placing the birth plan in a small basket of goodies makes it even more welcome.

before, and expectant women and their partners are involved in making more of those decisions than ever before. But how can you and your practitioner keep track of all those decisions—from how you'll manage the pain to who'll catch your emerging baby? Enter the birth plan.

A birth plan is just that—a plan (or more aptly, a wish list). In it, pregnant women and their partners can offer up their best-case birthing scenario: how they'd ideally like labor and delivery to play out if all goes according to "plan." Besides listing those parental preferences, the typical birth plan factors in what's practical, what's feasible, and what the practitioner and hospital or birthing center find acceptable (not everything on a birth plan may fly medically, obstetrically, or policywise). It isn't a contract but a written understanding between a patient and her practitioner and/or hospital or birthing center. Not only can a good birth plan deliver a better birth experience, it can head off unrealistic expectations, minimize disappointment, and eliminate major conflict and miscommunication between a birthing woman and her birth attendants. Some practitioners routinely ask an expectant couple to fill out a birth plan; others are happy to oblige if one is requested. A birth plan is also a springboard for dialogue between patient and practitioner.

Some birth plans cover just the basics; others are extremely detailed (down to the birthing room music and lighting). And because every expectant woman is different—not only in what she'd like out of the birth experience but what she can likely expect, given her particular medical and obstetrical background—a birth plan should be individualized (so don't fill yours out based on your friend's). Some of the issues you may want to tackle in your

Your Main Squeeze

Your baby might not be ready for delivery yet, but it isn't too soon to start getting your body—and your pelvic floor muscles, in particular—geared up for the big day. Never thought much about your pelvic muscles—or maybe never even realized you had any? It's time to start paying attention. They're the muscles that support your uterus, bladder, and bowels, and they're designed to stretch so your baby can come out. They're also the muscles that keep your urine from leaking when you cough or laugh (a skill set you're only likely to appreciate when it's gone, as can happen with postpartum incontinence). These multitalented muscles can also make for a much more satisfying sexual experience.

Luckily, there are exercises that can easily work these miracle muscles, whipping them into shape with minimal time and minimal effort (no workout clothes necessary, no visit to a gym required, and you don't even have to break a sweat). Just 5 minutes of these amazing exercises, called Kegels, three times a day and you'll tone your way to a long list of both short- and long-term benefits. Toned pelvic floor muscles can ease a host of pregnancy and postpartum symptoms from hemorrhoids to urinary and fecal incontinence. They can help you prevent an episiotomy or even a tear during delivery. Plus doing your Kegels faithfully during pregnancy will help your vagina snap back more gracefully after your baby's grand exit.

Ready to Kegel? Here's how: Tense the muscles around your vagina and anus and hold (as you would if you were trying to stop the flow of urine), working up to 10 seconds. Slowly release and repeat; shoot for three sets of 20 daily. Keep in mind when you Kegel that all your focus should be on those pelvic muscles—and not any others. If you feel your stomach tensing or your thighs or buttocks contracting, your pelvics aren't getting their full workout. Make this exercise your main squeeze during pregnancy (doing them each time you stop at a traffic light, while you check your e-mail, in line at the ATM, while waiting for the cashier to ring up your groceries, or while working at your desk), and you'll reap the benefits of stronger pelvic floor muscles. Try doing them during sex, too—both you and your partner will feel the difference (now that's a workout you can get excited about!).

---

birth plan, should you decide to fill one out, are listed below. You can use it as a general guideline, then flesh it out as needed (you can refer to the appropriate pages before making your decisions). For a more detailed list and sample birth plan, see the *What to Expect Pregnancy Journal and Organizer.*

- How far into your labor you would like to remain at home and at what point you would prefer to go to the hospital or birthing center

- Eating and/or drinking during active labor (page 369)

- Being out of bed (walking around or sitting up) during labor

- Personalizing the atmosphere with music, lighting, items from home

- The use of a still camera or video camera

- The use of a mirror so you can see the birth

- The use of an IV (intravenous fluid administration; page 372)

- The use of pain medication and the type of pain medication (page 301)

- External fetal monitoring (continuous or intermittent); internal fetal monitoring (page 372)

- The use of oxytocin to induce or augment contractions (page 368)

- Delivery positions (page 376)

- Use of warm compresses and perineal massage (pages 352 and 375)

- Episiotomy (page 374)

- Vacuum extractor or forceps use (page 375)

- Cesarean delivery (page 398)

- The presence of significant others (besides your spouse) during labor and/or at delivery

- The presence of older children at delivery or immediately after

- Suctioning of the newborn; suctioning by the father

- Holding the baby immediately after birth; breastfeeding immediately

- Postponing cutting the cord, weighing the baby, and/or administering eye drops until after you and your baby greet each other

- Having the father help with the delivery and/or cut the cord

- Cord blood banking (page 330)

You may also want to include some postpartum items on your birth plan, such as:

- Your presence at the weighing of the baby, the pediatric exam, and baby's first bath

- Baby feeding in the hospital (whether it will be controlled by the nursery's schedule or your baby's hunger; whether supplementary bottles and pacifiers can be avoided if you're breastfeeding)

- Circumcision (see *What to Expect the First Year*)

- Rooming-in (page 431)

- Other children visiting with you and/or with the new baby

- Postpartum medication or treatments for you or your baby

- The length of the hospital stay, barring complications (page 430)

Of course, the most important feature of a good birth plan is flexibility. Since childbirth—like most forces of nature—is unpredictable, the best-laid plans don't always go, well, according to plan. Though chances are very good that your plan can be carried out just the way you drew it up, there's always the chance that it won't. There is no way to predict precisely how labor and delivery will progress (or not progress) until those contractions start coming, so a birth plan you design in advance may not end up being obstetrically or

Don't Hold It In

Making a habit of not urinating when you feel the need increases the risk that your inflamed bladder may irritate the uterus and set off contractions. Not going when you've got the urge could also lead to a UTI, another cause of preterm contractions. So don't hold it in. When you gotta go, go . . . promptly.

Lifesaving Screenings for Newborns

Most babies are born healthy and stay that way. But a very small percentage of infants are born apparently healthy and then suddenly sicken. Luckily, there are ways to screen for such metabolic disorders. Most babies born in the U.S. live in states that require screening for at least 21 life-threatening disorders—and there is an effort under way to push all 50 states to screen for 29 universally recommended diseases. These include phenylketonuria (PKU), congenital hypothyroidism, congenital adrenal hyperplasia, biotinidase deficiency, maple syrup urine disease, galactosemia, homocystinuria, and sickle cell anemia.

If your state doesn't offer at least the core group of these tests, you can request that a private lab arrange testing. The lab will use blood that's collected in the hospital during your baby's routine heel stick (when drops of blood are drawn from baby's heel after a quick stick with a needle).

In the very unlikely event your baby screens positive for any of the disorders, your baby's pediatrician and a genetic specialist can verify the results and begin treatment, if necessary (there is a high rate of false positives, so any positive result should be followed up by retesting). Early diagnosis and intervention can make a tremendous difference in the prognosis. For more information on private lab screening and newborn screening in general, contact Baylor University Medical Center: (800) 4BAYLOR (422-9567); baylorhealth.com/medicalspecialties/metabolic/newbornscreening.htm; or Pediatrix Screening: (954) 384-0175; pediatrixscreening.com.

To find out if your state screens for the 29 conditions that the March of Dimes recommends, go to genes-r-us.uthscsa.edu/.

---

medically wise, and it may have to be adjusted at the last minute. After all, there's no greater priority than your well-being and your baby's—and if your birth plan doesn't end up being consistent with that priority, it'll have to take a backseat. A change of mind (yours) can also prompt a change of plan (you were dead set against having an epidural, but somewhere around 4 cm, you become dead set on having one).

Bottom line: Birth plans, though by no means necessary (you can definitely decide to go with the flow when it comes to childbirth, and you'll give birth with or without one), are a great option, one that more and more expectant parents are taking advantage of. To find out more, and to figure out whether a birth plan is right for you, talk it over with your practitioner at your next visit.

Glucose Screening Test

"My practitioner says I need to take a glucose screening test to check for gestational diabetes. Why would I need it, and what does the test involve?"

Don't feel too picked on. Almost all practitioners screen for gestational diabetes in almost all patients at about 24 to 28 weeks (though those at higher risk for gestational diabetes, including older or obese mothers or those with a family history of diabetes, are screened earlier in their pregnancies and more

Doulas: Best Medicine for Labor?

Think three's a crowd? For many couples, not when it comes to labor and delivery. More and more are opting to share their birth experience with a doula, a woman trained as a labor companion. And for good reason. Studies have shown that women supported by doulas are much less likely to require cesarean deliveries, induction, and pain relief. Births attended by doulas may also be shorter, with a lower rate of complications.

Doula is a term that comes from ancient Greece, where it was used to describe the most important female servant in the household, the one who probably helped mom out the most during childbirth. What exactly can a doula do for you and your birth experience? That depends on the doula you choose, at what point in your pregnancy you hire her, and what your preferences are. Some doulas become involved well before that first contraction strikes, helping with the design of a birth plan and easing prelabor jitters. Many, on request, come to the house to help a couple through early labor. Once at the hospital or birthing center, the doula takes on a variety of responsibilities, again depending on your needs and wishes. Typically, her primary role is as a continuous source of comfort, encouragement, and support (both emotional and physical) during labor. She'll serve as a soothing voice of experience (especially valuable if you're first-timers), help with relaxation techniques and breathing exercises, offer advice on labor positions, and do her share of massage, hand holding, pillow plumping, and bed adjusting. A doula can also act as a mediator and an advocate, ready to speak for you as needed, to translate medical terms and explain procedures, and to generally run interference with hospital personnel. She won't take the place of your coach (and a good doula won't make him feel like she's taking his place, either) or the nurse on duty; instead, she will augment their support and services (especially important if the nurse assigned to you has several other patients in labor at the same time or if labor is long and nurses come and go as shifts change). She will also likely be the only person (besides the coach)

often). So chances are the test your practitioner ordered is just routine.

And it's simple, too, especially if you have a sweet tooth. You'll be asked to drink a very sweet glucose drink, which usually tastes like flat orange soda, one hour before having some blood drawn; you don't have to be fasting when you do this. Most women chugalug the stuff with no problem and no side effects; a few, especially those who don't have a taste for sweet liquids, feel a little queasy afterward.

If the blood work comes back with elevated numbers, which suggests the possibility that you might not be producing enough insulin to process the extra glucose in your system, the next level of test—the glucose tolerance test—is ordered. This fasting three-hour test, which involves a higher-concentration glucose drink, is used to diagnose gestational diabetes.

Gestational diabetes occurs in about 4 to 7 percent of expectant mothers, which makes it one of the most common pregnancy complications. Fortunately, it's also one of the most easily managed. When blood sugar is closely controlled through diet, exercise, and, if necessary, who will stay by your side throughout labor and delivery—a friendly and familiar face from start to finish. And many doulas don't stop there. They can also offer support and advice postpartum on everything from breastfeeding to baby care.

Though an expectant father may fear that hiring a doula will relegate him to third-wheel status, this isn't the case. A good doula is also there to help your coach relax so he can help you relax. She'll be there to answer questions he might not feel comfortable broaching with a doctor or nurse. She'll be there to provide an extra set of hands when you need your legs and back massaged at the same time, or when you need both a refill on ice chips and help breathing through a contraction. She'll be an obliging and cooperative member of your labor team—ready to pitch in, but not to push dad aside and take over.

How do you locate a doula? Many birthing centers and hospitals keep lists of doulas, and so do some practitioners. Ask friends who've recently used a doula for recommendations, or check online for local doulas. Once you've tracked down a candidate, arrange a consultation before you hire her to make sure both of you are comfortable with her. Ask her about her experience, her training, what she will do and what she won't do, what her philosophies are about childbirth (if you're planning on asking for an epidural, for instance, you won't want to hire a doula who discourages the use of pain relief), whether she will be on call at all times and who covers for her if she isn't, whether she provides pregnancy and/or postpartum services, and what her fees are (some doulas command hefty fees, especially those in big cities). For more information or to locate a doula in your area, contact Doulas of North America: (888) 788-DONA (788-3662); dona.com.

An alternative to a doula, which could also be beneficial, is a female friend or relative who has gone through pregnancy and delivery herself and with whom you feel totally comfortable. The plus: Her services will be free. The drawback: She probably won't be quite as knowledgeable. One way to remedy that is having a "lay doula," a female friend who goes through four hours of training in doula techniques (ask if your hospital has such a training course). Researchers have found that a "lay doula" can provide the same benefits as a professional one.

medication, women with gestational diabetes are likely to have perfectly normal pregnancies and healthy babies. See page 546 for more.

A Low-Birthweight Baby

"I've been reading a lot about the high incidence of low-birthweight babies. Is there anything I can do to be sure I won't have one?"

Some cases of low birthweight are preventable, so you can do a lot— and, inasmuch as you're reading this book, chances are good you already are. Nationally, 8 of every 100 newborns are categorized as low birthweight (under 5 pounds 8 ounces, or 2,500 grams), and slightly more than 1 in 100 babies as very low birthweight (3 pounds 5 ounces, or 1,500 grams, or less). But that rate is much lower among women who are conscientious about both medical care and self-care (and are lucky enough to be able to afford the first and informed enough to do a good job on the second). Most of the common causes of low birthweight—use of tobacco, alcohol, or drugs (particularly

Signs of Preterm Labor

Though the chances of your baby arriving early are pretty low, it's a good idea for every expectant mom to be familiar with the signs of premature labor, since early detection can have a tremendous impact on outcome. Think of the following as information you'll probably never use but should know, just to be on the safe side. Read this list over, and if you experience any of these symptoms before 37 weeks, call your practitioner immediately:

■ Persistent cramps that are menstrual-like, with or without diarrhea, nausea, or indigestion

■ Regular painful contractions coming every 10 minutes (or sooner) that do not subside when you change positions (not to be confused with the Braxton Hicks contractions you might be already feeling, which don't indicate early labor; see page 311)

■ Constant lower back pain or pressure or a change in the nature of lower backache

■ A change in your vaginal discharge, particularly if it is watery or tinged or streaked pinkish or brownish with blood

■ An achiness or feeling of pressure in the pelvic floor, the thighs, or the groin

■ Leaking from your vagina (a steady trickle or a gush)

Keep in mind that you can have some or all of these symptoms and not be in labor (most pregnant women experience pelvic pressure or lower back pain at some point). In fact, the majority of women who have symptoms of preterm labor do not deliver early. But only your practitioner can tell for sure, so pick up the phone and call. After all, it's always best to play it safe.

For information on preterm labor risk factors and prevention, see pages 44–47. For information on the management of preterm labor, see page 557.

cocaine), poor nutrition, extreme emotional stress (but not normal stress levels), and inadequate prenatal care, for example—are preventable. Many others, such as chronic maternal illnesses, can be controlled by a good working partnership between the mother and her practitioner. A major cause—premature labor—can sometimes be prevented.

Of course, sometimes a baby is small at birth for reasons that no one can control: the mother's own low weight when she was born, for example, or an inadequate placenta, or a genetic disorder. A very short interval (less than nine months) between pregnancies may also be a factor. But even in these cases, excellent diet and

prenatal care can often compensate and tip the scales in baby's favor. And when a baby does turn out to be small, the top-notch medical care currently available gives even the very smallest an increasingly good chance of surviving and growing up healthy.

If you think you have real reason to worry about having a low-birthweight baby, share your concern with your practitioner. An exam and/or an ultrasound will probably reassure you that your fetus is growing at a normal pace. If it does turn out that your baby is on the very small side, steps can be taken to uncover the cause and, if possible, correct it. See page 550 for more information.

Easing Labor Pain

Let's face it. Those 15 or so hours it takes to birth a baby aren't called labor because it's a walk in the park. Labor (and delivery) is hard work—hard work that can hurt, big time. And if you actually consider what's going on down there, it's really no wonder that labor hurts. During childbirth, your uterus contracts over and over again to squeeze a relatively big baby through one relatively tight space (your cervix) and out through an even tighter one (your vagina, the same opening you once thought was too small for a tampon). Like they say, it's pain with a purpose—a really cute and cuddly purpose—yet it's pain nonetheless.

But while there may be no getting around the pain of labor altogether (unless you're scheduled for a cesarean delivery, in which case you'll be skipping labor and labor pain), there are plenty of ways to get through it. As a laboring mom, you can select from a wide menu of pain-relief options, both the medicinal kind and the nonmedicinal variety (and you can even opt for a combo from both columns). You can choose to go unmedicated throughout your entire labor or just through part of labor (like those easier first centimeters). You can turn to alternative medicine and nondrug approaches to manage the pain (acupuncture, hypnosis, or hydrotherapy, for instance). Or you can birth your baby with a little help—or a lot of help—from an analgesic, such as the very popular epidural (which leaves you with little or no pain during labor but allows you to remain awake during the entire process).

Which option is for you? To figure that out, look into them all. Read up on childbirth pain management (the section that follows covers the gamut). Talk to your practitioner. Get insights from friends who have recently labored. And then do some thinking. Remember that the right option for you might not be one option but a combination of several (reflexology with an epidural chaser, or a variety of relaxation techniques topped off with a round of acupuncture). Remember, too, the value of staying flexible—and not just so you can stretch yourself into some of those pushing positions you learned in childbirth class. After all, the option or options you settle on now may not sit well later, and may need to be adjusted midlabor (you were planning on an epidural but found you could handle the pain—or vice versa). Most of all, remember that (barring any obstetrical situation that would dictate how you labor and deliver), it's completely your choice to make—your birth, your way.

Managing Your Pain with Medications

When it comes to pain relief during labor, there's a wide variety of medications to choose from, including anesthetics (substances that produce loss of sensation or put you to sleep), analgesics (pain relievers), and ataraxics (tranquilizers). In most circumstances, it'll be up to you to select the pain medication you want to make your labor and delivery as comfortable as possible, though your choice may be limited depending on the stage of labor, whether it's an emergency situation, or your past health history or your present condition (and that of your baby) precludes a particular drug, and the anesthesiologist's preference and expertise.

Something else to keep in mind as you begin to explore your options: How effective a drug is in relieving pain will depend on how it affects you (different drugs affect different people differently), the dosage, and other factors. There's always a remote chance that a drug won't provide you with the relief you're looking for, or that it might not give you any at all. Most of the time, though, pain medications work exactly the way they are supposed to—offering up just what you (and your practitioner) ordered.

Here are the most commonly used labor and delivery pain medications:

Epidural. The epidural is the pain relief of choice for two thirds of all laboring women delivering at hospitals. The major reasons for the epidural's current surge in popularity are its relative safety (only a small amount of medication is needed to achieve the desired effect), its ease of administration, and its patient-friendly results (local pain relief in the lower part of the body that allows you to be awake during the birth and alert enough to greet your baby immediately after it). It's also considered safer for your baby than other anesthetics because the epidural is injected directly into the spine (technically, into the epidural space, which is located between the ligament that sheathes the vertebrae and the membrane that covers the spinal cord), which means the drug barely reaches the bloodstream (unlike other anesthetics). And even better news: An epidural can be given to you as soon as you ask for one—no need to wait until you're dilated a certain amount (3 or 4 cm, for instance). Studies show that even an early epidural doesn't increase the chances of a C-section as was once

believed, nor does it slow down labor significantly. And even if labor does slow down a bit with an epidural, your doctor can give you Pitocin (a synthetic version of oxytocin, the hormone that triggers contractions naturally) to help get your labor back up to speed again.

Here's what you can expect if you're having an epidural:

- Before the epidural is administered, an IV of fluids is started (this is done to prevent a drop in blood pressure, a side effect some women have with an epidural; fluids will keep your blood pressure from going too low).

- In some hospitals (policies vary), a catheter (tube) is inserted into the bladder just before or just after administration of the epidural and stays in place to drain urine while the epidural is in effect (since the medication may suppress the urge to urinate). In other hospitals, the bladder is just drained intermittently with a catheter as needed.

- Your lower and midback are wiped with an antiseptic solution and a small area of the back is numbed with a local anesthetic. A larger needle is placed through the numbed area into the epidural space of the spine, usually while you're lying on your side or sitting up and leaning over a table or being supported by your spouse, coach, or nurse. Some women feel a little pressure as the needle is inserted. Others feel a little tingling or a momentary shooting pain as the needle finds the correct spot. If you're lucky (and many women are), you might not feel a thing while the epidural is being administered. Besides, compared to the pain of contractions, any discomfort from a needle poke is likely to be pretty minimal.

- The needle is removed, leaving a fine, flexible catheter tube in place. The tube is taped to your back so you can move from side to side. Three to five minutes following the initial dose, the nerves of the uterus begin to numb. Usually after 10 minutes, you'll begin to feel the full effect (hopefully, sweet relief). The medication numbs the nerves in the entire lower part of the body, making it hard to feel any contractions at all (and that's the point).

- Your blood pressure will be checked frequently to make sure it's not dropping too low. IV fluids and lying on your side will help counteract a drop in blood pressure.

- Because an epidural is sometimes associated with slowing of the fetal heartbeat, continuous fetal monitoring is usually required as well. Though such fetal monitoring limits your movements somewhat, it allows your practitioner to monitor the baby's heartbeat and allows you to "see" the frequency and intensity of your contractions (because, ideally, you won't be feeling them).

Happily, there are few side effects with an epidural, though some women might experience numbness on one side of the body only (as opposed to complete pain relief). Epidurals also might not offer complete pain control if you're experiencing back labor (when the fetus is in a posterior position, with its head pressing against your back).

Combined spinal epidural (aka "walking epidural"). The combined spinal epidural delivers the same amount of pain relief as a traditional epidural does, but it uses a smaller amount of medication to reach that goal. Not all anesthesiologists or hospitals offer this type of epidural (ask your practitioner if it'll be available to you). The anesthesiologist will start you off with a shot of analgesic directly into the spinal fluid to help relieve some pain, but because the medication is

Pushing Without the Pain

Does pushing have to be a pain? Not always. In fact, many women find they can push very effectively with an epidural, relying on their coach or a nurse to tell them when a contraction is coming on so they can get busy pushing. But if pain-free pushing isn't getting you (or your baby) anywhere—with the lack of sensation hampering your efforts—the epidural can be stopped so you can feel the contractions. The medication can then be easily restarted after delivery to numb the repair of a tear.

delivered only in the spinal fluid, you'll still feel and be able to use the muscles in your legs (which is why it's called a walking epidural). When you feel you need more pain relief, more medication is placed into the epidural space (through a catheter that was inserted at the same time the spinal medication was administered). Though you'll be able to move your legs, they'll probably feel weak, so it'll be unlikely you'll actually want to walk around.

Spinal block (for cesarean delivery) or saddle block (for instrument-assisted vaginal delivery). These regional blocks, which are rarely used these days, are generally administered in a single dose just prior to delivery (in other words, if you didn't have an epidural during labor but want pain relief for the delivery, you'll get the fast-acting spinal block). Like the epidural, these blocks are administered with you sitting up or lying on your side while an anesthetic is injected into the fluid surrounding the spinal cord.

The side effects of spinal and saddle blocks are the same as for an epidural (a possible drop in blood pressure).

Pudendal block. Occasionally used to relieve early second-stage pain, a pudendal block is usually reserved for the vaginal delivery itself. Administered through a needle inserted into the vaginal area, the medication reduces pain in the region but not uterine discomfort. It's useful when forceps or vacuum extraction is used, and its effect can last through episiotomy (if needed) and repair of an episiotomy or tear.

General anesthesia. General anesthesia is rarely used for deliveries these days and only used in specific cases for emergency surgical births. An anesthesiologist in an operating/delivery room injects drugs into your IV that put you to sleep. You'll be awake during the preparations and unconscious for however long it takes to complete the delivery (usually a matter of minutes). When you come to, you may be groggy, disoriented, and restless. You may also have a cough and sore throat (due to the tube that's routinely inserted through the mouth into the throat) and experience nausea and vomiting.

The major downside to general anesthesia (besides the fact that mom has to miss the birth) is that it sedates the baby along with the mother. The medical team will minimize those sedative effects by administering the anesthesia as close to the actual birth as possible. That way the baby can be delivered before the anesthetic has reached him or her in amounts large enough to have an effect. The doctor might also tilt you to your side or give you oxygen to get more oxygen to the baby, minimizing the drug's temporary effect.

Demerol. Demerol is one of the most frequently used obstetrical analgesics. This shot (sometimes given in the buttocks) or IV-administered drug is used to dull the pain and relax the mother so she is better able to cope with contractions. It can be repeated every two to four hours, as needed. But not all women like the drowsy feeling Demerol imparts, and some find they are actually less able to cope with labor pains while under the effects of Demerol.

There may be some side effects (depending on a woman's sensitivity), including nausea, vomiting, and a drop in blood pressure. The effect Demerol will have on the newborn depends on the total dose and how close to delivery it has been administered. If it has been given too close to delivery, the baby may be sleepy and unable to suck; less frequently, respiration may be depressed and supplemental oxygen may be required. Any effects on the newborn are generally short-term and, if necessary, can be treated.

Demerol is not generally administered until labor is well established and false labor has been ruled out, but no later than two to three hours before delivery is expected.

Tranquilizers. These drugs (such as Phenergan and Vistaril) are used to calm and relax an extremely anxious mom-to-be so that she can participate more fully in childbirth. Tranquilizers can also enhance the effectiveness of analgesics such as Demerol. Like analgesics, tranquilizers are usually administered once labor is well established, and well before delivery. But they are occasionally used in early labor if a mother's anxiety is slowing down the progress of her labor. Reactions to the effects of tranquilizers vary. Some women welcome the gentle drowsiness; others find it interferes with their control and with their memory of this memorable experience. Dosage definitely makes a difference. A small dose may serve to relieve anxiety without impairing alertness. A larger dose may cause slurring of speech and dozing between contraction peaks, making it difficult to use prepared childbirth techniques. Though the risks to a fetus or newborn from tranquilizers are minimal, most practitioners prefer to stay away from tranquilizers unless they're really necessary. If you think you might be extremely anxious during labor, you may want to try learning about some nondrug relaxation techniques now (such as meditation, massage, hypnosis; see below), so you won't end up needing this kind of medication.

Managing Your Pain with CAM

Not every woman wants traditional pain medication, but most still want their labor to be as comfortable as possible. And that's where complementary and alternative medicine (CAM) therapies can come in. These days, it's not just CAM practitioners who are touting the benefits of these techniques. More and more traditional physicians are hopping on board the CAM bandwagon, too. Many recommend CAM techniques to their patients—either as an alternative to pain medication or as a relaxing supplement to it. Even

Just Breathe

Hoping to skip the meds but can't—or don't want to—CAM? Lamaze (or other kinds of natural childbirth techniques) can be very effective in managing the pain of contractions. See page 279 for more.

if you're sure there's an epidural with your name on it waiting at the hospital, you may want to explore the world of CAM, too. (And to explore it well before your due date, since many of the techniques take practice—or even classes—to perfect, and most take plenty of planning.) But remember to seek out CAM practitioners who are licensed and certified, not to mention ones who have plenty of experience with pregnancy, labor, and delivery.

Acupuncture and acupressure. Scientific studies now back up what the Chinese have known for thousands of years: Acupuncture and acupressure are effective forms of pain relief. Researchers have found that acupuncture, through the use of needles inserted in specific locations, triggers the release of several brain chemicals, including endorphins, which block pain signals, relieving labor pain (and maybe even helping boost labor progress). Acupressure works on the same principle as acupuncture, except that instead of poking you with needles, your practitioner will use finger pressure to stimulate the points. Acupressure on the center of the ball of the foot is said to help back labor. If you're planning to use either during labor, let your prenatal practitioner know that your CAM practitioner will be with you through labor.

Reflexology. Reflexologists believe that the internal organs can be accessed through points on the feet. By massaging the feet during childbirth, a reflexologist can relax the uterus and stimulate the pituitary gland, apparently reducing the pain of childbirth and even shortening the duration of labor. Some of the pressure points are so powerful that you should avoid stimulating them unless you *are* in labor.

Physical therapy. From massage and hot compresses to ice packs and intense counterpressure on your sore spots, physical therapy during labor can ease a lot of the pain you're feeling. Massage at the hands of a caring coach or doula or a skilled health professional can bring relaxing relief and can help diminish pain.

Hydrotherapy. There's nothing like a warm bath—especially one with jets kneading your sore spots and particularly if you're in labor. Settle into a jetted tub (or merely a soaking tub) for a session of hydrotherapy during your labor to reduce pain and relax you. Many hospitals and birthing centers now provide such tubs to labor—or even deliver—in.

Hypnobirthing. Though hypnosis won't mask your pain, numb your nerves, or quell contractions, it can get you so deeply relaxed (some women describe it as becoming like a floppy rag doll) that you are totally unaware of any discomfort. Hypnosis doesn't work for everyone; you have to be highly suggestible (some clues are having a long attention span, a rich imagination, and if you enjoy—or don't mind—being alone). Still, more and more women these days are seeking the help of a medically certified hypnotherapist (you'll want to shy away from someone without such credentials) to train them to get through labor by self-hypnosis; sometimes, you can have a hypnotherapist with you during the process. It's not something you can just start when that first contraction hits; you'll have to practice quite a bit during pregnancy to be able to achieve total relaxation, even with a certified therapist at your side (and while you're practicing, you can use hypnosis to get relief from pregnancy aches, pains, and stress, too). One big benefit of hypnobirthing is that while you're completely relaxed, you're also completely awake and aware of every

moment of your baby's birth. There are also no physical effects on the baby (or on you).

Distraction. Even if you're not the type to try hypnosis (or you didn't plan far enough ahead), you can still try to get your mind off the pain of labor by using distraction techniques. Anything—watching TV, listening to music, meditating—that takes your mind off the pain can decrease your perception of it. So can focusing on an object (an ultrasound picture of your baby, a soothing landscape, a photo of a favorite place) or doing visualization exercises (for example, picturing your baby being pushed gently by contractions, preparing to exit the uterus, excited and happy). Keeping your pain in perspective is also key to an easier labor. Staying rested, relaxed, and positive (remember that the pain of a contraction is actually accomplishing something—each one getting you closer to your baby—and keep telling yourself that it won't last forever) will help you stay more comfortable.

Transcutaneous electrical nerve stimulation (TENS). This technique uses electrodes that deliver low-voltage pulses to stimulate nerve pathways to the uterus and cervix, supposedly blocking pain. Studies aren't clear on whether TENS is really effective at reducing labor pain, but some do show that it leads to a shorter first-stage labor and less need for pain meds.

Making the Decision

You now have the lowdown on pain relief options for labor and delivery—the information you'll need to make an informed decision. But before you decide what's best for you and your baby, you should:

- Discuss the topic of pain relief and anesthesia with your practitioner long before labor begins. Your practitioner's expertise and experience make him or her an invaluable partner—though not usually the deciding vote—in the decision-making process. Well before your first contraction, find out what kinds of drugs or CAM techniques he or she uses most often, what side effects may be experienced, when he or she considers medication absolutely necessary, and when the option is yours.

- Consider keeping an open mind. Though it's smart to think ahead about what might be best for you under certain circumstances, it's impossible to predict what kind of labor and delivery you'll have, how you will respond to the contractions, and whether or not you'll want, need, or have to have medication. Even if you're absolutely convinced that you'll

want an epidural, you may not want to close the door completely to trying some CAM approaches—either first, or on the side. After all, your labor may turn out to be more manageable (or a lot shorter) than you'd thought. And even if you're sold on an all-med-free delivery, you may want to think about leaving the medication window open—even if it's just a crack—in case your labor turns out to be tougher than you'd bargained for.

Most important of all, remember, as you sort through those pain relief options, to keep your eye on the bottom line—a bottom line that has a really cute bottom. After all, no matter how you end up managing the pain of childbirth—and even if you don't end up managing it the way you planned to or the way you really hoped to—you'll still manage to give birth to your baby. And what could be a better bottom line than that?

The
Eighth
Month

Approximately 32 to 35 Weeks

I N THIS NEXT-TO-LAST MONTH, YOU may still be relishing every expectant moment, or you may be growing increasingly weary of, well, growing—and growing. Either way, you're sure to be preoccupied with—and super-excited about—the much-anticipated event: your baby's arrival. Of course, along with that heaping serving of excitement (the baby's almost here!), you and your partner are likely experiencing a side of trepidation (the baby's almost here!)—especially if this is your first foray into parenthood. Talking those very normal feelings through—and tapping into the insights of friends and family members who've preceded you into parenthood—will help you realize that everyone feels that way, particularly the first time around.

Your Baby This Month

Week 32 This week your baby is tipping the scales at almost 4 pounds and topping out at just about 19 inches. And growing isn't the only thing on the agenda these days. While you're busy getting everything ready for baby's arrival, baby's busy prepping for that big debut, too. In these last few weeks, it's all about practice, practice, practice, as he or she hones the skills needed to survive outside the womb, from swallowing and breathing to kicking and sucking. And speaking of sucking, your little one has been able to suck his or her thumb for a while now (okay, maybe it's not a survival skill, but it sure is cute). Another change this week: Your baby's skin is no longer see-through. As more and more fat accumulates under the skin, it's finally opaque (just like yours!).

Week 33 Baby's gaining weight almost as fast as you are these days (averaging out

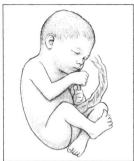

Your Baby, Month 8

to about half a pound a week), which puts the grand total so far at more than 4½ pounds. Still, your baby has plenty of growing up (and out) to do. He or she may grow a full inch this week alone and may come close to doubling in weight by D-day. And with that much baby inside your uterus now, your amniotic fluid level has maxed out (there's no room for more fluid now). Which explains why those pokes and kicks are sometimes extremely uncomfortable: There's less fluid to cushion the blows. Antibodies are also being passed from you to your baby as your little one continues to develop his or her own immune system. These antibodies will definitely come in handy on the outside and will protect your baby-to-be from many of those playground germs.

Week 34 Your baby could be as tall as 20 inches right now and weighs about 5 pounds. Got male (a male baby, that is)? If you do, then this is the week that his testicles are making their way down from his abdomen to their final destina-

tion: his scrotum. (About 3 to 4 percent of boys are born with undescended testicles, which is nothing to worry about; they usually make the trip down south before the first birthday.) And in other baby-related news, those tiny little fingernails have probably reached the tip of his or her fingers by this week, so make sure you have baby nail clippers on your shopping list!

Week 35 Your baby stands tall this week—if he or she could stand, that is—at about 20 inches, and continues to follow the ½-pound-a-week plan, weighing in at about 5½ big ones. While growth will taper off when it comes to height (the average full-termer is born at about 20 inches), your baby will continue to pack on the pounds up until delivery day. Something else he or she will be packing on in the few weeks that remain are brain cells. Brain development continues at a mind-boggling pace, making baby a little on the top-heavy side. And speaking of tops, it's likely your baby's bottom is. Most babies have settled into a head-down, bottoms-up position in Mom's pelvis by now, or will soon. That's a good thing, since it's easier on you if baby's head (the biggest part of his or her body) exits first during delivery. Here's another plus: Baby's head may be big, but it's still soft (at least, the skull is), allowing that tight squeeze through the birth canal to be a little less tight.

What You May Be Feeling

As always, remember that every pregnancy and every woman is different. You may experience all of these symptoms at one time or another, or only a few of them. Some may have continued from last month; others may be new. Still others may be hardly noticed because you've become so used to them. You may also have other, less common, symptoms. Here's what you might experience this month:

Physically

- Strong, regular fetal activity

- Increasing vaginal discharge

- Increased constipation

- Heartburn, indigestion, flatulence, bloating

- Occasional headaches, faintness, or dizziness

A Look Inside

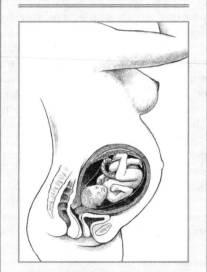

An interesting bit of pregnancy trivia: Measurement in centimeters from the top of your pubic bone to the top of your uterus roughly correlates with the number of weeks you're up to; so, at 34 weeks, your uterus measures close to 34 cm from the pubic bone.

- Nasal congestion and occasional nosebleeds; ear stuffiness

- Sensitive gums

- Leg cramps

- Backache

- Pelvic pressure and/or achiness

- Mild swelling of ankles and feet, and occasionally of hands and face

- Varicose veins of legs

- Hemorrhoids

- Itchy abdomen

- Protruding navel

- Stretch marks

- Increasing shortness of breath as the uterus crowds the lungs, which eases when the baby drops

- Difficulty sleeping

- Increasing "practice" (Braxton Hicks) contractions

- Increasing clumsiness

- Enlarged breasts

- Colostrum, leaking from nipples (though this premilk substance may not appear until after delivery)

Emotionally

- Increasing eagerness for the pregnancy to be over

- Apprehension about labor and delivery

- Increasing absentmindedness

- Trepidation about becoming a parent, if it's your first time

- Excitement—at the realization that it won't be long now

What You Can Expect at This Month's Checkup

After the 32nd week, your practitioner may ask you to come in every two weeks so your progress and your baby's can be more closely watched. You can expect the following to be checked, depending on your particular needs and your practitioner's style of practice:

- Weight and blood pressure

- Urine, for sugar and protein

- Fetal heartbeat

- Height of fundus (top of uterus)

- Size (you may get a rough weight estimate) and position of the fetus, by palpation (feeling from the outside)

- Feet and hands for swelling, and legs for varicose veins

- Group B strep test

- Symptoms you have been experiencing, especially unusual ones

- Questions and problems you want to discuss—have a list ready

What You May Be Wondering About

Braxton Hicks Contractions

"Every once in a while my uterus seems to bunch up and harden. What's going on?"

It's practicing. With delivery right around the corner, your body is warming up for the big day by flexing its muscles—literally. Those uterine calisthenics you're feeling are called Braxton Hicks contractions—practice-for-labor contractions that usually begin sometime after the 20th week of pregnancy (though they're more noticeable in the last few months of pregnancy). These rehearsal contractions (typically experienced earlier and with more intensity in women who've had a previous pregnancy) feel like a tightening sensation that begins at the top of your uterus and then spreads downward, lasting from 15 to 30 seconds, though they can sometimes last as long as two minutes or more.

If you check out your belly while you're having a Braxton Hicks, you might even be able to see what you're feeling; your usually round abdomen might appear pointy or strangely bunched up. Weird to watch, but normal.

Though Braxton Hicks contractions are not true labor, they may be difficult to distinguish from real labor—especially as they become more intense, which they often do as pregnancy draws to a close. And though they're not efficient enough to deliver your baby (even when they get really uncomfortable), they may give you a leg up on labor by getting effacement and early dilation of the cervix started when the time is right.

To relieve any discomfort you may feel during these contractions, try changing your position—lying down and relaxing if you've been on your feet, or getting up and walking around if you've been sitting. Be sure, too, that you're getting enough to drink. Dehydration (even minor dehydration) can sometimes cause contractions, including these practice ones. You can also use this labor rehearsal to practice your breathing exercises and the various other childbirth techniques you've learned, which can make it easier to deal with the real contractions when they do arrive.

If the contractions don't subside with a change in activity, and if they become progressively stronger and more regular, you may be in real labor, so be sure to put in a call to your practitioner. A good rule of thumb: If you have more than four Braxton Hicks in an hour, call your practitioner and let him or her know. If you're having a hard time distinguishing Braxton Hicks contractions from the real thing—especially if this is your first pregnancy and you've never experienced the real thing—read up about the different kinds of contractions on page 359 and give your practitioner a call, being sure to describe exactly what you're feeling.

Not-So-Funny Rib Tickling

"It feels as though my baby has his feet jammed up into my rib cage, and it really hurts."

In the later months, when fetuses run out of stretching room in their cramped quarters, the resourceful little creatures often do seem to find a snug niche for their feet between their mother's ribs, and that's one kind of rib tickling that doesn't tickle. Changing your own position may convince your baby to change his or hers. A gentle nudge from you or a few pelvic tilts may dislodge him. Or try relocating him with this exercise: Take a deep breath while you raise one arm over your head, then exhale while you drop your arm; repeat a few times with each arm.

If none of these tactics works, hang in there. When your little pain-in-the-ribs engages, or drops into your pelvis, which usually happens two or three weeks before delivery in first pregnancies (though often not until labor begins in subsequent ones), he probably won't be able to stretch his toes quite so high up.

Another reason for rib cage pain that you can't blame on your baby—at least not directly—comes from a loosening of the joints in the area, courtesy of pregnancy hormones. Acetaminophen (Tylenol) can help ease the ache, but also avoid heavy lifting, which can make it worse (and which you shouldn't be doing now anyway).

Shortness of Breath

"Sometimes I have trouble breathing, even when I'm not exerting any energy. Why is that happening to me? And does it mean my baby isn't getting enough oxygen?"

It's not surprising you're feeling a little spare on air these days. Your ever-expanding uterus is now crowding out all your other internal organs in an effort to provide spacious-enough accommodations for your ever-growing baby. Among those organs feeling the crunch are your lungs, which your uterus has compressed, limiting their ability to expand fully when you take a breath. This, teamed with the extra progesterone that has already been leaving you breathless for months, explains why a trip upstairs these days can make you feel as if you've just run a marathon (winded, big time). Fortunately, while this shortness of breath may feel very uncomfortable to you, it doesn't bother your baby in the least. He or she is kept well stocked with all the oxygen he or she needs through the placenta.

Choosing a Pediatrician

Choosing a pediatrician (or a family practitioner) is one of the most important decisions you'll make as a parent—and actually, you shouldn't wait until you become a parent to make it. Sifting through your choices and making your selection now, before your baby starts crying inexplicably at 3 A.M., will ensure that your transition to parenthood will be that much easier. It will also allow for an informed—not hasty—decision.

If you're not sure where to begin your search, ask your practitioner (if you've been happy with his or her care) or friends, neighbors, or coworkers who have young children for recommendations. Or contact the hospital or birthing center where you'll be delivering (you can call the labor and delivery floor or pediatrics, and ask a nurse on duty for some suggestions; no one gets a better look at doctors than nurses do). Of course, if you're on a health insurance plan that limits your choices, you'll have to choose from that list.

Once you've narrowed your choices down to two or three, call for consultations; most pediatricians or family practitioners will oblige. Bring a list of questions about issues that are important to you, such as office protocol (for instance, whether there are call-in hours for parents or when you can expect calls to be returned), breastfeeding support, circumcision, the use of antibiotics, whether the doctor handles all well-baby visits or whether they are typically handled by nurse-practitioners in the practice. Also important to know: Is the doctor board certified? Which hospital is the doctor affiliated with, and will he or she be able to care for the newborn in the hospital? For more questions to ask and issues to consider, check out the *What to Expect Pregnancy Journal and Organizer.*

Relief from that winded feeling usually arrives toward the end of pregnancy, when your baby drops into your pelvis in preparation for birth (in first pregnancies this generally occurs two to three weeks before delivery, in subsequent deliveries often not until labor begins). Until then, you may find it easier to breathe if you sit straight up instead of slumped over and sleep in a semi-propped-up position, bolstered by two or three pillows.

Sometimes breathlessness can be a sign that iron stores are low, so check in with your practitioner about it. Call immediately (or head to the ER) if shortness of breath is severe and accompanied by rapid breathing, blueness of the lips and fingertips, chest pain, and/or rapid pulse.

Lack of Bladder Control

"I watched a funny movie last night and I seemed to be leaking urine every time I laughed. Why is that?"

As if frequent bathroom runs weren't annoying enough lately, the third trimester has added another bladder issue to the mix: stress incontinence. This lack of bladder control—causing you to spring a small leak when you cough, sneeze, lift something heavy, or even laugh (though there's nothing funny about that)—is the result of the mounting pressure of the growing uterus on the bladder. Some women also experience urge incontinence, the sudden, overwhelming need to urinate (gotta go *now!*) during late pregnancy. Try these tips to help prevent or control stress or urge incontinence:

- Empty your bladder as completely as possible each time you pee by leaning forward.

- Practice your Kegel exercises. Being faithful to your Kegels will help strengthen the pelvic muscles and prevent or correct most cases of pregnancy-induced incontinence—plus, looking ahead, they'll also help prevent postpartum incontinence. For a Kegel how-to, see page 295.

- Do Kegels or cross your legs when you feel a cough, sneeze, or laugh coming on.

- Wear a panty liner if you need one, or you're afraid you'll need one. Graduate to a maxipad when leaks might be especially inconvenient.

- Stay as regular as you can, because impacted stool can put pressure on the bladder. Also, straining hard during bowel movements (as you're likely to do when you're constipated) can weaken pelvic floor muscles. For tips on fighting constipation, see page 173.

- If it's the urge that's driving you crazy (and sending you to the bathroom in a hurry all the time), try training your bladder. Urinate more frequently—about every 30 minutes to an hour—so that you go before you feel that uncontrollable need. After a week, try to gradually stretch the time between bathroom visits, adding 15 minutes more at a time.

- Continue drinking at least eight glasses of fluids a day, even if you experience stress incontinence or frequent urges. Limiting your fluid intake will not limit leaks and it may lead to UTIs and/or dehydration. Not only can either of these lead to a lot of other problems (including preterm contractions), but UTIs can exacerbate stress incontinence. See page 499 for tips on keeping your urinary tract healthy.

To be sure that the leak you've sprung is urine (which it almost certainly is) and not amniotic fluid, it's smart to initially give it the sniff test. If the liquid that has leaked doesn't smell like urine (which has an ammonia-like smell; amniotic fluid has a sweet smell), let your practitioner know as soon as possible.

How You're Carrying

"Everyone says I seem to be carrying small and low for the eighth month. My midwife says everything's fine, but what if my baby isn't growing the way she should be?"

The truth is, you can't tell a baby by her mom's belly. How you're carrying has much less to do with the bulk of your baby and much more to do with these factors:

- Your own bulk, shape, and bone structure. Bellies come in all sizes, just like expectant moms do. A petite woman may carry more compactly (small, low, and out in front) than a larger woman. On the other hand, some very overweight moms never seem to pop out much at all. That's because their babies have lots of growing room available in mom's already ample abdomen.

- Your muscle tone. A woman with very tight muscles may not pop as soon or as much as a woman with slacker muscles, particularly one who's already had a baby or two.

- The baby's position. How your fetus is positioned on the inside may also affect how big or small you look on the outside.

- Your weight gain. A bigger maternal weight gain doesn't necessarily predict a bigger baby, just a bigger mom.

The only assessments of a fetus's size that are worth paying attention to are medical ones—the ones you get from your practitioner at your prenatal visits, not the ones you get from your sister-in-law, your colleague at work, or perfect strangers in the supermarket checkout line. To evaluate your baby's progress more accurately at each prenatal visit, your practitioner won't just take a look at your belly. She'll routinely measure the height of your fundus (the top of the uterus) and palpate your abdomen to locate your baby's cute little body parts and estimate her size. Other tests, including ultrasound, may also be used as needed to approximate size.

Carrying Baby, Eighth Month

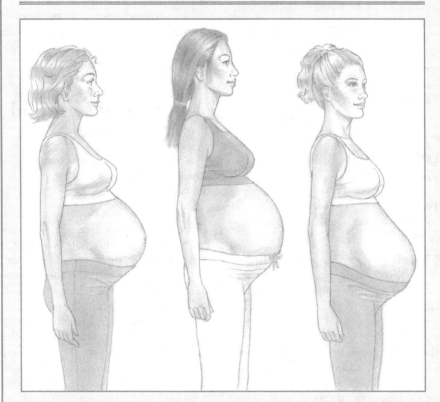

These are just three of the very different ways that a woman may carry near the end of her eighth month. The variations are even greater than earlier in pregnancy. Depending on the size and position of your baby, as well as your own size and weight gain, you may be carrying higher, lower, bigger, smaller, wider, or more compactly.

In other words, it's what's inside that counts—and apparently, what's inside your petite belly is a baby who's plenty big enough.

"Everyone says I'm having a boy because I'm all belly and no hips. I know that's probably an old wives' tale, but is there any truth to it at all?"

Predictions about the baby's sex—by old wives or others—have about a 50 percent chance of coming true. (Actually, a little better than that if a boy is predicted, since 105 boys are born for every 100 girls.) Good odds if you're placing a bet in Las Vegas; not necessarily good odds if you're basing your nursery theme and baby names on it.

That goes for "boy if you're carrying up front, girl if you're carrying wide," "girls make your nose grow, boys don't," and every other prediction not made from the pages of a baby's genetics report or from an ultrasound.

Your Size and Your Delivery

"I'm five feet tall and very petite. I'm afraid I'll have trouble delivering my baby."

When it comes to your ability to birth your baby, size matters— but inside size, not outside size. It's the size and shape of your pelvis in relation to the size of your baby's head that determines how difficult (or easy) your labor will be, not your height or your build. And just because you're extra petite doesn't necessarily mean you've got an extra-petite pelvis. A short, slight woman can have a roomier (or more accommodatingly configured) pelvis than a tall, full-figured woman.

How will you know what size your pelvis is (after all, it doesn't come with a label: small, medium, extra-large)? Your practitioner can make an educated guess about its size, usually using rough measurements taken at your first prenatal exam. If there's some concern that your baby's head is too large to fit through your pelvis while you're in labor, ultrasound may be used to get a better view (and measurement).

Of course, in general, the overall size of the pelvis, as of all bony structures, is smaller in people of smaller stature. Luckily, nature doesn't typically present an undersized woman with an oversized baby. Instead, newborns are usually pretty well matched to the size of their moms and their moms' pelvises at birth (though they may be destined for bigger things later on). And chances are, your baby will be just the right size for you.

Your Weight Gain and the Baby's Size

"I've gained so much weight that I'm afraid my baby will be very big and difficult to deliver."

Just because you've gained a lot of weight doesn't necessarily mean your baby has. Your baby's weight is determined by a number of variables: genetics, your own birthweight (if you were born large, your baby is more likely to be, too), your prepregnancy weight (heavier women tend to have heavier babies), and the kinds of foods you've gained the weight on. Depending on those variables, a 35- to 40-pound weight gain can yield a 6- or 7-pound baby and a 25-pound weight gain can net an 8-pounder. On average, however, the more substantial the weight gain, the bigger the baby.

By palpating your abdomen and measuring the height of your fundus (the top of the uterus), your practitioner will be able to give you some idea of your baby's size, though such guesstimates can be off by a pound or more. An ultrasound can gauge size more accurately, but it may be off the mark, too.

Even if your baby does turn out to be on the big side, that doesn't automatically predict a difficult delivery. Though a 6- or 7-pound baby often makes its way out faster than a 9- or 10-pounder, most women are able to deliver a large baby (or even an extra-large baby) vaginally and without complications. The determining factor, as in any delivery, is whether your baby's head (the largest part) can fit through your pelvis. See the previous question for more.

Baby's Position

"How can I tell which way my baby is facing? I want to make sure he's the right way for delivery."

Playing "name that bump" (trying to figure out which are shoulders, elbows, bottom) may be more entertaining than the best reality TV has to offer, but it's not the most accurate way of figuring out your baby's position. Your practitioner will be able to give you a better idea by palpating your abdomen for recognizable baby parts. The location of the baby's heartbeat is another clue to its position: If the baby's presentation is head first, the heartbeat will usually be heard in the lower half of your abdomen; it will be loudest if the baby's back is toward your front. If there's still some doubt, an ultrasound offers the most reliable view of your baby's position.

Still can't resist a round of your favorite evening pastime (or resist patting those round little parts)? Play away—and to make the game more interesting (and to help clue you in), try looking for these markers next time:

- The baby's back is usually a smooth, convex contour opposite a bunch of little irregularities, which are the "small parts"—hands, feet, elbows.

- In the eighth month, the head has usually settled near your pelvis; it is round, firm, and when pushed down bounces back without the rest of the body moving.

- The baby's bottom is a less regular shape, and softer, than the head.

Breech Baby

"At my last prenatal visit, my doctor said he felt my baby's head up near my ribs. Does that mean she's breech?"

Even as her accommodations become ever more cramped, your baby will still manage to perform some pretty remarkable gymnastics during the last weeks of gestation. In fact, although most fetuses settle into a head-down position between weeks 32 and 38 (breech

---

Turn, Baby, Turn

Some practitioners recommend simple exercises to help turn a breech baby into a delivery-friendly, heads-down position. Ask your practitioner whether you should be trying any of these at home: Rock back and forth a few times on your hands and knees several times a day, with your buttocks higher than your head; do pelvic tilts (see page 224); get on your knees (keep them slightly apart), and then bend over so your butt's up and your belly's almost touching the floor (stay in that position for 20 minutes three times a day if you can, for best results).

Face Forward

It's not just up or down that's important when it comes to the position of your baby—it's also front or back. If baby's facing your back, chin tucked onto his or her chest (as most babies end up positioned come delivery), you're in luck. This so-called occiput anterior position is ideal for birth because your baby's head is lined up to fit through your pelvis as easily and comfortably as possible, smallest head part first. If baby's facing your tummy (called occiput posterior, but also known by the much cuter nickname "sunny-side up"), it's a setup for back labor (see page 367) because his or her skull will be pressing on your spine. It also means your baby's exit might take a little longer.

As delivery day approaches, your practitioner will try to determine which way (front or back) your baby's head is facing—but if you're in a hurry to find out, you can look for these clues. When your baby is anterior (face toward your back), you'll feel your belly hard and smooth (that's your baby's back). If your little one is posterior, your tummy may look flatter and softer because your baby's arms and legs are facing forward, so there's no hard, smooth back to feel.

Do you think—or have you been told—that your baby is posterior? Don't worry about back labor yet. Most babies turn accommodatingly to the anterior position during labor. Some midwives recommend giving baby a nudge before labor begins by getting on all fours and doing pelvic rocks; whether these exercises can successfully flip a baby is unclear (research has yet to back it up, so to speak), but it certainly can't hurt. At the very least, it might help relieve any back pain you might be experiencing right now.

---

presentations occur in fewer than 5 percent of term pregnancies), some don't let on which end will ultimately be up until a few days before birth. Which means that just because your baby is bottoms down now doesn't mean that she will be breech when it comes time for delivery.

If your baby does stubbornly remain a breech as delivery approaches, you and your practitioner will discuss possible ways to attempt to turn your baby head down and the best method of delivery (see below).

"If my baby is breech, can anything be done to turn him?"

There are several ways to try to coax a bottoms-down baby heads up. On the low-tech side, your practitioner may recommend simple exercises, such as the ones described in the box, page 317. Another option (moxibustion) comes from the CAM camp and uses a form of acupuncture and burning herbs to help turn a stubborn fetus.

If your baby still seems determined not to budge, your practitioner may suggest a somewhat higher-tech, yet hands-on approach to manipulating your baby into the coveted heads-down position: external cephalic version (ECV). ECV is best performed around week 37 or 38 or very early in labor when the uterus is still relatively relaxed; some physicians prefer to attempt the procedure after an epidural has been given. Your practitioner (guided by ultrasound and usually in a hospital) will apply his or her hands to your abdomen (you'll feel some pressure, but probably no pain—especially if you've had an epidural) and try to gently

How Does Your Baby Lie?

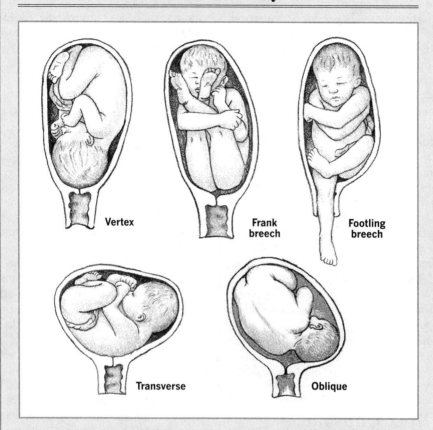

Vertex

Frank breech

Footling breech

Transverse

Oblique

Location, location, location—when it comes to delivery, a baby's location matters a lot. Most babies present head first, or in a vertex position. Breech presentations can come in many forms. A frank breech is when the baby is buttocks first, with his or her legs facing straight up and flat against the face. A footling breech is when one or both of the baby's legs are pointing down. A transverse lie is when the baby is lying sideways in the uterus. An oblique lie is when the baby's head is pointing toward mom's hip instead of toward the cervix.

turn your baby downward. Continuous monitoring will ensure that everything's okay while the maneuver's completed.

The chances of success are pretty high. About two thirds of all ECV attempts are successful (and the success rate is even higher for those who have delivered before, thanks to those laxer uterine and abdominal muscles). Some babies refuse to turn at all, and a small number of contrary fetuses turn and then flip back into a breech position.

"If my baby stays in a breech position, how will that affect labor and delivery? Will I still be able to try for a vaginal birth?"

Whether you'll be able to give vaginal birth a chance will depend on a variety of factors, including your practitioner's policy and your obstetrical situation. Most obs routinely perform a C-section when a baby's in a breech position (in fact, only 0.5 percent of breech babies end up arriving vaginally) because many studies have suggested it's a safer way to go. There are some doctors and midwives, however, who feel it's reasonable to attempt a vaginal delivery under some circumstances (such as when your baby is in a frank breech position and it's clear your pelvis is roomy enough to accommodate).

The bottom line if your baby remains bottom down: You'll need to be flexible in your childbirth plans. Even if your practitioner green-lights a trial of labor, it's just that—a trial. If your cervix dilates too slowly, if your baby doesn't move down the birth canal steadily, or if other problems come up, you'll likely wind up having a C-section. Talk the options over with your practitioner now so you'll be prepared for any possibility come delivery day.

Other Unusual Presentations

"My doctor said that my baby's in an oblique position—what's that and what does it mean for delivery?"

Babies can squirm their way into all kinds of unusual positions, and oblique is one of them. What this means is that your baby's head (though down) is pointed toward either of your hips, rather than squarely on your cervix. An oblique position makes a vaginal exit difficult, so your practitioner might do an external cephalic version (see page 318) to try to coax your baby's head straight down. Otherwise, he or she will probably opt for a C-section.

Yet another tight spot a baby can get into is a transverse position. This is when your baby's lying sideways, across your uterus, instead of vertically. Again, an ECV will be done to try and turn baby up and down. If that doesn't work, your baby will be delivered via cesarean.

Cesarean Delivery

"I was hoping for a vaginal birth, but my doctor just told me I'll probably have to have a cesarean. I'm really disappointed."

Even though it's still considered major surgery (and the happiest kind you can have), a cesarean is a very safe way to deliver, and in some cases, the safest way. It's also a more and more common way. Thirty percent of women are having C-sections these days, which means the chances that your baby will end up arriving via the surgical route are nearly 1 in 3, even if you don't have any predisposing factors.

That said, if you had your heart set on a vaginal delivery, the news that your baby may need to arrive surgically instead can be understandably disappointing. Visions of pushing your baby out the way nature intended—and perhaps the way you'd always pictured—can be displaced by concerns about the surgery, about being stuck in the hospital longer, about the tougher recovery, and about the scar that comes standard issue.

But here are some things to consider if your practitioner ultimately decides that your baby's best exit strategy is through your abdomen: Most hospitals now strive to make a cesarean delivery as family friendly as possible, with mom awake (but appropriately numb), dad in the room by her side, and a chance to take a good look at your baby and even do a little quick kissing and caressing right afterward if there's no medical reason to preclude it. (More serious cuddling and nursing usually have to wait until you're in recovery—after you've been stitched back up.) So a surgical birth experience may be more satisfying than you're imagining. And while the recovery will be longer and the scar unavoidable (though usually placed unobtrusively), you'll also be delivering with your perineum intact and your vaginal muscles unstretched. The plus side for baby in a cesarean delivery is purely cosmetic—and temporary; because there's no tight squeeze through the birth canal, he or she will have an initial edge in appearance over vaginally delivered babies (think round head, not pointy).

But by far the most important thing to keep in mind as your baby's arrival approaches: The best birth is the one that's safest—and when it's medically necessary, a cesarean birth is definitely safest.

And after all, any delivery that brings a healthy baby into the world and into your arms is a perfect delivery.

"Why does it seem everyone I know (my sister, my friends, plus just about every celebrity) is having C-sections these days?"

With cesarean rates in the United States at an all-time high (over 30 percent of women can expect to have a surgical delivery), just about everyone knows somebody who's had one. And if the past few years are any indication of future trends, you can expect those numbers to continue climbing—and to hear more and more C-section birth stories from the recently delivered around you.

Many factors contribute to these rising cesarean rates, including:

Safety. Cesarean delivery is extremely safe—for both mom and baby—especially with today's better technology (such as the fetal monitor and a variety

of other tests) that can more accurately indicate when a fetus is in trouble.

Bigger babies. With more expectant mothers exceeding the recommended weight gain of 25 to 35 pounds, and with the rate of gestational diabetes increasing, more large babies, who may be more difficult to deliver vaginally, are arriving.

Bigger moms. The C-section rate has also risen with the obesity rate. Being obese (or gaining too much weight during pregnancy) significantly increases a woman's chance of needing a C-section, partly because of other risk factors that accompany obesity (gestational diabetes, for instance), partly because obese women tend to have longer labors, and longer labors are more likely to end up on the operating table.

Older mothers. More and more women in their late 30s (and well into their 40s) are now able to have successful pregnancies, but they are more likely to require cesarean deliveries. The same is true of women with chronic health problems.

Repeat C-sections. Though VBAC (vaginal birth after cesarean; see page 325) is still considered a viable option in a few cases, fewer doctors and hospitals are allowing women to try one, and more are scheduling surgeries over a trial of labor.

Fewer instrumental deliveries. Fewer babies are being born with the help of vacuum extraction and even fewer with forceps, which means doctors are turning to surgical deliveries more often when they might have turned to instruments for help in the past.

Requests by moms. Since cesareans are so safe and can prevent the pain of labor while keeping the perineum neatly intact, some women—particularly those who've had one before—prefer them to vaginal deliveries and actually ask ahead for one (see page 323).

Be in the Know

The more you know, the better your birth experience will be. And that goes for a surgical birth experience, too. Here are a few topics you might want to bring up with your practitioner before the first contraction kicks in:

- If labor isn't progressing, will it be possible to try other alternatives before moving to a C-section—for example, oxytocin to stimulate contractions or squatting to make pushing more effective?

- If the baby is a breech, will attempts to turn the baby (using ECV or another technique) be tried first? Are there times when a breech vaginal birth might be possible?

- What kind of incision will likely be used?

- Can your coach be with you if you're awake? If you are asleep?

- Can your nurse-midwife or doula be with you, too?

- Will you and your spouse be able to hold the baby immediately after birth, and will you be able to nurse in the recovery room?

- If the baby doesn't need special care, can he or she room-in with you?

- How much recovery time will you need both in and out of the hospital? What physical discomforts and limitations can you expect?

To find out what you can expect at a cesarean delivery, see page 398.

Satisfaction. Family-friendly policies have made for a much more satisfying surgical birth experience. Since mom can be wide awake and alert during a cesarean section and family-friendlier hospital policies allow dad to be right alongside her, baby meet-and-greets can often take place right on the delivery table. What's more, a C-section is very quick, lasting a mere 10 minutes or less for the delivery itself (suturing mom back up takes about another 30 minutes).

Even with C-section rates as high as they are these days (and they're far lower for midwives, who attend only low-risk births), keep in mind that surgical deliveries still comprise the minority of births. After all, two out of three women can expect to deliver their babies vaginally.

"Do you generally know in advance that you are going to have a cesarean delivery, or is it usually last minute? What are the reasons you might have one?"

Some women won't find out whether they're having a C-section until they're well into labor, others will get the heads-up ahead of time. Different doctors follow different protocols when it comes to surgical deliveries. The most common reasons for a scheduled C-section include:

- A previous cesarean delivery, when the reason for it still exists (Mom has an abnormally-shaped pelvis, for example), or when a vertical incision was used before (instead of the more common low horizontal, which can better withstand the pressure of labor); a C-section is also called for when labor has to be induced in a woman who's already had a cesarean delivery

- When a fetus's head is believed to be too large to fit through mom's pelvis (cephalopelvic disproportion)

- Multiple births (almost all triplets or more are delivered by C-section; many twins are delivered by C-section)

- Breech or other unusual fetal presentation

- A fetal condition or illness (heart disease, diabetes, preeclampsia) in the mother that may make labor and vaginal delivery risky

- Maternal obesity

- An active herpes infection, especially a primary one, or an HIV infection

- Placenta previa (when the placenta partially or completely blocks the cervical opening) or placental abruption (when the placenta separates from the uterine wall too soon)

Sometimes the C-section decision isn't made until well into labor for reasons such as:

- Failure of labor to progress, such as when the cervix hasn't dilated quickly enough, or it's taking too long to push the baby out. (In most cases, physicians will try to give sluggish contractions a boost with oxytocin before resorting to a cesarean.)

- Fetal distress

- A prolapsed umbilical cord

- A ruptured uterus

If your practitioner says that a C-section will be necessary—or will probably be necessary—ask for a detailed explanation of the reasons. Ask, too, if any alternatives are open to you.

Elective Cesareans

"I've heard some women say they chose to have a C-section—is that something I should consider, too?"

Cesareans on demand may be more in demand than ever these days, but that doesn't mean you should sign up for yours. Opting for a surgical delivery when one isn't medically necessary isn't a decision you should take lightly (and definitely one you shouldn't base on trends). It deserves careful consideration—and plenty of discussion with your practitioner about the potential pros and cons.

Though you might have plenty of reasons for wanting a C-section, make sure you consider both sides of the equation. If you're . . .

. . . scared about the pain of a vaginal birth, keep in mind that electing to have a C-section isn't the only way to deliver without pain. There are many effective pain-relief options available to women having a vaginal birth (see page 302).

. . . worried about the aftereffects of a vaginal birth, like pelvic wear and tear or lax vaginal muscles, remember that regular pelvic floor exercises (aka Kegels) can significantly reduce the risk of those effects. What's more, a vaginal birth isn't any more likely to leave you with urinary incontinence issues than a C-section is (which means your baby's exit route doesn't impact the chances that you'll spring a leak postpartum).

. . . hoping to give birth when it's convenient for you, be sure you also consider the longer recovery time and hospital stay plus the increased risk from surgery for you and your baby if you select a C-section. That's not exactly convenient.

. . . going to have another baby, understand that opting for a C-section now

Scheduled Classes for Scheduled C's

Think a scheduled C-section means you won't have to schedule childbirth classes? Not so fast. Sure, you won't need to become an expert on breathing exercises or pushing techniques, but childbirth education classes still have plenty to offer you and your coach (including plenty on what to expect with a C-section—and with an epidural). Most classes also offer invaluable advice on taking care of your baby (which you'll have to master no matter which exit your baby takes), breastfeeding, and possibly getting back into shape postpartum. And don't tune out when the teacher's going over the labor breathing routine with the other students. You might find those skills come in handy postpartum when you're confronted with afterpains (as your uterus contracts back to its original size) or when baby's trying to feed off your painfully engorged breasts. Relaxation techniques also help all new moms (and dads).

may limit your options next time around. Some doctors and hospitals limit VBACs (vaginal births after cesarean) these days, which means you might not be able to choose a vaginal birth for your second baby, if you decide later on that C-sections aren't for you after all.

Something else to consider when contemplating a scheduled cesarean that's not medically necessary: The best time for your baby to make his or her exit from your uterus is when he or she is ready. When an elective delivery is planned, there's always the possibility that the baby will inadvertently be born too soon (particularly if the dates are off to begin with).

If, after careful consideration, you're still interested in signing up for an elective cesarean delivery, talk with your practitioner and decide together whether it's the choice that's right for you and your baby.

Repeat Cesareans

"I've had two cesareans and want to go for my third—and maybe my fourth child. Is there a limit on the number of C-sections you can have?"

Thinking of having lots of babies—but not sure whether you'll be allowed to make multiple trips to the hospital's happiest operating room? Chances are you'll be able to. Limits are no longer arbitrarily placed on the number of cesarean deliveries a woman can undergo, and having numerous cesareans is generally considered a much safer option than it once was. Just how safe depends on the type of incision made during the previous surgeries, as well as on the scars that are formed following the procedures, so discuss the particulars in your case with your practitioner.

Depending on how many incisions you've had, where you've had them, and how they've healed, multiple C-sections can put you at somewhat higher risk for certain complications. These include uterine rupture, placenta previa (a low-lying placenta), and placenta accreta (an abnormally attached placenta). So you'll need to be particularly alert for any bright red bleeding during your pregnancies, as well as the signs of oncoming labor (contractions, bloody show, ruptured membranes). If any of these occur, notify your practitioner right away.

Vaginal Birth After Cesarean (VBAC)

"I had my last baby by cesarean. I'm pregnant again and I'm wondering if I should try for a vaginal delivery this time."

The answer to your question depends on who you talk to. When it comes to determining whether it's safe for women to try for a VBAC (vaginal birth after cesarean; pronounced vee-back), the pendulum of opinions—expert or otherwise—continues to swing VBAC and forth. At one time, doctors and midwives were routinely encouraging pregnant women who'd had a C-section in the past to at least try for a vaginal birth (a trial of labor). But then came a study that warned of the risks (of uterine rupture or of the incision coming apart) if VBAC was attempted, leaving many pregnant women—and their practitioners—confused and unsure about what to do when it comes to childbirth after a C-section.

Looking at the statistics, though, your chances of having a successful VBAC are still pretty good. More than 60 percent of women who have had C-sections and who are candidates for a trial of labor are able to go through a normal labor and a vaginal delivery in subsequent deliveries. Even women who have had two cesarean deliveries have a good chance of being able to deliver vaginally, as long as the proper precautions are taken. And the study that caused the VBAC backlash actually showed that uterine rupture is really quite rare, happening only 1 percent of the time. What's more, that risk is only higher for certain women in certain circumstances, such as those who have a vertical uterine scar instead of a low transverse (95 percent of incisions are low transverse; check the records of your previous cesarean delivery to find out for sure which type of incision you had), or those whose labors are induced by prostaglandins or other hormonal stimulants (these make contractions stronger). Which means that a VBAC is worth a shot if your practitioner and hospital are willing (many hospitals have strict rules about who can or can't attempt a VBAC and some have stopped allowing VBACs altogether).

If you do decide you'd like to attempt a VBAC, you'll need to find a practitioner who backs you up on your decision (midwives are more open to VBACs and often more successful at making them work). Most important if you're pushing for pushing out your baby is to learn everything you can about VBAC, including what your options will be when it comes to pain relief (some physicians limit pain medications during VBAC, some offer epidurals). Keep in mind, too, that if your labor ends up having to be induced, your practitioner will likely veto VBAC.

If, despite all your best efforts, you end up having a repeat C-section, don't be disappointed. Remember that even the woman who has never had a cesarean before has a nearly 1 in 3 chance of needing one. Don't feel guilty, either, if you decide ahead of delivery (in consultation with your practitioner) that you'd rather schedule an elective second cesarean delivery than attempt VBAC. About a third of all C-sections are repeats, and many are actually performed at the request of the mother. Again, what's best for your baby—and best for you—is what matters.

"My ob is encouraging me to try for a VBAC, but I'm not sure why I should bother."

While your feelings definitely factor into the decision of whether or not to give VBAC a shot, your ob does have a point—and a point you might want to consider. The risks of a VBAC are very low, and a C-section, after all, is still major surgery. A vaginal birth means a shorter hospital stay, a lower risk of infection, no abdominal surgery, and a faster recovery—all good reasons to favor a VBAC. So it makes sense to weigh the pros and cons of VBAC and a repeat cesarean delivery before you make your decision.

If, after you've thought and talked it over, you're still convinced that VBAC's not for you, let your ob know your decision and your reasons—and schedule your cesarean delivery without feeling guilty.

Group B Strep

"My doctor is going to test me for group B strep infection. What does this mean?"

It means that your doctor's playing it safe, and when it comes to group B strep, safe is a very good way to play it.

Group B strep (GBS) is a bacterium that can be found in the vaginas of healthy women (and it's not related to group A strep, which causes the throat infection). In carriers (about 10 to 35 percent of all healthy women are carriers), it causes no problems at all. But in a newborn baby, who can pick it up while passing through the vagina during childbirth, GBS can cause very serious infection (though only 1 in every 200 babies born to GBS-positive mothers will be affected).

If you're a GBS carrier, you won't have any symptoms (that's a plus). But that also means you're unlikely to know you're a carrier (that's a minus—one that could potentially spell trouble for your baby come delivery). Which is why expectant moms are routinely tested for GBS between 35 and 37 weeks (testing done before 35 weeks isn't accurate in predicting who will be carrying GBS at the time of delivery). Coming soon to a hospital near you (though not yet widely available) is a rapid GBS test that can screen women during labor and provide results within the hour, which might make a test at 35 to 37 weeks unnecessary.

So how's the test currently done? It's performed like a Pap smear, using vaginal and rectal swabs. If you test positive (meaning you're a carrier), you'll be given IV antibiotics during labor—and this treatment completely eliminates any risk to your baby. (GBS can also show up in your urine during a routine pee-in-cup test at a prenatal checkup. If it does, it'll be treated right away with oral antibiotics.)

If your practitioner doesn't offer the GBS test during late pregnancy, you can request it. Even if you weren't tested but end up in labor with certain risk factors that point to GBS, your practitioner will just treat you with IV antibiotics to be sure you don't pass the infection on to your baby. If you've previously delivered a baby with GBS, your practitioner may also opt not to test you at 35 to 37 weeks and merely

---

Eat Up

Okay, you may be feeling like a cow these days, and that's all the more reason to keep grazing. Fitting your meals—and baby's nutrient shipments—into that uterus-cramped stomach of yours is likely getting more and more challenging. Which means that more than ever, the Six-Meal Solution is for you. So graze on, Mom.

proceed straight to treatment during labor.

Playing it safe through testing—and, if necessary, treatment—means that your baby will be safe from GBS. And that's a very good thing.

Taking Baths Now

"Is it okay for me to take a bath this far along into my pregnancy?"

Not only is it okay, but a warm bath can provide welcome relief from those late pregnancy aches and pains after a long day (and what day isn't long when you're eight months pregnant?). So hop—or rather, gingerly hoist yourself and your mountain of a belly—into the tub and enjoy a good soak.

If you're worried about bath-water entering your vagina (you may have heard that one through the pregnancy grapevine), don't be. Unless it's forced—as with douching or jumping into a pool, two things you shouldn't be doing anyway these days—water can't get where it shouldn't go. And even if a little water does make its way up, the cervical mucous plug that seals the entrance to the uterus effectively protects its precious contents from invading infectious organisms, should there be any floating around in your tub.

Even once you're in labor and the mucous plug is dislodged, you can still spend time in the bath. In fact, hydrotherapy during labor can provide welcome pain relief. You can even opt to give birth in a tub (see page 24).

One caveat when you're tubbing for two, especially this late in the pregnancy game: Make sure the tub has a nonslip surface or mat on the bottom so you don't take a tumble. And as always, avoid irritating bubble baths—as well as too-warm ones.

Driving Now

"I can barely fit behind the wheel. Should I still be driving?"

You can stay in the driver's seat as long as you fit there; moving the seat back and tilting the wheel up will help with that. Assuming you've got the room—and you're feeling up to it—driving short distances is fine up until delivery day.

Car trips lasting more than an hour, however, might be too exhausting late in pregnancy, no matter who's driving. If you must take a longer trip, be sure to shift around in your seat frequently and to stop every hour or two to get up and walk around. Doing some neck and back stretches may also keep you more comfortable.

Don't, however, try to drive yourself to the hospital while in labor (a really strong contraction may prove dangerous on the road). And don't forget the most important road rule on any car trip, whether you are driver or passenger (and even if you're a passenger being driven to the hospital or birthing center in labor): Buckle up.

Traveling Now

"I may have to make an important business trip this month. Is it safe for me to travel this late in pregnancy, or should I cancel?"

Before you schedule your trip, schedule a call or visit to your practitioner. Different practitioners have differing points of view on last-trimester travel. Whether yours will encourage you or discourage you from hitting the road—or the rails or the skies—at this point in your pregnancy will probably depend on that point of view, as well as on several other factors. Most important is the kind of pregnancy you've been having: You're more likely to get the green light if yours has been uncomplicated. How far along you are (most practitioners advise against flying after the 36th week) and whether you are at any increased risk at all for premature labor will weigh into the recommendation, too. Also very important is how you've been feeling. Pregnancy symptoms that multiply as the months pass also tend to multiply as the miles pass; traveling can lead to increased backache and fatigue, aggravated varicose veins and hemorrhoids, and added emotional and physical stress. Other considerations include how far and for how long you will be traveling (and how long you will actually be in transit), how demanding the trip will be physically and emotionally, as well as how necessary the trip is (optional trips or trips that can be easily postponed until well after delivery may not be worth making now). If you're traveling by air, you'll also need to factor in the restrictions—if any—of the airline you choose. Some will not let you travel in the ninth month without a letter from your practitioner affirming that you are not in imminent danger of going into labor while in flight; others are more lenient.

If your practitioner gives you the go-ahead, there are still plenty of other arrangements you'll need to make besides the travel ones. See page 250 for tips to ensure happy (and safer and more comfortable) trails for the pregnant you. Getting plenty of rest will be especially important. But most critical will be making sure you have the name, phone number, and address of a recommended practitioner (and the hospital or birthing center where he or she delivers) at your destination—one, of course, whose services will be covered by your insurance plan should you end up requiring them. If you're traveling a long distance,

you may also want to consider the possibility of bringing along your spouse on the remote chance that if you do end up going into labor at your destination, at least you won't have to deliver without him.

Making Love Now

"I'm confused. I hear a lot of contradictory information about whether sex in the last weeks of pregnancy is safe—and whether it triggers labor."

It's not like there hasn't been a lot of research done about sex in late pregnancy. It's just that most of it is conflicting, leaving you and all your very pregnant peers unsure of how to proceed—that is, if you're still in the mood to proceed. It is widely believed that neither intercourse nor orgasm alone triggers labor unless conditions are ripe, though many impatient-to-deliver couples have enjoyed trying to prove otherwise. If conditions are ripe, it's been theorized, the prostaglandins in semen might be able to help get the labor party started. But even that's not a sure thing—or a theory you can necessarily bank on taking you to the birthing room, even under the right, ripe conditions. In fact, one study found that low-risk women who had sex in the final weeks of pregnancy actually carried their babies slightly longer than those who abstained from sex during that time. Are you confused yet?

Based on what's known, most physicians and midwives allow patients with normal pregnancies to make love right up until delivery day. And most couples apparently can do so without any problems arising, so to speak.

Check with your practitioner to see what the latest consensus is and what's safe in your situation. If you get a green light (chances are, you will), then by all means hit the sheets—if you have the will and the energy (and the gymnastic skills that might be necessary at this point). If the light is red (and it probably will be if you are at high risk for premature delivery, have placenta previa, or are experiencing unexplained bleeding), try getting intimate in other ways. While you still have some evenings to yourselves, rendezvous for a romantic candlelit dinner or a starlit stroll. Cuddle while you watch TV, or soap each other in the shower. Or use massage as the medium. Or do everything but—use your hands and your mouths to your heart's content, assuming your practitioner hasn't red-lighted orgasm for you. This may not quite satisfy like the real thing, but try to remember you have a whole lifetime of lovemaking ahead—though the pickings may continue to be slim in that department at least until baby's sleeping through the night.

Your Twosome

"The baby isn't even born yet, and already my relationship with my husband seems to be changing. We're both so wrapped up in the birth and the baby, instead of in each other, the way we used to be."

Babies bring a lot of things when they arrive in a couple's lives—joy, excitement, and a lot of dirty diapers, for starters. But they also bring change—and considering they're only pint-size, they bring a whole bunch of change.

Not surprisingly, your relationship with your spouse is one place where you'll notice that change, and it sounds like you've glimpsed it already. And that's actually a really good thing. When baby makes three, your twosome is bound to undergo some shifting of dynamics and reshuffling of priorities. But this predictable upheaval is usu-

ally less stressful—and easier to adapt to—when a couple begins the natural and inevitable evolution of their relationship during pregnancy. In other words, the changes to your relationship are more likely to represent a change for the better if they begin before baby's arrival. Couples who don't anticipate at least some disruption of romance-as-usual—who don't realize that wine and roses will often give way to spit-up and strained carrots, that lovemaking marathons will place (well) behind baby-rocking marathons, that three's not always as cozy as two, at least not in the same way—often find the reality of life with a demanding newborn harder to handle.

So think ahead, plan ahead—and be ready for change. But as you get yourselves into nurture mode, don't forget that baby won't be the only one who'll need nurturing. As normal—and healthy—as it is to be wrapped up in the pregnancy and your expected extra-special delivery, it's also important to reserve some emotional energy for the relationship that created that bundle of joy in the first place. Now is the time to learn to combine the care and feeding of your baby with the care and feeding of your marriage. While you're busily feathering your nest, make the effort to regularly reinforce romance. At least once a week, do something together that has nothing to do with childbirth or babies. See a movie, have dinner out, play miniature golf, hit the flea market. While you're out shopping for tiny onesies, buy a little something special (and unexpected) for your other special someone. Or surprise him with a pair of tickets for a show or a game you know he'd love to see. At dinner, spend at least some time asking about his day, talking about yours, discussing the day's headlines, reminiscing about your first date, dreaming about a

Considering Cord Blood Banking

As if you don't have enough to think about before baby's born, here's another decision you'll have to make: Should you save your baby's umbilical cord blood—and if so, how?

Cord blood harvesting, a painless procedure that takes less than five minutes and is done after the cord has been clamped and cut, is completely safe for mother and child (as long as the cord is not clamped and cut prematurely). A newborn's cord blood contains stem cells that in some cases can be used to treat certain immune system disorders or blood diseases. And research is under way to determine if these stem cells can also be useful in treating other conditions, such as diabetes, cerebral palsey, even heart disease.

There are two ways to store the blood: You can pay for private storage or you can donate the blood to a public storage bank. Private storage can be expensive, and the benefits for low-risk families—in other words, those who do not have any familial immune disorders—are not completely clear yet.

For these reasons, ACOG recommends doctors present the pros and cons of cord blood banking, and the American Academy of Pediatrics (AAP) doesn't recommend *private* cord blood storage unless a family member has a medical condition that might be helped by a stem cell transplant now or in the near future. These conditions include leukemia, lymphoma, and neuroblastoma; sickle cell anemia, aplastic anemia, and thalassemia illness; Gaucher disease and Hurler syndrome; Wiskott-Aldrich syndrome; and severe hemoglobinopathy. The AAP does, however, support parents donating the cord blood to a bank for general use by the public. This costs the donor nothing and could save a life.

Investigate your family's medical history to see if private cord blood banking makes sense for you. Or if you feel the potential future benefits are worth the cost, no matter what your family history, sign up for private banking (see below). You can also talk the cord blood options over with your practitioner.

For general information on cord blood banking, visit parentsguidecordblood .com. For information on donating cord blood, contact the International Cord Blood Registry at (650) 635-1452, cordblooddonor.org; or the National Marrow Donor Program at (800) MARROW2 (627-7692), marrow.org. For private banking options, contact the Cord Blood Registry at (888) 932-6568, cordblood.com; or ViaCord at (877) 535-4148, viacord.com.

---

second honeymoon (even if it won't be in the cards for many moons), all without mentioning the b-word. Bring massage oil to bed now and then, and rub each other the right way; even if you're not in the mood for sex—or it's seeming too much like hard work these days—any kind of touching can keep you close. None of this flame fanning will make the upcoming wonderful event any less anticipated, but it will remind you both that there's more to life than Lamaze and layettes.

Keeping this very important thought in mind now will make it easier to keep the love light burning later when you're taking turns walking the floor at 2 A.M. And that love light, after all, is what will make the cozy nest you're busily preparing for your baby—and the one you'll soon be sharing as a family of three—a happy and secure one.

Breastfeeding

For the past 30-odd weeks, you've likely seen (and felt) your breasts grow . . . and grow . . . and grow. If you've given any thought to what's going on underneath those giant cups you've now traded up for, you probably know that your breasts aren't growing randomly but are gearing up for one of nature's most important jobs: baby feeding.

It's clear that your breasts are already on board with breastfeeding. Whether you are, too, or whether you're still weighing your baby-feeding options, you'll probably want to learn more about this amazing process, a process that turns breasts (your breasts!) into the perfect purveyors of the world's most perfect infant food. You'll get some valuable highlights and insights here, but for much more on breastfeeding (from the why-to's to the how-to's), see *What to Expect the First Year.*

Why Breast Is Best

Just as goat's milk is the ideal food for kids (goat kids, that is), and cow's milk is the best meal for young calves, your human breast milk is the perfect meal for your human newborn. Here are the reasons why:

It's custom-made. Tailored to meet the nutritional needs of human infants, breast milk contains at least 100 ingredients that aren't found in cow's milk and that can't be precisely replicated in commercial formulas. The protein in breast milk is mostly lactalbumin, which is more nutritious and digestible than the major protein component of cow's milk, caseinogen, which is what formula is made from. The amount of fat in the two milks is similar, but the fat in mother's milk is more easily broken down and used by a baby. Infants also have an easier time absorbing the important micronutrients in breast milk than in cow's milk.

It's safe. You can be sure that the milk served up directly from your breast isn't improperly prepared, contaminated, tampered with, or spoiled. It never gets pulled from the shelves or overstays its sell-by date.

It's a tummy soother. Nursed babies are almost never constipated, thanks to the easier digestibility of breast milk. They also rarely have diarrhea, since breast milk seems both to destroy some diarrhea-causing organisms and to encourage the growth of beneficial flora in the digestive tract, which further discourage digestive upset. On a purely aesthetic note, the bowel movements of a breastfed baby are sweeter smelling (at least until solids are introduced). They're also less apt to cause diaper rash.

It's a fat flattener. Not only is breastfeeding less likely to cause overweight infants, but having been nursed for at least six months (or better, at least a year) appears to be related to lower rates of obesity later in life. It may also be linked to lower cholesterol readings in adulthood.

It's a brain booster. Breastfeeding appears to slightly increase a child's IQ. This may be related not only to the brain-building fatty acids (DHA) it contains, but to the closeness and mother-baby interaction that is built into breastfeeding, which naturally fosters intellectual development.

It keeps allergies on hold. Virtually no baby is allergic to breast milk (though once in a while an infant can have an allergic reaction to a certain food or foods in mom's diet, including cow's milk). On the other hand, beta-lacto-globulin, a substance contained in cow's milk, can trigger an allergic response, with a variety of possible symptoms ranging from mild to severe. Soy milk formulas, which are often substituted when an infant is allergic to cow's milk, stray even further in composition from what nature intended and can also cause an allergic reaction. Studies show, too, that breastfed infants are less likely to get childhood asthma than those babies fed formula.

It's an infection preventer. Breastfed babies are less subject not only to diarrhea but to infections of all kinds—including UTIs and ear infections. In fact, a number of studies suggest that a very wide range of diseases may be somewhat lower in breastfed children, including bacterial meningitis, SIDS, diabetes, some childhood cancers, Crohn's disease, and other chronic digestive diseases. Protection is partially provided by the transfer of immune factors in breast milk and in the premilk substance, colostrum.

It builds stronger mouths. Because nursing at the breast requires more effort than sucking on a bottle, breastfeeding may encourage optimum development of jaws, teeth, and palate. Also, recent studies show that babies who are breastfed are less likely to get cavities later on in childhood than those who are not.

It expands the taste buds early on. Want to raise an adventurous eater? Start at the breast. Developing those little taste buds on breast milk, which takes on the flavor of whatever you've been eating, may acclimate a baby early on to a world of flavors. Researchers have found that

nursed babies are less likely to be timid in their tastes than their formula-fed peers once they graduate to the high chair—which means they may be more likely to open wide to that spoonful of yams (or that forkful of curried chicken) later on.

Breastfeeding offers a pile of perks for Mom, too:

Convenience. Breastfeeding requires no advance planning, packing, or equipment; it's always available (at the park, on an airplane, in the middle of the night), at just the right temperature. When you're nursing, you can pack up the baby and hit the road without having to pack up and lug around bottles, nipples, cleaning supplies, and so on; your breasts will always come along for the ride (you can't forget to pack them). You can also skip 2 A.M. trips to the kitchen for a formula refill; late-night feedings require nothing more complicated than an easy-access nightie and a cozy, sleepy snuggle with your little one. When you and baby aren't together (if you work outside the home, for instance), milk can be expressed in advance and stored in the freezer for bottle-feedings as needed.

Economy. Breast milk is free, and so is its delivery system.

Speedy recovery. When baby sucks on your breasts, it triggers the release of the hormone oxytocin, which helps speed the shrinking of the uterus back to its prepregnant size and may decrease the flow of lochia (postpartum vaginal bleeding), which means less blood loss. Nursing also enforces rest periods for you—particularly important, as you'll discover, during the first six postpartum weeks.

Speedy return to prepregnancy shape. And speaking of shrinking, all those extra calories your baby is draining out of you means that even though you'll

Prepping for Breastfeeding

Luckily, nature has worked out all the details, so there's not much you'll need to do to get ready for breastfeeding while you're still expecting (other than read up as much as you can). Some lactation experts recommend that during the last months of pregnancy you skip the soap on your nipples and areolas—just rinse with water, instead (it's not like they get that dirty, anyway). Soap tends to dry the nipples, which may lead to cracking and soreness early in breastfeeding. If your breasts are dry or itchy, a mild cream or lotion may feel soothing, but avoid getting it on the nipple or areola. If your nipples are dry, you can apply a lanolin-based cream such as Lansinoh.

The no-prep-necessary rule applies even to women with small or flat nipples. Flat nipples don't need to be prepped for nursing with breast shells, hand manipulation, or a manual breast pump during pregnancy. Not only are these prepping techniques often less effective than no treatment, but they can do more harm than good. The shells, besides being embarrassingly conspicuous, can cause sweating and rashes. Hand manipulation and pumping can stimulate contractions and, occasionally, even trigger breast infection.

One possible exception: You may want to think about planning ahead if your nipples are inverted (in other words, they retract when you squeeze the areola), which can make nursing a little trickier. Breast shells may help draw nipples out, but you probably won't want to use them frequently, for the reasons above. Ask your practitioner for the name of a lactation consultant who may be able to advise you, or contact your local La Leche League.

---

be adding more calories to your diet to make milk, you won't be piling on the pounds—and you might start seeing that waistline of yours sooner.

Period postponement. Your period will be slower to return, and who could complain about that? But unless you want your children very closely spaced—or enjoy surprises—you should *not* rely on breastfeeding as your only form of contraception. Most mothers who exclusively breastfeed—and whose babies are not sucking often on pacifiers—are probably protected for a few postpartum months. But they can begin menstruating as early as four months after giving birth and may be fertile before that first period.

Bone building. Nursing can improve mineralization in your bones after wean-ing and may reduce the risk of hip fracture after menopause, assuming you're taking in enough calcium to fill your needs and milk-making requirements.

Health benefits. Feeding your baby via the breast can reduce your risk of some cancers down the road. Women who breastfeed have a lower risk of developing ovarian cancer and breast cancer. Nursing also seems to reduce your risk of developing type 2 diabetes.

The biggest and best bonus. Breastfeeding brings you and your baby together, skin to skin, eye to eye, at least six to eight times a day. The emotional gratification, the intimacy, the sharing of love and pleasure, can not only be very fulfilling and make for a strong mother-child relationship, but it may also enhance your baby's brain development. (A note to mothers

The Breast: Sexual or Practical?

Or can it be both? If you think about it, having two or even more roles in life is not unusual—even roles that are very different, that require different skill sets and different attitudes (lover and mother, for example). You can look at the different roles of the breast—one sexual and one practical—in the same way: Each is important; neither is mutually exclusive. You can have one and the other, too (and in fact, breastfeeding makes lots of women—and their partners—feel especially sensuous). In deciding whether or not to breastfeed, keep this in mind.

of twins: All the advantages of breastfeeding are doubled for you. See page 447 for tips on tandem breastfeeding.)

For more information on breastfeeding, contact your local La Leche League, (800) La Leche (525-3243), or visit LLLUSA.org.

Why Some Opt for the Bottle

Maybe you've decided that breastfeeding definitely isn't for you. Or maybe there's a reason you won't be able to breastfeed, at least not exclusively. Don't feel guilty about choosing the bottle over the breast (or even combining the two; see page 336). Here are some of the pros of bottle-feeding:

More shared responsibility. Bottle-feeding allows dad to share the feeding responsibilities and its bonding benefits more

easily. (Although the father of a breastfed baby can derive the same benefits, assuming his baby will take a bottle at all, by feeding a bottle of expressed mother's milk, as well as by taking charge of other baby-care activities, such as bathing, changing, and rocking.)

More freedom. Bottle-feeding doesn't tie a mom down to her baby. She's able to work outside the home without worrying about pumping and storing milk. She can travel a few days without the baby, even sleep through the night, because someone else can feed her baby. (Of course, these options are also open to breastfeeding moms who express milk or supplement with formula.)

Potentially, more romance. Bottle-feeding doesn't interfere with a couple's sex life (except when baby wakes up for a feeding at the wrong time). Breastfeeding can, to some extent. First, because lactation hormones can keep the vagina relatively dry (though vaginal lubricants can remedy the problem); and second, because leaky breasts during lovemaking can be a cold shower for some couples. For bottle-feeding couples, the breasts can play their strictly sensual role rather than their utilitarian one.

Fewer limitations on your diet. Bottle-feeding doesn't cramp your eating style. You can eat all the spicy foods and cabbage you want (though many babies don't object to these tastes in breast milk, and some actually lap them up), you can have a daily glass of wine or a cocktail without factoring in the next feeding, and you don't have to worry about as many nutritional requirements.

No public displays. If you're uncomfortable about the possibility of nursing in public, breastfeeding may be hard to imagine. That hangup, though, is often quickly hung up; many women who opt to try breastfeeding soon find it becomes second nature (and easy to accomplish discreetly), even in the most public places.

Less stress. Some women worry that they're too impatient or tense by nature to breastfeed. Given a try, you may find, however, that nursing is actually very relaxing: a stress-buster, not a stress-inducer (at least once it's well established).

Making the Choice to Breastfeed

For more and more women today, the choice is clear. Some know they'll opt for breast over bottle long before they even decide to become pregnant. Others, who never gave it much thought before pregnancy, choose breastfeeding once they've read up on its many benefits. Some women teeter on the brink of indecision right through pregnancy and even delivery. A few women, convinced that nursing isn't for them, still can't shake the nagging feeling that they ought to do it anyway.

Undecided? Here's a suggestion: Try it—you may like it. You can always quit if you don't, but at least you will have cleared up those nagging doubts. Best of all, you and your baby will have reaped some of the most important benefits of breastfeeding, if only for a brief time.

Nursing After Breast Surgery

Many women who have had breast reductions are able to breastfeed, though most don't produce enough milk to nurse exclusively. Whether you will be able to breastfeed your baby—and how much you'll need to supplement your milk supply with formula—will depend at least in part on how the procedure was performed. Check with your surgeon. If care was taken to preserve milk ducts and nerve pathways, chances are good that you'll be able to produce at least some milk. (The same applies if you had breast surgery because of breast cancer or because of fibrocystic breasts.)

If your surgeon is reassuring, increase your chances of success by reading up on breastfeeding and working with a lactation consultant who is familiar with the challenges of nursing after a breast reduction. Closely monitoring your baby's intake (by keeping an eye on growth and the number of dirty and wet diapers) will be especially important. If you don't end up making enough milk, supplement with bottles of formula (do the combo). Also consider using a nursing supplementation system, which allows you to breastfeed and supplement with formula at the same time and can encourage milk production while ensuring that your baby gets enough to eat. Remember, any amount of breastfeeding—even if it doesn't turn out to be baby's only or even primary source of nutrition—is beneficial. Visit bfar.org for more information on breastfeeding after reduction.

Breast augmentation is far less likely to interfere with breastfeeding than a breast reduction, but it depends on the technique, the incision, and the reason why it was done. While many women with implants are able to nurse exclusively, a significant minority may not produce enough milk. To make sure your supply meets your baby's demand, you'll need to keep close tabs on his or her growth and the number of dirty and wet diapers accumulated daily.

Got Pierced?

You're all set to nurse your baby-to-be, but there's one wrinkle—or rather, one ring, or one stud—that you're not sure what to do with. If you have a nipple piercing, good news: No evidence shows that nipple piercing has any effect on a woman's ability to breastfeed. But experts (in both the lactation and the piercing businesses) agree that you should remove any nipple jewelry before you nurse your baby. This is not only due to the potential for infection for you; it's also because the jewelry could pose a choking hazard for your baby or injure his or her tender gums, tongue, or palate during feedings.

But do be sure to give breastfeeding a fair trial. The first few weeks can be challenging, even for the most enthusiastic breastfeeders, and are always a learning process (though getting help from a lactation consultant or a sister or friend who has breastfed could make things easier if you're having a hard time). A full month, or even six weeks, of nursing is generally needed to establish a successful feeding relationship and give a mom the chance to figure out whether breast is best for her.

Mixing Breast and Bottle

Some women who choose to breastfeed find—for one reason or another—that they can't or don't want to do it exclusively. Maybe exclusive breastfeeding doesn't turn out to be practical in the context of their lifestyle (too many business trips away from home or a job

that otherwise makes pumping a logistical nightmare). Maybe it proves to be too physically challenging. Fortunately, neither breastfeeding nor bottle-feeding is an all-or-nothing proposition—and for some women, combining the two is a compromise that works. If you choose to do the combo, keep in mind that you'll need to wait until breastfeeding is well established (at least two to three weeks) before introducing formula. For more information on combining breast and bottle, see *What to Expect the First Year.*

When You Can't or Shouldn't Breastfeed

Unfortunately, the option of breastfeeding isn't open to every new mother. Some women can't or shouldn't nurse their newborns. The reasons may be emotional or physical, due to the mother's health or the baby's, temporary (in which case breastfeeding can sometimes begin later on) or long term. The most common maternal factors that may prevent or interfere with breastfeeding include:

- Serious debilitating illness (such as cardiac or kidney impairment, or severe anemia) or extreme underweight, though some women manage to overcome the obstacles and breastfeed their babies.

- Serious infection, such as active untreated tuberculosis; during treatment, breasts can be pumped so a supply will be established once breastfeeding resumes.

- Chronic conditions that require medications that pass into the breast milk and might be harmful to the baby, such as antithyroid, anticancer, or antihypertensive drugs or mood-altering drugs, such as lithium, tranquilizers, or sedatives. If you take any kind of medication, check with your physician if you're considering breastfeeding. In some cases, a change of medication or spacing of doses may make breastfeeding possible. A temporary need for medication, such as penicillin, even at the time you begin nursing, doesn't usually have to interfere with breastfeeding. Women who need antibiotics during labor or due to a breast infection (mastitis) can continue to breastfeed while on the medication.

■ Exposure to certain toxic chemicals in the workplace; check with OSHA (see page 194).

■ Alcohol abuse. An occasional drink is okay, but too much alcohol can cause problems for a nursing baby.

■ Drug abuse, including the use of tranquilizers, cocaine, heroin, methadone, or marijuana.

■ AIDS, or HIV infection, which can be transmitted via body fluids, including breast milk.

Some conditions in the newborn may make breastfeeding difficult, but not (with the right lactation support) impossible. They include:

■ A premature or very small baby, who may have difficulty sucking or latching on properly. A preemie who is sick and has to spend time in the NICU (neonatal intensive care unit) also may not be able to nurse, though you can pump to establish a good milk supply and feed the breast milk to the baby with the help of the hospital staff.

■ Disorders such as lactose intolerance or PKU in which neither human nor cow's milk can be digested. In the case of PKU, babies can be breastfed if they also receive supplemental phenylalanine free formula; with lactose intolerance (which is extremely rare at birth),

When Father Knows Breast

It only takes two to breastfeed, but it often takes three to make it happen. Researchers have found that when fathers are supportive of breastfeeding, moms are likely to give it a try 96 percent of the time; when dads are ambivalent, only about 26 percent give it a try. What's more, say researchers, keeping dad in the breastfeeding loop (by providing him with lots of nursing know-how so he can better support you) can help extend the length of time you end up breastfeeding—plus it could make nursing easier overall. Dads: Take note, and join the breastfeeding team!

mother's milk can be treated with lactase to make it digestible.

■ Cleft lip or other mouth deformities that interfere with sucking. Though the success of breastfeeding depends somewhat on the type of defect, with special help, nursing is usually possible. (Babies with cleft palates won't be able to breastfeed but will still be able to be fed pumped breast milk.)

Very rarely, the milk supply isn't adequate, perhaps because of insufficient glandular tissue in the breast, and breastfeeding just doesn't work—no matter how hard mother and baby work at it.

If you end up not being able to nurse your baby—even if you very much wanted to—there's no reason to add guilt to your disappointment. In fact, it's important that you don't, to avoid letting those feelings interfere with the very important process of getting to know and love your baby—a process that by no means must include breastfeeding.

CHAPTER 14

The
Ninth
Month

Approximately 36 to 40 Weeks

FINALLY, THE MONTH YOU'VE BEEN waiting for, working toward, and possibly worrying about just a little bit is here at long last. Chances are you're at once very ready (to hold that baby . . . to see your toes again . . . to sleep on your stomach!) and not ready at all. Still, despite the inevitable flurry of activity (more practitioner appointments, a layette to shop for, projects to finish at work, paint colors to pick for baby's room), you may find that the ninth month seems like the longest month of all. Except, of course, if you don't deliver by your due date. In that case, it's the tenth month that's the longest.

Your Baby This Month

Week 36 Weighing about 6 pounds and measuring somewhere around 20 inches tall, your baby is almost ready to be served up into your arms. Right now, most of baby's systems (from circulatory to musculoskeletal) are just about equipped for life on the outside. Though the digestive system is ready to roll, too, it hasn't really gotten a work-out yet. Remember, up until this point, your baby's nutrition has been arriving via the umbilical cord—no digestion necessary. But that's soon to change. As soon as baby takes his or her first suckle at your breast (or suck from the bottle), that digestive system will be jump-started—and those diapers will start filling.

Week 37 Here's some exciting news: If your baby were born today, he or she would be considered full term. Mind you, that doesn't mean he or she is finished growing—or getting ready for life on the outside. Still gaining weight at about a half pound a week, the average fetus this age weighs about 6½ pounds (though size varies quite a bit from fetus to fetus, as it does from newborn to newborn). Fat continues to accumulate on your baby, forming kissable dimples in those cute elbows, knees, and shoulders, and adorable creases and folds in the neck and wrists. To keep busy until the big debut, your baby is practicing to make perfect: inhaling and exhaling amniotic fluid (to get the lungs ready for that first breath), sucking on his or her thumb (to prepare for that first suckle), blinking, and pivoting from side to side (which explains why yesterday you felt that sweet little butt on the left side and today it's taken a turn to the right).

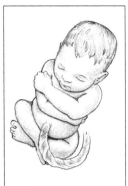

Your Baby, Month 9

Week 38 Hitting the growth charts at close to 7 pounds and the 20-inch mark (give or take an inch or two), your little one isn't so little anymore. In fact, baby's big enough for the big time—and the big day. With only two (or four, max) weeks left in utero, all systems are (almost) go. To finish getting ready for his or her close-up (and all those photo ops), baby has a few last-minute details to take care of, like shedding that skin-protecting vernix and lanugo. And producing more surfactant, which will prevent the air sacs in the lungs from sticking to each other when your baby begins to breathe—something he or she will be doing very soon. Baby will be here before you know it!

Week 39 Not much to report this week, at least in the height and weight department. Fortunately for you and your overstretched skin (and aching back), baby's growth has slowed down—or even taken a hiatus until after delivery. On average, a baby this week still weighs in at around 7 or 8 pounds and measures up at 19 to 21 inches (though yours may be a little bigger or smaller). Still, progress is being made in some other areas, especially baby's brain, which is growing and developing up a storm (at a rapid pace that will continue during the first three years of life). What's more, your baby's pink skin has turned white or whitish (no matter what skin your baby will ultimately be in, since pigmentation doesn't occur until soon after birth). A development that you may have noticed by now if this is your first pregnancy: Baby's head might have dropped into your pelvis. This change of baby's locale might make for easier breathing (and less heartburn), but could also make it harder for you to walk (make that to waddle).

Week 40 Congratulations! You've reached the official end of your pregnancy (and perhaps the end of your rope). For the record, your baby is fully full term and could weigh in anywhere between the 6- and 9-pound mark and measure anywhere from 19 to 22 inches, though some perfectly healthy babies check in smaller or bigger than that. You may notice when your baby emerges that he or she (and you'll know for sure at that momentous moment which) is still curled into the fetal position, even though the fetal days are over. That's just sheer force of habit (after spending nine months in the cramped confines of your uterus, your baby doesn't yet realize there's room to spread out now) and comfort (that snug-as-a-bug position feels good). When you do meet your new arrival, be sure to say hello—and more. Though it's your first face-to-face, your baby will recognize the sound of your voice—and that of dad's. And if he or she doesn't arrive on time (choosing to ignore the due date you've marked in red on your calendar), you're in good—though anxious—company. About half of all pregnancies proceed past the 40-week mark, though, thankfully, your practitioner will probably not let yours continue beyond 42 weeks.

Weeks 41–42 Looks like baby has opted for a late checkout. Fewer than 5 percent of babies are actually born on their due date—and around 50 percent decide to overstay their welcome in Hotel Uterus,

thriving well into the tenth month (though you may have lost that "thriving" feeling long ago). Remember, too, that most of the time an overdue baby isn't overdue at all—it's just that the due date was off. Less often, a baby may be truly postmature. When a postmature baby does make a debut, it's often with dry, cracked, peeling, loose, and wrinkled skin (all completely temporary). That's because the protective vernix was shed in the weeks before, in anticipation of a delivery date that's since come and gone. An "older" fetus will also have longer nails, possibly longer hair, and definitely little or none of that baby fuzz (lanugo) at all. They are also more alert and open-eyed (after all, they're older and wiser). Just to be sure all is well, your practitioner will likely monitor an overdue baby closely through nonstress tests and checks of the amniotic fluid or biophysical profiles.

What You May Be Feeling

You may experience all of these symptoms at one time or another, or only a few of them. Some may have continued from last month; others may be new. Still others may hardly be noticed because you are used to them and/or because they are eclipsed by new and more exciting signs indicating that labor may not be far off:

Physically

- Changes in fetal activity (more squirming and less kicking, as your baby has progressively less room to move around)

- Vaginal discharge becomes heavier and contains more mucus, which may

be streaked red with blood or tinged brown or pink after intercourse or a pelvic exam or as your cervix begins to dilate

- Constipation

- Heartburn, indigestion, flatulence, bloating

- Occasional headaches, faintness, dizziness

- Nasal congestion and occasional nosebleeds; ear stuffiness

- Sensitive gums

- Leg cramps at night

- Increased backache and heaviness

A Look Inside

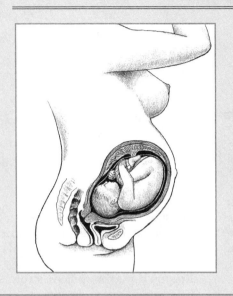

Your uterus is right under your ribs now, and your measurements aren't really changing that much from week to week anymore. The top of your uterus is around 38 to 40 cm from the top of your pubic bone. Your weight gain slows down or even stops as D-day approaches. Your abdominal skin is stretched as far as you think it can go, and you're probably waddling more now than ever, possibly because the baby has dropped in anticipation of impending labor.

- Buttock and pelvic discomfort and achiness

- Increased swelling of ankles and feet, and occasionally of hands and face

- Itchy abdomen, protruding navel

- Stretch marks

- Varicose veins in your legs

- Hemorrhoids

- Easier breathing after the baby drops

- More frequent urination after the baby drops, since there's pressure on the bladder once again

- Increased difficulty sleeping

- More frequent and more intense Braxton Hicks contractions (some may be painful)

- Increasing clumsiness and difficulty getting around

- Colostrum, leaking from nipples (though this premilk substance may not appear until after delivery)

- Extra fatigue or extra energy (nesting syndrome), or alternating periods of each

- Increase in appetite or loss of appetite

Emotionally

- More excitement, more anxiety, more apprehension, more absentmindedness

- Relief that you're almost there

- Irritability and oversensitivity (especially with people who keep saying "Are you still around?")

- Impatience and restlessness

- Dreaming and fantasizing about the baby

What You Can Expect at This Month's Checkup

You'll be spending more time than ever at your practitioner's office this month (stock up on some good waiting-room reading if you've already plowed through the office collection), with appointments scheduled weekly. These visits will be more interesting—the practitioner will estimate baby's size and may even venture a prediction about how close you are to delivery—with the excitement growing as you approach the big day. In general, you can expect your practitioner to check the following, though there may be variations, depending on your particular needs and your practitioner's style of practice:

■ Your weight (gain generally slows down or stops)

■ Your blood pressure (it may be slightly higher than it was at midpregnancy)

■ Your urine, for sugar and protein

■ Your feet and hands for swelling, and legs for varicose veins

■ Your cervix (the neck of your uterus), by internal examination, to see if effacement (thinning) and dilation (opening) have begun

■ The height of the fundus

■ The fetal heartbeat

■ Fetal size (you may get a rough weight estimate), presentation (head or buttocks first), position (front or rear facing), and descent (is presenting part engaged?) by palpation (feeling with the hands)

■ Questions and concerns you want to discuss, particularly those related to labor and delivery—have a list ready. Include frequency and duration of Braxton Hicks contractions, if you've noticed any, and other symptoms you have been experiencing, especially unusual ones.

You can also expect to receive a labor and delivery protocol (when to call if you think you are in labor, when to plan on heading to the hospital or birthing center) from your practitioner; if you don't, be sure to ask for these instructions.

What You May Be Wondering About

Urinary Frequency— Again

"During the last few days, it seems like I'm in the bathroom constantly. Is it normal to be urinating this frequently now?"

Having a little first-trimester déjà vu? That's because your uterus is right back where it started: down low in your pelvis, pressing squarely on your bladder. And this time, the weight of your uterus is significantly greater, which means the pressure on your bladder is greater, too—as is that need to pee. So you go, girl—again, and again, and again. As long as frequency isn't accompanied by signs of infection (see page 498), it's completely normal. Don't be tempted to cut back on fluids in an attempt to cut back on your trips to the bathroom—your body needs those fluids more than ever. And, as always, go as soon as you feel the urge (and can find a bathroom).

Leaky Breasts

"A friend of mine says she had milk leaking from her breasts in the ninth month; I don't. Does this mean I won't have any milk?"

Milk isn't made until baby's ready to drink it—and that's not until three to four days after delivery. What your friend was leaking was colostrum, a thin, yellowish fluid that is the precursor to mature breast milk. Colostrum is chock-full of antibodies to protect a newborn baby and has more protein and less fat and milk sugar (the better to digest it) than the breast milk that arrives later.

Some, but far from all, women leak this phenomenal fluid toward the end of their pregnancies. But even women who don't experience leakage of colostrum are still producing it. Not leaking, but still curious? Squeezing your areola may allow you to express a few drops (but don't squeeze with a vengeance—that'll only result in sore nipples). Still can't get any? Don't worry. Your baby will be able to net what he or she needs when the time comes (if you plan to breastfeed). Not leaking isn't a sign that your supply won't ultimately keep up with demand.

If you are leaking colostrum, it's probably just a few drops. But if you're leaking more than that, you may want to consider wearing nursing pads in your bra to protect your clothes (and to prevent potentially embarrassing moments). And you might as well get used to the wet T-shirt look, since this is just a glimpse of leaky breasts—and wet bras, nightgowns, and shirts—to come.

Spotting Now

"Right after my husband and I made love this morning, I began to spot a little. Does this mean that labor is beginning?"

Don't order the birth announcements yet. Pinkish-stained or red-streaked mucus appearing soon after intercourse or a vaginal examination, or brownish-tinged mucus or brownish spotting appearing within 48 hours after the same, is usually just a normal result of the sensitive cervix being bruised or manipulated, not a sign that labor's about to start up. But pinkish- or brownish-tinged or bloody mucus accompanied by contractions or other signs of oncoming labor, whether it follows intercourse or not, could be signaling the start of labor (see page 359).

If you notice bright red bleeding or persistent red spotting after intercourse—or any time, for that matter—check in with your practitioner.

Water Breaking in Public

"I'm really worried that my water will break in public."

Most women worry about springing an amniotic leak—especially a public one—late in pregnancy, but few ever do. Contrary to popular pregnancy belief, your "water" (more accurately, your membranes) isn't likely to "break" (more accurately, rupture) before labor begins. In fact, more than 85 percent of women enter the birthing room with their membranes fully intact. And even if you end up being among the 15 percent who do spring a prelabor leak, you won't have to fear a public puddle at your feet. Unless you're lying down (something you probably don't do much in public anyway), amniotic

Baby's Crying Already?

The most joyous sound a new parent hears is that first cry the baby makes after he or she is born. But would you believe that your little one is already crying inside you? It's true, according to researchers, who found that third-trimester fetuses show crying behaviors—quivering chin, open mouth, deep inhalations and exhalations, and startle responses—when a loud noise and vibration were sounded near the mom's belly. It's known that the crying reflex is well developed even in premature infants, so it's not surprising that babies are perfecting this skill long before they're ready to emerge (and it explains why they're so good at crying once they come out!).

fluid is less likely to go with the flow, and more likely to come out as a slow trickle—or at most a small gush. That's because when you're upright (standing, walking, even sitting), your baby's head acts like a cork in a bottle, blocking the opening of the uterus and keeping most of the amniotic fluid in. In other words, it's probable that the forecast for the rest of your pregnant future will remain "mainly dry."

Something else to keep in mind: If you do actually experience a noticeable public gush of fluid, you can be sure that no one around you will stare, point, or chuckle. Instead, they will either offer you help or discreetly ignore you. After all, no one is likely to overlook the fact that you're pregnant, so it's just as unlikely they'll mistake amniotic fluid for anything else.

The bright side of a water break (in public or at home) is that it's usually followed by labor, typically within 24 hours. If labor doesn't start spontaneously within that time, your practitioner will probably start it for you. Which means your baby's arrival will be just a day away, either way.

Though it really isn't necessary, wearing a panty liner or maxipad in the last weeks may give you a sense of security, as well as keep you fresh as your vaginal discharge increases. You also might want to place heavy towels, a plastic sheet, or hospital bed pads under your sheets in the last few weeks, just in case your water breaks in the middle of the night.

Baby Dropping

"If I'm past my 38th week and haven't dropped, does it mean I'm going to be late?"

Just because your baby doesn't seem to be making his or her way toward the exit doesn't mean that exit will be late. "Dropping," also called "lightening," is what happens when a baby descends into mom's pelvic cavity, a sign that the presenting part (first part out, usually the head) is engaged in the upper portion of the bony pelvis. In first pregnancies, dropping generally takes place two to four weeks before delivery. In women who have had children previously, it usually doesn't happen until they go into labor. But as with almost every aspect of pregnancy, exceptions to the rule are the rule. You can drop four weeks before your due date and deliver two weeks late, or you can go into labor without having dropped at all. You can even drop and then undrop. Your baby's head can appear to settle in and then float up again (meaning it's not really fixed in place yet).

Often, dropping is obvious. You might not only see the difference (your belly seems lower—perhaps a lot lower—and tilted farther forward), you might feel the difference, too. As the upward pressure of the uterus on your diaphragm is relieved, you can breathe more easily, literally. With your stomach less crowded, you can eat more easily, too—and finish up your meals without a side of heartburn and indigestion. Of course, these welcome changes are often offset by a new set of discomforts, including pressure on the bladder (which will send you to the bathroom more frequently, again), the pelvic joints (which will make it harder to walk . . . or waddle), and the perineal area (sometimes causing pain); sharp little shocks or twinges on the pelvic floor (thanks to baby's head pressing hard on it); and a sense of being off-balance (because your center of gravity has shifted once more).

It is possible, however, for baby to drop unnoticed. For instance, if you were carrying low to begin with, your pregnant profile might not change noticeably after dropping. Or if you never experience difficulty breathing or getting a full meal down, or if you always urinate frequently, you might not detect any obvious difference.

Your practitioner will rely on two more indicators to figure out whether or not your baby's head is engaged: First, he or she will do an internal exam to see whether the presenting part—ideally the head—is in the pelvis; second, he or she will feel that part externally (by pressing on your belly) to determine whether it is fixed in position or still "floating" free.

How far the presenting part has progressed through the pelvis is measured in "stations," each a centimeter long. A fully engaged baby is said to be at "zero station"; that is, the fetal head has descended to the level of the prominent bony landmarks on either side of the midpelvis. A baby who has just begun to descend may be at –4 or –5 station. Once delivery begins, the head continues on through the pelvis past 0 to +1, +2, and so on, until it begins to "crown" at the external vaginal opening at +5. Though a woman who goes into labor at 0 station probably has less pushing ahead than the woman at –3, this isn't invariably true, since station isn't the only factor affecting the progression of labor.

Though the engagement of the fetal head strongly suggests that the baby can get through the pelvis without difficulty, it's no guarantee. Conversely, a fetus that is still free floating going into labor isn't necessarily going to have trouble negotiating the exit. And in fact, the majority of fetuses that haven't yet engaged when labor begins come through the pelvis smoothly. This is particularly true in moms who have already delivered one or more babies.

Changes in Baby's Movements

"My baby used to kick so vigorously, and I can still feel him moving, but he seems less active now."

When you first heard from your baby, way back in the fifth month or so, there was ample room in the uterus for acrobatics, kickboxing, and punching. Now that conditions are getting a little cramped, his gymnastics are curtailed. In this uterine straitjacket, there is little room for anything more than turning, twisting, and wiggling—which is probably what you've been feeling. And once your baby's head is firmly engaged in your pelvis, he will be even less mobile. But this late in the game, it's not important what kind of fetal

Going Down?

You may be in for a surprise—and a treat—at one of this month's weigh-ins. Most expectant moms who reach the end of pregnancy also reach the end of pregnancy weight gain. Instead of watching the numbers on the scale go up (and up), you may start seeing those numbers go nowhere—or even go down—over the last few weeks. What's up (or rather, down) with that? After all, your baby isn't losing weight—and your ankles (not to mention your hips) are still plenty puffy, thank you very much. What's happening, actually, is perfectly normal. In fact, this weight gain standstill (or downward trend) is one way that your body gets ready for labor. Amniotic fluid starts to decrease (less water equals less weight), and loose bowels (common as labor approaches) can also send the numbers down, as can all that sweating you're doing (especially if you've been nesting overtime). And if you think this weight loss is exciting, wait until delivery day. That's when you'll experience your biggest one-day weight-loss total ever!

movement you feel (or even if it's only on one side), as long as you feel some every day. If, however, you feel no activity (see next question) or a sudden spurt of very panicky, frantic, jerky, or violent activity, check with your practitioner.

"I've hardly felt the baby kick at all this afternoon. What does that mean?"

Chances are your baby has settled down for a nap (older fetuses, like newborns, have periodic interludes of deep sleep) or that you've been too busy or too active to notice any movements. For reassurance, check for activity using the test on page 289. You may want to repeat this test routinely twice a day throughout the last trimester. Ten or more movements during each test period mean that your baby's activity level is normal. Fewer suggest that medical evaluation might be necessary to determine the cause of the inactivity, so contact your practitioner if that's the case. Though a baby who is relatively inactive in the womb can be perfectly healthy, inactivity at this point sometimes indicates fetal distress. Picking up this distress early and taking steps to intervene can often prevent serious consequences.

"I've read that fetal movements are supposed to slow down as delivery approaches. My baby seems as active as ever."

Every baby's different, even before he or she is born—especially when it comes to activity levels, and particularly as delivery day approaches. While some babies move a bit less as they get ready to arrive, others keep up an energetic pace right until it's time for that first face-to-face. In late pregnancy, there is generally a gradual decline in the number of movements, probably related to tighter quarters, a decrease in amniotic fluid, and improved fetal coordination. But unless you're counting every single movement, you're not likely to notice a big difference.

Nesting Instinct

"I've heard about the nesting instinct. Is it pregnancy legend, or is it for real?"

The need to nest can be as real and as powerful an instinct for some humans as it is for our feathered and four-legged friends. If you've ever witnessed the birth of puppies or kittens, you've probably noticed how restless the laboring mother becomes just before delivery—frantically running back and forth, furiously shredding papers in a corner, and finally, when she feels all is in order, settling into the spot where she will give birth. Many expectant mothers do experience the uncontrollable urge to ready their nests, too, just prior to childbirth. For some it's subtle. All of a sudden, it becomes vitally important to clean out and restock the refrigerator and make sure there's a six-month supply of toilet paper in the house. For others, this unusual burst of manic energy plays itself out in behavior that is dramatic, sometimes irrational, and often funny (at least, to those watching it)—cleaning every crevice of the nursery with a toothbrush, rearranging the contents of the kitchen cabinets alphabetically,

washing everything that isn't tied down or being worn, or folding and refolding baby's clothes for hours on end.

Though it isn't a reliable predictor of when labor will begin, nesting usually intensifies as the big moment approaches—perhaps as a response to increased adrenaline circulating in an expectant mom's system. Keep in mind, however, that not all women experience the nesting instinct, and that those who don't are just as successful in bearing and caring for their nestlings as those who do. The urge to slump in front of the television during the last few weeks of pregnancy is as common as the urge to clean out closets, and just as understandable. Make that more understandable.

If a nesting urge does strike, make sure it's tempered by common sense. Suppress that overwhelming urge to paint the baby's nursery yourself; let someone else climb the ladder with the bucket and roller while you oversee

Getting Ready

These days, it almost goes without saying that becoming educated about childbirth is one of the best ways to prepare for this momentous experience. So by all means make sure you and your coach are as educated as you can be: Read the next chapter, along with any other materials on labor and delivery you can get your hands on; watch DVDs; take a childbirth class together. But don't let your preparedness stop there. Be as prepared for matters practical and aesthetic, and plan, too, for your entertainment. Consider, for example: Are you interested in having the event videotaped (if that's allowed where you're delivering), or will a few photos suffice? Will music

soothe your soul when your soul needs it most, or will you prefer some peace and quiet? What will distract you best between contractions—playing poker with your partner or solitaire on your cell phone, checking e-mail on your laptop, or watching reruns of your favorite sitcoms on TV? (Of course, also be prepared for the possibility that once those contractions begin, you may have little patience for distractions.) Don't forget to include the materials you'll need for the activities you've planned (including batteries for that camera, plus your phone charger) in the suitcase you'll be taking to the hospital or birthing center (see page 356 for a complete packing list).

How Is Baby Doing?

As your pregnancy nears its end (yes, it *will* end), your practitioner will be keeping a closer eye on your health and that of your baby—especially once you pass the 40-week mark. That's because 40 weeks is the optimum uterine stay for babies; those who stick around much longer can face potential challenges (becoming too big to arrive vaginally, experiencing a decline in their placenta's function, or a dip in amniotic fluid levels). Luckily, your practitioner can tap into plenty of tests and assessments of fetal well-being to make sure all's well and will end well:

Kick counts. Your record of fetal movements (see page 289), though not foolproof, can provide some indication of how your baby is doing. Ten movements an hour is usually reassuring. If you don't notice enough activity, other tests are then performed.

The nonstress test (NST). You'll be hooked up to a fetal monitor (the same kind that's used during labor) in your practitioner's office to measure the baby's heart rate and response to movement. You will be holding a clicker contraption (like a buzzer on a game show), and each time you feel the baby move, you'll click it. The monitoring goes on for 20 to 40 minutes and is able to detect if the fetus is under any stress.

Fetal acoustical stimulation (FAS) or vibroacoustic stimulation (VAS). This nonstress test, in which a sound-and-vibration-producing instrument is placed on the mother's abdomen to determine the fetus's response to sound or vibrations, is useful if there's a question about how to interpret a standard NST.

The contraction stress test (CST) or oxytocin challenge test (OCT). If the results of a nonstress test are unclear, your practitioner may order a stress test. This test, done at a hospital, tests how the baby responds to the "stress" of uterine contractions to get some idea of how the baby will handle full-blown labor. In this somewhat more complex and time-consuming test (it may take a number of hours), you're hooked up to a fetal monitor. If contractions are not occurring on their own, you'll be given a low-dose IV of oxytocin (or you'll be asked to stimulate your nipples) to jump-

---

from a comfy chair. Don't let over-zealous home cleaning exhaust you, either—you'll need energy reserves for both labor and a new baby. Most important of all, keep the limitations of your species in mind. Although you may share this nesting instinct with members of the animal kingdom, you are still only human—and you can't expect to get everything done before that little bundle of joy arrives at your nest.

When You Will Deliver

"I just had an internal exam and the doctor said I'll probably be going into labor very soon. Can she really tell exactly how close I am?"

Your practitioner can make a prediction about when you'll give birth, but it's still just an educated guess—just as your original due date was. There are clues that labor is getting closer, which start the contractions. How the fetus responds to contractions indicates its probable condition and that of the placenta. This rough simulation of the conditions of labor can, if the results are unequivocal, allow a prediction to be made about whether or not the fetus can safely remain in the uterus and whether it can meet the strenuous demands of true labor.

A biophysical profile (BPP). A BPP generally evaluates, through the use of ultrasound, four aspects of life in the uterus: fetal breathing, fetal movement, fetal tone (the ability of your baby to flex a finger or toe), and amniotic fluid volume. When all these are normal, the baby is probably doing fine. If any of these are unclear, further testing (such as a CST or a VAS) will be given to provide a more accurate picture of the baby's condition.

The "modified" biophysical profile. The "modified" biophysical profile combines the NST with an evaluation of the quantity of amniotic fluid. A low level of amniotic fluid may indicate that the fetus is not producing enough urine and the placenta may not be functioning up to par. If the fetus reacts appropriately to the nonstress test and levels of amniotic fluid are adequate, it's likely that all is well.

Umbilical artery Doppler velocimetry. This test uses ultrasound to look at the flow of blood through the umbilical artery. A weak, absent, or reverse flow indicates the fetus is not getting adequate nourishment and probably not growing well.

Other tests of fetal well-being. These include regular ultrasound exams to document fetal growth; amniotic fluid sampling (through amniocentesis); fetal electrocardiography or other tests (to assess the fetal heart); and fetal scalp stimulation (which tests how a fetus reacts to pressure on, or pinching of, the scalp).

Most of the time, fetuses pass these tests with flying colors, which means they can continue to stay put until they're good and ready to make their debuts. Rarely, the test results can be labeled "nonreasurring," which really isn't as unreassuring as it sounds. Because these tests yield plenty of false positives, a nonreassuring result doesn't definitely diagnose distress, but it will mean that your practitioner will continue to test your baby, and if it turns out that there's any indication of fetal distress, will induce your labor. (For information on labor induction, see page 368.)

a practitioner looks for beginning in the ninth month, both by palpating the abdomen and doing an internal exam. Has lightening or engagement taken place? What level, or station, has the baby's presenting part descended to? Have effacement (thinning of the cervix) and dilation (opening of the cervix) begun? Has the cervix begun to soften and move to the front of the vagina (another indicator that labor is getting closer) or is it still firm and positioned to the back?

But "soon" can mean anywhere from an hour to three weeks or more. A practitioner's prediction of "you'll be in labor by this evening" could segue into a half month more of pregnancy, whereas a forecast of "labor's weeks away" could be followed hours later by birth. The fact is that engagement, effacement, and dilation can occur gradually, over a period of weeks or even a month or more in some women—and overnight in others. Which means that these clues

Do-It-Yourself Labor Induction?

So what happens if you're overdue, and still as pregnant as ever (make that more pregnant than ever), with your baby showing no signs of budging? Should you just let nature take its course, no matter how long that course takes? Or should you take matters into your own hands, and try some do-it-yourself labor induction techniques? And if you do take matters into your own hands, will it even work? While there are plenty of natural methods you can use to try to bring on labor (and plenty of old wives' tales to go along with them), it's hard to prove that any of them will do the trick. Some women swear by them, but none of the home-grown methods passed from mom-to-be to mom-to-be has been documented as consistently effective. That's probably at least partly due to the fact that when they do appear to work, it's difficult to establish whether they actually worked—or whether labor, coincidentally, started on its own at the same time.

Still, if you're at the end of your rope (and who isn't by 40 weeks?), you might want to give these a try:

Walking. It has been suggested that walking can help ease the baby into the pelvis, thanks perhaps to the force of gravity or the swaying (or waddling) of your hips. Once your baby puts pressure on the cervix—literally—labor just might get going. If it turns out that your stroll doesn't jump-start labor, you'll be no worse for the wear. In fact, you might be in better shape for labor, whenever it actually does begin.

Sex. Sure you're the size of a small hippo, but hopping (make that hoisting yourself) into bed with your partner may be an effective way to mix business with pleasure. Or not. Some research shows that semen (which contains prostaglandins) can stimulate contractions, while other research has found that women who continue to have sex late in pregnancy might carry their babies even longer than those who abstain.

are far from sure bets when it comes to pinpointing the start of labor.

So feel free to pack your bags, but don't keep the car running. Like every pregnant woman who preceded you into the birthing room, you will still have to play the waiting game, knowing for certain only that your day, or night, will come—sometime.

The Overdue Baby

"I'm a week overdue. Is it possible that I might never go into labor on my own?"

The magic date is circled in red on the calendar; every day of the 40 weeks that precede it is crossed off with great anticipation. Then, at long last, the big day arrives—and, as in about half of all pregnancies, the baby doesn't. Anticipation dissolves into discouragement. The stroller and crib sit empty for yet another day. And then a week. And then, in about 10 percent of pregnancies, most often those of first-time mothers, two weeks. Will this pregnancy never end?

Though women who have reached the 42nd week might find it hard to believe, no pregnancy on record ever went on forever, even before the advent

The bottom line? Go for your bottom lines, if you're game to try (and get a good laugh while you're at it). After all, it may be the last time in a long time that you'll actually be able (or willing) to have sex. If getting busy brings on labor, great—if it doesn't, still great.

Other natural methods have potential drawbacks (even though they've been passed down from midwives to old wives to new doctors). So before you try these at home, discuss them with your practitioner first:

Nipple stimulation. Interested in some nipple tweaking (ouch)? How about some nipple twisting (double ouch)? Stimulating your nipples for a few hours a day (yes, hours) can release your own natural oxytocin and bring on contractions. But here's the caveat: Nipple stimulation—as enticing as hours of it may sound (or not)—can lead to painfully long and strong uterine contractions. So unless your practitioner advises it and is monitoring your progress, you may want to think four times—twice for each nipple—before you or your spouse attempt nipple stimulation.

Castor oil. Hoping to sip your way into labor with a castor oil cocktail? Women have been passing down this yucky-tasting tradition for generations on the theory that this powerful laxative will stimulate your bowels, which in turn will stimulate your uterus into contracting. The caveat for this one: Castor oil (even mixed with a more appetizing drink) can cause diarrhea, severe cramping, and even vomiting. Before you chug-a-lug, be sure you're game to begin labor that way.

Herbal teas and remedies. Raspberry leaf tea, black cohosh—these herbal remedies might be just what your grandmother orders to bring on labor, but since no studies have been done to establish the safety of any herbal treatments as labor inducers, don't use any without getting the green light from your practitioner first.

And while you're pondering the effectiveness of the do-it-yourself methods, remind yourself that you *will* go into labor—either on your own or with a little help from your practitioner—in a week or two.

of labor induction. Studies show that about 70 percent of apparent post-term pregnancies aren't post-term at all. They are only believed to be late because of a miscalculation of the time of conception, usually thanks to irregular ovulation or a woman's uncertainty about the exact date of her last period. And in fact, when early ultrasound examination is used to confirm the due date, diagnoses of post-term pregnancy drop dramatically from the long-held estimate of 10 percent to about 2 percent.

Even if you do end up among those 2 percent of women who are truly over-due, your practitioner won't let your pregnancy pass the 42-week mark. In fact, most practitioners won't even let a pregnancy continue that long, choosing instead to induce by the time your baby has clocked in 41 uterine weeks. And, of course, if at any point test results show that the placenta is no longer doing its job well or that the amniotic fluid levels have dipped too low—or if there are any other signs that baby might not be thriving—your practitioner will take action, and depending on the situation, either induce labor or perform a cesarean delivery. Which means that even if you don't end up going into labor on your own, you won't be pregnant forever.

"I've heard that overdue babies don't continue to thrive. I just passed my 40th week—does that mean my baby should be delivered?"

Just because your pregnancy has exceeded those 40 allotted weeks doesn't necessarily mean that your baby has worn out his or her uterine welcome—or that a speedy exit is called for. Many babies actually continue to grow and thrive well into the tenth month. But when a pregnancy goes post-term (technically, at the 42-week mark), the once ideal environment in a womb can become less hospitable. The aging placenta can fail to supply enough nutrition and oxygen, and production of amniotic fluid can drop off.

Babies born after spending time in such an inhospitable environment are called postmature. Their skin is dry, cracked, peeling, loose, and wrinkled, having already shed the cheesy vernix coating that previously protected it. Being "older" than other new arrivals, they have longer nails and more hair, and are generally open-eyed and alert. Because they are usually larger than term babies, with wider head circumferences, and because they may sometimes be in distress, postmature babies are more likely to be delivered by cesarean. They may also need some special care in the neonatal intensive care nursery for a short time after birth. So, though the majority of post-term babies arrive home a little later than scheduled, they arrive completely healthy.

To prevent postmaturity, many practitioners choose to induce labor

Massage It, Mama

Got nothing but time on your hands as you wait for baby's arrival? Put your hands (or a special someone else's hands) to good use—and give yourself a rub. Perineal massage can help gently stretch a first timer's perineum (that area of skin between your vagina and rectum), which in turn can minimize the "stinging" that occurs when baby's head crowns during childbirth. And here's another plus you'll appreciate: It may also help you avoid an episiotomy and tearing, according to some experts.

Here's how to give your perineum the right rub: With clean hands (and short nails) insert your thumbs or index fingers (lubricated with a little K-Y jelly if you'd like) inside your vagina. Press down (toward your rectum) and slide your fingers across the bottom and sides of your perineum. Repeat daily during the last weeks of pregnancy,

five minutes (or longer) each time. Not in the mood for a perineal massage? It's certainly not something you have to do. Don't bother if you don't feel comfortable with the concept, it seems too weird, or you just don't have the time. Though anecdotal evidence has long supported its effectiveness, clinical research has not yet backed it up. Even without the rubbing, your body will still stretch when the time comes. And don't bother with perineal massage if you've already popped out a baby or two. Your perineum doesn't need, and probably won't benefit from, the extra stretching.

One word to the wise: If you do go the massage route, proceed gently. The last thing you want to do right before labor is to pull too hard, scratch yourself, or irritate the sensitive skin down there. Bottom line: Massage with care.

when it's certain that a pregnancy is past 41 weeks and the cervix is found to be ripe (soft and ready to dilate) or sooner if there are complications of any kind. Other practitioners may choose to wait it out a bit longer, performing one or more assessment tests (see box, page 348) to see if the baby is still doing well in the uterus, and repeating these tests once or twice a week until labor begins. Ask your practitioner what game plan he or she usually goes with when a baby's late.

Of course, chances are good your baby will decide to check out of your womb sooner than later—and without any prompting.

Inviting Others to the Birth

"I'm really excited about having my baby and I want to share the experience with my sisters and best friends—and, of course, my mom. Would it be weird to have them all in the birthing room with me and my husband?"

Someone's having a birth day party (your baby, in fact), and if you're like more and more moms-to-be, the guest list is getting longer and longer. There's definitely nothing weird about wanting to have those who are closest to you by your side on the big day—and, in fact, it's a trend that's gaining popularity in birthing circles.

Why is more merrier for some women on labor day? For one, the widespread use of epidurals has made labor less laborious for many. With little or no pain to deal with—or breathe through—there's more opportunity to socialize (plus, it's a lot easier to be in a party mood if you're not groaning and panting). For another, hospitals and birthing centers are also enabling the

Foods to Bring It On?

Hungry for labor? Ready to do—or eat—anything that might trigger that first real contraction? Though there's no science backing them up, plenty of old wives (or old friends) will tell you about a last supper that ended with a trip down labor lane. Among the often heard: If your stomach can take the heat, dip into something spicy. Or order something that gets your bowels—and hopefully your uterus—in an uproar (a crate of bran muffins, chased down by a bucket of prune juice, perhaps?). Not in the mood for something so stimulating? Some women swear by eggplant, tomatoes, and balsamic vinegar (not necessarily together); others say pineapple buys a ticket on the Labor Express. Whatever you dig into, remember that unless your baby and your body are ready to take the labor plunge, it's unlikely that dinner's going to pull the trigger.

maternity mob, making some birthing rooms bigger (more equipped to handle the overflow of guests) and more comfortable (complete with sofas and extra chairs for visitors to plop down on while they're waiting for the headliner to make his or her debut). Some even have Internet access to keep guests busy when there's a break in the action. Policies have become more lenient, too—and at some hospitals and birthing centers, even open door (for as many as can fit in the door, that is). And having a gaggle of girlfriends and relatives may be just what the doctor—

Sounds Like a Plan

How far along in labor should you be before calling your practitioner? Should you call if your water breaks? How can you make contact if the contractions start outside of regular office hours? Should you call first and then head for the hospital or birthing center? Or the other way around?

Don't wait until labor starts to get the answers to these important questions. Discuss all of these and other labor logistics with your practitioner at your next appointment, and write down all the pertinent info; otherwise, you'll be sure to forget the instructions once those contractions kick in.

Also, be sure you know the best route to your place of delivery, roughly how long it will take to get there at various times of the day, and what kind of transportation is available if you don't have someone to drive you (don't plan on driving yourself). And if there are other children at home, or an elderly relative, or a pet, be sure you've made plans for their care in advance.

Keep a copy of all the above information in the bag you're likely to be using and in the suitcase you've packed, as well as on your refrigerator door or bedside table.

---

or midwife—ordered, too. Many practitioners reason that having more distraction, support, and back-rubbing hands makes a mom-to-be happier and more relaxed during labor—always a good thing, whether it's a medicated birth or not.

Clearly, there are lots of good reasons why you might want an encouraging entourage in the birthing room with you. Still, there are a few caveats to consider before you issue the invites: You'll have to get the medical-powers-that-be to sign off on your guest list (not all practitioners are mob friendly, and some hospitals cap the number of guests you're allowed). You'll also have to be sure your spouse is on board with the guest list (remember, even though you'll be doing most of the work, both of you are co-hosting the party, and he won't want to be relegated to B-list). Think about, too, whether you'll really be comfortable with so many eyes on you during

a very private moment (there will be moaning, grunting, peeing, probably a little pooping—and you will be half-naked). Something else to ponder: Will those you've invited (your brother, your father-in-law, for example) be comfortable with what you're inviting them to view—and might their discomfort put you on edge when you most need to be relaxed? Will you want everyone standing around chatting when you're craving peace and quiet (and rest)? Will you feel obligated to entertain your guests when you need to be focused on birthing your baby?

If you decide you'd like the company, just remember to put flexibility on the list, too. Remember (and remind your guests) that there's always the possibility your intended uneventful vaginal birth may turn into an unexpected C-section, in which case only the expectant dad will be allowed to follow the party into the OR. Or that you'll decide—say somewhere around the second hour of pushing—that you're not up to guests anymore and they might be shown to the door for delivery. (And if you do end up regretting your decision to invite a crowd, don't worry about hurting anyone's feelings by sending the guests packing; as a woman in labor, your feelings are the only ones that matter.)

Not feeling like inviting a crowd? Don't let trends—or pushy relatives—guilt you into a full birthing room. What feels right for you and your spouse is the right decision.

Another Long Labor?

"I had a 30-hour labor my first time around and finally delivered after three hours of pushing. Though we both came out of it fine, I dread going through that again."

Anyone brave enough to go back into the ring after such a challenging first round deserves a break. And chances are good that you'll get one. Of course, though the odds of an easier childbirth are significantly improved the second time around, there are no sure bets in labor and delivery rooms. Your baby's position or other factors may alter these odds. Short of a crystal ball, there's no way to predict precisely what will happen this time around.

But second and subsequent labors and deliveries are usually easier and shorter than first ones—often dramatically so. Less resistance will be met from your now-roomier birth canal and your laxer muscles, and though the process won't be effortless—it rarely is—it probably will seem like less of an ordeal. The most marked difference may be in the amount of pushing you have to do; second babies often pop out in a matter of minutes rather than hours.

Mothering

"Now that the baby's almost here, I'm beginning to worry about how I'm going to take care of her. I've never even held a newborn before."

Most women aren't born mothers—any more than men are born fathers—instinctively knowing how to soothe a crying baby, change a diaper, or give a bath. Motherhood—parenthood, for that matter—is a learned art, one that requires plenty of practice to make perfect (or actually, near-perfect—since there's no such thing as a perfect parent).

Time was, women routinely practiced on other people's babies, caring for younger siblings or other infants in the family or the neighborhood, before they had their own. These days, though, many women—just like you—have never held a newborn until they hold their own. Their training for motherhood comes on the job, with a little help from parenting books, magazines, and websites, and, if they're lucky enough to find one locally, from a baby-care class. Which means that for the first week or two—and often much longer—a new mom can feel out of her element as the baby does more crying than sleeping, the diapers leak, and many tears are shed over the "no-tears" shampoo (on both sides of the bottle).

Slowly but surely—one dirty diaper, one marathon feeding session, one sleepless night at a time—every new mom (even the greenest) begins to feel like an old pro. Trepidation turns to assurance. The baby she was afraid to hold (won't it break?) is now cradled casually in her left arm while her right pays bills online or pushes the vacuum cleaner. She can dispense vitamin drops, give baths, and slip squirming arms and legs into onesies in her sleep—literally, sometimes. As she hits her maternal stride and settles into

What to Take to the Hospital or Birthing Center

Though you could show up with just your belly and your insurance card, traveling that empty-handed to the hospital or birthing center probably isn't the best idea. Traveling light, however, is (no need to lug a huge suitcase along with that big belly), so pack only what you think you'll really use or need. Be sure to pack that bag early (so you won't be turning the house upside down for your iPod when the contractions are coming five minutes apart) with as many—or as few—of the following as you'd like:

For the Labor or Birthing Room

- This book and *The What to Expect Pregnancy Journal and Organizer,* which has ample room for labor-and-delivery and meet-the-baby note keeping. A pen and pad may also be useful for jotting down questions and answers on procedures and on your condition and your baby's; instructions for when you go home; and the names of staff members who have taken care of you.

- Several copies of your birth plan, if you're using one (see page 294).

- A watch with a second hand for timing contractions. Better yet, make sure your coach is wearing one at all times during the last few weeks of your pregnancy.

- An MP3 player, iPod, or CD player, along with some of your favorite tunes, if music soothes and relaxes you.

- A camera and/or video equipment, if you don't trust your memory to capture the moment (and if the hospital or birthing center rules allow media coverage of births—most do). Don't forget extra batteries and/or chargers.

- Entertainment: a laptop, a Sudoku or crossword book, a handheld video game player, knitting, or whatever diversions you think will keep you from focusing too much on your labor.

- Favorite lotions, oils, or anything else you like for massages.

- A tennis ball or back massager, for firm countermassage, should lower backache be a problem.

- A pillow of your own to make you more comfortable during and after labor.

- Sugarless lollipops or candies to keep your mouth moist.

- A toothbrush, toothpaste, and mouthwash (you may find yourself desperate for a freshen-up after eight hours or so).

- Heavy socks, should your feet become cold.

a somewhat predictable rhythm, parenting an infant becomes second nature. She starts to feel like the mom she is, and—difficult though it may be to imagine right now—you will, too.

Though nothing can make those first days with a first baby a cinch, starting the learning process before your newborn is placed in your arms (and in your round-the-clock care) can make them seem a little less overwhelming. Any of the following can help moms- (and dads-) to-be ease into their new roles: visiting a newborn nursery and viewing the most

- Comfortable slippers with nonskid bottoms, in case you feel like doing some walking during labor, and so you can do some strolling in the halls later, between baby feedings.

- A scrunchie, clip, or hairband, if your hair is long, to keep it out of your face and tangle free. A hairbrush, too, if you think it'll come in handy.

- A couple of sandwiches or other snacks for your coach, so he won't have to leave your side when his stomach starts growling.

- A change of clothes for your coach, for comfort's sake and if he plans to sleep over in the hospital.

- A cell phone and charger (though you might not be allowed to use a cell in the room).

For Postpartum

- A robe and/or nightgowns/pj's, if you'd rather wear your own than the hospital's. Make sure it opens in the front if you'll be breastfeeding. Keep in mind, however, that though pretty nightgowns or comfy pj's can boost your spirits, they may get bled on and stained.

- Toiletries, including shampoo and conditioner, body wash, deodorant, hand mirror, makeup, and any other essentials of beauty and hygiene.

- Your favorite brand of maxipads, though the hospital will also provide some (skip the tampons).

- A couple of changes of underwear and a nursing bra.

- All the entertainment listed above, plus books (including a baby-name book if that decision's still up in the air).

- A supply of snacks: trail mix, soy chips, cereal bars, and other healthy treats to keep you from starving when the hospital food doesn't cut it or hunger strikes between meals.

- A list of phone numbers of family and friends to call with the good news; a phone card or calling card number in case you have no cell phone reception or the hospital doesn't allow cell phone usage.

- A going-home outfit for you, keeping in mind that you'll still be sporting a sizable belly (you'll probably look like you're at least five or six months pregnant right after the birth; plan accordingly).

- A going-home outfit for baby: a kimono or stretchie, T-shirt, booties, a receiving blanket, and a heavy bunting or blanket if it's cold; diapers will probably be provided by the hospital, but bring along an extra, just in case.

- Infant car seat. Most hospitals will not let you leave with the baby unless he or she is safely strapped into an approved rear-facing infant car seat. Besides, it's the law.

---

recent arrivals; holding, diapering, and soothing a friend's or family member's infant; reading up on a baby's first year; visiting first-year websites and message boards (no one can teach you more about being a mom than another mom; check out whattoexpect.com) and watching a DVD or taking a class in baby care (and baby CPR). For even more reassurance, talk to friends who have recently become parents. You'll be relieved to know that just about everybody comes into the job with the same new-mom (or new-dad) jitters.

Fill 'Er Up

Your kitchen, that is. Though shopping for strollers, diapers, and pint-size clothing understandably has been your priority these days, don't forget to take a time-out at the market. Even with swollen ankles and a super-size belly weighing you down, grocery and staple shopping is easier nine months pregnant than it will be again for a long time—so take advantage and stock up now so you won't have to later with baby (and car seat, and diaper bag) in tow. Fill your pantry, fridge, and freezer to the brim with healthy foods that are easy to serve—cheese sticks, individual containers of yogurt, frozen fruit bars, frozen fruit for making smoothies, cereal, granola bars, soups, dried fruit and nuts. Don't forget the paper products, too (you'll be using paper towels by the crateful, and disposable plates and cups can fill in when you don't get around to emptying the dishwasher). And while you're in the kitchen—and have the time—cook up some extra servings of your favorite freezer-friendly foods (lasagna, mini meatloaves, chili, pancakes, muffins), and store them in clearly marked single-meal containers in the freezer. They'll be ready to pop in the microwave when you're pooped (and hungry) postpartum.

ALL ABOUT

Prelabor, False Labor, Real Labor

It always seems so simple on TV. Somewhere around 3 A.M., the pregnant woman sits up in bed, puts a knowing hand on her belly, and reaches over to rouse her sleeping husband with a calm, almost serene, "Honey, it's time."

But how, you wonder, does this woman know it's time? How does she recognize labor with such cool, clinical confidence when she's never been in labor before? What makes her so sure she's not going to get to the hospital, be examined by the resident, found to be nowhere near her time, and be sent home, amid snickers from the night shift, just as pregnant as when she arrived? The script, of course.

On our side of the screen (with no script in hand), we're more likely to awaken at 3 A.M. with complete uncer-

tainty. Are these really labor pains or just more Braxton Hicks? Should I turn on the light and start timing? Should I bother to wake my spouse? Do I drag my practitioner out of bed at 1 A.M. to report what might really be false labor? If I do and it isn't time, will I turn out to be the pregnant woman who cried "labor" once too often, and will anybody take me seriously when it's for real? Or will I be the only woman in my childbirth class not to recognize labor? Will I leave for the hospital too late, maybe giving birth in the back of a taxicab (and ending up on the evening news)? The questions multiply faster than the contractions.

The fact is that most women, worry though they might, don't end up misjudging the onset of their labor. The vast majority, thanks to instinct, luck, or no-doubt-about-it killer contractions, show up at the hospital or birthing center neither too early nor too late, but at just about the right time. Still, there's no reason to leave your judgment up to chance. Becoming familiar in advance with the signs of prelabor, false labor, and real labor will help allay the concerns and clear up the confusion when those contractions (or are they?) begin.

Prelabor Symptoms

Before there's labor, there's prelabor—a sort of preshow that sets things up before the main event. The physical changes of prelabor can precede real labor by a full month or more—or by only an hour or so. Prelabor is characterized by the beginning of cervical effacement and dilation, which your practitioner can confirm on examination, as well as by a wide variety of related signs that you may notice yourself:

Dropping. Usually somewhere between two and four weeks before labor starts in first-time mothers, the fetus begins to settle down into the pelvis. This milestone is rarely reached in second or later births until labor is about to kick off.

Sensations of increasing pressure in the pelvis and rectum. Crampiness (similar to menstrual cramps) and groin pain are common—and particularly likely in second and later pregnancies. Persistent low backache may also be present.

Loss of weight or no gain. Weight gain might slow down in the ninth month; as labor approaches, you might even lose a bit of weight, up to 2 or 3 pounds.

A change in energy levels. Some ninth-monthers find that they are increasingly exhausted. Others experience energy spurts. An uncontrollable urge to scrub floors and clean out closets has been related to the "nesting instinct," in which the female of the species—that's you—prepares the nest for the impending arrival (see page 346).

A change in vaginal discharge. If you've been keeping track, you may find that your discharge increases and thickens.

Loss of the mucous plug. As the cervix begins to thin and open, the "cork" of mucus that seals the opening of the uterus becomes dislodged (see page 362). This gelatinous chunk of mucus can be passed through the vagina a week or two before the first real contractions, or just as labor begins.

Pink, or bloody, show. As the cervix effaces and dilates, capillaries frequently rupture, tinting the mucus pink or streaking it with blood (see page 363). This "show" usually means labor will start within 24 hours—though it could be as much as several days away.

Intensification of Braxton Hicks contractions. These practice contractions (see page 311) may become more frequent and stronger, even painful.

Diarrhea. Some women experience loose bowel movements just before labor starts.

False Labor Symptoms

Is it or isn't it? Real labor probably has not begun if:

■ Contractions are not at all regular and don't increase in frequency or severity. Real contractions won't necessarily fall into a neat textbook pattern, but they will become more intense and more frequent over time.

■ Contractions subside if you walk around or change your position (though this can sometimes be the case in early "real" labor, too).

■ Show, if any, is brownish. This kind of discharge is often the result of an internal exam or intercourse within the past 48 hours.

■ Fetal movements intensify briefly with contractions. (Let your practitioner know right away if activity becomes frantic or jerky.)

Keep in mind that false labor (though it isn't the real thing) isn't a waste of time—even if you've driven all the way to the hospital or birthing center. It's your body's way of getting pumped, primed, and prepped for the main event, so when the time comes, it'll be ready—whether you are or not.

Real Labor Symptoms

No one knows exactly what triggers real labor (and more women are concerned with "when" than "why"), but it's believed that a combination of factors are involved. This very intricate process begins with the fetus, whose brain sets off a relay of chemical messages (which probably translate into something like, "Mom, let me out of here!") that kick off a chain reaction of hormones in the mother. These hormonal changes in turn pave the way for the work of prostaglandins and oxytocin, substances that trigger contractions when all labor systems are "go."

You'll know that the contractions of prelabor have been replaced by true labor if:

■ The contractions intensify, rather than ease up, with activity and aren't relieved by a change in position.

■ Contractions become progressively more frequent and painful, and gen-erally (but not always) more regular. Every contraction won't necessarily be more painful or longer (they usually last about 30 to 70 seconds) than the last one, but the intensity does build up as real labor progresses. Frequency doesn't always increase in regular, perfectly even intervals, either—but it does increase.

■ Early contractions feel like gastroin-testinal upset, or like heavy menstrual cramps, or like lower abdominal pressure. Pain may be just in the lower abdomen or in the lower back and abdomen, and it may also radiate down into the legs (particularly the upper thighs). Location, however, is not as reliable an indication, because false labor contractions may also be felt in these places.

■ You have show and it's pinkish or blood-streaked.

In 15 percent of labors, the water breaks—in a gush or a trickle—before labor begins. But in many others, the membranes rupture spontaneously during labor, or are ruptured artificially by the practitioner.

When to Call the Practitioner

Your practitioner has likely told you when to call if you think you're in labor (when contractions are five to seven minutes apart, for instance). Don't wait for perfectly even intervals; they may never come. If you're not sure you're in real labor—but the contractions are coming pretty regularly—call anyway. Your practitioner will probably be able to tell from the sound of your voice, as you talk through a contraction, whether it's the real thing—but only if you don't try to cover up the pain in the name of good phone manners. Even if you've checked and rechecked the above lists and you're still unsure, call your practitioner. Don't feel guilty about waking him or her in the middle of the night (people who deliver babies for a living don't expect to work only 9 to 5) or be embarrassed if it turns out to be a false alarm (you wouldn't be the first expectant mom to misjudge her labor signs, and you won't be the last). Don't assume that if you're not sure it's real labor, it isn't. Err on the side of caution and call.

Also call your practitioner immediately if contractions are increasingly strong but your due date is still weeks

---

Ready or Not

To make sure you're ready for your baby's arrival when he or she is ready to arrive, start reading up now about labor and delivery in the next chapter.

---

away, if your water breaks but labor hasn't begun, if your water breaks and it has a greenish-brown tint, if you notice bright red blood, or if you feel the umbilical cord slip into your cervix or vagina.

Labor and Delivery

ARE YOU COUNTING DOWN THE days? Eager to see your feet again? Desperate to sleep on your stomach—or just plain desperate to sleep? Don't worry—the end (of pregnancy) is near. And as you contemplate that happy moment—when your baby will finally be in your arms instead of inside your belly—you're probably also giving a lot of thought to (and coming up with a lot of questions about) the process that will make that moment possible: labor and delivery. When will labor start, you're likely wondering? More important, when will it end? Will I be able to handle the pain? Will I need an epidural (and when can I have one)? A fetal moni-

tor? An episiotomy? What if I want to labor—and deliver—while squatting? Without any meds? What if I don't make any progress? What if I progress so quickly that I don't make it to the hospital or birthing center in time?

Armed with answers to these (and other) questions—plus the support of your partner and your birth attendants (doctors, midwives, nurses, doulas, and others)—you'll be prepared for just about anything that labor and delivery might bring your way. Just remember the most important thing that labor and delivery will bring your way (even if nothing else goes according to plan): that beautiful new baby of yours.

What You May Be Wondering About

Mucous Plug

"I think I lost my mucous plug. Should I call my doctor?"

Don't send out for the champagne just yet. The mucous plug—the clear, globby, gelatinous blob-like barrier that has corked your cervix throughout

your pregnancy—occasionally becomes dislodged as dilation and effacement begin. Some women notice the passage of the mucous plug (what exactly *is* that in the toilet?); others don't (especially if you're the flush-and-rush type). Though the passage of the plug is a sign that your body's preparing for the big day, it's not a reliable signal the big day has arrived—or even that it's around the corner. At this point, labor could be one or two days, or even weeks, away, with your cervix continuing to open gradually over that time. In other words, there's no need to call your practitioner or frantically pack your bags just yet.

No plug in your pants or your toilet? Not to worry. Many women don't lose it ahead of time (and others overlook it), and that doesn't predict anything about the eventual progress of labor.

Bloody Show

"I have a pink mucousy discharge. Does it mean labor's about to start?"

Sounds like it's bloody show time—and happily, this particular production is a preview of labor, not of a gory horror movie. Passing that bloody show, a mucous discharge tinged pink or brown with blood, is usually a sign that the blood vessels in the cervix are rupturing as it dilates and effaces and the process that leads to delivery is well under way (and that's something to applaud!). Once the bloody show has made its debut in your underwear or on the toilet paper, chances are your baby's arrival is just a day or two away. But since labor is a process with an erratic timetable, you'll be kept in suspense until the first true contractions strike.

If your discharge should suddenly become bright red, contact your practitioner right away.

Your Water Breaking

"I woke up in the middle of the night with a wet bed. Did I lose control of my bladder, or did my water break?"

A sniff of your sheets will probably clue you in. If the wet spot smells sort of sweet (not like urine, which has the harsher odor of ammonia), it's likely to be amniotic fluid. Another clue that the membranes surrounding your baby and containing the amniotic fluid he or she's been living in for nine months have probably ruptured: You continue leaking the pale, straw-colored fluid (which won't run dry because it continues to be produced until delivery, replacing itself every few hours). Another test: You can try to stem the flow of the fluid by squeezing your pelvic muscles (Kegel exercises). If the flow stops, it's urine. If it doesn't, it's amniotic fluid.

You are more likely to notice the leaking while you are lying down; it usually stops, or at least slows, when you stand up or sit down, since the baby's head acts as a cork, blocking the flow temporarily. The leakage is heavier—whether you're sitting or standing—if the break in the membranes is down near the cervix than if it is higher up.

Your practitioner has probably given you a set of instructions to follow if your water breaks. If you don't remember the instructions or have any doubts about how to proceed—call, night or day.

"My water just broke, but I haven't had any contractions. When is labor going to start, and what should I do in the meantime?"

It's likely that labor's on the way—and soon. Most women whose membranes rupture before labor begins can expect to feel the first contraction within 12 hours of that first trickle; most others can expect to feel it within 24 hours.

About 1 in 10, however, find that labor takes a little longer to get going. To prevent infection through the ruptured amniotic sac (the longer it takes for labor to get going, the greater the risk), most practitioners induce labor within 24 hours of a rupture, if a mom-to-be is at or near her due date, though a few induce as early as six hours after. Many women who have experienced a rupture actually welcome a sooner-than-later induction, preferring it to 24 hours of wet waiting.

The first thing to do if you experience a trickle or flow of fluid from your vagina—besides grab a towel and a box of maxipads—is call your practitioner (unless he or she has instructed otherwise). In the meantime, keep the vaginal area as clean as possible to avoid infection. Don't have sex (not that there's much chance you'd want to right now), use a pad (not a tampon) to absorb the flow, don't try to do your own internal exam, and, as always, wipe from front to back when you use the toilet.

Rarely, when the membranes rupture prematurely and the baby's presenting part is not yet engaged in the pelvis (more likely when the baby is breech or preterm), the umbilical cord can become "prolapsed"—it is swept into the cervix, or even down into the vagina, with the gush of amniotic fluid. If you can see a loop of umbilical cord at your vaginal opening, or think you feel something inside your vagina, call 911. For more on what to do if the cord is prolapsed, see page 565.

Darkened Amniotic Fluid

"My membranes ruptured, and the fluid isn't clear—it's greenish brown. What does this mean?"

Your amniotic fluid is probably stained with meconium, a greenish-brown substance that is actually your baby's first bowel movement. Ordinarily, meconium is passed after birth as the baby's first stool. But sometimes—such as when the fetus has been under stress in the womb, and more often when it is past its due date—the meconium is passed before birth into the amniotic fluid.

Meconium staining alone is not a sure sign of fetal distress, but because it suggests the possibility of distress, notify your practitioner right away. He or she will likely want to get labor started (if contractions aren't already in full swing) and will monitor your baby very closely throughout labor.

Low Amniotic Fluid During Labor

"My doctor said that my amniotic fluid is low and she needs to supplement it. Should I be concerned?"

Usually, nature keeps the uterus well stocked with a self-replenishing supply of amniotic fluid. Fortunately, even when levels do run low during labor, medical science can step in and supplement that natural source with a saline solution pumped directly into the amniotic sac through a catheter inserted through the cervix into the uterus. This procedure, called amnioinfusion, can significantly reduce the possibility that a surgical delivery will become necessary due to fetal distress.

Irregular Contractions

"In childbirth class we were told not to go to the hospital until the contractions were regular and five minutes apart. Mine are less than five minutes apart, but they aren't at all regular. I don't know what to do."

Just as no two women have exactly the same pregnancies, no two women have exactly the same labors. The labor often described in books, in childbirth education classes, and by practitioners is what is typical—close to what many women can expect. But far from every labor is true-to-textbook, with contractions regularly spaced and predictably progressive.

If you're having strong, long (20 to 60 seconds), frequent (mostly 5 to 7 minutes apart or less) contractions, even if they vary considerably in length and time elapsed between them, don't wait for them to become regular before calling your practitioner or heading for the hospital or birthing center—no matter what you've heard or read. It's possible your contractions are about as regular as they're going to get and you're well into the active phase of your labor.

Calling Your Practitioner During Labor

"I just started getting contractions and they're coming every three or four minutes. I feel silly calling my doctor, who said we should spend the first several hours of labor at home."

Better silly than sorry. It's true that most first-time mothers-to-be (whose labors are generally slow-going at first, with a gradual buildup of contractions) can safely count on spending the first several hours at home, leisurely finishing up their packing and their baby prep. But it doesn't sound like your labor's fitting that typical first-timer pattern. If your contractions have started off strong—lasting at least 45 seconds and coming more frequently than every 5 minutes—your first several hours of labor may very well be your last (and if you're not a first-timer, your labor may be on an even faster track). Chances are that much of the first stage of labor has

passed painlessly and your cervix has dilated significantly during that time. This means that not calling your practitioner, chancing a dramatic dash to the hospital or birthing center at the last minute—or not getting there in time—might be considerably sillier than picking up the phone now.

So by all means call. When you do, be clear and specific about the frequency, duration, and strength of your contractions. Since your practitioner is used to judging the phase of labor in part by the sound of a woman's voice as she talks through a contraction, don't try to downplay your discomfort, put on a brave front, or keep a calm tone when you describe what you're experiencing. Let the contractions speak for themselves, as loudly as they need to.

If you feel you're ready but your practitioner doesn't seem to think so, ask if you can go to the hospital/birthing center or to your practitioner's office and have your progress checked. Take your bag along just in case, but be ready to turn around and go home if you've only just begun to dilate—or if nothing's going on at all.

Not Getting to the Hospital in Time

"I'm afraid that I won't get to the hospital in time."

Fortunately, most of those sudden deliveries you've heard about take place in the movies and on TV. In real life, deliveries, especially those of first-time mothers, rarely occur without ample warning. But once in a great while, a woman who has had no labor pains, or just erratic ones, suddenly feels an overwhelming urge to bear down; often she mistakes it for a need to go to the bathroom.

Emergency Delivery if You're Alone

You'll almost certainly never need the following instructions—but just in case, keep them handy.

1. Try to remain calm. You can do this.

2. Call 911 (or your local emergency number) for the emergency medical service. Ask them to call your practitioner.

3. Find a neighbor or someone else to help, if possible.

4. Start panting to keep yourself from pushing.

5. Wash your hands and the vaginal area, if you can.

6. Spread some clean towels, newspapers, or sheets on a bed, sofa, or the floor, and lie down to await help (unlock the door so help can get in easily).

7. If despite your panting the baby starts to arrive before help does, gently ease him or her out by pushing each time you feel the urge.

8. As the top of the baby's head begins to appear, pant or blow (do not push), and apply very gentle counterpressure to your perineum to keep the head from popping out suddenly. Let the head emerge gradually—don't pull it out. If there is a loop of umbilical cord around the baby's neck, hook a finger under it and gently work it over the baby's head.

9. Next, take the head gently in two hands and press it very slightly downward (do not pull), pushing the baby out at the same time, to deliver the front shoulder. As the upper arm appears, lift the head carefully, feeling for the rear shoulder to deliver. Once the shoulders are free, the rest of your baby should slip out easily.

10. Place the baby on your abdomen or, if the cord is long enough (don't tug at it), on your chest. Quickly wrap the baby in blankets, towels, or anything else that's clean.

11. Wipe baby's mouth and nose with a clean cloth. If help hasn't arrived and the baby isn't breathing or crying, rub his or her back, keeping the head lower than the feet. If breathing still hasn't started, clear out the mouth some more with a clean finger and give two quick and extremely gentle puffs of air into his or her nose and mouth.

12. Don't try to pull the placenta out. But if it emerges on its own before emergency assitance arrives, wrap it in towels or newspaper, and keep it elevated above the level of the baby, if possible. There is no need to try to cut the cord.

13. Keep yourself and your baby warm and comfortable until help arrives.

As remote as the possibility is that this will happen to you, it's a good idea for both you and your coach to become familiar with the basics of an emergency delivery (see boxes, above and on page 370). Once that's done, relax, knowing that a sudden and quick delivery is an extremely remote possibility.

Having a Short Labor

"I always hear about women who have really short labors. How common are they?"

While they make for really good labor stories, not all of the short labors you've heard about are as short as they seemed. Often, an expectant mom who appears to have a quickie labor has actually been having painless contractions for hours, days, even weeks, contractions that have been dilating her cervix gradually. By the time she finally feels one, she's well into the final stage of labor.

That said, occasionally the cervix dilates very rapidly, accomplishing in a matter of minutes what the average cervix (particularly a first-time mom's cervix) takes hours to do. And happily, even with this abrupt, or precipitous, kind of labor (one that takes three hours or less from start to finish), there is usually no risk to the baby.

If your labor seems to start with a bang—with contractions strong and close together—get to the hospital or birthing center quickly (so you and your baby can be monitored closely). Medication may be helpful in slowing contractions a bit and easing the pressure on your baby and on your own body.

Back Labor

"The pain in my lower back since my contractions began is so bad that I don't see how I'll be able to make it through labor."

What you're probably experiencing is known in the birthing business as "back labor." Technically, back labor occurs when the fetus is in a posterior position, with its face up and the back of its head pressing against your sacrum, or the back of your pelvis. (Ironically, this position is nicknamed "sunny-side up" in birthing circles—though there's nothing cheerful about back labor.) It's possible, however, to experience back labor when the baby isn't in this position or to continue to experience it after the baby has turned

to a head-to-the-front position—possibly because the area has already become a focus of tension.

When you're having this kind of pain—which often doesn't let up between contractions and can become excruciating during them—the cause doesn't matter much. How to relieve it, even slightly, does. If you're opting to have an epidural, go for it (there's no need to wait, especially if you're in a lot of pain). It's possible that you might need a higher dose than usual to get full comfort from the back labor pain, so let the anesthesiologist know about it. Other options (such as narcotics) also offer pain relief. If you'd like to stay med free, several measures may help relieve the discomfort of back labor; all are at least worth trying:

Taking the pressure off. Try changing your position. Walk around (though this may not be possible once contractions are coming fast and furious), crouch or squat, get down on all fours, do whatever is most comfortable and least painful for you. If you feel you can't move and would prefer to be lying down, lie on your side, with your back well rounded—in a sort of fetal position.

Heat or cold. Have your coach (or doula or nurse) use warm compresses, a heating pad, or ice packs or cold compresses—whichever soothes best. Or alternate heat and cold.

Counterpressure and massage. Have your coach experiment with different ways of applying pressure to the area of greatest pain, or to adjacent areas, to find one or more that seem to help. He can try his knuckles, the heel of one hand reinforced by pressure from the other hand on top of it, a tennis ball, or a back massager, using direct pressure or a firm circular motion. Pressure or a firm massage can be applied while you're sitting or while you're lying on your side. Cream, oil, or powder can be applied periodically to reduce possible irritation.

Reflexology. For back labor, this therapy involves applying strong finger pressure just below the center of the ball of the foot.

Other alternative pain relievers. Hydrotherapy can definitely ease the pain somewhat. If you've had some experience with meditation, visualization, or self-hypnosis for pain, try these, too. They often work, and they certainly couldn't hurt. Acupuncture can also help, but you'll have to arrange ahead of time to have a therapist on call when you go into labor.

Labor Induction

"My doctor wants to induce labor. But I'm not overdue yet and I thought induction was only for overdue babies."

Sometimes Mother Nature needs a little help making a mother out of a pregnant woman. About 20 percent of pregnancies end up needing that kick in the maternity pants, and though a lot of the time induction is necessary because a baby is overdue, there are many other reasons why your practitioner might feel that nature needs a nudge, such as:

- Your membranes have ruptured and contractions have not started on their own within 24 hours (though some practitioners induce much sooner).

- Tests suggest that your uterus is no longer a healthy home for your baby because the placenta is no longer functioning optimally or amniotic fluid levels are low, or for another reason.

- Tests suggest that the baby isn't thriving and is mature enough to be delivered.

- You have a complication, such as preeclampsia or gestational diabetes, or a chronic or acute illness, that makes it risky to continue your pregnancy.

- There's a concern that you might not make it to the hospital or birthing center on time once labor has started, either because you live a long distance away or because you've had a previous very short labor.

If you're still unsure about your doctor's reasons for inducing labor, ask for a better explanation. To find out all you'll need to know about the induction process, keep reading.

"How does induction work?"

Induction, like naturally triggered labor, is a process—and sometimes a pretty long process. But unlike naturally triggered labor, your body will be getting some help with the heavy lifting if you're induced. Labor induction usually involves a number of steps (though you won't necessarily go through all of them):

- First, your cervix will need to be ripened (or softened) so that labor can begin. If you arrive with a ripe cervix, great—you'll probably move right on to the next step. If your cervix is not dilated, not effaced, and not soft at all, your practitioner will likely administer a hormonal substance such as prostaglandin E in the form of a vaginal gel (or a vaginal suppository in tablet form) to get things started. In this painless procedure, a syringe is used to place the gel in the vagina close to your cervix. After a few hours or longer of letting the gel do its work, you'll be checked to see if your cervix is getting softer and beginning to efface and dilate. If it isn't, a second dose of the prostaglandin gel is administered. In many cases, the gel is enough to get contractions and labor started. If your cervix is ripe enough but contractions have not begun, the induction process continues. (Note: Some practitioners use mechanical agents to ripen the cervix, such as a catheter with an inflatable balloon, graduated dilators to gently stretch the cervix, or even a botanical—called Laminaria japonicum—that, when inserted, gradually opens the cervix as it absorbs fluid around it.)

- If the amniotic sac is still intact, your practitioner may strip the membranes by swiping a finger across the fine membranes that connect the amniotic sac to the uterus to release prostaglandin (this process isn't always pain free, and while it isn't meant to break your water, it sometimes does). Or he or she may artificially rupture your membranes (see page 373) to try to get labor started.

- If neither the prostaglandin nor the stripping or rupturing of the membranes has brought on regular contractions, your practitioner will slowly administer intravenous Pitocin, a synthetic form of the hormone oxytocin (which is produced naturally by the body throughout pregnancy and also plays an important role in labor), until contractions are well established. The drug misoprostol, given through the vagina, might be used as an alternative to other ripening and induction techniques. Some research shows giving misoprostol decreases the amount of oxytocin needed and shortens labor.

- Your baby will be continuously monitored to assess how he or she is dealing with labor. You'll also be monitored to make sure the drug isn't overstimulating your uterus, triggering contractions that are too long or powerful. If that happens, the rate of infusion

can be reduced or the process can be discontinued entirely. Once your contractions are in full swing, the oxytocin may be stopped or the dose decreased, and your labor should progress just as a noninduced labor does.

- If, after 8 to 12 hours of oxytocin administration, labor hasn't begun or progressed, your practitioner might stop the induction process to give you a chance to rest before trying again or, depending on the circumstances, the procedure may be stopped in favor of a cesarean delivery.

Eating and Drinking During Labor

"I've heard conflicting stories about whether it's okay to eat and drink during labor."

Should eating be on the agenda when you're in labor? That depends on who you're talking to. Some practitioners red-light all food and drink during labor, on the theory that food in the digestive tract might be aspirated, or "breathed in," should emergency general anesthesia be necessary. These practitioners usually okay ice chips only, supplemented as needed by intravenous fluids. Many other practitioners do allow liquids and light solids (read: no stuffed-crust pizza) during a low-risk labor, reasoning that a woman in labor needs both fluids and calories to stay strong and do her best work, and that the risk of aspiration (which only exists if general anesthesia is used, and it rarely is except in emergency situations) is extremely low: 7 in 10 million births. Their position has even been backed up by research, which shows that women who are allowed to eat and drink during labor have shorter labors by an average of 90 minutes, are less likely to need

Emergency Delivery: Tips for the Coach

At Home or in the Office

1. Try to remain calm while at the same time comforting and reassuring the mother. Remember, even if you don't know the first thing about delivering a baby, a mother's body and her baby can do most of the job on their own.

2. Call 911 (or your local emergency number) for the emergency medical service; ask them to call the practitioner.

3. Have the mother start panting, to keep from pushing.

4. If there's time, wash your hands and the vaginal area with soap and water (use an antibacterial product, if you have one handy).

5. If there is time, place the mother on the bed (or desk or table) so her buttocks are slightly hanging off, her hands under her thighs to keep them elevated. If available, a couple of chairs can support her feet. A few pillows or cushions under her shoulders and head will help to raise her to a semi-sitting position, which can aid delivery. If you are awaiting emergency help and the baby's head hasn't appeared, having the mother lie flat may slow delivery until help arrives.

Protect delivery surfaces, if possible, with a plastic tablecloth, shower curtain, newspapers, towels, or similar material. A dishpan or basin can be placed under the mother's vagina to catch the amniotic fluid and blood.

6. If there's no time to get to a bed or table, place newspapers or clean towels or folded clothing under the mother's buttocks. Protect delivery surfaces, if possible, as described in number 5.

7. As the top of the baby's head begins to appear, instruct the mother to pant or blow (not push), and apply very gentle counterpressure to her perineum (the area between the vagina and the anus) to keep the head from popping out suddenly. Let the head emerge gradually—never pull it out. If there is a loop of umbilical cord around the baby's neck, hook a finger under it and gently work it over the baby's head.

8. Next, take the head gently in two hands and press it very slightly downward (do not pull), asking the mother to push at the same time, to deliver the front shoulder. As the upper arm appears, lift the head carefully, watching for the rear shoulder to deliver. Once the shoulders are free, the rest of the baby should slip out easily.

9. Place the baby on the mother's abdomen or, if the cord is long enough (don't tug at it), on her chest. Quickly wrap the baby in blankets, towels, or anything else that's clean.

---

oxytocin to speed up labor, require fewer pain medications, and have babies with higher Apgar scores than women who fast. Check with your practitioner to find out what will and won't be on the menu for you during labor.

Even if your practitioner gives you the go-ahead on eating, chances are you won't be in the market for a major meal once the contractions begin in earnest (and besides, you'll be pretty distracted). After all, labor can really spoil your appetite. Still, an occasional light, easy-to-digest snack during the early hours of labor—Popsicles, Jell-O, applesauce, cooked fruit, plain pasta, toast with jam, or clear broth are ideal choices—may help keep your energy

10. Wipe baby's mouth and nose with a clean cloth. If help hasn't arrived and the baby isn't breathing or crying, rub his or her back, keeping the head lower than the feet. If breathing still hasn't started, clear out the mouth some more with a clean finger, and give two quick and extremely gentle puffs of air into his or her nose and mouth.

11. Don't try to pull the placenta out. But if it emerges on its own before emergency assistance arrives, wrap it in towels or newspaper, and keep it elevated above the level of the baby, if possible. There is no need to try to cut the cord.

12. Keep both mother and baby warm and comfortable until help arrives.

En Route to the Hospital

If you're in your car and delivery is imminent, pull over to a safe area. If you have a cell phone with you, call for help. If not, turn on your hazard warning lights or turn signal. If someone stops to help, ask him or her to call 911 or the local emergency medical service. If you're in a cab, ask the driver to radio or use his cell phone to call for help.

If possible, help the mother into the back of the car. Place a coat, jacket, or blanket under her. Then, if help has not arrived, proceed as for a home delivery. As soon as the baby is born, proceed to the nearest hospital.

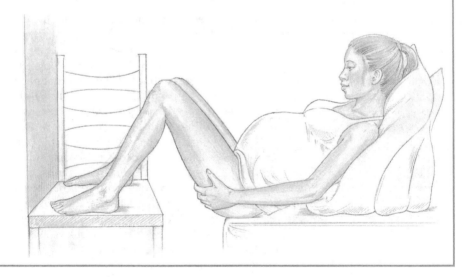

up at a time when you need it most (you probably won't be able to, or won't want to, eat during the later parts of active labor). When deciding—with your practitioner's help—what to eat and when, also keep in mind that labor can make you feel pretty nauseous. Some women throw up as labor progresses, even if they haven't been eating.

Whether you can chow down or not during labor, your coach definitely can—and should (you don't want him weak from hunger when you need him most). Remind him to have a meal before you head off to the hospital or birthing center (his mind's probably on your belly, not his) and to pack a bunch of snacks to take along so he won't have to leave your side when his stomach starts growling.

Routine IV

"Is it true that I'll be hooked up to an IV as soon as I'm admitted into the hospital when I'm in labor?"

That depends a lot on the policies of the hospital you'll be delivering in. In some hospitals, it's routine to give all women in labor an IV, a flexible catheter placed in your vein (usually in the back of your hand or lower arm) to drip in fluids and medication. The reason is precautionary—to prevent dehydration, as well as to save a step later on in case an emergency arises that necessitates medication (there's already a line in place to administer drugs—no extra poking or prodding required). Other hospitals and practitioners omit routine IVs and instead wait until there is a clear need before hooking you up. Check your practitioner's policy in advance, and if you strongly object to having a routine IV, say so. It may be possible to hold off until the need, if any, comes up.

You'll definitely get an IV if an epidural is on the agenda. IV fluids are routinely administered before and during the placement of an epidural to reduce the chance of a drop in blood pressure, a common side effect of this pain relief route. The IV also allows for easier administration of Pitocin should labor need to be augmented.

If you end up with a routine IV or an IV with epidural that you were hoping to avoid, you'll probably find it's not all that intrusive. The IV is only slightly uncomfortable as the needle is inserted and after that should barely be noticed. When it's hung on a movable stand, you can take it with you to the bathroom or on a stroll down the hall. If you very

strongly don't want an IV but hospital policy dictates that you receive one, ask your practitioner whether a heparin lock might be an option for you.

With a heparin lock, a catheter is placed in the vein, a drop of the blood-thinning medication heparin is added to prevent clotting, and the catheter is locked off. This option gives the hospital staff access to an open vein should an emergency arise but doesn't hook you up to an IV pole unnecessarily—a good compromise in certain situations.

Fetal Monitoring

"Will I have to be hooked up to a fetal monitor the whole time I'm in labor? What's the point of it anyway?"

For someone who's spent the first nine months of his or her life floating peacefully in a warm and comforting amniotic bath, the trip through the narrow confines of the maternal pelvis will be no joyride. Your baby will be squeezed, compressed, pushed, and molded with every contraction. And though most babies sail through the birth canal without a problem, others find the stress of being squeezed, compressed, pushed, and molded too difficult, and they respond with decelerations in heart rate, rapid or slowed-down movement, or other signs of fetal distress. A fetal monitor assesses how your baby is handling the stresses of labor by gauging the response of its heartbeat to the contractions of the uterus.

But does that assessment need to be continuous? Most experts say no, citing research showing that for low-risk women with unmedicated deliveries, intermittent fetal heart checks using a Doppler or fetal monitor are an effective way to assess a baby's condition. So if you fit in that category, you probably won't have to be attached to a fetal monitor for the entire duration of your labor. If, however, you're being induced, have an epidural, or have certain risk factors (such as meconium staining), you're most likely going to be hooked up to an electronic fetal monitor throughout your labor.

There are three types of continuous fetal monitoring:

External monitoring. In this type of monitoring, used most frequently, two devices are strapped to the abdomen. One, an ultrasound transducer, picks up the fetal heartbeat. The other, a pressure-sensitive gauge, measures the intensity and duration of uterine contractions. Both are connected to a monitor, and the measurements are recorded on a digital and paper readout. When you're connected to an external monitor, you'll be able to move around in your bed or on a chair nearby, but you won't have complete freedom of movement, unless telemetry monitoring is being used (see this page).

During the second (pushing) stage of labor, when contractions may come so fast and furious that it's hard to know when to push and when to hold back, the monitor can be used to accurately signal the beginning and end of each contraction. Or the use of the monitor may be all but abandoned during this stage, so as not to interfere with your concentration. In this case, your baby's heart rate will be checked periodically with a Doppler.

Internal monitoring. When more accurate results are required—such as when there is reason to suspect fetal distress—an internal monitor may be used. In this type of monitoring, a tiny electrode is inserted through your vagina onto your baby's scalp, and a catheter is placed in your uterus or an external pressure gauge is strapped to your abdomen to measure the strength of your contrac-

tions. Though internal monitoring gives a slightly more accurate record of the baby's heart rate and your contractions than an external monitor, it's only used when necessary (since its use comes with a slight risk of infection). Your baby may have a small bruise or scratch where the electrode was attached, but it'll heal in a few days. You'll be more limited in your movement with an internal monitor, but you'll still be able to move from side to side.

Telemetry monitoring. Available only in some hospitals, this type of monitoring uses a transmitter on your thigh to transmit the baby's heart tones (via radio waves) to the nurse's station—allowing you to take a lap or two around the hallway while still having constant monitoring.

Be aware that with both internal and external types of monitoring, false alarms are common. The machine can start beeping loudly if the transducer has slipped out of place, if the baby has shifted positions, if the monitor isn't working right, or if contractions have suddenly picked up in intensity. Your practitioner will take all these factors and others into account before concluding that your baby really is in trouble. If the abnormal readings do continue, several other assessments can be performed (such as fetal scalp stimulation) to determine the cause of the distress. If fetal distress is confirmed, then cesarean delivery is usually called for.

Artificial Rupture of Membranes

"I'm afraid that if my water doesn't break on its own, the doctor will have to rupture the membranes artificially. Won't that hurt?"

Most women actually don't feel a thing when their membranes are artificially ruptured, particularly if they're already in labor (there are far more significant pains to cope with then). If you do experience a little discomfort, it'll more likely be from the introduction into the vagina of the Amniohook (the long plastic device that looks like a sharp-pointed crochet hook and is used to perform the procedure) than from the rupture itself. Chances are, all you'll really notice is a gush of water, followed soon—at least that's the hope—by harder and faster contractions that will get your baby moving. Artificial rupture of the membranes is also performed to allow for other procedures, such as internal fetal monitoring, when necessary.

Though the latest research seems to indicate that artificially rupturing the membranes doesn't shorten the length of labor or decrease the need for Pitocin, many practitioners still turn to artificial rupture in an attempt to help move a sluggish labor along. If there's no compelling reason to rupture them (labor's moving along just fine), you and your practitioner may decide to hold off and let them rupture naturally. Occasionally, membranes stay stubbornly intact throughout delivery (the baby arrives with the bag of waters still surrounding him or her, which means it will need to be ruptured right after birth), and that's fine, too.

An Episiotomy

"I heard episiotomies aren't routine anymore. Is that true?"

Happily, you've heard right. An episiotomy—a surgical cut in your perineum (the muscular area between your vagina and your anus) to enlarge the vaginal opening just before the baby's head emerges—is no longer performed routinely at delivery. These days, in fact,

midwives and most doctors rarely make the cut without a good reason.

It wasn't always that way. The episiotomy was once thought to prevent spontaneous tearing of the perineum and postpartum urinary and fecal incontinence, as well as reduce the risk in the newborn of birth trauma (from the baby's head pushing long and hard against the perineum). But it's now known that infants fare just fine without an episiotomy, and mothers, too, seem to do better without it. An average total labor doesn't seem to be any longer, and mothers often experience less blood loss, less infection, and less perineal pain after delivery without an episiotomy (though you can still have blood loss and infection with a tear). What's more, research has shown that episiotomies are more likely than spontaneous tears to turn into serious third- or fourth-degree tears (those that go close to or through the rectum, sometimes causing fecal incontinence).

But while routine episiotomies are no longer recommended, there is still a place for them in certain birth scenarios. Episiotomies may be indicated when a baby is large and needs a roomier exit route, when the baby needs to be delivered rapidly, when forceps or vacuum delivery need to be performed, or for the relief of shoulder dystocia (a shoulder gets stuck in the birth canal during delivery).

If you do need an episiotomy, you'll get an injection (if there's time) of local pain relief before the cut, though you may not need a local if you're already anesthetized from an epidural or if your perineum is thinned out and already numb from the pressure of your baby's head during crowning. Your practitioner will then take surgical scissors and make either a median (also called midline) incision (a cut made directly toward the rectum) or a mediolateral incision (which slants away from the rectum).

After delivery of your baby and the placenta, the practitioner will stitch up the cut (you'll get a shot of local pain medication if you didn't receive one before or if your epidural has worn off).

To reduce the possibility that you'll need an episiotomy and to ease delivery without one, some midwives recommend perineal massage (see page 352) for a few weeks before your due date if you're a first-time mom. (If you've delivered vaginally before, you're already stretched, so do-ahead massage probably won't accomplish much.) During labor, the following can also help: warm compresses to lessen perineal discomfort, perineal massage, standing or squatting and exhaling or grunting while pushing to facilitate stretching of the perineum. During the pushing phase, your practitioner will probably use perineal support—applying gentle counterpressure to the perineum so your baby's head doesn't push out too quickly and cause an unnecessary tear.

If you haven't already, discuss the episiotomy issue with your practitioner. It's very likely he or she will agree that the procedure should not be performed unless there's a good reason. Document your feelings about episiotomies in your birth plan, too, if you like. But keep in mind that, very occasionally, episiotomies do turn out to be necessary, and the final decision should be made in the delivery or birthing room—when that cute little head is crowning.

Forceps

"How likely will it be that I'll need forceps during delivery?"

Pretty unlikely these days. Forceps—long curved tong-like devices designed to help a baby make his or her descent down the birth canal—are used in only a very small percentage of deliveries (vacuum extraction is more common; see next question). But if your practitioner does decide to use forceps, rest assured; they are as safe as a C-section or vacuum extraction when used correctly by an experienced practitioner (many younger doctors have not been trained in their use, and some are reluctant to use them).

Forceps are considered when a laboring mom is just plain exhausted or if she has a heart condition or very high blood pressure that might make strenuous pushing harmful to her health. They might also be used if the baby needs to be delivered in a hurry because of fetal distress (assuming the baby is in a favorable position—for example, close to crowning) or if the baby's in an unfavorable position during the pushing stage (the forceps can be used to rotate the baby's head to facilitate the birth).

Your cervix will have to be fully dilated, your bladder empty, and your membranes ruptured before forceps are used. Then you'll be numbed with a local anesthetic (unless you already have an epidural in place). You'll also likely receive an episiotomy to enlarge the vaginal opening to allow for placement of the forceps. The curved tongs of the forceps will then be cradled one at a time around the temples of the baby's crowning head, locked into position, and used to gently deliver the baby. There may be some bruising or swelling on the baby's scalp from the forceps, but it will usually go away within a few days after birth.

If your practitioner attempts delivery with forceps, but the attempt is unsuccessful, you'll likely undergo a C-section.

Vacuum Extraction

"My friend's ob used a vacuum extractor to help deliver her baby. Is that the same as forceps?"

It does the same job. The vacuum extractor is a plastic cup placed on the baby's head, and it uses gentle suction to help guide him or her out of the birth canal. The suction prevents the baby's head from moving back up the birth canal between contractions and can be used to help mom out while she is pushing during contractions. Vacuum extraction is used in about 5 percent of deliveries and offers a good alternative to both forceps and C-section under the right circumstances.

Your practitioner would use vacuum extraction for the same reason forceps would be used during delivery (see previous question). Vacuum deliveries are associated with less trauma to the vagina (and possibly a lower chance of needing an episiotomy) and less need for local anesthesia than forceps, which is another reason why more practitioners opt for them over forceps these days.

Babies born with vacuum extraction experience some swelling on the scalp, but it usually isn't serious, doesn't require treatment, and goes away within a few days. As with forceps, if the vac-

uum extractor isn't working successfully to help deliver the baby, a cesarean delivery is recommended.

If during delivery your doctor suggests the need for vacuum extraction to speed things up, you might want to ask if you can rest for several contractions (time permitting) before trying again; such a break might give you the second wind you need to push your baby out effectively. You can also try changing your position: Get up on all fours, or squat; the force of gravity might shift the baby's head.

Before you go into labor, ask your practitioner any questions you have about the possible use of vacuum extraction (or forceps). The more you know, the better prepared you'll be for anything that comes your way during childbirth.

Labor Positions

"I know you're not supposed to lie flat on your back during labor. But what position is best?"

There's no need to take labor lying down, and in fact, lying flat on your back is probably the least efficient way to birth your baby: first because you're not enlisting gravity's help to get your baby out, and second because there's the risk of compressing major blood vessels (and possibly interfering with blood flow to the fetus) when you're on your back. Expectant mothers are encouraged to labor in any other position that feels comfortable, and to change their position as often as they can (and want to). Getting a move on during labor, as well as varying your position often, not only eases discomfort but may also yield speedier results.

You can choose from any of the following labor and delivery postures (or variations of these):

Vacuum Extractor

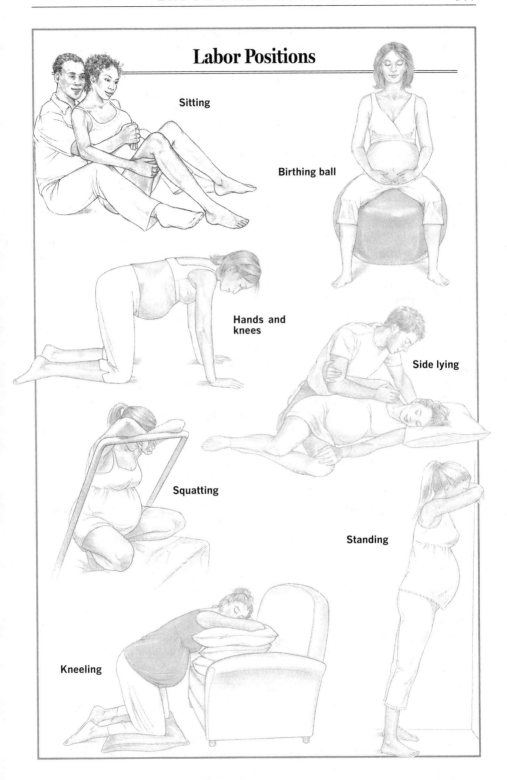

Labor Positions

Sitting

Birthing ball

Hands and knees

Side lying

Squatting

Standing

Kneeling

Standing or walking. Getting vertical not only helps relieve the pain of contractions but also takes advantage of gravity, which may allow your pelvis to open and your baby to move down into your birth canal. While it's unlikely you'll be heading for the track once contractions are coming fast and furious, walking (or just leaning against a wall or your coach) during the early stages of labor can be an effective move.

Rocking. Sure, your baby's not even born yet, but he or she will still enjoy a little rocking—as will you, especially when those contractions start coming. Slip into a chair or remain upright, and sway back and forth. The rocking motion may allow your pelvis to move and encourage the baby to descend. And again, staying upright allows you to use the force of gravity to help in the process.

Squatting. You probably won't be able to stand and deliver, but once you get closer to the pushing phase of childbirth, you might want to consider squatting. There's a reason why women have delivered their babies in a squatting position for centuries: It works. Squatting allows the pelvis to open wide, giving your baby more room to move on down. You can use your partner for squatting support (you'll probably be a little wobbly, so you'll need all the support you can get), or you can use a squatting bar, which is often attached to the birthing bed (leaning on the bar will keep your legs from tiring out as you squat).

Birthing balls. Sitting or leaning on one of these large exercise balls can help open up your pelvis—and it's a lot easier than squatting for long periods.

Sitting. Whether in bed (the back of the birthing bed can be raised so you're almost sitting upright), in your partner's arms, or on a birthing ball, sitting can ease the pain of contractions and may allow gravity to help bring your baby down into the birth canal. You might also consider a birthing chair, if one is available, which is specifically designed to support a woman in a sitting or squatting position during delivery and, theoretically, speed labor. Another plus: Moms get to see more of the birth in this position.

Kneeling. Got back labor? Kneeling over a chair or over your spouse's shoulders is a great position when the back of the baby's head is pushing against your spine. It encourages the baby to move forward, taking that load off your back. Even if you don't have back labor, kneeling can be an effective labor and delivery position. Because kneeling allows you to shift and transfer some of the pressure toward the lower spine while you push your baby out, it seems to reduce childbirth pain even more than sitting does.

Hands and knees. Getting on all fours is another way to cope more comfortably with back labor—and to help get that puppy out faster. This position allows you to do pelvic tilts for comfort, while giving your spouse or doula access to your back for massage and counterpressure. You might even consider delivering in this position (no matter what kind of labor you're having), since it opens up the pelvis and uses gravity to coax baby down.

Side lying. Too tired to sit? Or squat? Just need to lie down? Lying on your side is much better than lying on your back, since it doesn't compress the major veins in your body. It's also a good delivery option, helping to slow a too-fast birth as well as easing the pain of some contractions.

Remember that the best labor position is the one that's best for you. And what's best in the early stages of labor might make you miserable when you're in the throes of transition, so change positions as often—or as little—as you want. If you're being continuously monitored, your positions are somewhat limited. It'll be hard to walk, for instance—but you'll have no problem squatting, rocking, sitting, getting on your hands and knees, or lying on your side. Even if you have an epidural, sitting, side lying, or rocking are options available to you.

Being Stretched by Childbirth

"I'm concerned about stretching during delivery. Will my vagina ever be the same again?"

Mother Nature definitely had mothers in mind when she thought up vaginas. Their incredible elasticity and accordion-like folds allow this amazing organ to open up for childbirth (and the passage of that 7- or 8-pound baby) and then—over a period of weeks following delivery—return to close to original size. In other words, your vagina's definitely designed to take it.

The perineum is also elastic but less so than the vagina. Massage during the months prior to delivery may help increase its elasticity and reduce stretching (though don't go overboard; see page 352). Likewise, exercising the pelvic muscles with Kegels during this period may enhance their elasticity, strengthen them, and speed their return to normal tone.

Most women find that the slight increase in vaginal roominess typically experienced postpartum is imperceptible and doesn't interfere at all with sexual enjoyment. For those who were previously too snug, that extra room can be a real plus—making sex more of a pleasure and in some cases, literally,

Apgar Score

The Apgar score is your baby's first test, and it's a way to quickly evaluate your newborn's condition. At one minute and again at five minutes after birth, a nurse, midwife, or doctor check the infant's Appearance (color), Pulse (heartbeat), Grimace (reflex), Activity (muscle tone), and Respiration. Babies who score above 6, which most babies do, are fine. Those who score between 4 and 6 often need resuscitation, which generally includes suctioning their airways and administering oxygen. Those who score under 4 require more dramatic lifesaving techniques.

less of a pain. Very occasionally, however, in a woman who was "just right" before, childbirth does stretch the vagina enough that sexual satisfaction decreases. Often, the vaginal muscles tighten up again in time. Doing Kegels faithfully and frequently helps speed that process. If six months after delivery you still find that your vagina's too slack for comfort, talk to your doctor about other possible treatments.

The Sight of Blood

"The sight of blood makes me feel faint. I'm not sure if I'll be able to handle watching my delivery."

Here's some good news for the squeamish. First of all, there isn't all that much blood during childbirth— not much more than you see when you've got your period. Second, you're not really a spectator at your delivery; you'll be a very active participant, putting every ounce of your concentration and energy into pushing your baby those last few inches. Caught up in the excitement and anticipation (and, let's face it, the pain and fatigue), you're unlikely to notice, much less be unsettled by, any bleeding. If you ask friends who are new mothers, few will be able to tell you just how much blood, if any, there was at their deliveries.

If you still feel strongly that you don't want to see any blood, simply keep your eyes off the mirror at the moment of birth (and look away, too,

if an episiotomy is performed). Instead, just look down past your belly for a good view of your baby as he or she emerges. From this vantage point, virtually no blood will be visible. But before you decide to opt out of watching your own delivery, watch someone else's by viewing a childbirth DVD. You'll probably be much more amazed than horrified.

Some fathers, too, worry about how they'll handle viewing the birth. If your spouse is anxious about this aspect of delivery, have him read page 483.

have him read page 483.

ALL ABOUT
Childbirth

Delivering a baby is the challenge of a lifetime, but it's also an emotional and physical rush like no other. It's an experience that you may be looking ahead to with trepidation (and maybe a little dread), but that you'll

likely look back on—once it's all said, done, and delivered—with nothing but the purest joy (and maybe a little relief).

Fortunately, you won't be going it alone. In addition to the support of

Stages and Phases of Childbirth

Childbirth progresses in three stages: labor, delivery of the baby, and delivery of the placenta. Unless labor is cut short (or eliminated) by a C-section, all women go through the labor stage, which includes early labor, active labor, and transitional labor. The timing and intensity of the contractions can help pinpoint which phase of labor you're in at any particular time, and so can some of the symptoms you're experiencing along the way. Periodic internal exams will confirm the progress.

Stage One: Labor

Phase 1: Early (Latent)—thinning (effacement) and opening (dilation) of the cervix to 3 cm; contractions are 30 to 45 seconds long, 20 minutes apart or less.

Phase 2: Active—dilation of cervix to 7 cm; contractions are 40 to 60 seconds long, coming 3 to 4 minutes apart.

Phase 3: Transitional—dilation of cervix to 10 cm (fully dilated); contractions are 60 to 90 seconds long, about 2 to 3 minutes apart.

Stage Two: Delivery of the baby

Stage Three: Delivery of the placenta

your coach, you'll have plenty of medical professionals on the scene, too. But even with all that expertise in your camp, it'll help to have some know-how of your own.

After nine months at it—graduating from queasiness and bloating to heartburn and backache—you almost certainly know what to expect when you're expecting by now. But what should you expect when you're laboring and delivering?

That's actually hard to predict (make that impossible). Like every pregnancy before it, every labor and delivery is different. But just as it was comforting to know what you might expect during those months of growing your baby, it'll be comforting to have a general idea of what you might have in store for you during those hours of childbirth. Even if it turns out to be nothing like you expected (with the exception of that very happy and cuddly ending).

Stage One: Labor

Phase 1: Early Labor

This phase is usually the longest and, fortunately, the least intense phase of labor. Over a period of hours, days, or weeks (often without noticeable or bothersome contractions), or over a period of two to six hours of no-doubt-about-it contractions, your cervix will efface (thin out) and dilate (open) to 3 cm.

Contractions in this phase usually last 30 to 45 seconds, though they can be shorter. They are mild to moderately strong, may be regular or irregular (around 20 minutes apart, more or less), and become progressively closer together, but not necessarily in a consistent pattern.

During early labor, you might experience any or all of the following:

- Backache (either constant or with each contraction)
- Menstrual-like cramps
- Lower abdominal pressure
- Indigestion
- Diarrhea
- A sensation of warmth in the abdomen
- Bloody show (blood-tinged mucus)
- Rupture of the amniotic membranes (your water will break), though it's more likely that they'll rupture sometime during active labor.

Emotionally, you may feel excitement, relief, anticipation, uncertainty, anxiety, fear; some women are relaxed and chatty, others tense and apprehensive.

For the Record

Instead of grabbing the nearest piece of scrap paper to write down the timing of your contractions, flip open to the childbirth journal in *The What to Expect Pregnancy Journal and Organizer* to record all the info about your contractions and your labor experience (or better yet, have your spouse jot it down). This way you'll have a keepsake to help you remember the event—not that you'd ever forget.

What You Can Do. Of course you're excited (and nervous), but it's important to relax—or at least try to relax. This could take a while.

- If it's nighttime, try to sleep (you might not be able to later, when the contractions are coming fast and furious). If you can't sleep—what with all the adrenaline pumping—get up and do things around the house that will distract you. Cook a few more dishes to add to your freezer stash, fold some baby clothes, do the rest of the laundry so you can come home to an empty hamper (it'll fill up again soon enough), or log on to your favorite message board to see if anyone else is in the same boat. If it's daytime, go about your usual routine, as long as it doesn't take you far from home (don't go anywhere without your cell phone). If you're at work, you might want to head home (it's not like you're going to get anything done anyway). If you have nothing planned, find something relaxing to keep you occupied. Take a walk, watch TV, e-mail friends and family, finish packing your bag.

- Alert the media. Okay, maybe not the media (yet)—but you'll definitely want to put your spouse on alert if he's not with you. He probably doesn't have to rush to your side just yet if he's at work—unless he really wants to—since there's not much for him to do this early on. If you have hired a doula, it would be a good idea to issue a bulletin to her, too.

- Eat a light snack or meal if you're hungry (broth, toast with jam, plain pasta or rice, Jell-O, a Popsicle, pudding, a banana, or something else your practitioner has suggested)—now's the best time to stock up on energy foods. But don't eat heavily, and avoid hard-to-digest foods (burgers, potato chips).

You may also want to skip anything acidic, such as orange juice or lemonade. And definitely drink some water—it's important to stay hydrated.

- Make yourself comfortable. Take a warm shower; use a heating pad if your back is aching; take acetaminophen (Tylenol) if your practitioner approves. Don't take aspirin or ibuprofen (Advil, Motrin).

- Time contractions (from the beginning of one to the beginning of the next) for half an hour if they seem to be getting closer than 10 minutes apart and periodically even if they don't. But don't be a constant clock-watcher.

- Remember to pee often, even if you're not feeling the urge to. A full bladder could slow down the progress of labor.

- Use relaxation techniques if they help, but don't start any breathing exercises yet or you'll become bored and exhausted long before you really need them.

For the Coach: What You Can Do. If you're around during this phase, here are some ways you can help out. If a doula's also on site, she can share in any or all of these:

- Practice timing contractions. The interval between contractions is timed from the beginning of one to the beginning of the next. Time them periodically, and keep a record. When they are coming less than 10 minutes apart, time them more frequently.

- Spread the calm. During this early phase of labor, your most important function is to keep your partner relaxed. And the best way to do this is to keep yourself relaxed, both inside and out. Your own anxiety can be passed on to her without your real-

Call Your Practitioner If...

Your practitioner probably told you not to call until you're in more active labor, but may have suggested that you call early on if labor begins during the day or if your membranes rupture. Definitely call immediately, however, if your membranes rupture and the amniotic fluid is murky or greenish, if you have any bright red vaginal bleeding, or if you feel no fetal activity (it may be hard to notice because you are distracted by contractions, so try the test on page 289). Although you may not feel like it, it's best if you—not your coach—make the call and talk to your practitioner. A lot can be lost in third-party translations.

izing it, and it can be communicated not just through words but through touch—or even expressions (so no tensed-up foreheads, please). Doing relaxation exercises together or giving her a gentle, unhurried massage may help. It's too soon, however, to have her begin using breathing exercises. For now, just breathe.

■ Offer comfort, reassurance, and support. She'll need them from now on.

■ Keep your sense of humor, and help her keep hers; time flies, after all, when you're having fun. It'll be easier to laugh now than when contractions are coming fast and hard (she probably won't find very much of anything funny then).

■ Try distraction. Suggest activities that will help keep both your minds off her labor: playing video games, watching a silly sitcom or reality show, checking out celebrity birthday sites to see who baby might be celebrating with next year, baking something for the postpartum freezer stash, taking short strolls.

■ Keep up your own strength so you'll be able to reinforce hers. Eat periodically but empathetically (don't go wolfing down a Big Mac when she's sticking to pudding). Prepare a sandwich to take along to the hospital or birthing center, but avoid anything with a strong or lingering odor. She won't be in the mood to be sniffing bologna or onions on your breath.

Phase 2: Active Labor

The active phase of labor is usually shorter than the first, lasting an average of 2 to 3½ hours (with, again, a wide range considered normal). The contractions are more concentrated now, accomplishing more in less time, and they're also increasingly more intense (in other words, painful). As they become stronger, longer (40 to 60 seconds, with a distinct peak about halfway through), and more frequent (generally 3 to 4 minutes apart, though the pattern may not be regular), the cervix dilates to 7 cm. With fewer breaks in the action, there's less opportunity to rest between contractions.

You'll likely be in the hospital or birthing center by now, and you can expect to feel all or some of the following (though you won't feel pain if you've had an epidural):

■ Increasing pain and discomfort with contractions (you may not be able to talk through them now).

■ Increasing backache.

■ Leg discomfort or heaviness.

On to the Hospital or Birthing Center

Sometime near the end of the early phase or the beginning of the active phase (probably when your contractions are five minutes apart or less, sooner if you live far from the hospital or if this isn't your first baby), your practitioner will tell you to pick up your bag and get going. Getting to the hospital or birthing center will be easier if your coach is reachable anywhere, anytime by cell phone or beeper and can get to you quickly (do not try to drive yourself to the hospital or birthing center; take a taxi or ask a friend to drive you if your coach can't be reached); you've planned your route in advance; are familiar with parking regulations (if parking is likely to be a problem, taking a cab may be more sensible); and know which entrance will get you to the obstetrical floor most quickly. En route, recline the front seat as far back as is comfortable, if you'd like (remember to fasten your seatbelt). If you have chills, bring along a blanket to cover you.

Once you reach the hospital or birthing center, you can probably expect something like the following:

- To get registered: If you've preregistered (and it's best if you have), the admission process will be quick and easy; if you're in active labor and in no mood to answer questions, your coach can take care of it. If you haven't preregistered, you (or better yet, your coach) will have to go through a more lengthy process, so be prepared to fill out a bunch of forms and answer a lot of questions.

- Once on the labor and delivery floor, a nurse will take you to your room (most likely a labor, delivery, and recovery room, or LDR). Sometimes, you may be brought first to a triage (assessment) room, where your cervix will be checked, your baby's heart rate assessed, and your contractions monitored for some time to see if you're actively in labor or not. In some hospitals or birthing centers, your coach and other family members may be asked to wait outside while you are being admitted and prepped. Speak up if you'd rather your coach stay by your side; most hospitals or birthing centers are

- Fatigue.

- Increasing bloody show.

- Rupture of the membranes (if they haven't earlier), or they might be ruptured artificially now.

Emotionally, you may feel restless and find it more difficult to relax; or your concentration may become more intense, and you may become completely absorbed in your labor efforts. Your confidence may begin to waver ("How will I make it through?"), along with your patience ("Will this labor never end?"), or you may feel excited and encouraged that things are really starting to happen. Whatever your feelings, they're normal—just get ready to start getting "active."

During active labor, assuming all is progressing normally and safely, the hospital or birthing center staff will leave you alone (or stay out of your way, but in your room), checking and monitoring you as needed, but also allowing you to work through your labor with your coach and other support people without interference. You can expect them to:

flexible. (Note to the coach: This is a good time to make a few priority phone calls or to get a snack if you haven't brought one. If you aren't called into the room within 20 minutes or so, remind someone at the nurses' station that you're waiting. Be prepared for the possibility that you will be asked to put on a clean gown over your clothes.)

- Your nurse will take a brief history, asking, among other things, when the contractions started, how far apart they are, whether your membranes have ruptured, and, possibly, when and what you last ate.

- Your nurse will ask for your signature (or your spouse's) on routine consent forms.

- Your nurse will give you a hospital gown to change into and might request a urine sample. She will check your pulse, blood pressure, respiration, and temperature; look for leaking amniotic fluid, bleeding, or bloody show; listen to the fetal heartbeat with a Doppler or hook you up to a fetal monitor, if this is deemed necessary. She may also evaluate the fetus and its position.

- Depending on the policies of your practitioner and the hospital or birthing center (and, ideally, your preferences), an IV may be started.

- Your nurse, your practitioner, or a staff doctor or midwife will examine you internally to see how dilated and effaced your cervix is (if it wasn't already checked). If your membranes haven't ruptured spontaneously and you are at least 3 or 4 cm dilated (many practitioners prefer to wait until the cervix has dilated to 5 cm), your membranes may be artificially ruptured—unless you and your practitioner have decided to leave them intact until they break on their own or until later in labor. The procedure is generally painless; all you'll feel is a warm gush of fluid.

If you have any questions—about hospital or birthing center policy, about your condition, about your practitioner's plans—that haven't been answered before, now is the time for you or your coach to ask them. Your coach can also take this opportunity to hand a copy of your birth plan, if you have one, to the birth attendants.

- Take your blood pressure.

- Monitor your baby with a Doppler or fetal monitor.

- Time and monitor the strength of your contractions.

- Evaluate the quantity and quality of bloody discharge.

- Get an IV going if you're going to want an epidural.

- Possibly try to augment your labor if it's progressing very slowly by the use of Pitocin or by artificially ruptur-

ing the membranes (if they are still intact).

- Periodically examine you internally to check how labor is progressing and how dilated and effaced your cervix is.

- Administer pain relief if you choose to have some.

They'll also be able to answer any questions you might have (don't be shy about asking or having your coach ask) and provide additional support as you go through labor.

Are Things Slowing Down?

There's probably nothing you want more than to keep things moving along when it comes to labor. And making good progress during labor—which happens most of the time—requires three main components: strong uterine contractions that effectively dilate the cervix, a baby that is in position for an easy exit, and a pelvis that is sufficiently roomy to permit the passage of the baby. But, in some cases, labor doesn't progress by the book, because the cervix takes its time dilating, the baby takes longer than expected to descend through the pelvis, or pushing isn't getting you (or your baby) anywhere.

Sometimes, contractions slow down after an epidural kicks in, too. But keep in mind that expectations for the progress of labor are different for those who have an epidural (first and second stage may take longer, and that's typically nothing to worry about).

To get a stalled labor back up and running, there are a number of steps your practitioner (and you) can take:

- If you're in early labor and your cervix just isn't dilating or effacing, your practitioner may suggest some activity (such as walking) or just the opposite (sleep and rest, possibly aided by relaxation techniques). This will also help rule out false labor (the contractions of false labor usually subside with activity or a nap).

- If you're still not dilating or effacing as quickly as expected, your practitioner may try to rev things up by administering Pitocin (oxytocin), prostaglandin E, or another labor stimulator. He or she might even suggest a labor booster that you can take into your own hands (or your coach's): nipple stimulation.

- If you're already in the active phase of labor, but your cervix is dilating very slowly (less than 1 to 1.2 cm of dilation per hour in women having their first babies, and 1.5 cm per hour in those who've had previous deliveries), or if your baby isn't moving down the birth canal at a rate of more than 1 cm per hour in women having their first babies, or 2 cm per hour in others, your practitioner may rupture your membranes and/or continue administering oxytocin.

- If you end up pushing more than two hours (if you're a first-time mother who hasn't had an epidural) or three hours (if you have had an epidural), your practitioner will reassess your baby's position, see how you're feeling, perhaps attempt to birth your baby using vacuum extraction or (less likely) forceps, or decide to do a cesarean delivery.

To keep the ball (and the baby) rolling throughout labor, remember to urinate periodically, because a full bladder can interfere with the baby's descent. (If you have an epidural, chances are your bladder is being emptied by a catheter.) Full bowels may do the same, so if you haven't moved your bowels in 24 hours, give it a try. You might also try to nudge a sluggish labor along by utilizing gravity (sitting upright, squatting, standing, or walking). Ditto for trying to push along the pushing stage. A semi-sitting or semi-squatting position may be most effective for delivery.

Most physicians perform a C-section after 24 hours of active labor (sometimes sooner) if sufficient progress has not been made by that time; some will wait longer, as long as both mother and baby are doing well.

What You Can Do. It's all about your comfort now. So:

- Don't hesitate to ask your coach for whatever you need to get and stay as comfortable as possible, whether it's a back rub to ease the ache or a damp washcloth to cool your face. Speaking up will be important. Remember, as much as he's going to want to help, he's going to have a hard time anticipating your needs, especially if this is his first time.

- Start your breathing exercises, if you plan to use them, as soon as contractions become too strong to talk through. Didn't plan ahead and practice? Ask the nurse or doula for some simple breathing suggestions. Remember to do whatever relaxes you and makes you feel more comfortable. If the exercises aren't working for you, don't feel obligated to stick with them.

- If you'd like some pain relief, now's a good time to ask for it. An epidural can be given as early as you feel you need it.

- If you're laboring without pain relief, try to relax between contractions. This will become increasingly difficult as they come more frequently, but it will also become increasingly important as your energy reserves are taxed. Use the relaxation techniques you learned in childbirth class or try the one on page 142.

- Stay hydrated. With your practitioner's green light, drink clear beverages frequently to replace fluids and to keep your mouth moist. If you're hungry, and again, if you have your practitioner's okay, have a light snack (another Popsicle, for example). If your practitioner doesn't allow anything else by mouth, sucking on ice chips can serve to refresh.

Don't Hyperventilate

With all the breathing going on during labor, some women start to hyperventilate or overbreathe, causing low levels of carbon dioxide in the blood. If you feel dizzy or lightheaded, have blurred vision or a tingling and numbness of your fingers and toes, let your coach, a nurse, your practitioner, or your doula know. They'll give you a paper bag to breathe into (or suggest you breathe into your cupped hands). A few inhales and exhales will get you feeling better in no time.

- Stay on the move if you can (you won't be able to get around much if you have an epidural). Walk around, if possible, or at least change positions as needed. (See page 377 for suggested labor positions.)

- Pee periodically. Because of tremendous pelvic pressure, you may not notice the need to empty your bladder, but a full bladder can keep you from making the progress you'll definitely want to be making. No need to trek to the bathroom if you have an epidural (not that you could anyway), because you've probably been given a catheter to empty your bladder.

For the Coach: What You Can Do. If a doula is present, she can help out with many of these. Discuss ahead of time who will do what for your laboring spouse.

- Hand a copy of the birth plan to each nurse or other attendant at the birth, so everyone's on the same page about preferences. If the shift changes, make sure the new nurses receive a copy.

- If mom wants medication, let the nurse or practitioner know. Respect whatever decision she makes—to continue unmedicated or to go for pain relief.

- Take your cues from her. Whatever mom wants, mom should get. Keep in mind that what she'll want may change from moment to moment (the TV blaring one second, no TV the next). Ditto for her mood and her reaction to you. Don't take it personally if she doesn't respond to, doesn't appreciate—or is even annoyed by—your attempts to comfort her. Ease up, if that's what she seems to prefer—but be prepared to step it up 10 minutes later, if she wants. Remember that your role is important, even if you sometimes feel superfluous or in the way. She'll appreciate you in the morning (or whenever it's all over).

- Set the mood. If possible, keep the door to the room closed, the lights low, and the room quiet to promote a relaxed and restful atmosphere. Soft music may also help (unless she'd rather watch TV; remember, she's the boss). Continue encouraging relaxation techniques between contractions and breathing with her through the contractions—but don't push if she's not into them or if pushing the relaxation agenda is starting to stress her out. If distractions seem to help her, turn to cards or handheld video games, light conversation, or TV. But distract her only as much as she seems to want to be distracted.

- Pump her up. Reassure her and praise her efforts (unless your verbal reassurance is making her more edgy), and avoid criticism of any kind (even the constructive type). Be her cheerleader (but keep it low-key—she probably won't appreciate full-on exuberance). Particularly if progress is slow, suggest that she take her labor one contraction at a time, and remind her that each pain brings her closer to seeing the baby. If she finds your cheers irritating, however, skip them. Stick to sympathy if that's what she seems to need.

- Keep track of the contractions. If she's on a monitor, ask the practitioner or the nurse to show you how to read it. Later, when contractions are coming one on top of the other, you can announce each new contraction as it begins—unless she starts to find that annoying. (The monitor may detect the tensing of the uterus before she can, and can let her know when she's having one if she can't feel them, thanks to an epidural.) You can also encourage your spouse through those tough contractions by telling her when each peak is ending. If there is no monitor, ask a nurse to show you how to recognize the arrival and departure of contractions with your hand on her abdomen (unless she doesn't want it there).

- Massage her abdomen or back, or use counterpressure or any other techniques you've learned, to make her more comfortable. Let her tell you what kind of stroking or touching or massage helps. If she prefers not to be touched at all, then it might be best to comfort her verbally. Remember, what feels good one moment might irk her the next, and vice versa.

- Remind her to take a bathroom break at least once an hour if she doesn't have a catheter. She might not feel the urge, but a full bladder can stand in the way of labor progress.

- Suggest a change of position periodically; take her for a hallway walk, if that's possible.

- Be the ice man. Find out where the ice machine is, and keep those chips coming. If she's allowed to sip on fluids or snack on light foods, offer them periodically. Popsicles may be especially refreshing; ask the nurse if there's a stash you can help yourself to.

- Keep her cool. Use a damp washcloth, wrung out in cold water, to help cool her body and face; refresh it often.

- If her feet are cold, offer to get out a pair of socks and put them on her (reaching her feet isn't easy for her).

- Be her voice and her ears. She has enough going on, so lighten her load. Serve as her go-between with medical personnel as much as possible. Intercept questions from them that you can answer, and ask for explanations of procedures, equipment, and use of medication, so you'll be able to tell her what's happening. For instance, now might be the time to find out if a mirror will be provided so she can view the delivery. Be her advocate when necessary, but try to fight her battles quietly, perhaps outside the room, so she won't be disturbed.

Phase 3: Transitional Labor

Transition is the most demanding phase of labor but, fortunately, typically the quickest. Suddenly, the intensity of the contractions picks up. They become very strong, 2 to 3 minutes apart, and 60 to 90 seconds long, with very intense peaks that last for most of the contraction. Some women, particularly women who have given birth before, experience multiple peaks. You may feel as though the contractions never disappear completely and you can't completely relax between them. The final 3 cm of dilation, to a full 10 cm, will probably take place in a very short time: on average, 15 minutes to an hour, though it can also take as long as 3 hours.

You'll feel plenty when you're in transition (unless, of course, you're numbed by an epidural or other pain relief), and may experience some or all of the following:

- More intense pain with contractions

- Strong pressure in the lower back and/ or perineum

- Rectal pressure, with or without an urge to push or move your bowels (you might even feel the urge to grunt—so let it out!)

- An increase in your bloody show as more capillaries in the cervix rupture

- Feeling very warm and sweaty or chilled and shaky (or you might alternate between the two)

- Crampy legs that may tremble uncontrollably

- Nausea and/or vomiting

- Drowsiness between contractions as oxygen is diverted from your brain to the site of the delivery

- A tightening sensation in your throat or chest

- Exhaustion

Emotionally, you may feel vulnerable and overwhelmed, as though you're reaching the end of your rope. In addition to frustration over not being able to push yet, you may feel discouraged, irritable, disoriented, restless, and may have difficulty concentrating and relaxing (it might seem impossible to do either). You may also find excitement reaching a fever pitch in the midst of all the stress. Your baby's almost here!

What You Can Do. Hang in there. By the end of this phase, which is not far off, your cervix will be fully dilated, and it'll be time to begin pushing your baby out. Instead of thinking about the work ahead, try to think about how far you've come.

- Continue to use breathing techniques if they help. If you feel the urge to push, resist. Pant or blow instead, unless you've been instructed otherwise. Pushing against a cervix that isn't completely dilated can cause it to swell, which can delay delivery.

- If you don't want anybody to touch you unnecessarily, if your coach's once comforting hands now irritate you, don't hesitate to let him know.

- Try to relax between contractions (as much as is possible) with slow, deep, rhythmic breathing.

- Keep your eye on the prize: That bundle of joy will soon be arriving in your arms.

When you're a full 10 cm dilated, you'll be moved to the delivery room, if you aren't already there. Or, if you're in a birthing bed, the foot of the bed will simply be removed to prepare for delivery.

For the Coach: What You Can Do. Again, the doula, if one is present, can share these comforting techniques with you:

- If your laboring spouse has an epidural or other kind of pain relief, ask her if she needs another dose. Transition can be quite painful, and if her epidural is wearing off, she won't be a happy camper. If it is, let the nurses or the practitioner know. If mom's continuing unmedicated, she'll need you more now than ever (read on).

- Be there, but give her space if she seems to want it. Often, women in transition don't like being touched—but, as always, take your cues from her. Abdominal massage may be especially offensive now, though counterpressure applied to the small of her back may continue to provide some relief for back pain. Be prepared to back off—even from her back—as directed.

- Don't waste words. Now's not the time for small talk, and probably not for jokes, either. Offer quiet comfort, and help her with instructions that are brief and direct.

- Offer lots of encouragement, unless she prefers you to keep quiet. At this moment, eye contact or touch may communicate more expressively than words.

- Breathe with her through every contraction if it seems to help her through them.

- Help her rest and relax between contractions, touching her abdomen lightly to show her when a contraction is over. Remind her to use slow, rhythmic breathing in between contractions, if she can.

- If her contractions seem to be getting closer and/or she feels the urge to push—and she hasn't been examined recently—let the nurse or practitioner know. She may be fully dilated.

- Offer her ice chips or a sip of water frequently, and mop her brow with a cool damp cloth often. If she's chilly, offer her a blanket or a pair of socks.

- Stay focused on the payoff you're both about to get. It's been a long haul, but it won't be long before the pushing begins—and that anticipated bundle arrives in your arms.

Stage Two: Pushing and Delivery

Up until this point, your active participation in the birth of your child has been negligible. Though you've definitely taken the brunt of the abuse in the proceedings, your cervix and uterus (and baby) have done most of the work. But now that dilation is complete, your help is needed to push the baby the remainder of the way through the birth canal and out. Pushing and delivery generally take between half an hour and an hour, but can sometimes be accomplished in 10 (or even fewer) short minutes or in 2, 3, or even more very long hours.

The contractions of the second stage are usually more regular than the contractions of transition. They are still about 60 to 90 seconds in duration but sometimes further apart (usually about 2 to 5 minutes) and possibly less painful, though sometimes they are more intense. There now should be a well-defined rest period between them, though you may still have trouble recognizing the onset of each contraction.

Common in the second stage (though you'll definitely feel a lot less—and you may not feel anything at all—if you've had an epidural):

- Pain with the contractions, though possibly not as much

- An overwhelming urge to push (though not every woman feels it, especially if she's had an epidural)

- Tremendous rectal pressure (ditto)

- A burst of renewed energy (a second wind) or fatigue

- Very visible contractions, with your uterus rising noticeably with each

- An increase in bloody show

- A tingling, stretching, burning, or stinging sensation at the vagina as your baby's head emerges (it's called the "ring of fire" for good reason)

- A slippery wet feeling as your baby emerges

Emotionally, you may feel relieved that you can now start pushing (though some women feel embarrassed, inhibited, or scared); you may also feel exhilarated and excited or, if the pushing stretches on for much more than an hour, frustrated or overwhelmed. In a prolonged second stage, you may find your preoccupation is less with seeing the baby than with getting the ordeal over with (and that's perfectly understandable—and normal).

What You Can Do. It's time to get this baby out. So get into a pushing position (which one will depend on the bed, chair, or tub you're in, your practitioner's preferences, and, hopefully, what's most comfortable and effective for you). A semi-sitting or semi-squatting position is often the best because it enlists the aid of gravity in the birthing process and may afford you more pushing power. Tucking your chin to your chest when you're in this position will help you focus your pushes to where they need to be. Sometimes, if the pushing isn't moving your baby down the birth canal, it may be helpful to change positions. If you've been semi-inclined, for example, you might want to get up on all fours or try squatting.

Once you're ready to begin pushing, give it all you've got. The more efficiently you push and the more energy you pack into the effort, the more quickly your baby will make the trip

A Baby Is Born

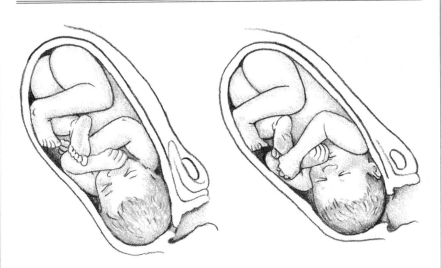

1. The cervix has thinned (effaced) somewhat but has not begun to dilate much.

2. The cervix has fully dilated and the baby's head has begun to press into the birth canal (vagina).

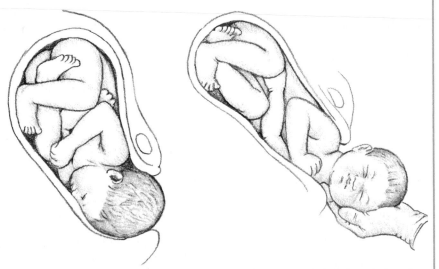

3. To allow the narrowest diameter of the baby's head to fit through the mother's pelvis, the baby usually turns sometime during labor. Here, the slightly molded head has crowned.

4. The head, the baby's broadest part, is out. The rest of the delivery should proceed quickly and smoothly.

through the birth canal. Frantic, disorganized pushing wastes energy and accomplishes little. Keep these pushing pointers in mind:

- Relax your body and your thighs and then push as if you're having a bowel movement (the biggest one of your life). Focus your energy on your vagina and rectum, not your upper body (which could result in chest pain after delivery) and not your face (straining with your face could leave you with black-and-blue marks on your cheeks and bloodshot eyes, not to mention do nothing to help get your baby out).

- Speaking of bowel movements, since you're bearing down on the whole perineal area, anything that's in your rectum may be pushed out, too; trying to avoid this while you're pushing can slow your progress. Don't let inhibition or embarrassment break the pushing rhythm. A little involuntary pooping (or passage of urine) is experienced by nearly everyone during delivery. No one else in the room will think twice about it, and neither should you. Pads will immediately whisk away anything that comes out.

- Take a few deep breaths while the contraction is building so you can gear up for pushing. As the contraction peaks, take a deep breath and then push with all your might—holding your breath if you want or exhaling as you push, whatever feels right to you. If you'd like the nurses or your coach to guide you by counting to 10 while you push, that's fine. But if you find it breaks your rhythm or isn't helpful, ask them not to. There is no magic formula when it comes to how long each push should last or how many times you should push with each contraction—the most important

thing is to do what comes naturally. You may feel as many as five urges to bear down, with each push lasting just seconds—or you may feel the urge to bear down just twice, but with each push lasting longer. Follow those urges, and you'll deliver your baby. Actually, you'll deliver your baby even if you don't follow your urges or if you find you don't have any urges at all. Pushing doesn't come naturally for every woman, and if it doesn't for you, your practitioner, nurse, or doula can help direct your efforts, and redirect them if you lose your concentration.

- Don't become frustrated if you see the baby's head crown and then disappear again. Birthing is a two-steps-forward, one-step-backward proposition. Just remember, you are moving in the right direction.

- Rest between contractions. If you're really exhausted, especially when the pushing stage drags on, your practitioner may suggest that you not push for several contractions so you can rebuild your strength.

- Stop pushing when you're instructed to (as you may be, to keep the baby's head from being born too rapidly). If you're feeling the urge to push, pant or blow instead.

- Remember to keep an eye on the mirror (if one is available) once there's something to look at. Seeing your baby's head crown (and reaching down and touching it) may give you the inspiration to push when the pushing gets tough. Besides, unless your coach is videotaping, there won't be any replays to watch.

While you're pushing, the nurses and/or your practitioner will give you support and direction; continue to monitor your baby's heartbeat, with either

A First Look at Baby

Those who expect their babies to arrive as round and smooth as a Botticelli cherub may be in for a shock. Nine months of soaking in an amniotic bath and a dozen or so hours of compression in a contracting uterus and cramped birth canal take their toll on a newborn's appearance. Those babies who arrived via cesarean delivery have a temporary edge as far as appearance goes.

Fortunately, most of the less-than-lovely newborn characteristics that follow are temporary. One morning, a couple of weeks after you've brought your wrinkled, slightly scrawny, puffy-eyed bundle home from the hospital, you'll wake to find that a beautiful cherub has taken its place in the crib.

Oddly shaped head. At birth, the infant's head is, proportionately, the largest part of the body, with a circumference as large as his or her chest. As your baby grows, the rest of the body will catch up. Often, the head has molded to fit through Mom's pelvis, giving it an odd, possibly pointed "cone" shape. Pressing against an inadequately dilated cervix can further distort the head by raising a lump. The lump will disappear in a day or two, the molding within two weeks, at which point your baby's head will begin to take on that cherubic roundness.

Newborn hair. The hair that covers the baby's head at birth may have little resemblance to the hair the baby will have later. Some newborns are virtually bald, some have thick manes, but most have a light cap of soft hair. All eventually lose their newborn hair (though this may happen so gradually that you don't notice), and it will be replaced by new growth, possibly of a different color and texture.

Vernix caseosa coating. The cheesy substance that coats the fetus in the uterus is believed to protect the skin from the long exposure to the amniotic fluid. Premature babies have quite a bit of this coating at birth; on-time babies just a little; postmature babies have almost none, except possibly in the folds of their skin and under their fingernails.

Swelling of the genitals. This can occur in both male and female new-

---

a Doppler or fetal monitor; and prepare for delivery by spreading sterile drapes and arranging instruments, donning surgical garments and gloves, and sponging your perineal area with antiseptic (though midwives generally just don gloves and do no draping). They'll also perform an episiotomy if necessary, or use vacuum extraction or, less likely, forceps if necessary.

Once your baby's head emerges, your practitioner will suction your baby's nose and mouth to remove excess mucus, then assist the shoulders and torso out. You usually only have to give one more small push to help with that— the head was the hard part, and the rest slides out pretty easily. The umbilical cord will be clamped (usually after it stops pulsating) and cut—either by the practitioner or by your coach—and your baby will be handed to you or placed on your belly. (If you've arranged for cord blood collection, it will be done now.) This is a great time for some caressing and skin-to-skin contact, so lift up your gown and bring baby close. In case you need a reason to do that, studies show borns. The breasts of newborns, male and female, may also be swollen (occasionally even engorged, secreting a white or pink substance nicknamed "witch's milk") due to stimulation by maternal hormones. The hormones may also stimulate a milky-white, even blood-tinged, vaginal secretion in girls. These effects are normal and disappear in a week to 10 days.

Puffy eyes. Swelling around the newborn's eyes, normal for someone who's been soaking in amniotic fluid for nine months and then squeezed through a narrow birth canal, may be exacerbated by the ointment used to protect the eyes from infection. It disappears within a few days. Caucasian babies' eyes are often, but not always, a slate blue, no matter what color they will be later on. In babies of color, the eyes are usually brown at birth.

Skin. Your baby's skin will appear pink, white, or even grayish at birth (even if it will eventually turn brown or black). That's because pigmentation doesn't show up until a few hours after birth. A variety of rashes, tiny "pimples," and whiteheads may also mar your baby's skin thanks to maternal hormones, but all are temporary. You may also notice skin dryness and cracking, due to first-time exposure to air; these, too, will pass.

Lanugo. Fine downy hair, called lanugo, may cover the shoulders, back, forehead, and temples of full-term babies. This will usually be shed by the end of the first week. Such hair can be more abundant, and will last longer, in a premature baby and may be gone in a postmature one.

Birthmarks. A reddish blotch at the base of the skull, on the eyelid, or on the forehead, called a salmon patch, is very common, especially in Caucasian newborns. Mongolian spots—bluish-gray pigmentation of the deep skin layer that can appear on the back, buttocks, and sometimes the arms and thighs—are more common in Asians, southern Europeans, and blacks. These markings eventually disappear, usually by the time a child is 4 years old. Hemangiomas, elevated strawberry-colored birthmarks, vary from tiny to about quarter size or even larger. They eventually fade to a mottled pearly gray, then often disappear entirely. Coffee-with-cream colored (café-au-lait) spots can appear anywhere on the body; they are usually inconspicuous and don't fade.

that infants who have skin-to-skin contact with their mothers just after delivery sleep longer and are calmer hours later.

What's next for your baby? The nurses and/or a pediatrician will evaluate his or her condition, and rate it on the Apgar scale at one minute and five minutes after birth (see box, page 379); give a brisk, stimulating, and drying rubdown; possibly take the baby's footprints for a keepsake; attach an identifying band to your wrist and to your baby's ankle; administer nonirritating eye ointment to your newborn to prevent infection (you can ask that the ointment be administered after you've had time to cuddle with your newborn); weigh, then wrap the baby to prevent heat loss. (In some hospitals and birthing centers, some of these procedures may be omitted; in others, many will be attended to later, so you can have more time to bond with your newborn.)

Then you'll get your baby back (assuming all is well) and you may, if you wish to, begin breastfeeding (but don't worry if you and/or your baby don't catch on immediately; see Getting Started Breastfeeding, page 435).

Sometime after that, it's off to the nursery for baby (if you've delivered in a hospital) for a more complete pediatric exam and some routine protective procedures (including a heel stick and a hepatitis B shot). Once your baby's temperature is stable, he or she will get a first bath, which you (and/or dad) may be able to help give. If you have rooming-in, your baby will be returned as soon as possible and tucked into a bassinet next to your bed.

For the Coach: What You Can Do. Once again, these responsibilities can be shared with a doula.

- Continue giving comfort and support (a whispered "I love you" can be more valuable to her during the pushing stage than anything else), but don't feel hurt if the object of your efforts doesn't seem to notice you're there. Her energies are necessarily focused elsewhere.

- Help her relax between the contractions—with soothing words, a cool cloth applied to forehead, neck, and shoulders, and, if feasible, back massage or counterpressure to help ease backache.

- Continue to supply ice chips or fluids to moisten her mouth as needed. She's likely to be parched from all that pushing.

- Support her back while she's pushing, if necessary; hold her hand, wipe her brow—or do whatever else seems to help her. If she slips out of position, help her back into it.

- Periodically point out her progress. As the baby begins to crown, remind her to keep an eye on the mirror so she can have visual confirmation of what she is accomplishing. When she's not looking, or if there's no mirror, give her inch-by-inch descriptions. Take her hand and touch baby's head together for renewed inspiration.

- If you're offered the opportunity to catch your baby as he or she emerges or, later, to cut the cord, don't be afraid. Both are relatively easy jobs, and you'll get step-by-step directions and backup from the attendants. You should know, however, that the cord can't be snipped like a piece of string. It's tougher than you may think.

Stage Three: Delivery of the Placenta

The worst is over, and the best has already come. All that remains is tying up the loose ends, so to speak. During this final stage of childbirth (which generally lasts anywhere from five minutes to half an hour or more), the placenta, which has been your baby's life support inside the womb, will be delivered. You will continue to have mild contractions approximately a minute in duration, though you may not feel them (after all, you're preoccupied with your newborn!). The squeezing of the uterus separates the placenta from the uterine wall and moves it down into the lower segment of the uterus or into the vagina so it can be expelled.

Your practitioner will help deliver the placenta by either pulling the cord gently with one hand while pressing and kneading your uterus with the other or exerting downward pressure on the top of the uterus, asking you to push at the appropriate time. You might get some Pitocin (oxytocin) via injection or in your IV to encourage uterine contractions, which will speed expulsion of the placenta, help shrink the uterus back to size, and minimize bleeding. Once the placenta is out, your practitioner will examine it to make sure it's intact. If it isn't, he or she will inspect your uterus manually for placental fragments and remove any that remain.

Now that the work of labor and delivery is done, you may feel overwhelmingly exhausted or, conversely, experience a burst of renewed energy. If you've been deprived of food and drink, you are likely to be very thirsty and, especially if labor has been long, hungry. Some women experience chills in this stage; all experience a bloody vaginal discharge (called lochia) comparable to a heavy menstrual period.

How will you feel emotionally after you've delivered your baby? Every woman reacts a little differently, and your reaction is normal for you. Your first emotional response may be joy, but it's just as likely to be a sense of relief. You may be exhilarated and talkative, elated and excited, a little impatient at having to push out the placenta or submit to the repair of an episiotomy or a tear, or so in awe of what you're cuddling in your arms (or so beat, or a little bit of both) that you don't notice. You may feel a closeness to your spouse and an immediate bond with your new baby, or (and this is just as normal) you may feel somewhat detached (who is this stranger sniffing at my breast?), even a little resentful—particularly if the delivery was a difficult one (so this is the little person who made me suffer so much!). No matter what your response

now, you will come to love your baby intensely. These things just sometimes take time. (For more on bonding, see page 430.)

What You Can Do.

- Have a good cuddle with your new arrival! Once the cord is cut, you'll have a chance to breastfeed or just do some snuggling. Speak up, too. Since your baby will recognize your voice, cooing, singing, or whispered words will be especially comforting (it's a strange new world, and you'll be able to help baby make some sense out of it). Under some circumstances, your baby may be kept in a heated bassinet for a while or be held by your coach while the placenta is being delivered—but not to worry, there's plenty of time for baby bonding.

- Spend some time bonding with your coach, too—and enjoying your cozy new threesome.

- Help deliver the placenta, if necessary, by pushing when directed. Some women don't even have to push at all for the placenta to arrive. Your practitioner will let you know what to do, if anything.

- Hang in there during repair of any episiotomy or tears.

- Take pride in your accomplishment!

All that's left to do, then, is for your practitioner to stitch up any tear (if you're not already numbed, you'll get a local anesthetic) and clean you up. You'll likely get an ice pack to put on your perineum to minimize swelling—do ask for one if it's not offered. The nurse will also help you put on a maxipad or add some thick pads under your bottom (remember, you'll be bleeding a lot). Once you're feeling up to it, you'll be transferred to a postpartum room (unless you've delivered in an LDRP—a labor, delivery, recovery, and postpartum—room, in which case you'll get to stay put).

For the Coach: What You Can Do. If a doula is present, she can continue to help out, concentrating on the more practical aspects of postdelivery care while you spend some quality time with the two stars of the show.

- Offer some well-earned words of praise to the new mom—and congratulate yourself, too, for a job well done.

- Begin bonding with your little one—with some holding and cuddling, and by doing soft singing or talking. Remember, your baby has heard your voice a lot during his or her stay in the uterus and is familiar with its sound. Hearing it now will bring comfort in this strange new environment.

- Don't forget to do some cuddling and bonding with the new mom, too.

- Ask for an ice pack to soothe her perineal area, if the nurse doesn't offer one.

- Ask for some juice for the new mom; she may be very thirsty. After she's been rehydrated, and if both of you are in the mood, break out the bubbly—champagne or sparkling cider if you brought some along.

- If you've brought along the necessary equipment, take baby's first photos or capture your amazing newborn on video.

Cesarean Delivery

You won't be able to participate actively at a cesarean delivery the way you would at a vaginal one, and some would consider that a definite plus. Instead of huffing, puffing, and pushing your baby into the world, you'll get to lie back and let everybody else do all the heavy lifting. In fact, your most important contribution to your baby's cesarean birth will be preparation: The more you know, the more comfortable you'll feel. Which is why it's a good idea to look this section over ahead of time, even if you're not having a planned cesarean.

Thanks to regional anesthesia and the liberalization of hospital regulations, most women (and their coaches) are able to be spectators at their cesarean deliveries. Because they aren't preoccupied with pushing or pain, they're often able to relax (at least to some degree) and marvel at the birth. This is what you can expect in a typical cesarean birth:

- An IV infusion will be started (if it isn't already in) to provide speedy access if additional medications or fluids are needed.

- Anesthesia will be administered: either an epidural or a spinal block (both of which numb the lower part of your body but don't knock you out). In rare emergency situations, when a baby must be delivered immediately, a general anesthetic (which does put you to sleep) may be used.

- Your abdomen will be washed down with an antiseptic solution. A catheter (a narrow tube) will be inserted into your bladder to keep it empty and out of the surgeon's way.

- Sterile drapes will be arranged around your exposed abdomen. A screen will be put up at about shoulder level so you won't have to see the incision being made.

- If your coach is going to attend the delivery, he will be suited up in sterile garb. He will sit near your head so that he can give you emotional support and hold your hand; he may have the option of viewing the actual surgery.

- If yours is an emergency cesarean, things may move very quickly. Try to stay calm and focused in the face of all that activity, and don't let it worry you—that's just the way things work in a hospital sometimes.

- Once the physician is certain that the anesthetic has taken effect, an incision (usually a horizontal bikini cut) is made in the lower abdomen, just above the pubic hairline. You may feel a sensation of being "unzipped" but no pain.

- A second incision is then made, this time in your uterus. The amniotic sac is opened, and, if it hasn't already ruptured, the fluid is suctioned out; you may hear a sort of gurgling or swooshing sound.

- The baby is then eased out, usually while an assistant presses on the uterus. With an epidural (though not likely with a spinal block), you will probably feel some pulling and tugging sensations, as well as some pressure. If you're eager to see your baby's arrival, ask the doctor if the screen can be lowered slightly, which will allow you to see the actual birth but not the more graphic details.

- Your baby's nose and mouth are then suctioned; you'll hear the first cry, the cord will be quickly clamped and cut, and you'll be allowed a quick glimpse of your newborn.

- While the baby is getting the same routine attention that a vaginally delivered infant receives, the doctor will remove the placenta.

- Now the doctor will quickly do a routine check of your reproductive organs and stitch up the incisions that were made. The uterine incision will be repaired with absorbable stitches, which do not have to be removed. The abdominal incision may be closed with either stitches or surgical staples.

- An injection of oxytocin may be given intramuscularly or into your IV, to help contract the uterus and control bleeding. IV antibiotics may be given to minimize the chances of infection.

You may have some cuddling time in the delivery room, but a lot will depend on your condition and the baby's, as well as hospital rules. If you can't hold your baby, perhaps your spouse can. If he or she has to be whisked away to the NICU nursery, don't let it get you down. This is standard in many hospitals following a cesarean delivery and is more likely to indicate a precaution than a problem with your baby's condition. And as far as bonding is concerned, later can be just as good as sooner—so not to worry if the snuggles have to wait a little while.

Congratulations—You've done it . . .
Now relax and enjoy your new baby!

PART 3

Twins, Triplets & More

When You're Expecting Multiples

Expecting More Than One

HAVE TWO (OR MORE) PAS-sengers aboard the mother ship? Even if you'd been hoping for multiples, your first response to the news that you're carrying more than one can be all over the emotional map—ranging from disbelief to joy, from excitement to

Seeing Double—Everywhere?

If it looks like multiples are multiplying these days, it's because they are. In fact, about 3 percent of babies in the United States are now born in sets of two, three, or more, with the majority (about 95 percent) of these multiple births comprised of twins. At least twice as amazing, the number of twin births has jumped more than 50 percent in recent years, and higher-order multiple births (triplets and more) has risen an astonishing 400 percent.

So what's up with this multiple-baby boom? The surge in older moms has a lot to do with it. Moms over the age

of 35 are naturally more likely to drop more than one egg at ovulation (thanks to greater hormone fluctuations, specifically FSH, or follicle-stimulating hormone), upping the odds of having twins. Another factor is the increase in fertility treatments (also more common among older moms), which multiplies the chances of a multiple pregnancy. And yet another surprising factor, say some experts, might be the increase in obesity. Women with prepregnancy BMIs higher than 30 are significantly more likely to have fraternal twins than women with lower BMIs.

trepidation (make that fear). And in between all the whoops of delight and buckets of tears will come the questions: Will the babies be healthy? Will I be healthy? Will I be able to stick with my regular practitioner, or will I have to see a specialist? How much food will I have to eat, and how much weight do I have to gain? Will there be enough room inside of me for two babies? Will there be enough room in my house for two babies? Will I be able to carry them to term? Will I have to go on bed rest? Will giving birth be twice as hard?

Carrying one baby comes with its share of challenges and changes; carrying more than one—well, you've probably already done the math. But not to worry. You're up for it—or at least you will be once you're armed with the information in this chapter (and the support of your partner and your practitioner). So sit back (comfortably, while you still can) and get ready for your marvelous multiple pregnancy.

What You May Be Wondering About

Detecting a Multiple Pregnancy

"I just found out I'm pregnant and I have a feeling it's twins. How will I find out for sure?"

Gone are the days when multiples took their parents by surprise in the delivery room. Today, most parents-to-be of multiples discover the exciting news pretty early on. Here's how:

Ultrasound. The proof is in the picture—the ultrasound picture, that is. If you're looking for indisputable confirmation that you're carrying more than one baby, an ultrasound is the best way to get it. Even an early first-trimester ultrasound done at six to eight weeks (which you're very likely to have if your blood hCG level is high or if you've conceived using fertility treatments, though some practitioners also do them routinely) can sometimes detect multiples. But if you want to be absolutely sure you're seeing double, you'll want to look to an ultrasound done after the 12th week (because very early ultrasounds don't always uncover both babies).

Doppler. The beat goes on . . . and on. Your practitioner can usually pick up a baby's heartbeat sometime after the ninth week. And though it's hard to distinguish two heartbeats with just a Doppler, if your practitioner is an experienced listener and thinks he or she detects two distinct beats, there's a good chance that you're carrying multiples (an ultrasound will confirm the news).

Hormone levels. The pregnancy hormone hCG is detectable in your urine about 10 days postconception, and its level rises rapidly throughout the first trimester. Sometimes (but not always), a higher-than-usual hCG level may indicate multiple fetuses. That said, the range of normal hCG levels for twins also falls within the normal range for singletons, so an elevated level of hCG does not, in and of itself, indicate a multiple pregnancy.

Fraternal or Identical?

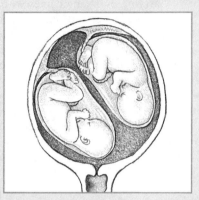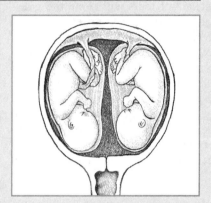

Fraternal twins (left), which result from two eggs being fertilized at the same time, each have their own placenta. Identical twins (right), which come from one fertilized egg that splits and then develops into two separate embryos, may share a placenta or—depending on when the egg splits—may each have their own.

Fraternal twins are the more common type of twin, with your chances of having fraternal twins increasing with your age and the number of children you have. Your chance of having twins in general increases if you have twins in your family on your mother's side.

Test results. An unusually high (positive) result on the triple (or quad) screen (see page 63) in the second trimester can sometimes indicate a multiple pregnancy.

Your measurements. Not surprisingly, the more babies, the bigger the uterus. At each visit, your practitioner feels for the height of the fundus (the top of your uterus) to measure that growth. Measuring larger than would be expected for gestational age may be a sign that you have more than one baby on board (but not always; see page 162).

Bottom line on your hunch: Lots of clues can point to a multiple pregnancy (including your mom-to-be instincts), but only an ultrasound can tell you for sure. Check with your practitioner.

Choosing a Practitioner

"I just found out I'm having twins. Can I use my regular ob-gyn, or do I need to see a specialist?"

If you're happy with your practitioner, there's no reason to trade in for a specialist's care just because you have two babies to care for. (Just make sure you are really happy with your practitioner, since you'll be spending more time with him or her during your twin pregnancy—more babies equals more office visits). Even if your regular practitioner is a midwife, you'll likely be able to continue seeing her as long as you also have a physician on board for regular checkups and for delivery.

Do you like your regular ob but also like the idea of extra-careful care? Many ob-gyn practices send patients who are pregnant with multiples to a specialist for periodic consultations—a good compromise if you'd like to combine the familiar comfort of your practitioner's care with the expertise of a specialist's. Moms-to-be of multiples who have specific special needs (such as advanced age, history of miscarriage, or a chronic health condition) may want to consider switching to a maternal-fetal medicine specialist (also known as a perinatologist). Talk that possibility over with your practitioner if your pregnancy falls into a higher risk category.

When choosing a practitioner for your multiple pregnancy, you'll also need to factor in his or her hospital affiliation. Ideally, you'll want a facility with the ability to care for premature babies (one with a neonatal intensive care unit) in case your bundles arrive early, as multiples often do.

Also ask about the practitioner's policy on topics specifically related to multiple births: Will you be induced at 37 or 38 weeks as a matter of course, or will you have the option of carrying beyond that time frame if all is going well? Will a vaginal birth be possible, or does the practitioner routinely deliver multiples via cesarean delivery? Will you be able to give birth in an LDR (labor and delivery room), or is it routine to deliver multiples in an OR as a precautionary measure?

For more general information about choosing a practitioner, see page 21.

Pregnancy Symptoms

"I've heard that when you're pregnant with twins, your pregnancy symptoms are worse than with just one baby. Is that true?"

Twice the babies sometimes spell twice the pregnancy discomforts, but not always. Every multiple preg-

nancy, like every singleton pregnancy, is different. An expectant mom of one may suffer enough morning sickness for two, while a mom-to-be of multiples might sail through her pregnancy without a single queasy day. The same with other symptoms, too.

But though you shouldn't expect a double dose of morning sickness (or heartburn, or leg cramps, or varicose veins), you can't count it out. The miseries do, on average, multiply in a multiple pregnancy, and that's not surprising given the extra weight you'll be carrying around and the extra hormones you're already generating. Among the symptoms that might be—but won't necessarily be—exponentially exacerbated when you're expecting twins or more:

- Morning sickness. Nausea and vomiting can be worse in a multiple pregnancy, thanks to—among other things—the higher levels of hormones circulating in a mom's system. Morning sickness can also start earlier and last longer.

- Other tummy troubles. Hello, heartburn, indigestion, and constipation. More gastric crowding (and more gastric overloading, since moms of multiples are eating for three or more) can lead to an increase in the kinds of digestive discomforts pregnancy's known for.

- Fatigue. This is a no-brainer: The more weight you're dragging around, the more you're likely to drag. Fatigue can also increase with the extra energy an expectant mom of multiples expends (your body has to work twice as hard to grow two babies). Sleep deprivation can also wear you out (it's difficult enough to settle down with a watermelon-size belly, let alone one that's the size of two watermelons).

- All those other physical discomforts. Every pregnancy comes with its share of aches and pains; your twin pregnancy might just come with a little more than its share. Toting that extra baby can translate to extra backache, pelvic twinges, crampiness, swollen ankles, varicose veins, you name it. Breathing for three or more can also seem an extra effort, especially as your babies get big enough to push up on your lungs.

■ Fetal movement. Though every pregnant woman might feel at some point that she's expecting an octopus, the eight limbs you'll be carrying will really pack a punch. Make that many punches, and kicks.

Whether your pregnancy ends up bestowing you with double the discomforts or not, one thing's for sure—it'll also bestow you with twice the rewards. Not bad, for nine months' work.

Eating Well with Multiples

"I'm committed to eating well now that I'm pregnant with triplets, but I'm not sure what that means—eating three times as much?"

Belly up to the buffet table, Mom— feeding four means it's always time to chow down. While you won't literally have to quadruple your daily intake (any more than a woman expecting a single baby has to double it), you will need to do some serious eating in the months to come. Moms-to-be of multiples should indulge in an extra 150 to 300 calories a day per fetus, doctor's orders (good news if you're looking for a license to eat, not so good news if queasiness or tummy crowding has your appetite cramped). Which translates to an extra 300 to 600 calories if you're carrying twins, an extra 450 to 900 calories for triplets (if you've started out with

an average prepregnancy weight). But before you take that extra allotment as a free pass to Burritoville (extra guacamole for Baby A; extra sour cream for Baby B; refried beans for Baby C), think again. The quality of what you eat will be just as important as the quantity. In fact, good nutrition during a multiple pregnancy has an even greater impact on baby birthweight than it does during a singleton pregnancy.

So just how do you eat well when you're expecting more than one? Check out the Pregnancy Diet (see Chapter 5) and:

Keep it small. The bigger your belly gets, the smaller you'll want your meals to stay. Not only will grazing on five or six healthy mini meals and snacks ease your digestive overload (and your tummy crowding), but it'll keep your energy up—while delivering the same nutritional bottom line as three squares.

Make your calories count. Pick foods that pack plenty of nutrients into small servings. Studies show that a high-calorie diet that's also high in nutrients significantly improves your chances of having healthy full-term babies. Wasting too much of that premium space on junk food, on the other hand, means you'll have less room for nutritious food.

Go for extra nutrients. Not surprisingly, your need for nutrients multiplies with each baby—which means you'll have to tack on some extra servings to your Daily Dozen (see page 93). It's usually recommended that women carrying multiples get one extra serving of protein, one extra serving of calcium, and one extra serving of whole grains. Be sure to ask your practitioner what he or she recommends in your case.

Pump up the iron. Another nutrient you'll need to ramp up is iron, which helps your body manufacture red blood cells (you'll need lots of those for the increased blood your multiple-baby factory will be using) and helps keep you from becoming anemic, which often happens in multiple pregnancies. Red meat, dried fruit, pumpkin seeds, and spinach are great sources of iron (you can find more iron-rich foods on page 100). Your prenatal vitamin and possibly a separate iron supplement should fill in the rest; ask your practitioner.

Keep the water flowing. Dehydration can lead to preterm labor (something moms-to-be of multiples are already at risk for), so make sure you drink at least eight 8-ounce glasses of liquid a day.

For more information on eating well for multiples, check out *What to Expect: Eating Well When You're Expecting.*

Weight Gain

"I know I'm supposed to gain more weight with twins, but just how much more?"

Get ready to gain. Most practitioners advise a woman expecting twins to gain 35 to 45 pounds and a woman expecting triplets to gain an average of 50 pounds (a little less if you were over-weight prepregnancy; a little more if you were underweight). Sounds like a piece of cake, right? Or maybe two pieces of cake (or heck, maybe the whole cake). But the reality is, gaining enough weight isn't always as easy as it seems when you've got two—or more—on board. In fact, a variety of challenges you may face throughout your pregnancy can keep the numbers on the scale from climbing fast enough.

Standing between you and weight gain in the first trimester might be nausea, which can make it difficult to get food down—and then keep it down. Eating tiny amounts of comforting (and, hopefully, sometimes nutritious) food throughout the day can help get you through those probably queasy months. Aim for a pound-a-week gain through the first trimester, but if you find you can't gain that much, or have trouble gaining any at all, relax. You can have fun catching up later. Just be sure to take your prenatal vitamin and stay hydrated.

Use the second trimester (which will probably be your most comfortable one—and the easiest one for you to do some serious chowing down in) as your chance to load up on the nutrition your babies need to grow. If you gained no weight during the first trimester (or

What to Gain When You're Gaining for Two or More

Pregnancy Status	First-Trimester Weight Gain	Second-Trimester Weight Gain	Third-Trimester Weight Gain	Total Weight Gain
Underweight with Twins	4–6 pounds	19–23 pounds	17–21 pounds	40–50 pounds
Normal to Overweight with Twins	3–4 pounds	19–22 pounds	13–19 pounds	35–45 pounds
Triplets	4–5 pounds	30+ pounds	11–15 pounds	45+ pounds

Multiple Time Line

Already counting down your 40 weeks? You might not have to count that high after all. A twin pregnancy may be considered full-term a full 3 weeks earlier, at 37 weeks, which is certainly reason to celebrate (3 weeks less of puffiness, heartburn—and waiting!). But just as 95 percent of all singletons fail to arrive on their due date, multiples keep their moms and dads (and practitioners) guessing, too. They might just stay put until 39 weeks (or longer)—or they might make their appearance before they've clocked in the full 37 weeks. In fact, the average multiple pregnancy lasts 35½ weeks.

If your babies do end up overstaying their 37-week term, your practitioner may elect to induce at 38 weeks, depending on how they're doing and how you're doing, as well as his or her practice preferences. Be sure to have an end-game discussion with your practitioner long before the end is near, because many differ on how they typically handle the late stages of a multiple pregnancy.

if you lost weight due to severe nausea and vomiting), your practitioner may want you to gain 1½ to 2 pounds per week during this period for twins or 2 to 2½ per week for triplets. (If you've been gaining steadily through the first trimester, you'll only have to aim for 1½ pounds a week for twins or 2 per week for triplets.) That may seem like a lot of weight in a short time, and you're right—it is. But it's weight that's important to gain. Supercharge your eating plan with extra servings of protein, calcium, and whole grains. Heartburn and

indigestion starting to cramp your eating style? Spread your nutrients out over those six (or more) mini meals.

As you head into the home stretch (aka, the third trimester), reach for a goal of 1½ to 2 pounds per week through your seventh month. By 32 weeks, your babies may be 4 pounds each, which won't leave much room in your crowded-out stomach for food. Still, even though you'll be feeling plenty bulky already, your babies will have to bulk up quite a bit more—and they'll appreciate the nutrition a well-balanced diet provides. So focus on quality over quantity, and expect to taper down to a pound a week or less in the eighth month and just a pound or so total during the ninth. (This makes more sense when you remember that most multiple pregnancies don't make it to 40 weeks.)

Exercise

"I'm a runner, but now that I'm pregnant with twins, can I keep on exercising?"

Exercise can benefit most pregnancies, but when you're staying fit for three, you'll have to work out with care. If your practitioner green-lights exercise during the first and second trimesters (do be sure to ask), he or she will probably steer you toward more gentle options than running. You'll definitely be advised to avoid any workout that puts a lot of downward pressure on your cervix or raises your body temperature significantly. ACOG recommends that moms-to-be of multiples stay away from high-impact aerobic exercise (which would include running) because it can increase the risk of preterm labor for them. This holds true for experienced runners, too.

Looking for a more sensible fitness routine for the three of you? Good options include swimming or pregnancy water aerobics, stretching, prenatal yoga, light weight training, and riding a stationary bicycle, all exercises that don't require you to be on your feet while you do them. And don't forget your Kegels, the anywhere-anytime exercise designed to strengthen your pelvic floor (which needs extra reinforcement when there are extra babies inside).

No matter what you're doing during your workout, if the exertion is causing Braxton Hicks contractions or any other red flags listed on page 223, stop immediately, rest, drink some water, and call your practitioner if they don't subside in 20 minutes or more.

Mixed Feelings

"Everybody thinks it's so exciting that we're going to have twins, except us. We're disappointed and scared. What's wrong with us?"

Absolutely nothing. Prenatal daydreams don't usually include two cribs, two high chairs, two strollers, or two babies. You prepare yourself psychologically, as well as physically and financially, for the arrival of one baby—and when you suddenly discover you're having two, feelings of disappointment aren't unusual. Neither is trepidation. The impending responsibilities of caring for one new infant are plenty daunting without having them doubled.

While some expectant parents are happy to hear they're expecting more than one, others take some time getting used to the news. It's just as common to feel initial shock as initial joy—to experience a sense of loss for the intimacy and normalcy of the one-on-one relationship you'd have with a single baby but can't immediately see yourselves having with two. Instead of picturing yourselves rocking, feeding, and cuddling that one baby, you may have a hard time coming to terms with the thought of life with two

newborns. You may also be flooded by conflicted emotions—first asking "Why us?" then feeling guilty about questioning your double blessing (especially if becoming pregnant was a struggle to begin with). All of these feelings (and the others you might be experiencing) are a completely normal reaction to the news that your pregnancy and your lives are taking an unexpected and very special turn.

So accept the fact that you're ambivalent about the dual arrivals, and don't saddle yourselves with guilt (since your feelings are normal and understandable, there's absolutely nothing to feel guilty about). Instead, use the months before delivery to get used to the idea that you'll be having twins (believe it or not, you will get used to it—and you will become happy about it!). Talk openly and honestly to each other (the more you let your feelings out, the less they'll weigh you down and the faster you'll work through them). Talk to anyone you know who has twins, and if you don't know anyone, seek them out through groups and message boards. Sharing your feelings with others who've felt them, and recognizing that you're not the first expectant parents to experience them, will help you accept and, in time, become excited about this pregnancy and the two beautiful babies you'll be holding one day soon. Twins, you'll find, may be double the effort at first, but they're also double the pleasure down the road.

Insensitive Comments

"I can't believe it, but when I told my friends that we're expecting twins, one of them said to me, 'Better you than me.' I thought she'd be happy for me—why would she make such a nasty comment?"

That might be the first insensitive comment you've been ambushed by during your multiple pregnancy,

Multiple Connections

As a multiples mother-to-be, you're about to join a special club already filled with thousands of women just like you—women who are also expecting double the delight and, no doubt, experiencing double the anxiety. Never been a joiner? Membership in this particular club does come with plenty of rewards. By talking to other moms-to-be of multiples, you'll be able to share your fears, your joy, your symptoms, your funny stories (the ones nobody else would get) with women who know just how you're feeling. You'll also be able to score reassuring advice from other expectant moms who have more than one on the way (as well as from those who've already had their multi-stork delivery). Join a discussion group online (check out whattoexpect.com for a multiples message board) or ask your practitioner to hook you up with other pregnant-with-multiples women in his or her practice and start your own group. There are also national organizations that can provide you with contact information for local clubs, including the National Organization of Mothers of Twins Clubs, nomotc.org, or you can use an online search engine to find a local multiples chapter. You can also check out online sites that cater specifically to parents of multiples: mothersofmultiples.com; twinstuff.com.

but it probably won't be the last. From coworkers to family members to friends to those perfect (make that not-so-perfect) strangers in the supermarket, you'll be amazed at the remarkably rude things people feel completely comfortable saying to an expectant mom of multiples, ranging from "Wow, you're so huge—you must have a litter in there!" to "Boy, you're in for it!" to "I could never manage more than one at a time."

What's up with the lack of tact? The truth is, many people don't know how to react to the news that you're carrying multiples. Sure, a simple "Congratulations!" might be in order, but most people assume that twins are special (they are) and therefore need to be recognized with a "special" comment. Curious about what it must be like to be pregnant with twins, in awe of what you'll be going through once they're born, they're clueless about the right response—so they dish out the completely wrong one. Their intentions are good, but their follow-through stinks.

The best way to react to the rudeness? Don't take it personally, and don't take it too seriously. Realize that even as your friend opened her mouth and inserted her foot, she was almost certainly trying to wish you well (and she probably has no idea that she offended you, so try not to take offense). Remember, too, that you're the best spokeswoman for moms of twins everywhere—and you'll have lots of chances to spread the wonderful word on multiples.

"People keep on asking me if twins run in my family or if I had fertility treatment. I'm not ashamed that I conceived my babies using a fertility drug, but it's also not something I want to share with strangers."

A pregnant woman brings out the nosy like no one else, but a woman expecting multiples becomes everybody's business. Suddenly, your pregnancy goes public—with people you hardly know (or don't know at all) prying into your personal life (and bedroom habits) and prodding you for personal information without thinking twice. But that's just the point—these people aren't really thinking twice—or even once. They're not asking to be intrusive, they're just curious (multiples are fascinating stuff, after all), and they haven't been educated in the fine art of twin etiquette. If you're open to spilling the juicy details, then by all means, go for it ("Well, first we tried Clomid, and when that didn't work we tried IVF, which means that my husband and I went to a fertility clinic . . ."). By the time you're halfway done with your story, the questioner will probably be bored to tears and looking for the nearest exit. Or, you can try one of these responses the next time someone asks about the conception of your twins:

- "They were a big surprise." This can be true whether you've conceived with or without fertility help.

- "Twins run in the family—now." This will shut them up while keeping them guessing.

- "We had sex twice in one night." Who hasn't at some point? Even if the last time was on your honeymoon, it's not a lie—and it'll be the end of the line for their line of questioning.

- "They were conceived with love." Well, that's a given, no matter what— and where do they go from there?

- "Why do you ask?" If they're TTC (trying to conceive) themselves, then maybe it'll open up a conversation that could help them (infertility can be a lonely road, as you probably know). If not, it could stop them in their nosy tracks. After all, they're not nearly as interested in talking about their own lives as they are about yours.

Not in the mood for a witty retort— or to even respond at all (especially after you've been asked the same question five times in a single day)? There's nothing wrong with letting the questioner know that the answer is none of her business, which it isn't. "That's a personal matter" says it all.

Safety in Numbers

"We'd barely adjusted to the fact that I was pregnant when we found out I'm carrying twins. Are there any extra risks for them, or for me?"

Extra babies do come with some extra risks, but not as many as you'd think. In fact, not all twin pregnancies are classified as "high risk" (though higher-order multiples definitely fall into that category), and most expectant mothers of multiples can expect to have relatively uneventful pregnancies (at least in terms of complications). Plus, entering your twin pregnancy armed with a little knowledge about the potential risks and complications can help you avoid many, and will prepare you should you encounter any. So relax (twin pregnancies are really safe), but read up.

For the babies, the potential risks include:

Early delivery. Multiples tend to arrive earlier than singletons. More than half of twins (59 percent of them), most triplets (93 percent), and practically all quadruplets are born premature. While women pregnant with only one fetus deliver, on average, at 39 weeks, twin delivery, on average, occurs at 35 to 36 weeks. Triplets usually come (again, on average) at 32 weeks, and quadruplets at 30 weeks. (Keep in mind that term for twins is considered 37 weeks, not 40.) After all, as cozy as it can be for your little ones in the uterus, it can also get pretty crowded as they grow. Be sure you know the signs of premature labor, and don't hesitate to call your practitioner right away if you're experiencing any of them (see page 300).

Low birthweight. Since many multiple pregnancies end early, most babies born of multiple pregnancies arrive weighing less than 5½ pounds, which is considered low birthweight. Most 5-pounders end up doing just fine healthwise, thanks to advances in caring for these small newborns, but babies born weighing less than 3 pounds are at increased risk for health complications as newborns, as well as for long-term disabilities. Making sure your prenatal health is in top-notch condition

and your diet contains plenty of nutrients (including the right amount of calories) can help get your babies to a bigger birthweight. (See *What to Expect the First Year* for more on premature babies.)

Twin-to-Twin Transfusion Syndrome (TTTS). This in utero condition, which happens in about 15 percent of identical twin pregnancies in which the placenta is shared (fraternal twins are almost never affected because they never share a placenta), occurs when blood vessels in their shared placenta cross, resulting in one baby getting too much blood flow and the other too little. This condition is dangerous for the babies, though not to the mother. If it's detected in your pregnancy,

Multiple Benefits

Good news! There's never been a safer time to conceive, carry, and give birth to more than one baby, and for lots of reassuring reasons. Here's what you have going for you as a mom-to-be of multiples these days:

- A heads-up. Since the discovery that you're carrying multiples almost always comes early on in pregnancy these days, you've got extra time for planning and preparing for your babies, plus plenty of time to get the best possible prenatal care. And good prenatal care is the ticket to a healthy pregnancy—doubly so in a multiple pregnancy.

- Lots more practitioner visits. Good prenatal care starts with more frequent practitioner visits. You'll likely be seen every two to three weeks (rather than every four) up until your seventh month and more frequently after that. And those visits may get more in-depth as your preg-

nancy progresses. You'll get all the tests singleton moms get, but you may also get internal exams earlier than a singleton mom-to-be would get (to check for signs of preterm labor).

- Pictures, pictures, pictures. Of your babies, that is. You'll get extra ultrasounds to monitor your babies and make sure their development and growth is on track and the pregnancy is healthy. Which means extra reassurance, plus extra pictures for your baby book.

- Extra attention. Good prenatal care also means extra attention to your health to reduce your risk of certain pregnancy complications (like hypertension, anemia, placenta abruption, and preterm labor, which are all more common in multiple pregnancies). With all that extra attention, any problem that develops will be treated quickly.

your practitioner may opt to use amnio-centesis to drain off excess fluid, which improves blood flow in the placenta and reduces the risk of preterm labor. Laser surgery to seal off the connection between the blood vessels is another option your practitioner may use. If you're dealing with TTTS, check out fetalhope.org for more information and resources.

A multiple pregnancy can also impact the health of the mother-to-be:

Preeclampsia. The more babies you're carrying, the more placenta you've got on board. This added placenta (along with the added hormones that come with two babies) can sometimes lead to high blood pressure, which may in turn progress to preeclampsia. Preeclampsia affects one in four mothers of twins and usually is caught early, thanks to careful monitoring by your practitioner. For more on the condition and treatment options, see page 548.

Gestational diabetes. Expectant multiple moms are slightly more likely to have gestational diabetes than a singleton mom. That's probably because higher hormone levels can interfere with a mother's ability to process insulin. Diet can usually control (or even prevent) this condition, but sometimes extra insulin is needed (see page 546 for more).

Placental problems. Women pregnant with multiples are at a somewhat higher risk for complications such as placenta previa (low-lying placenta) or placental abruption (premature separation of the placenta). Fortunately, careful monitoring (which you'll be getting) can detect previa long before it poses any significant risk. Abruption can't be detected before it happens, but because your pregnancy is being carefully watched, steps can be taken to avoid further complications should an abruption occur.

Bed Rest

"Will I have to be on bed rest just because I'm carrying twins?"

To bed rest or not to bed rest? That is the question many moms-to-be of multiples ask, and many practitioners don't always have an easy answer. That's because there really isn't an easy answer. The obstetrical jury is still out on whether bed rest helps prevent the kinds of complications sometimes associated with a multiple pregnancy (such as preterm labor and preeclampsia). So in the meantime, until more is known, some practitioners prescribe it in some cases. The more babies in a pregnancy, the more likely it will be prescribed, since the risk of complications increases with each additional fetus.

Be sure to have a discussion with your practitioner early in your pregnancy about his or her philosophy on bed rest. Some practitioners prescribe it routinely for all expectant mothers of multiples (often beginning between 24 and 28 weeks); more and more do it on a case-by-case basis, taking a wait-and-see approach.

If you are put on bed rest, see page 571 for tips on coping with it. And keep in mind that even if you aren't sent to bed, your practitioner will probably still advise you to take it easy, cut back on work, and stay off your feet as much as possible during the latter half of your pregnancy—so get ready to rest up.

Vanishing Twin Syndrome

"I've heard of vanishing twin syndrome. What is it?"

Detecting multiple pregnancies early using ultrasound technology has many benefits, because the sooner you and your practitioner discover you've got two (or more) babies to care for, the better care you'll be able to get. But there's sometimes a downside to knowing so soon. Identifying twin pregnancies earlier than ever also reveals losses that went undetected before the days of early ultrasound.

The loss of one twin during pregnancy can occur in the first trimester (often before the mother even knows she's carrying twins) or, less commonly, later in the pregnancy. During a first-trimester loss, the tissue of the miscarried twin is usually reabsorbed by the mother. This phenomenon, called vanishing twin syndrome, occurs in about 20 to 30 percent of multiple pregnancies. Documentation of vanishing twin syndrome has grown significantly over the past few decades, as early ultrasounds—the only way to be sure early in pregnancy that you're carrying twins—have become routine. Researchers report more cases of vanishing twin syndrome in women older than 30, though that may be because older mothers in general have higher rates of multiple pregnan-

cies, especially with the use of fertility treatments.

There are rarely any symptoms when the early loss of one twin occurs, though some mothers experience mild cramping, bleeding, or pelvic pain, similar to a miscarriage (though none of those symptoms is a sure sign of such a loss). Decreasing hormone levels (as detected by blood tests) may also indicate that one fetus has been miscarried.

The good news is that when vanishing twin syndrome occurs in the first trimester, the mother usually goes on to experience a normal pregnancy and delivers the single healthy baby without complication or intervention. In the much less likely case that a twin dies in the second or third trimester, the remaining baby may be at an increased risk of intrauterine growth restriction, and the mother may be at risk of preterm labor, infection, or bleeding. The remaining baby would then be watched carefully and the rest of the pregnancy monitored for complications.

For help coping with the loss of a twin in utero, see page 583.

For help coping with the loss of a twin in utero, see page 583.

ALL ABOUT

Multiple Childbirth

You're probably spending a lot of time wondering (okay, maybe you've been obsessing) about the day you'll actually give birth to your bundles of joy. Every delivery day is an unforgettable one, but if you're carrying twins (or more), yours probably won't be the typical birth story you've heard from moms who've delivered just one. Not surprisingly, things can get a little more complicated when you've got two babies or more heading for the exit—and a lot more interesting.

Will your labor and delivery be twice the effort? What will be the ideal way to deliver your multiple newborns into your two arms? The answers can depend on a lot of factors, such as fetal position, your health, the safety of the babies, and so on. Multiple births have more variables—and more surprises—than single births. But since you'll be getting two (or more) for the price of one labor, your multiple childbirth will be a pretty good deal no matter how it ends up playing out. And remember that whatever route your babies take from your snug womb to your even snugger embrace, the best way is the one that is the healthiest and safest for them—and for you.

Laboring with Twins or More

How will your labor differ from the labor of a mother-of-one? Here are a few ways:

- It could be shorter. Will you have to endure double the pain to end up cuddling double the pleasure? Nope. In fact, when it comes to labor, you're likely to catch a really nice break (for once). The first stage of labor is often shorter with multiples—which means that it may take less time to get to the point where you can start pushing, if you'll be delivering vaginally. The catch? You'll be hitting the harder part of labor sooner.

- Or it could be longer. Because a multiples mom's uterus is overstretched, contractions are sometimes weaker. And weaker contractions could mean that it might take longer to become fully dilated.

- It'll be watched more closely. Because your medical team will have to be twice as careful during your multiple delivery, you'll be monitored more during labor than most moms of singletons. Throughout labor, you'll likely be attached to two (or more) fetal monitors so your practitioner can see how each baby is responding to your contractions. Early on, the babies' heartbeats may be monitored with external belt monitors; this could allow you to go off the monitors periodically so you can walk around or hit the whirlpool tub to help ease your pain (if you're so

inclined). In the latter stages of labor, Baby A (the one closest to the exit) may be monitored internally with a scalp electrode while Baby B is still monitored externally. This will put an end to any wandering because you'll be tethered to a machine (but by this time, you may be well past the point of wanting to move around anyway). Be sure to discuss fetal monitoring and how it will affect your mobility with your practitioner.

- You'll probably have an epidural. If you've had your heart set on one anyway, you'll be happy to hear that epidurals are strongly encouraged—or even required—with multiple deliveries, in case an emergency C-section becomes necessary to deliver one or all of your babies. If you'd like to avoid an epidural, talk to your practitioner, because practitioner and hospital policies differ on this topic.

- You'll probably deliver in an operating room. Most hospitals require this, just to be on the safe side (and in case an emergency C-section becomes necessary), so ask ahead. Chances are you'll be able to labor in one of those comfy rooms with the pretty curtains and relaxing prints, but when it's time to push, you'll likely be wheeled into the OR.

Twin Timing

Just how far apart will your multiples be born? With vaginal deliveries, most babies are born 10 to 30 minutes apart. With C-sections, it can be just seconds, or up to a minute or two, between births.

Position, Position, Position

Quick . . . flip a coin. Heads (up) or tails (down)? Or maybe a combination of both? How multiples will end up at delivery time (and how you'll end up delivering) is anybody's guess. Here's a look at the possible ways your twins may be presenting and the likely delivery scenarios for each situation.

Vertex/vertex. This is the most cooperative position that twins can wind up in on delivery day, and they wind up in it about 40 percent of the time. If both your babies are vertex (heads down), you'll likely be able to go into labor naturally and attempt a vaginal birth. Keep in mind, however, that even perfectly positioned singletons sometimes need to be delivered by C-section. This goes double for twins.

Vertex/breech. The second best-case scenario if you're hoping for a vaginal birth for your twins is the vertex/breech setup. This means that if Baby A is head down and well positioned for delivery, it may be possible for your practitioner to manipulate Baby B from the breech position to vertex after Baby A is born. This can be done either by applying manual pressure to your abdomen (external version) or literally reaching inside your uterus to turn Baby B (internal version). The internal version sounds much more complicated than it is; because Baby A has essentially warmed up and stretched out the birth canal already, the procedure's over pretty quickly. If Baby B remains stubbornly breech, your practitioner may do a breech extraction, in which your baby is pulled feet first right out the door.

Breech/vertex or breech/breech. If Baby A is breech or if both your babies are bottoms down, your physician will almost certainly recommend a C-section. Though external version is commonplace for breech singletons (and can work in the above-mentioned vertex/breech multiple pregnancy), it's considered too risky in this scenario.

Baby A oblique. Who knew there were so many positions for babies to lie in? When Baby A is oblique, it means his or her head is pointed down, but toward either of your hips rather than squarely on your cervix. In a singleton pregnancy with oblique presentation, a practitioner would probably try external version to bring the baby's head where it needs to be (facing the exit), but that's risky with twins. In this case, two things can happen: An oblique presentation can correct itself as contractions progress, resulting in a vaginal birth, or more likely, your practitioner will recommend a C-section to avoid a long, drawn-out labor that may or may not lead to a vaginal birth.

Transverse/transverse. In this setup, both babies are lying horizontally across your uterus. A double transverse almost always results in a C-section.

Delivering Twins

Here's what you can expect when delivering your twins:

Vaginal delivery. About half of all twins born these days come into the world the old-fashioned way, but that doesn't mean the birthing experience is the same as it is for singleton moms. Once you're fully dilated, delivery of Baby A may be a cinch ("Three pushes was all it took!") or a protracted ordeal ("It took three hours!"). Though that latter scenario is far from a given, some research has shown that the pushing phase (stage two) is usually longer in a twin delivery than in a singleton delivery. The second twin in a vaginal delivery usually comes within 10 to 30 minutes of the first, and most mothers report that delivering Baby B is a snap compared to Baby A. Depending on the position of Baby B, he or she may need some help from the doctor, who can either reach in and move the baby into the birth canal (internal version) or use vacuum extraction to speed the delivery. The possibility of this kind of intervention is yet another reason why many doctors strongly recommend epidurals for multiple moms. (An arm reaching up into your uterus to pull out a baby isn't pretty without pain meds.)

Mixed delivery. In rare cases (very rare cases), Baby B must be delivered by C-section after Baby A has been delivered vaginally. This is usually done only when an emergency situation has come up that puts Baby B at risk, such as placental abruption or cord prolapse. (Those all-important fetal monitors tell your doctor just how well Baby B is doing after Baby A's arrival.) A mixed delivery is not fun for mom; in the moment, of course, it can be very scary, and after the babies are born, it means recovery from both a vaginal birth and major abdominal surgery, a big double ouch. But when it's necessary, it can be a baby-saving procedure, well worth the added recovery time.

Planned C-section. A scheduled C-section is discussed with your doctor in advance and a date is set. Possible reasons for this plan include a previous C-section (a VBAC is not common practice for multiples), placenta previa or other obstetrical or medical issues, or fetal positions that make vaginal delivery unsafe. With most planned C-sections, your spouse, partner, or coach can accompany you into the operating room, where you will probably be given a spinal block—a pumped-up version of the epidural used to block pain

Recovery from a Multiple Delivery

Besides having your hands twice as full, your recovery from a multiple delivery will be very similar to that of a singleton delivery, so be sure to read through Chapters 17 and 18. You can also expect these postpartum differences:

- It'll likely take longer for your belly to return to normal size (it was stretched out more, after all). You'll likely have more extra skin to contend with, too, after all that stretching.

- You may experience more lochia (vaginal bleeding) for a longer period of time. That's because more blood was stored up in your uterus during your pregnancy, and it all has to go now.

- Getting back into shape will take longer—mostly because you were probably pretty inactive for the last three months of your pregnancy (no matter how physically fit, or not, you were before your pregnancy).

- You'll be achier for longer because of all the extra weight you carried around during pregnancy. Not to mention all the extra carrying around you'll be doing after delivery.

Breastfeeding for Two Is Good for Mom, Too

You probably already know that breastfeeding is the best for your babies (see page 447 for tips on breastfeeding multiples). But did you know that it also does your postpartum body good? Breastfeeding releases hormones (oxytocin) that help your uterus contract to its normal size (and remember, yours was especially stretched). This in turn will also stem the flow of lochia, so you'll lose less blood. And if you're concerned about losing weight, just consider those little nurslings to be nature's liposuction machines: Breastfeeding two babies will burn fat and calories twice as fast, which means you'll also have license to continue eating more. Nurse three (or more) and the calorie bonuses multiply.

If your newborns are in the NICU, you probably won't be able to nurse them directly at first, but they'll benefit greatly from the ideal nutrition only you can provide (especially if they're preemies). So cozy up to an electric pump (they can likely be fed with the expressed milk), and continue pumping until they're released and ready to cozy up to your breasts.

in a vaginal birth. You may be surprised by how fast it all goes after you're numb: Baby A's and Baby B's birth times will be separated by anywhere from seconds to just a minute or two.

Unplanned C-section. An unplanned C-section is the other possible way your babies might enter the world. In this case, you may walk into your usual weekly prenatal appointment and find out that you're going to meet your babies the same day. Best to be prepared, so in those later weeks of pregnancy, be sure to get your bag packed and ready to go. Reasons for a surprise cesarean delivery include such conditions as intrauterine growth restriction (where the babies run out of room to grow) or a sharp rise in your blood pressure (preeclampsia). Another unplanned C-section scenario may arise if you labor for a very long time and don't progress at all. A uterus holding 10 or more pounds of babies may be too stretched to contract effectively, so a cesarean delivery might be the only way out.

Delivering Triplets

Wondering if your triplets are destined to take the abdominal route out? Cesarean delivery is most often used for triplets—not only because it's usually safest, but because C-sections are more common in high-risk deliveries (a category triplets always fall into) and because they're more common among older moms (who give birth to the majority of triplets). But some doctors say that vaginal delivery can be an option if Triplet A (the one nearest the "exit") is in a head-down presentation and there are no other complicating factors (such as preeclampsia in the mother or fetal distress in one or more of the babies). In some rare cases, the first baby or the first and second may be delivered vaginally, and the final one may require a cesarean delivery. Of course, more important than having all three of your babies exit vaginally is having all four of you leaving the delivery room in good condition—and any route to that outcome will be a successful one.

PART 4

After the Baby Is Born

CHAPTER 17

Postpartum: The First Week

ONGRATULATIONS! THE MOMENT you've awaited for 40 (or so) weeks has finally arrived. You've put months of pregnancy and long hours of childbirth behind you, and you're officially a mother, with a new bundle of joy in your arms instead of in your belly. But the transition from pregnancy to postpartum comes with more than just a baby. It also comes with a variety of new symptoms (good-bye pregnancy aches, pains, and discomforts, hello postpartum ones) and a variety of new questions (Why am I sweating so much? Why am I having contractions if I've already delivered? Will I ever be able to sit again? Why do I still look six months pregnant? Whose breasts are these anyway?). Hopefully, you'll have a chance to read up on these and many more pertinent postpartum topics in advance. Once you're on full-time mom duty, finding the time to read anything (never mind use the toilet) won't be easy.

What You May Be Feeling

During the first week postpartum, depending on the type of delivery you had (easy or difficult, vaginal or cesarean) and other individual factors, you may experience all, or only some, of the following:

Physically

- Vaginal bleeding (lochia) similar to your period

- Abdominal cramps (afterpains) as your uterus contracts

- Exhaustion

- Perineal discomfort, pain, numbness, if you had a vaginal delivery (especially if you had stitches)

- Some perineal discomfort if you had a C-section

- Pain around the incision and, later, numbness in the area, if you had a C-section (especially a first one)

- Discomfort sitting and walking if you had an episiotomy, a repair of a tear, or a cesarean delivery

- Difficulty urinating for a day or two

- Constipation; discomfort with bowel movements for the first few days

- Hemorrhoids, continued from pregnancy, or new from pushing

- All-over achiness, especially if you did a lot of pushing

- Bloodshot eyes; black-and-blue marks around eyes, on cheeks, elsewhere, from too-vigorous pushing

- Sweating, and lots of it, particularly at night

- Breast discomfort and engorgement beginning around the third or fourth day postpartum

- Sore or cracked nipples, if you're breastfeeding

Emotionally

- Elation, blues, or swings between the two

- New-mom jitters; trepidation about caring for your new baby, especially if you're a first timer

- Frustration, if you're having a hard time getting started breastfeeding

- A feeling of being overwhelmed by the physical, emotional, and logistical challenges facing you

- Excitement about starting your new life with your new baby

What You May Be Wondering About

Bleeding

"I expected some bleeding after delivery, but when I got out of bed for the first time and saw the blood running down my legs, I was a little freaked out."

Grab a pile of pads, and relax. This discharge of leftover blood, mucus, and tissue from your uterus, known as lochia, is normally as heavy as (and often heavier than) a menstrual period for the first three to ten postpartum days. It may total up to 2 cups before it begins to taper off, and at times it may seem pretty profuse. A sudden gush when you stand up in the first few days is normal—it's just the flow that accumulates when you've been lying down or sitting. Because blood and an occasional blood clot are the predominant ingredients of lochia during the immediate postpartum period, your discharge can be quite red for anywhere from five days to three weeks, gradually turning to a watery pink, then to brown, and finally to a yellowish white. Maxipads, not tampons, should be used to absorb the flow, which may continue on and off for just a couple of weeks or as long as six weeks.

In some women, light bleeding continues for three months. The flow is different for everyone.

Breastfeeding—and/or intravenous Pitocin (oxytocin), which is routinely ordered by some doctors following delivery—may reduce the flow of lochia by encouraging uterine contractions. These postdelivery contractions help shrink the uterus back to its normal size more quickly while pinching off exposed blood vessels at the site where the placenta separated from the uterus. For more about these contractions, see the next question.

If you're in the hospital or birthing center and you think your bleeding may be excessive, notify a nurse. If you experience what seems to be abnormally heavy bleeding (see page 569) once you're home, call your practitioner without delay; if you can't reach him or her, go to the emergency room (in the hospital where you delivered, if possible).

Afterpains

"I've been having crampy pains in my abdomen, especially when I'm nursing. What's that about?"

Thought you'd felt the last of those contractions? Unfortunately, they don't end immediately with delivery—and neither does the discomfort they cause. Those so-called afterpains are triggered by the contractions of the uterus as it shrinks (from about 2⅓ pounds to just a couple of ounces) and makes its normal descent back into the pelvis following the birth of your baby. You can keep track of the shrinking size of your uterus by pressing lightly below your navel. By the end of six weeks, you probably won't feel it at all.

Afterpains can definitely be a pain, but they do good work. Besides helping the uterus find its way back to its usual size and location, those contractions help slow normal postpartum bleeding. They're likely to be more of a pain in women whose uterine muscles are lacking in tone because of previous births or excessive stretching (as with a multiple pregnancy). Afterpains can be more pronounced during nursing, when contraction-stimulating oxytocin is released (a good thing, actually, since it means your uterus is shrinking faster) and/or if you've had intravenous Pitocin (oxytocin) following delivery.

The pains should subside naturally within four to seven days. In the meantime, acetaminophen (Tylenol) should provide relief. If it doesn't, or if the pains persist for more than a week, see your practitioner to rule out other postpartum problems, including infection.

Perineal Pain

"I didn't have an episiotomy, and I didn't tear. Why am I so sore down below?"

You can't expect some 7 pounds of baby to pass unnoticed. Even if your perineum was left neatly intact during the baby's arrival, that area has still been stretched, bruised, and generally traumatized, and discomfort, ranging from mild to not so mild, is the very normal result. The pain may be worse when you cough or sneeze, and you may even find that it hurts to sit down for a few days. You can try the same tips given in the next answer for women with post-tear pain.

It's also possible that in pushing your baby out, you developed hemorrhoids and, possibly, anal fissures, which can range from uncomfortable to extremely painful. See page 272 for tips on dealing with hemorrhoids.

"I tore during delivery and now I'm incredibly sore. Could my stitches be infected?"

Everyone who delivers vaginally (and sometimes those who have a lengthy labor before delivering via cesarean) can expect some perineal pain. But, not surprisingly, that pain's likely to be compounded if the perineum was torn or surgically cut (aka an episiotomy). Like any freshly repaired wound, the site of a laceration or episiotomy will take time to heal, usually 7 to 10 days. Pain alone during this time, unless it is very severe, is not an indication that you've developed an infection.

What's more, infection (though possible) is really very unlikely if your perineal area has been well cared for since delivery. While you're in the hospital or birthing center, a nurse will check your perineum at least once daily to be certain there is no inflammation or other indication of infection. She'll also instruct you in postpartum perineal hygiene, which is important in preventing infection not only of the repair site but of the genital tract as well (germs can get around). For this reason, the same precautions apply for those who delivered completely intact. Here's the self-care plan for a healthy postpartum perineum:

- Use a fresh maxipad at least every four to six hours.

- Pour or squirt warm water (or an antiseptic solution, if one was recommended by your practitioner or nurse) over your perineum while you pee to ease burning, and after you're done on the toilet, to keep the area clean. Pat dry with gauze pads or with the paper wipes that come with some hospital-provided sanitary pads, always from front to back. Gently does it—no rubbing.

- Keep your hands off the area until healing is complete.

Though discomfort is likely to be greater if you've had a repair (with itchiness around the stitches possibly accompanying soreness), the suggestions below will likely be welcome no matter how you delivered. To relieve perineal pain:

Ice it. To reduce swelling and bring soothing relief, use chilled witch hazel pads, a surgical glove filled with crushed ice, or a maxipad with a built-in cold pack, applied to the site every couple of hours during the first 24 hours following delivery.

Heat it. Warm sitz baths (a bath in which only your hips and buttocks are submerged) for 20 minutes a few times a day or hot compresses will ease discomfort.

Numb it. Use local anesthetics in the form of sprays, creams, ointments, or pads recommended by your practitioner. Acetaminophen (Tylenol) may also help.

Keep off it. To keep the pressure off your sore perineum, lie on your side when possible, and avoid long periods of standing or sitting. Sitting on a pillow (especially one with an opening in the center) or inflated tube (usually marketed to hemorrhoid sufferers) may also help, as can tightening your buttocks before sitting.

Keep it loose. Tight clothing, especially underwear, can rub and irritate the area, plus slow healing. Let your perineum breathe as much as possible (for now, favor baggy sweats over spandex leggings).

Exercise it. Kegel exercises, done as frequently as possible after delivery and right through the postpartum period, will stimulate circulation to the area, promoting healing and improving muscle tone. Don't worry if you can't feel yourself doing the Kegels; the area will be numb right after delivery. Feeling

When to Call Your Practitioner Postpartum

Few women feel their physical (or emotional) best after delivering a baby—that's just par for postpartum. Especially in the first six weeks after delivery, experiencing a variety of aches, pains, and other uncomfortable (or unpleasant) symptoms is common. Fortunately, what isn't common is having a serious complication. Still, it's smart to be in the know. That's why all recent deliverees should be aware of symptoms that might point to a postpartum problem, just in case. Call your practitioner without delay if you experience any of the following:

- Bleeding that saturates more than one pad an hour for more than a few hours. If you can't reach your practitioner immediately, call your local emergency room and have the triage nurse assess you over the phone. He or she will be able to tell you whether or not you should come into the ER. While waiting or en route to the ER, if necessary, lie down and keep an ice pack (or a ziplock plastic bag filled with ice cubes and a couple of paper towels to absorb the melting ice) on your lower abdomen (directly over your uterus, if you can locate it).

- Large amounts of *bright red* bleeding any time after the first postpartum week. But don't worry about light menstrual-like bleeding for up to 6 weeks (in some women as many as 12) or a flow that increases when you're more active or when you're nursing.

- Bleeding that has a foul odor. It should smell like a normal menstrual flow.

- Numerous or large (lemon-size or larger) clots in the vaginal bleeding. Occasional small clots in the first few days, however, are normal.

will return to the perineum gradually over the next few weeks—and in the meantime, the work's being done even if you can't feel it.

If your perineum becomes very red, very painful, and swollen, or if you detect an unpleasant odor, you may have developed an infection. Call your practitioner.

Delivery Bruises

"I look more like I've been in a boxing ring than in a birthing room. How come?"

Look and feel like you've taken a beating? That's normal postpartum. After all, you probably worked harder birthing your child than most boxers work in the ring, even though you were only facing a 7- or 8-pounder. Thanks—or no thanks—to powerful contractions and strenuous pushing (especially if you were pushing with your face and chest instead of your lower body), you might be sporting a variety of unwelcome delivery souvenirs. These may include black or bloodshot eyes (dark glasses will do a cover-up job in public until your eyes return to normal, and cold compresses for 10 minutes several times a day may help speed that return) and bruises, ranging from tiny dots on the cheek to larger black-and-blue marks on the face or upper chest area. You may also be bringing home soreness in your chest

- A complete absence of bleeding during the first few postpartum days

- Pain or discomfort, with or without swelling, in the lower abdominal area beyond the first few days after delivery

- Persistent pain in the perineal area, beyond the first few days

- After the first 24 hours, a temperature of over 100°F for more than a day

- Severe dizziness

- Nausea and vomiting

- Localized pain, swelling, redness, heat, and tenderness in a breast once engorgement has subsided, which could be signs of mastitis or breast infection. Begin home treatment (page 446) while waiting to reach your practitioner.

- Localized swelling and/or redness, heat, and oozing at the site of a C-section incision

- After the first 24 hours, difficult urination; excessive pain or burning when urinating; a frequent urge to urinate that yields little result; scanty and/or dark urine. Drink plenty of water while trying to reach your practitioner.

- Sharp chest pain (not chest achiness, which is the usual result of strenuous pushing); rapid breath or heartbeat; blueness of fingertips or lips

- Localized pain, tenderness, and warmth in your calf or thigh, with or without redness, swelling, and pain when you flex your foot. Rest, with your leg elevated, while you try to reach your practitioner.

- Depression that affects your ability to cope or that doesn't subside after a few days; feelings of anger toward your baby, particularly if those feelings are accompanied by violent urges. See page 458 for more on postpartum depression.

and/or difficulty taking a deep breath, due to strained chest muscles (hot baths, showers, or a heating pad may ease it), pain and tenderness in the area of your tailbone (heat and massage may help), and/or general all-over achiness (again, heat may help).

Difficulty Urinating

"It's been several hours since I gave birth, and I haven't been able to pee."

Peeing doesn't come easily for most women during the first 24 postpartum hours. Some women feel no urge at all; others feel the urge but are unable to satisfy it. Still others manage to uri-

nate, but with accompanying pain and burning. There are a host of reasons why basic bladder function often becomes too much like hard work after delivery:

- The holding capacity of the bladder increases because it suddenly has more room to expand—thus your need to pee may be less frequent than it was during pregnancy.

- The bladder may have been traumatized or bruised during delivery. Temporarily paralyzed, it may not send the necessary signals of urgency even when it's full.

- Having had an epidural may decrease the sensitivity of the bladder or your alertness to its signals.

- Pain in the perineal area may cause reflex spasms in the urethra (the tube through which the urine exits), making urination difficult. Swelling of the perineum may also stand between you and an easy pee.

- The sensitivity of the site of a tear or episiotomy repair can cause burning and/or pain with urination. Burning may be alleviated somewhat by standing astride the toilet while urinating so the flow comes straight down, without touching sore spots. Squirting warm water on the area while you pee can also decrease discomfort (use the squirt bottle the nurse probably gave you; ask for one if she didn't).

- Dehydration, especially if you didn't do any drinking during a long labor, and didn't receive any IV fluids.

- Any number of psychological factors may keep you from going with the flow: fear of pain, lack of privacy, embarrassment or discomfort over using a bedpan or needing assistance at the toilet.

As difficult as peeing may be after delivery, it's essential that you empty your bladder within six to eight hours to avoid urinary tract infection, loss of muscle tone in the bladder from overdistension, and bleeding (because an overfull bladder can get in the way of your uterus as it attempts the normal postpartum contractions that staunch bleeding). Therefore, the nurse will ask you frequently after delivery if you've accomplished this important goal. She may even request that you make that first postpartum pee into a container or bedpan, so she can measure your output, and may palpate your bladder to make sure it's not distended. To help get things flowing:

- Be sure you're drinking plenty of fluids: What goes in is more likely to go out. Plus, you lost a lot during delivery.

- Take a walk. Getting up out of bed and going for a slow stroll as soon after delivery as you're able will help get your bladder (and your bowels) moving.

- If you're uncomfortable with an audience (and who isn't?), have the nurse wait outside while you urinate. She can come back in when you've finished and give you a demonstration of perineal hygiene, if she hasn't already.

- If you're too weak to walk to the bathroom and you have to use a bedpan, ask for some warm water to pour over the perineal area (which may stimulate the urge). It will also help to sit on the pan, instead of lying on it. Privacy, again, will be key to success.

- Warm your perineal area in a sitz bath or chill it with ice packs, whichever seems to induce urgency for you.

- Turn the water on while you try. Running water in the sink really does encourage your own faucet to flow.

If all efforts fail and you haven't peed within eight hours or so after delivery, your practitioner may order a catheter (a tube inserted into your urethra) to empty your bladder—another good incentive to try the methods above.

After 24 hours, the problem of too little generally becomes one of too much. Most new moms usually begin urinating frequently and plentifully as the excess fluids of pregnancy are excreted. If you're still having trouble peeing, or if output is scant during the next few days, it's possible you have a urinary tract infection (see page 498 for signs and symptoms of a UTI).

"I can't seem to control my urine. It just leaks out."

The physical stress of childbirth can put a lot of things temporarily out of commission, including the bladder. Either it can't let go of the urine—or it lets go of it too easily, as in your case. Such leakage (called urinary incontinence) occurs because of loss of muscle tone in the perineal area. Kegel exercises, which are recommended for every postpartum mom anyway, can help restore the tone and help you regain control over the flow of urine. See page 454 for more tips on dealing with incontinence; if it continues, consult your practitioner.

That First Bowel Movement

"I delivered two days ago and I haven't had a bowel movement yet. I've actually felt the urge, but I've been too afraid of opening my stitches to try."

The passage of the first postpartum bowel movement is a milestone every newly delivered woman is anxious to put behind her (so to speak). And the longer it takes you to get past that milestone, the more anxious—and the more uncomfortable—you're likely to become.

Several physiological factors may interfere with the return of bowel-business-as-usual after delivery. For one thing, the abdominal muscles that assist in elimination have been stretched during childbirth, making them flaccid and sometimes temporarily ineffective. For another, the bowel itself may have taken a beating during delivery, leaving it sluggish. And, of course, it may have been emptied before or during delivery (remember that diarrhea you had prelabor? The poop that you squeezed out during pushing?), and probably stayed pretty empty because you didn't eat much solid food during labor.

But perhaps the most potent inhibitors of postpartum bowel activity are psychological: worry about pain; the unfounded fear that you'll split open any stitches; concern that you'll make your hemorrhoids worse; the natural embarrassment over lack of privacy in the hospital or birthing center; and the pressure to "perform," which often makes performance all the more elusive.

Just because postpartum constipation is common, though, doesn't mean you can't fight it. Here are some steps you can take to get things moving again:

Don't worry. Nothing will keep you from moving your bowels more effectively than worrying about moving your bowels. Don't worry about opening the stitches—you won't. Finally, don't worry if it takes a few days to get things moving—that's okay, too.

Request roughage. If you're still in the hospital or birthing center, select as many whole grains (especially bran cereal) and fresh fruits and vegetables from the menu as you can. Since those pickings may be slim, supplement with bowel-stimulating food brought in from outside, such as apples and pears, raisins and other dried fruit, nuts, seeds, and bran muffins. If you're home, make sure you're eating regularly and well—and that you're getting your fill of fiber. As much as you can, stay away from bowel-clogging foods (like those gift boxes of chocolates that are likely piling up on your bedstand or coffee table—tempting but, sadly, constipating).

Keep the liquids coming. Not only do you need to compensate for fluids you lost during labor and delivery, you need to take in additional liquids to help soften stool if you're clogged up. Water's always a winner, but you may also find apple or prune juice especially effective. Hot water with lemon can also do the trick.

Chew, chew, chew. Chewing gum stimulates digestive reflexes for some people and could get your system back to normal, so grab a stick of gum.

Get off your bottom. An inactive body encourages inactive bowels. You won't be running laps the day after delivery, but you will be able to take short strolls up and down the halls. Kegel exercises, which can be practiced in bed almost immediately after delivery, will help tone up not only the perineum but also the rectum. At home, take walks with baby; also, see page 465 for postpartum exercise ideas.

Don't strain. Straining won't break open any stitches you have, but it can lead to or aggravate hemorrhoids. If you already have hemorrhoids, you may find relief with sitz baths, topical anesthetics, witch hazel pads, suppositories, or hot or cold compresses.

Use stool softeners. Many hospitals send women home with both a stool softener and a laxative, for good reason. Both can help get you going.

The first few bowel movements may be a pain to pass, literally. But fear not. As stools soften and you become more regular, the discomfort will ease and eventually end—and moving your bowels will become second nature once again.

Excessive Sweating

"I've been waking up at night soaked with sweat. Is this normal?"

It's messy, but it's normal. New moms are sweaty moms, and for a couple of good reasons. For one thing, your hormone levels are dropping—reflecting the fact that you're no longer pregnant, as you might have noticed. For another, perspiration (like frequent urination) is your body's way of ridding itself of pregnancy-accumulated fluids after delivery—something you're bound to be happy about. Something you might not be happy with is how uncomfortable that perspiration might make you, and how long it might continue. Some women keep sweating up a storm for several weeks or more. If you do most of your perspiring at night, as most new moms do, covering your pillow with an absorbent towel may help you sleep better (it'll also help protect your pillow).

Don't sweat the sweat—it's normal. Do make sure, though, that you're drinking enough fluids to compensate for the ones you're losing, especially if you're breastfeeding but even if you're not.

Fever

"I've just come home from the hospital and I'm running a fever of about 101°F. Should I call my doctor?"

It's always a good idea to keep your practitioner in the loop if you're not feeling well right after giving birth. A fever on the third or fourth postpartum day could possibly be a sign of postpartum infection, but it could also be caused by a nonpostpartum-related illness. Fever can also occasionally be caused by the combination of excitement and exhaustion that's common in the early postpartum period. A brief low-grade fever (less than 100°F) occasionally accompanies engorgement when your milk first comes in, and it's nothing to worry about. But as a precaution, report to your practitioner any fever over 100°F that lasts more than a day during the first three postpartum weeks or that lasts more than a few hours if it's a higher fever—even if it's accompanied by obvious cold or flu symptoms or vomiting—so that its cause can be determined and any necessary treatment started.

Engorged Breasts

"My milk finally came in, leaving my breasts three times their normal size—and so hard and painful that I can't put on a bra. Is this what I have to look forward to until I wean my baby?"

Just when you thought your breasts couldn't get any bigger, they do. That first milk delivery arrives, leaving your breasts swollen, painfully tender, throbbing, granite hard—and sometimes seriously, frighteningly gigantic. To make matters more uncomfortable and inconvenient, this engorgement (which can extend all the way to the armpits) can make nursing painful for you and, if your nipples are flattened by the swelling, frustrating for your baby. The longer it takes for you and your baby to hook up for your first nursing sessions, the worse the engorgement is likely to be.

Happily, though, it won't last long. Engorgement, and all its miserable effects, gradually lessens once a well-coordinated milk supply-and-demand system is established, typically within a matter of days. Nipple soreness, too—which usually peaks at about the 20th feeding, if you're keeping count—generally diminishes rapidly as the nipples toughen up. And with proper care (see page 444), so does the nipple cracking and bleeding some women also experience.

Until nursing becomes second nature for your breasts—and completely painless for you—there are some steps you can take to ease the discomfort and speed the establishment of a good milk supply (read all about it starting on page 435).

Women who have an easy time getting started with breastfeeding (especially second timers) may not experience very much engorgement at all. As long as baby's getting those milk deliveries, that's normal, too.

Engorgement if You're Not Breastfeeding

"I'm not nursing. I've heard that drying up the milk can be painful."

Your breasts are programmed to fill (or make that overfill) with milk around the third or fourth postpartum day, whether you plan to use that milk to feed your baby or not. This engorgement can be uncomfortable, even painful—but it's only temporary.

Milk is produced by your breasts only as needed. If the milk isn't used, production stops. Though sporadic leaking may continue for several days, or even weeks, severe engorgement shouldn't last more than 12 to 24 hours. During this time, ice packs, mild pain relievers, and a supportive bra may help. Avoid nipple stimulation, expressing milk, or hot showers, all of which stimulate milk production and keep that painful cycle going longer.

Where's the Breast Milk?

"It's been two days since I delivered, and nothing comes out of my breasts when I squeeze them, not even colostrum. Is my baby going to starve?"

Not only is your baby not starving, he isn't even hungry yet. Babies aren't born with a big appetite or with immediate nutritional needs. And by the time your baby begins to hunger for a breastful of milk (on the third or fourth

Should I Stay or Should I Go Now?

Wondering when you'll be able to bring baby home? How long you and your baby stay in the hospital will depend on the kind of delivery you had, your condition, and your baby's condition. By federal law, you have the right to expect your insurer to pay for a 48-hour stay following a normal vaginal delivery and 96 hours following a cesarean delivery. If both you and your baby are in fine shape and you're eager to get home, you may be able to arrange with your practitioner for an early discharge. In that case, plan on having a home nurse visit (your insurance plan may pay for it) or taking your newborn for an office visit to the doctor within a few days, just to be sure no problems have cropped up. The baby's weight and general condition will be assessed (including a check for jaundice). There should also be an evaluation of how feeding is going—keeping and bringing along a feeding diary will help.

If you do stay the full 48 or 96 hours, take advantage of the opportunity to rest as much as possible. You'll need that energy stash for when you get home.

day postpartum), you'll undoubtedly be able to serve it up.

Which isn't to say that your breasts are empty now. Colostrum, which provides your baby with enough nourishment (for now) and with important antibodies his or her own body can't yet produce (and also helps empty baby's digestive system of excess mucus and his or her bowels of meconium), is definitely present in the tiny amounts necessary. A

teaspoon or so per feeding is all your baby needs at this point. But until the third or fourth postpartum day, when your breasts begin to swell and feel full (indicating the milk has come in), it's not that easy to express by hand. A day-old baby, eager to suckle, is better equipped to extract this premilk than you are.

Bonding

"I expected to bond with my baby as soon as she was born, but I'm not feeling anything at all. Is something wrong with me?"

Moments after delivery, you're handed your long-anticipated bundle of joy, and she's more beautiful and more perfect than you ever dared to imagine. She looks up at you and your eyes lock in a heady gaze, forging an instant maternal-child bond. As you cradle her tiny form, breathe in her sweetness, cover her soft face with kisses, you feel emotions you never knew you had, and they overwhelm you in their intensity. You're a mom in love.

And most likely, you were dreaming—or, at least, pregnant daydreaming. Birthing-room scenes like this one are the stuff dreams—and sappy commercials—are made of, but they don't play out for a lot of new moms. A possibly more-realistic scenario: After a long, hard labor that's left you physically and emotionally drained, a wrinkled, puffy, red-faced stranger is placed in your awkward arms, and the first thing you notice is that she doesn't quite resemble the chubby-cheeked cherub you'd been expecting. The second thing you notice is that she doesn't stop squalling. The third, that you have no idea how to make her stop squalling. You struggle to nurse her, but she's uncooperative; you try to socialize with her, but she's more interested in squalling than in sleeping—and frankly, at this point, so are you. And you can't help wondering (after you've woken up): "Have I missed my opportunity to bond with her?"

Absolutely, positively not. The process of bonding is different for every parent and every baby, and it doesn't come with a use-by date. Though some moms bond faster than others with their newborns—maybe because they've had experience with infants before, their expectations are more realistic, their labors were easier, or their babies are more responsive—few find that attachment forming with super glue speed. The bonds that last a lifetime don't form overnight. They form gradually, over time—something you and your baby have lots of ahead of you.

So give yourself that time—time to get used to being a mother (it's a major adjustment, after all) and time to get to know your baby, who, let's face it, is a newcomer in your life. Meet your baby's basic needs (and your own), and you'll find that love connection forming—one day (and one cuddle) at a time. And speaking of cuddles, bring 'em on. The more nurturing you do, the more like a nurturer you'll feel. Though it may not seem like it's coming naturally at first, the more time you spend cuddling, caressing, feeding, massaging, singing to, cooing to, and talking to your baby—the more time you spend skin to skin and face to face—the more natural it will start feeling, and the closer you'll become. Believe it or not, before you know it, you'll feel like the mother you are (really!), bound to your baby by the kind of love you've dreamed of.

"My new son was premature and was rushed to the NICU right away. The doctors say he'll be there for at least two weeks. Will it be too late for good bonding when he gets out?"

Not at all. Sure, having a chance to bond right after birth—to make contact, skin to skin, eye to eye—is wonderful. It's first step in the development of a lasting parent-child connection. But it's only the first step. And this step doesn't have to take place at delivery. It can take place hours or days later in a hospital bed, or through the portholes of an incubator, or even weeks later at home.

And luckily, you'll be able to touch, talk to, or possibly hold your baby even while he's in the NICU. Most hospitals not only allow parent-child contact in such situations, they encourage it. Talk to the nurse in charge of the NICU and see how you can best get close to your newborn during this trying time. For more on the care of premature babies, see *What to Expect the First Year.*

Keep in mind, too, that even moms and dads who have a chance to bond in the birthing room don't necessarily feel that instant attachment (see the previous question). Love that lasts a lifetime takes time to develop—time that you and your baby will start having together soon.

Rooming-In

"Having the baby room in with me sounded like a great idea when I was pregnant. But back then I had no idea how tired I was going to be. What kind of mother would I be, though, if I asked the nurse to take her?"

You would be a very human mother. You've just completed one of life's greatest challenges, childbirth, and are about to begin an even greater one, child rearing. Needing a little bit of rest in between is completely normal—and completely understandable.

Full-time rooming-in is a wonderful option in family-centered maternity care, giving new parents the chance to start getting to know their new arrival from minute one. But it's not a requirement, and it's not for everyone. Some women handle it easily, of course—maybe because their deliveries were a breeze or because they came on the job with previous newborn experience. For them, an inconsolable infant at 3 A.M. may not be a joy, but it's not a nightmare, either. However, for a new mom who's been without sleep for more hours than she can count, who's drained from labor and delivery, and who's never been closer to a baby than a diaper ad (sound familiar?), such predawn bouts can leave her feeling overwhelmed and underprepared.

If you're happy having your baby room with you, great. But if you committed to this sleeping arrangement only to realize you'd really rather get some sleep, don't feel you can't opt out. Partial rooming-in (during the day but not at night) may be a good compromise for you. Or you might prefer to get a good night's sleep the first night and start rooming-in on the second. Just make sure that baby is brought to you for feedings—and not given any supplementary bottles—if you're nursing.

Be flexible. Focus on the quality of the time you spend with your baby in the hospital rather than the quantity, and don't feel guilty about factoring your own needs into the equation. Round-the-clock rooming-in will begin soon enough at home. Get the rest you need now and you'll be better equipped to handle it later.

Recovery from a Cesarean Delivery

"What will my recovery from a C-section be like?"

Recovery from a C-section is similar to recovery from any abdominal surgery, with a delightful difference:

Instead of losing an old gallbladder or appendix, you gain a brand-new baby.

Of course, there's another difference, arguably less delightful. In addition to recovering from surgery, you'll also be recovering from childbirth. Except for a neatly intact perineum, you'll experience all the same postpartum discomforts over the next weeks (lucky you!) that you would have had if you'd delivered vaginally: afterpains, lochia, perineal discomfort (if you went through a lengthy labor before the surgery), breast engorgement, fatigue, hormonal changes, and excessive perspiration, to name a few.

As for your surgical recovery, you can expect the following in the recovery room:

Pain around your incision. Once the anesthesia wears off, your wound, like any wound, is going to hurt—though just how much depends on many factors, including your personal pain threshold and how many cesarean deliveries you've had (the first is usually the most uncomfortable). You will probably be given pain relief medication as needed, which may make you feel woozy or drugged. It will also allow you to get some needed sleep. You don't have to be concerned if you're nursing; the medication won't pass into your colostrum, and by the time your milk comes in, you probably won't need any heavy painkillers. If the pain continues for weeks, as it sometimes does, you can safely rely on over-the-counter pain relief. Ask your practitioner for a recommendation and dosing. To encourage healing, also try to avoid heavy lifting for the first few weeks after the surgery.

Possible nausea, with or without vomiting. This isn't always an aftereffect of the surgery, but if it is, you may be given an anti-nausea medication.

Exhaustion. You're likely to feel somewhat weak after surgery, partly due to blood loss, partly due to the anesthetic. If you went through some hours of labor before the surgery, you'll feel even more beat. You might also feel emotionally spent (after all, you did just have a baby—and surgery), especially if the C-section wasn't planned.

Regular evaluations of your condition. A nurse will periodically check your vital signs (temperature, blood pressure, pulse, respiration), your urinary output and vaginal bleeding, the dressing on your incision, and the firmness and level of your uterus (as it shrinks in size and makes its way back into the pelvis). She will also check your IV and urinary catheter.

Once you have been moved to your room, you can expect:

More checking. The nurse will continue to monitor your condition.

Removal of the urinary catheter. This will probably take place shortly after surgery. Urination may be difficult, so try the tips on page 426. If they don't work, the catheter may be reinserted until you can pee by yourself.

Encouragement to exercise. Before you're out of bed, you'll be encouraged to wiggle your toes, flex your feet to stretch your calf muscles, push against the end of the bed with your feet, and turn from side to side. You can also try the exercises on pages 466 and 467. They're intended to improve circulation, especially in your legs, and prevent the development of blood clots. (But be prepared for some of them to be quite uncomfortable, at least for the first 24 hours or so.)

To get up between 8 and 24 hours after surgery. With the help of a nurse, you'll sit up first, supported by the raised head of the bed. Then, using your hands for support, you'll slide your legs over the side of the bed and dangle them for a few minutes. Then, slowly, you'll be helped to step down on the floor, your hands still on the bed. If you feel dizzy (which is normal), sit right back down. Steady yourself for a few more minutes before taking a couple of steps, and then take them slowly; the first few may be extremely painful. Though you may need help the first few times you get up, this difficulty in getting around is temporary. In fact, you may soon find yourself more mobile than the vaginal deliveree next door—and you will probably have the edge when it comes to sitting.

A slow return to a normal diet. While it used to be routine (and still is in some hospitals and with some physicians) to keep women on IV fluids for the first 24 hours after a cesarean delivery and limit them to clear liquids for a day or two after that, starting up on solids much sooner may be a better bet. Research has shown that women who start back on solids earlier (gradually, but beginning as early as four to eight hours post-op) have that first bowel movement earlier and are generally ready to be released from the hospital 24 hours sooner than those kept on fluids only. Procedures may vary from hospital to hospital and from physician to physician; your condition after the surgery may also play a part in deciding when to pull the plug on the IV and when to pull out the silverware. Keep in mind, too, that reintroduction of solids will come in stages. You'll start with fluids by mouth, moving on next to something soft and easily tolerated (like Jell-O), and on (slowly) from there. But your diet will have to stay on the bland and easily digested side for at least a few days; don't even think about having someone smuggle in a burger yet. Once you're back on solids, don't forget to push the fluids, too—especially if you're breastfeeding.

Referred shoulder pain. Irritation of the diaphragm, caused by small amounts of blood in your belly, can cause a few hours of sharp shoulder pain following surgery. A pain reliever may help.

Probably constipation. Since the anesthesia and the surgery (plus your limited diet) may slow your bowels down, it may be a few days until you pass that first movement, and that's normal. You may also experience some painful gassiness because of the constipation. A stool softener, suppository, or other mild laxative may be prescribed to help move things along, especially if you're uncomfortable. The tips on page 427 may help, too.

Abdominal discomfort. As your digestive tract (temporarily put out of commission by surgery) begins to function again, trapped gas can cause considerable pain, especially when it presses against your incision line. The discomfort may be worse when you laugh, cough, or sneeze. Ask the nurse or doctor to suggest some possible remedies. A suppository may help release the gas, as may strolling up and down the hall. Lying on your side or on your back, your knees drawn up, taking deep breaths while holding your incision can also bring some relief.

To spend time with your baby. You'll be encouraged to cuddle and feed your baby as soon as possible (if you're nursing, place the baby on a pillow over your incision or lie on your side while nursing). And yes, you can even lift your baby. Hospital regulations and your condition permitting, you'll probably be able to have modified or full rooming-in; having your spouse bunking with you, too, will be a big help. Don't push the rooming-in agenda, though, if you're not up to it—or just want some rest.

Removal of stitches. If your stitches or staples aren't self-absorbing, they will be removed about four or five days after delivery. The procedure isn't very painful, although you may have some discomfort. When the dressing is off, take a good look at the incision with the nurse or doctor; ask how soon you can expect the area to heal, which changes will be normal, and which might require medical attention.

In most cases, you can expect to go home about two to four days postpartum. But you'll still have to take it easy, and you'll continue to need help both with baby care and self-care. Try to have someone with you at all times during the first couple of weeks.

Coming Home with Baby

"In the hospital, the nurses changed my baby's diaper, gave him a bath, and told me when to nurse him. Now that I'm home with him, I feel underprepared and overwhelmed."

It's true that babies aren't born with how-to's written on their cute, dimply bottoms (wouldn't that be convenient?). Fortunately, they do typically come home from the hospital with instructions from the staff about feeding, bathing, and changing diapers. Already lost those? Or maybe they ended up smeared with mustardy poop the first time you tried to change baby's diaper while simultaneously trying to read the instructions for changing baby's diaper? Not to worry; there's a wealth of information out there to help you tackle your new job as new parent both in books and online. Plus, you've probably already scheduled the first visit to the pediatrician, where you'll be armed with even more information—not to mention answers to the 3,000 questions you've managed to accumulate (that is, if you remember to write them down and bring them along).

Of course, it takes more than know-how to make a parenting expert out of a new parent. It takes patience, perseverance, and practice, practice, practice. Luckily, babies are forgiving as you learn. They don't care if you put the diaper on backward or forgot to wash behind their ears at bath time. They're also not shy about giving you feedback: They'll definitely let you know if they're hungry, tired, or if you've made the bathwater too cold (though at first you may not be able to tell which complaint is which). Best of all, since your baby's never had another mom to compare you with, you definitely stack up really well in his book. In fact, you're the best he's ever had.

Still suffering from a crumbling of confidence? What might help most—besides the passing of time and the accumulation of experience—is to know that you're in good company. Every mom (even those seasoned pros you doubt-less eye with envy) feels in over her head in those early weeks, especially when postpartum exhaustion—teamed with nightly sleep deprivation and the recovery from childbirth—is taking its toll on her, body and soul. So cut yourself plenty of slack (and while you're at it, cut yourself a piece of cheese and maybe a slice of bread, too—low blood sugar can contribute to that overwhelmed feeling), and give yourself plenty of time to adjust and to get with the parenting program. Pretty soon (sooner than you think), the everyday challenges of baby care won't be so challenging anymore. In fact, they'll come so naturally, you'll be able to do them in your sleep (and will often feel as though you are). You'll be diapering, feeding, burping, and soothing with the best of them—with one arm tied behind your back (or at least, one arm folding laundry, catching up on e-mail, reading a book, spooning cereal into your mouth, or otherwise multitasking). You'll be a mother. And mothers, in case you haven't heard, can do anything.

Getting Started Breastfeeding

There's nothing more natural than nursing a baby, right? Well, not always, at least not right away. Babies are born to nurse, but they're not necessarily born knowing how to nurse. Ditto for moms. The breasts are standard issue, they fill with milk automatically, but knowing how to position them effectively in baby's mouth, well, that's a learned art.

Truth is, while breastfeeding is a natural process, it's a natural process that doesn't necessarily come naturally—or quickly—to some mothers and babies. Sometimes there are physical factors that foil those first few attempts; at other times it's just a simple lack of experience on the part of both participants. But whatever might be keeping your baby and your breasts apart, it won't be long before they're in perfect sync. Some of the most mutually satisfying breast-baby relationships begin with several days—or even weeks—of fumbling, bungled efforts, and tears on both sides.

Learning as much as you can about breastfeeding ahead of time—including how to deal with those inevitable setbacks—can help speed that mutual adjustment. Doing lots of reading up or even taking a prenatal class in breastfeeding will be invaluable, as will the following:

■ Get off to an early start. Right in the birthing room is ideal, if that's possible (see Breastfeeding Basics for a how-to, page 438.) Let your practitioner know that you'd like to begin breastfeeding as soon after delivery as you can (and while you're at it, write down that request in your birth plan, if you're using one). Don't be disappointed if either you or baby (or both of you) isn't up to nursing right away. That doesn't mean you won't be able to start successfully later. And keep in mind that even the earliest of starts won't guarantee a smooth first nursing experience. You both have a lot to learn.

■ Keep the nursing team together. Arrange for full or partial rooming-in, if you feel up to it, so you'll be ready to nurse when baby's ready. If you'd rather rest between feedings—you've earned it—ask for a demand-feeding schedule (your baby will be brought to you when he or she is hungry).

■ Enlist as much help as you can. Ideally, a lactation specialist will join you during at least a couple of your first baby feedings to provide hands-on instruction, helpful hints, and perhaps some reading materials. If this service isn't offered to you, ask if a lactation consultant or a nurse who is knowledgeable about breastfeeding can observe your technique and redirect you if you and your baby aren't on target. If you leave the hospital or birthing center before getting this help, your technique should be evaluated by some-

one with breastfeeding expertise—the baby's doctor, a home nurse, or an outside lactation consultant—within a few days. You can also find empathy, advice, and referrals to lactation consultants by calling your local La Leche League chapter. Or contact the International Lactation Consultant Association (ILCA), (919) 861-5577, ilca.org, for a lactation consultant in your area.

■ Don't let well-wishers get in the way. Consider limiting visitors (maybe even to just your spouse) while you and baby are getting the hang of breastfeeding. As anxious as you are to show your new arrival off, you'll need to maintain a relaxed atmosphere—and complete concentration—during those learning-to-nurse sessions.

■ Be patient if your baby gets off to a slow start. He or she may be just as tuckered out from delivery as you are, maybe even more so. Newborn babies are sleepy babies, and yours is likely to be especially drowsy and sluggish at the breast if you received anesthesia or had a prolonged, difficult labor. That's no problem because newborns need little nourishment during the first few days of life. By the time your baby starts needing some serious chow, he or she will be ready to do some serious chowing down. What babies do need even early on, though, is nurturing. Cuddling at the breast is just as important as suckling.

■ Keep your baby bottle-free. Make sure your baby's appetite and sucking instinct aren't sabotaged between nursings by well-meaning nurses wielding bottles of formula or sugar water. First, because it doesn't take much to satisfy a newborn's tender appetite. If your baby is given even a small supplementary feeding in the nursery, he or she will be too full for your breast when it's time to nurse. If your baby doesn't nurse, your breasts won't be stimulated to produce milk, and a vicious cycle—one that interferes with the establishment of a good demand-and-supply system—can begin. Second, because a rubber nipple requires less effort, your baby's sucking reflex may become lazy when a bottle's offered. Faced with the greater challenge of tackling the breast, baby may just give up. Pacifiers might also interfere with nursing (though not in all cases). So issue orders—through your baby's doctor—that, as recommended by the American Academy of Pediatrics, supplementary feedings and pacifiers should not be given to your baby in the nursery unless medically necessary.

- Nurse on demand. And if the demand isn't there yet, nurse frequently anyway, getting in at least 8 to 12 feedings a day. Not only will this keep your baby happy, it will stimulate milk production and increase your milk supply to meet his or her growing demand. Imposing a four-hour feeding schedule, on the other hand, can worsen breast engorgement early on and result in a baby who's not getting enough to eat later.

- Nurse without limits. It used to be thought that keeping initial feedings short (five minutes on each breast) would prevent sore nipples by toughening them up gradually. Sore nipples, however, result from improper positioning of the baby on the breast and have little to do with the length of the feeding. Most newborns require 10 to 45 minutes to complete a feeding (it's not as easy as it looks). As long as your positioning is correct, there's no need to put time limits on nursing sessions.

Nursing and the NICU Baby

If your baby has to be in the neonatal intensive care unit (NICU) for any reason and can't go home with you, don't give up on breastfeeding. Babies who are premature or have other problems do better on breast milk, even when they're not ready to tackle a breast. Talk to your baby's neonatologist and the nurse in charge to see how you can best feed your baby in this situation. If you can't nurse directly, perhaps you can pump milk to be given to your baby via tube feeding or bottle. If even this isn't possible, see if you can keep pumping milk to keep your supply up until your baby is ready to feed from you directly.

- Go for empty. Ideally, at least one breast should be "emptied" at each feeding—and this is actually more important than being sure that baby feeds from both breasts. When a breast isn't sufficiently drained, baby doesn't get to the hind milk, which comes at the end of a feeding and contains more of the calories baby needs to gain weight than the milk that comes first (foremilk is baby's thirst quencher; hind milk's the body builder). Hind milk is also more satiating, which means it keeps baby's tank fuller longer. So don't pull the plug just because your baby has fed for 15 minutes on breast number one—wait until he or she seems ready to quit. Then offer the second breast, but don't force it. Remember to start the next feeding on the breast that baby nursed from last and didn't empty completely.

Breastfeeding Basics

1. Pick a quiet location. Until you and baby have breastfeeding down pat, set yourselves up in an area that has few distractions and a low noise level.

2. Have a beverage at your side so you can drink as baby drinks. Avoid anything hot (which could scald you or your baby if it spilled); if you're not thirsting for a cold drink, opt instead for something lukewarm. Add a healthy snack, if it's been a while since your last meal.

3. As you become more comfortable with breastfeeding, you can keep a book or magazine handy to keep you busy during marathon feeding sessions. (But don't forget to put your reading matter down periodically so you can interact with your nursing infant.) In the early weeks, turning on the TV could be too distracting. So can talking on the phone; turn down the ringer and let voice mail pick up messages—or have someone else answer.

4. Get comfy. If you're sitting up, a pillow across your lap can help raise your baby to a comfortable height. Make sure, too, that your arms are propped up on a pillow or chair arms. Trying to hold 6 to 8 pounds without support can lead to arm cramps and pain. And put up your legs, if you can.

5. Position your baby on his or her side, facing your nipple. Make sure baby's whole body is facing you—tummy to tummy—with ear, shoulder, and hip in a straight line. You don't want your baby's head turned to the side; rather, it should be straight in line with his or her body. (Imagine how difficult it would be for you to drink and swallow while turning your head to the side. It's the same for your baby.) Proper positioning is essential to prevent nipple soreness and other breastfeeding problems.

Lactation specialists recommend two nursing positions during the first few weeks. The first is called the crossover hold: Hold your baby's head with the opposite hand (if nursing on the right breast, hold your baby with your left hand). Rest your hand between your baby's shoulder blades, your thumb behind one ear, your other fingers behind the other ear. Using your other hand, cup your breast, placing your thumb above your nipple and areola (the dark area) at the spot where your baby's nose will touch your breast. Your index finger should be at the spot where your baby's chin will touch the breast. *Lightly* compress your breast so your nipple points slightly toward your baby's nose. You are now ready to have baby latch on (see step 6).

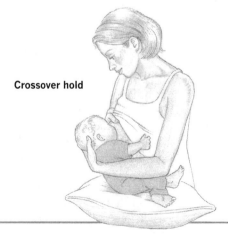

Crossover hold

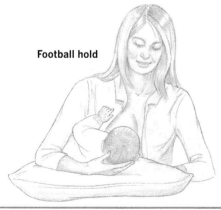

Football hold

The second position is called the football hold. This position, also called the clutch hold, is especially useful if you've had a C-section and want to avoid placing your baby against your abdomen; or if your breasts are large; or if your baby is small or premature; or if you are nursing twins: Position your baby at your side in a semisitting position facing you, with his or her legs under your arm (your right arm if you're nursing on the right breast). Support your baby's head with your right hand and cup your breast as you would for the crossover hold.

As soon as you're more comfortable with nursing, you can add the cradle hold, in which your baby's head rests in the crook of your arm, and the side-lying hold, in which you and your baby lie on your sides, tummy to tummy. This position is a good choice when you're nursing in the middle of the night.

6. Gently tickle your baby's lips with your nipple until his or her mouth is opened very wide, like a yawn. Some lactation specialists suggest directing your nipple toward your baby's nose and then down to the upper lip to get your baby to open his or her mouth very wide. This prevents the lower lip from getting tucked in during nursing. If your baby turns his or her head away, gently stroke his or her cheek on the side nearest you. The rooting reflex will make baby turn his or her head toward your breast.

7. Once that little mouth is opened wide, move your baby closer. Do not move your breast toward your baby. Many latching-on problems occur because mom is hunched over baby, trying to shove breast into mouth. Instead, keep your back straight and bring your baby to your breast.

8. Don't stuff your nipple in an unwilling mouth; let your baby take the initiative. It might take a couple of attempts before your baby opens his or her mouth wide enough to latch on properly.

9. Be sure baby latches on to both the nipple and the areola that surrounds it. Sucking on just the nipple won't compress the milk glands and can cause soreness and cracking. Also be sure that it's the nipple and areola that the baby is busily milking. Some infants are so eager to suck that they will latch on to any part of the breast (even if no milk is delivered), causing a painful bruise.

10. If your breast is blocking your baby's nose, *lightly* depress the breast with your finger. Elevating baby slightly may also help provide a little breathing room. But as you maneuver, be sure not to loosen his or her grip on the areola.

11. Check for swallowing. You can be sure that milk is flowing if there is a strong, steady, rhythmic motion visible in your baby's cheek.

12. If your baby has finished suckling but is still holding on to the breast, pulling it out abruptly can cause injury to your nipple. Instead, break the suction first by depressing the breast or by putting your finger into the corner of the baby's mouth to let in some air.

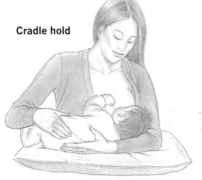

Cradle hold

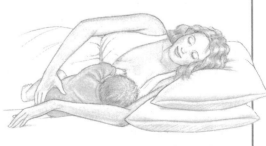

Side-lying hold

Keeping Track

To be sure each breast gets a chance to be stimulated, use a reminder such as a notation in your breastfeeding journal, a small scrunchie looped around your bra strap, or a bracelet on your wrist to indicate which side you nursed from last. At your next feeding, just start with the other side (and switch the scrunchie or bracelet to the other side, too).

- Don't let sleeping babies lie if it means that they'll sleep through a feeding. Some babies, especially in the first few days of life, may not wake often enough for nourishment. If it's been three hours since your newborn last fed, then it's time for a wake-up call. Here's one way to accomplish this. First, unwrap your baby if he or she is swaddled or heavily dressed; the cool air will help begin the waking process. Then try sitting baby up, one hand supporting the back and the other holding the chin, and rub the back gently. Massaging the arms and legs or dabbing a little cool water on the forehead may help, too. The moment baby stirs, quickly adopt the nursing position. Or lay your sleeping baby on your bare chest. Babies have a keen sense of smell, and the aroma of your breast may awaken him or her.

- Don't try to feed a screaming baby. Ideally, you will feed your baby when he or she first shows signs of hunger or interest in sucking, which might include mouthing his or her hands or rooting around for the nipple, or just being particularly alert. Try not to wait until frantic crying—a late indication of hunger—begins. But if the frenzy has started, do some rocking and soothing before you put baby to breast. Or offer your finger to suck on until baby calms down. After all, it's hard enough for an inexperienced suckler to find the nipple when calm; when your newborn has worked up to a full-fledged frenzy, it may be impossible.

- Stay calm. Start out as relaxed as you can, and try to stay that way no matter how frustrating the nursing episode becomes. If you've allowed visitors, send them packing 15 minutes before a feeding, and use that time to chill out a little. Do some relaxation exercises before you begin (see page 142) or tune in to some soft music. As you nurse, try to keep your cool. Tension not only hampers milk letdown (your breasts' way of making your milk available for suckling), it can generate stress in your baby (infants are extremely sensitive to mom's moods). An anxious baby can't nurse effectively.

- Keep track. Once your milk comes in and until breastfeeding is well established, keep a running written record of baby's feedings (when they begin and end) as well as of wet and soiled diapers produced each day. While that may sound obsessive, it'll really help give you a good sense of how breastfeeding is going—and also makes it possible for you to report progress to your baby's doctor more accurately (you will be asked). Continue to strive for at least 8 to 12 feedings in each 24-hour period, but never force your baby to suckle. Though the length of feedings may vary considerably, once engorgement and nipple soreness have leveled off, they'll average about half an hour each, usually divided between both breasts (though sometimes a baby will turn away or fall asleep before latching on to breast number two, which is fine as long as number one has been drained well). Your baby's weight gain and diaper record will give you an even clearer picture of baby's intake. There should be at least six wet diapers (the urine should appear clear and not dark yellow) and at least three bowel movements over a 24-hour period. No matter how long baby is suckling, if weight gain and output are satisfactory, you can assume the intake is, too.

Engorgement: When the Milk Comes In

Just when you and your baby seem to be getting the hang of this whole nursing thing, milk gets in the way. Up until now, your baby has been easily extracting tiny amounts of colostrum (premilk), and your breasts have been easily handling the workload. Then it happens, suddenly and without warning: Your milk comes in. Within a few hours, your breasts become swollen, hard, and painful. Nursing from them can become frustrating for baby and seriously uncomfortable for you.

Fortunately, this miserable chapter in breastfeeding history is usually pretty brief, often lasting no more than 24 to 48 hours (though it can occasionally linger as long as a week). While it lasts, here are a variety of ways of relieving engorgement and the discomfort that comes with it:

- Heat it. Use heat briefly to help soften the areola and encourage letdown at the beginning of a nursing session. To do this, place a washcloth dipped in warm, not hot, water on just the areola, or lean it into a bowl of warm water.

- Massage it. You can also encourage milk flow by gently massaging the breast your baby is suckling.

- Cool it. Use ice packs after nursing to reduce engorgement. And although it may sound a little strange and look even stranger, chilled cabbage leaves may also prove soothing (use large outer leaves and make an opening in the center of each for your nipple; rinse and pat dry before applying).

- Dress for it. Wear a well-fitting nursing bra (with wide straps and no plastic lining) around the clock. Pressure against your sore and engorged breasts can hurt, however, so make sure the bra is not too tight. And wear loose clothing that doesn't rub against your sensitive breasts.

- Keep at it. Don't be tempted to skip or skimp on a feeding because of pain. The less your baby sucks, the more engorged your breasts will become—and the more you'll hurt.

Next Stop: Easy Street

Hit a breastfeeding bump or two? Stick with nursing and you'll soon be cruising down Easy Street (as you'll find out, once you get the hang of it, there's no easier way to feed a baby). In the meantime, get the help you need to fix any rough spots you've been facing—either from the tips here or from a lactation consultant. Also, don't let the bumps with a first baby discourage you from nursing your next. Thanks to mom's previous experience (and that of her breasts), nursing is typically second nature with second (and subsequent) babies, making engorgement, nipple soreness, and other problems a lot less common.

The Breastfeeding Diet

It's the couch potato's dream—burning up the calories of a 5-mile run without leaving your lounge chair. And guess what? That dream is your reality now that you're breastfeeding your little Tater Tot. It's true. Milk production burns 500 calories a day, which means that you'll get to eat an extra 500 calories a day (up from your prepregnancy numbers—not your pregnancy allotment) to meet that need.

Hello, potato chips? Not exactly. Quality matters as much as quantity (remember, you're still—sort of—eating for two). The good news is that you're probably an old pro at eating well, what with all the practice you've had for the past nine months. The even better news is that eating well while breastfeeding is very much like eating well while expecting, but with (best news of all) more relaxed recommendations. Plus, while calories definitely count, you still won't need to count them. Just follow the Breastfeeding Diet as best you can:

What to eat. As always, eating well is about getting the right balance of good—and good for you—food. Try to include the following each day while you're breastfeeding:

- Protein: 3 servings

- Calcium: 5 servings (that's up 1 serving from your pregnancy requirement of 4)

- Iron-rich foods: 1 or more servings

- Vitamin C: 2 servings

- Green leafy and yellow vegetables, yellow fruits: 3 to 4 servings

- Other fruits and veggies: 1 or more servings

- Whole-grain and other complex carbohydrates: 3 or more servings

- High-fat foods: moderate amounts —you don't need as much as you did during pregnancy

- At least 8 glasses of water, juice, or other noncaffeinated, nonalcoholic beverages

- DHA-rich foods to promote baby's brain growth (look for this fabulous fat in wild salmon, sardines, walnuts, flaxseed oil, as well as DHA-enriched eggs)

- Prenatal vitamin daily

- Take matters into your own hands. Hand-express a bit of milk from each breast before nursing to lessen the engorgement. This will get your milk flowing, and soften the nipple so your baby can get a better hold on it.

- Switch it. Change nursing positions from one feeding to the next (try the football hold at one feeding, the cradle hold at the next; see page 438). This will ensure that all the milk ducts are being emptied and may help ease the ouch of engorgement.

- Get some relief. For severe pain, take acetaminophen (Tylenol) or another mild pain reliever prescribed by your practitioner.

Leaking Milk

The first few weeks of nursing can be very wet ones. Milk may leak, drip,

You may need to increase your caloric intake as your baby grows bigger and hungrier, or decrease it if you supplement nursing with formula and/or solids, or if you have considerable fat reserves you'd like to begin burning.

What not to eat. When you're breastfeeding, you have a lot more menu options than you did while you were expecting—served up with some caveats. It's fine to pop open the cork on that pinot noir you've been pining for (or flip the top on that ale you've been aching for). But drink within limits (a couple of glasses a week, preferably taken right after you nurse, rather than before, to allow a few hours for the alcohol to metabolize and for far less to reach your baby). Time to pick up your coffee habit where you left off? Depends on how hefty your habit was. More than a cup or two of joe can make junior jittery and keep you both from getting any sleep. And though it's safe to reel in the sushi again, continue to avoid high-mercury fish, such as shark, tilefish, and mackerel, and to limit those that may contain moderate amounts of that heavy metal.

What to watch out for. If you have a family history of allergies, check with the doctor to see if you should avoid peanuts and foods that contain them (and possibly other highly allergic foods). Also watch out for herbs, even some seemingly innocuous herbal teas. Stick to reliable brands and choose flavors that are considered safe during lactation, including orange spice, peppermint, raspberry, red bush, chamomile, and rosehip. Read labels carefully to make sure other herbs haven't been added to the brew, and drink them only in moderation. And when it comes to sugar substitutes, sucralose (Splenda) or aspartame are considered better bets than saccharine.

What to watch for in your baby. A few moms find that their own diet affects their babies' tummies and temperaments. While what you eat does indeed change the taste and smell of your milk (that happens for all mothers), this is actually a good thing since it exposes your baby to many different flavors. But some babies can occasionally be sensitive to certain foods that end up in mom's milk. If you suspect that something in your diet is turning baby off his or her feed (or turning his or her tummy), try eliminating the food for a few days to gauge the response. Some of the more common troublemakers are cow's milk, eggs, fish, citrus fruits, nuts, and wheat.

For more information on what to eat when you're breastfeeding, see *What to Expect: Eating Well When You're Expecting.*

or even spray from your breasts, and it can happen at any time, anywhere, without warning. All of a sudden, you'll feel the tingle of letdown—and before you can grab a nursing pad or a sweater to cover up with, you'll look down to see the telltale circle of dampness that gives new meaning to the term "wet T-shirt."

Besides those inopportune and public moments ("So that's why the delivery guy was looking at me funny . . ."), you might find yourself springing spontane-ous leaks when you're sleeping or taking a warm shower, when you hear your baby cry, when you think about or talk about your baby. Milk may drip from one breast while you nurse from the other, and if your baby has settled into a somewhat regular feeding schedule, your breasts may be dripping with anticipation before baby latches on.

Though it may be uncomfortable, unpleasant, and endlessly embarrassing, this side effect of breastfeeding is

Medication and Lactation

Many medications are known to be safe for use while you're breastfeeding; others are known not to be; and the scientific jury's still out on the rest. But just as you did while you were expecting, check all medications (prescription or over-the-counter) with your practitioner and your baby's pediatrician before taking them, and be sure any physician who prescribes a new medication knows that you're nursing. Keep in mind that it's usually best to take medication just after a feeding, so that levels in your milk will be lowest when you nurse next time.

completely normal and very common, particularly in the early weeks. (Not leaking at all or leaking only a little can be just as normal, and in fact, many second-time mothers might notice that their breasts leak less than they did the first time around.) In most cases, as breastfeeding becomes established, the system eventually settles down and leaking lessens considerably. In the meantime, while you may not be able to turn off that leaky faucet, you may be able to make living with it a little less messy:

■ Stock up on nursing pads. If you're a leaker, you'll find that in the first postpartum weeks, you'll be changing your nursing pads as often as you nurse—sometimes even more frequently. Keep in mind that, like a diaper, they should be changed whenever they become wet. Make sure you use pads that don't have a plastic or waterproof liner; they'll just trap moisture and lead to irritated nipples. Some women prefer the disposable variety,

while others like the feel of the reusable cotton ones.

■ Protect your bed. If you find you're leaking a lot at night, use extra nursing pads, or place a large towel under you while you sleep. The last thing you'll want to be doing now is changing your sheets every day or, worse, shopping for a new mattress.

■ Don't pump to prevent leaking. Extra pumping won't control the leak; on the contrary, the more you stimulate your breasts, the more milk they'll produce, and the more leaking you'll have to contend with.

■ Try to stop the overflow. Once nursing is well established and your milk production has leveled off, you can try to stop the leaking by pressing your nipples (though probably not in public) or holding your arms against your breasts when you feel a leak coming on. Don't, however, do this in the first few weeks because it may inhibit milk letdown and can lead to a clogged milk duct.

Sore Nipples

Tender nipples can make nursing a miserable—and frustrating— experience. Fortunately, most women don't stay sore long; their nipples toughen up quickly and breastfeeding soon becomes a completely painless pleasure. But some women, especially those who have "barracuda babies" (babies with a vigorous suck) or who have been positioning their newborns incorrectly at their breasts, continue to experience soreness and cracking. To ease the discomfort so you can start enjoying breastfeeding:

■ Position the right way. Be sure your baby is correctly positioned, facing your breast (see box, page 438). Vary your nursing position so a different part of the areola is compressed at each feeding, but always keep baby facing your breasts.

- Let your nipples breathe (try this at home). Expose sore or cracked nipples to the air briefly after each feeding. Protect them from clothing that rubs and other irritations, and if you're really sore, you might want to consider surrounding them with a cushion of air by wearing breast shells (not shields).

- Keep them dry. Change nursing pads as soon as they become damp. Also, make sure the nursing pads don't have a plastic liner, which will only trap moisture. If you live in a humid climate, wave a blow dryer, set on warm, across each breast (about 6 to 8 inches away) for two or three minutes (no more) after feedings. This is very comforting, if slightly difficult to explain should someone walk in while you're doing it.

- Heal with milk. Breast milk can actually help heal sore nipples. So let whatever milk is left on the breast after a feeding dry there, instead of wiping it away. Or express a few drops of milk at the end of a feeding and rub it on your nipples, letting your nipples dry before you put your bra back on.

- Rub it on. Nipples are naturally protected and lubricated by sweat glands and skin oils. But using a commercial preparation of modified lanolin can prevent and/or heal nipple cracking. After nursing, apply ultrapurified medical-grade lanolin, such as Lansinoh, but avoid petroleum-based products and petroleum jelly itself (Vaseline), as well as other oily products. Wash nipples only with water—never with soap, alcohol, or wipes—whether your nipples are sore or not. Your baby is already protected from your germs, and the milk itself is clean.

- Try tea for two. Wet regular tea bags with cool water and place them on your sore nipples. The properties in the tea may help soothe and heal them.

- Treat them equally. Don't favor one breast because it is less sore or because the nipple isn't cracked; the only way to toughen up nipples is to use them. Plus, for both breasts to become good producers, they both have to get equal stimulation time.

  If one nipple is a lot more sore than the other, nurse from the less tender one first because the baby will suck more vigorously when he or she is hungry. Try to do this only as long as you absolutely have to—and for no more than a few days—because it could keep the sore breast from getting the stimulation it needs and ultimately affect your milk supply. Fortunately, the worst of the soreness shouldn't continue longer than this (if it does, contact a lactation consultant; improper positioning may be the problem).

- Chill out before feeding. Relaxation will enhance the letdown of milk (which will mean that baby won't have to suck as hard), while tension will inhibit it.

- Seek relief. Take acetaminophen (Tylenol) before you nurse to ease soreness.

- Keep a watch. If your nipples are cracked, be especially alert to signs of breast infection (see next page), which can occur when germs enter a milk duct through a crack in the nipple.

When Breastfeeding Gets Bumpy

Once nursing is established, it's usually a smooth ride until baby's weaned. But once in a while, there's a bump or two along the way, among them:

Clogged milk ducts. Sometimes a milk duct clogs, causing milk to back up. This condition—characterized by a small, red, and tender lump on the breast—can lead to infection, so it's important to resolve it quickly. The best way to do this is to offer the affected breast first and let your baby empty it as completely as possible. If baby doesn't finish the job, express any remaining milk by hand or with a breast pump. Keep pressure off the duct by making sure your bra is not too tight (avoiding underwires for now may help) and by varying nursing positions to put pressure on different ducts. Applying hot packs or warm compresses before nursing and gentle massage may also be helpful (baby's chin, if correctly positioned, can provide a clogged duct with an excellent massage). Do not use this time to wean the baby because discontinuing nursing now will only compound the clog.

Breast infection. A more serious and less common complication of breastfeeding is mastitis, or breast infection, which can develop in one or both breasts, most often during the early postpartum period (though it can occur anytime during breastfeeding). The factors that can combine to cause mastitis are failure to drain breasts of milk at each nursing, germs (usually from baby's mouth) gaining entrance into the milk ducts through a crack in the nipple, and lowered resistance in mom due to stress and fatigue.

The most common symptoms of mastitis are severe soreness or pain, hardness, redness, heat, and swelling of the breast, with flulike symptoms—generalized chills and a fever of about 101°F to 102°F. If you develop such symptoms, contact your doctor right away. Prompt medical treatment is necessary and may include bed rest, antibiotics, pain relievers, increased fluid intake, and moist heat applications. You should begin to feel drastically better within 36 to 48 hours after beginning the antibiotics. If you don't, let your practitioner know; he or she may need to prescribe a different type of antibiotic.

Continue to nurse during treatment. Since the baby's germs probably caused the infection in the first place, they won't be harmful. The antibiotics prescribed for the infection will be safe, too. And draining the breast will help prevent clogged milk ducts. Nurse (if you can; it may be quite painful) on the infected breast, and express whatever baby doesn't finish with a pump. If the pain is so bad that you can't nurse, try hand pumping or using a manual breast pump on your breasts (whichever hurts less) while lying in a tub of warm water with your breasts floating comfortably; you can let the milk drip into the water. (Don't use an electric pump in the tub.)

Delay in treating mastitis or discontinuing treatment too soon could lead to the development of a breast abscess, the symptoms of which include excruciating, throbbing pain; localized swelling, tenderness, and heat in the area of the abscess; and temperature swings between 100°F and 103°F. Treatment includes antibiotics and, generally, surgical drainage. The drain may stay in place after surgery. Breastfeeding on that breast usually can't continue in most cases, but you can keep nursing with the other breast until you wean your baby.

Breastfeeding After a Cesarean Delivery

How soon you can breastfeed your newborn after a surgical delivery will depend on how you feel and how your baby is doing. If you're both in good shape, you can probably introduce baby to breast in the recovery room shortly after the surgery is completed. If you're groggy from general anesthesia or your baby needs immediate care in the nursery, this first nursing session may have to wait. If after 12 hours you still haven't been able to get together with your baby, ask about using a pump to express your premilk (colostrum) and get lactation started.

You'll probably find breastfeeding after a C-section uncomfortable at first. It will be less so if you try to avoid putting pressure on the incision with one of these techniques: Place a pillow on your lap under the baby; lie on your side; or use the football hold (page 438), again supported by a pillow, to nurse. Both the afterpains you experience as you nurse and the soreness at the site of the incision are normal and will lessen in the days ahead.

Breastfeeding Multiples

Breastfeeding, like just about every aspect of caring for newborn multiples, seems as though it will be at least twice as challenging. However, once you've fallen into the rhythm of nursing your multiples (and you will!), you'll find that it's not only possible but doubly (or even triply) rewarding. To successfully nurse twins and more, you should:

Eat well—and eat up. Fulfill all the dietary recommendations for lactating mothers (see the Breastfeeding Diet, page 442),

---

Bottle Baby

Chose the bottle, or the combo? Getting started bottle-feeding is usually a lot easier than getting started breastfeeding (especially because formula comes with instructions, but breasts don't). But there's still plenty to learn, and you can read all about it in *What to Expect the First Year.*

---

with these additions: 400 to 500 calories above your prepregnancy needs for each baby you are nursing (you may need to increase your caloric intake as the babies grow bigger and hungrier or decrease it if you supplement nursing with formula and/or solids, or if you have considerable fat reserves you would like to burn); an additional serving of protein (for a total of four) and an additional serving of calcium (six total) or the equivalent in calcium supplements.

Pump it up. If your babies are in the NICU and are still too small to breastfeed, or if you need some extra help getting your supply stimulated in the early going, consider using an electric double pump. Later, pumping will allow you to get a few precious extra hours of sleep while someone else feeds the babies. Don't get discouraged if the pump doesn't get you going—no pump can empty a breast as well as a baby can. But regular stimulation from a pump (and your babies) will pump up your milk supply eventually.

Nurse two at a time (or not). You've got two breasts and two (or more) mouths to feed. Are you up to feeding two babies at once? You just might be, especially with a little help (like from oversize nursing

Tandem Nursing

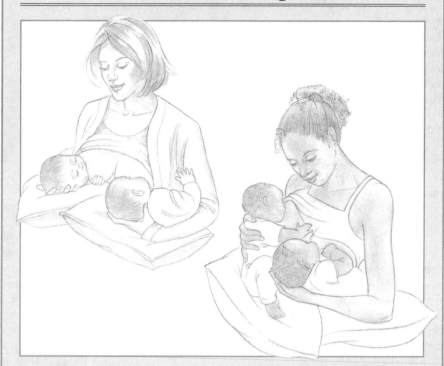

Some mothers of multiples prefer to nurse one baby at a time, finding it easier and more satisfying. Others would rather not spend all day breastfeeding and find that nursing two babies simultaneously saves time and works well. Here are two positions you can use while nursing two at the same time: (1) Position both babies in the football (or clutch) hold. Use pillows to support your babies' heads. (2) Combine the cradle hold and the football hold, again using pillows for support and experimenting until both you and your babies are comfortable.

pillows for twins). An obvious—and big—advantage of tandem nursing two babies is that you don't spend all day and night nursing (first Baby A, now Baby B, and back to Baby A, and so on). To nurse two at the same time, position both babies on the pillow first, and then latch them on (or you can ask someone to hand the babies to you one at a time, especially while you're still getting used to the juggling act).

If tandem nursing doesn't appeal to you, don't do it. You can bottle-feed one (using either pumped milk or formula, if you're supplementing) while nursing the other (and then switch off), or nurse one baby after the other. Some babies are very efficient, taking a full feed in only 10 or 15 minutes. If this is the case with yours, count your little blessings—you won't spend any more time nursing than the average tandem feeder.

Got three (or more) babies to feed? Breastfeeding triplets (and even quads) is possible, too. Nurse two at a time, and then nurse the third one afterward, remembering to switch off which baby gets solo suckling time. For more information on breastfeeding higher-order multiples, check out mostonline.org or tripletconnection.org.

Enlist twice as much help. Get as much help as you can with housework, meal prep, and infant care, to con- serve the energy you need to fuel milk production.

Treat each diner differently. Even identical twins have different personalities, appetites, and nursing patterns. So try to tune into the needs of each. And keep extra-careful records to make sure each baby is well fed at each feeding.

Give both breasts a workout. Switch breasts for each baby at each feeding so both breasts are stimulated equally.

Give It Time

So you've been a mom for a week (with the stretch marks, postpartum pains, and bags under your eyes to prove it), and by now you may be wondering: When am I going to feel like one? When will I be able to accomplish latch-on without 20 minutes of fumbling? Or finally get the hang of burping? Or stop worrying about breaking the baby every time I pick her up? When will I be able to coo without feeling like an awkward idiot? When will I figure out which cries mean what—and how to respond to any of them? How do I put on a diaper so it doesn't leak? Get the onesie over baby's head without a struggle? Shampoo that little patch of hair without dripping soap into those tender eyes? When will the job that nature just signed me up for start coming naturally?

The truth is, giving birth makes you a mother, but it doesn't necessarily make you feel like a mother. Only time spent on this sometimes bewildering, sometimes overwhelming, always amazing job will do that. The day-to-day (and night-to-night) of parenting is never easy, but it absolutely, positively gets easier.

So cut yourself some slack, pat yourself on the back, and give yourself time, Mom. Which, by the way, you are.

CHAPTER 18

Postpartum: The First 6 Weeks

B Y NOW YOU'RE PROBABLY EITHER settling into your new life as a fledgling mom or figuring out how to juggle new baby care with the demands of older children. Almost certainly, much of your daily—and nightly—attention is focused on that recently arrived little bundle. Babies, after all, don't take care of themselves. But that doesn't mean you should neglect your own care (yes, moms have needs, too!).

Though most of your questions and concerns are likely to be baby-related right now, you're sure to have some that are a little more mommy-centric, too, from the state of your emotions ("Will I ever stop crying during insurance commercials?"), to the state of your sexual union ("Will I ever want to do 'it' again?"), to the state of your waist ("Will I ever be able to wear jeans that zip?"). The answers: yes, yes, and yes—just give it time.

What You May Be Feeling

The first six weeks postpartum are considered a "recovery" period. Even if you sailed through your pregnancy and had the easiest labor and delivery on record (and especially if you didn't), your body has still been stretched and stressed to the max—and

it needs a chance to regroup. Every new mom, like every expectant one, is different—so all will make that recovery at a different rate, with a different collection of postpartum symptoms. Depending on the type of delivery you had, how much help you have at home, and a variety of other individual factors, you may experience all, or only some, of the following:

Physically

- Continued period-like vaginal discharge (lochia), first dark red, then pink, turning brownish, then yellowish white

- Fatigue

- Some continuing pain, discomfort, and numbness in the perineum, if you had a vaginal delivery (especially if you had stitches) or labored before having a cesarean delivery

- Diminishing incision pain, continuing numbness, if you had a C-section (especially if it was your first)

- Gradual easing of constipation and, hopefully, hemorrhoids

- Gradual slimming of your belly as your uterus recedes into the pelvis

- Gradual weight loss

- Gradual decrease in swelling

- Breast discomfort and nipple soreness until breastfeeding is well established

- Backache (from weak abdominal muscles and from carrying baby)

- Joint pain (from joints loosened during pregnancy in preparation for delivery)

- Achiness in arms and neck (from carrying and feeding baby)

- Hair loss

Emotionally

- Elation, moodiness, or swings between the two

- A sense of being overwhelmed, a growing feeling of confidence, or swings between the two

- Little interest in sex or, less commonly, stepped-up desire

What You Can Expect at Your Postpartum Checkup

Your practitioner will probably schedule you for a checkup four to six weeks postpartum. (If you had a cesarean delivery, you may be asked to come in at about three weeks postpartum to have your incision looked at.) During your postpartum visit, you can expect the following to be checked, though the exact rundown of the visit will vary depending on what your particular needs are and your practitioner's style of practice. Don't forget to write down all the questions that are sure to come up (and that you're sure to forget if you don't write them down).

- Blood pressure

- Weight, which may possibly be down by about 17 to 20 pounds

- Your uterus, to see if it has returned to prepregnant shape, size, and location

- Your cervix, which will be on its way back to its prepregnant state but will still be somewhat engorged

- Your vagina, which will have contracted and regained much of its muscle tone

- The episiotomy or laceration repair site, if any; or, if you had a cesarean delivery, the site of your incision

- Your breasts

- Hemorrhoids or varicose veins, if you have either

- Questions or problems you want to discuss—have a list ready

At this visit, your practitioner will also discuss with you the method of birth control that you're planning to use (if you're planning not to get pregnant again immediately, that is). If you plan on using a diaphragm and your cervix has recovered, you will be fitted for one (toss your old one, because it won't fit properly anymore); if you're not fully healed, you may have to use condoms until you can be refitted. Birth control pills may be prescribed now, too, though if you're breastfeeding, your oral contraceptive options will be limited to those that are safe during lactation, such as the progesterone-only mini pill. For more on birth control options, see *What to Expect the First Year.*

What You May Be Wondering About

Exhaustion

"I knew I'd be tired after giving birth, but I haven't gotten any sleep in more than four weeks, and I'm so exhausted, it's not funny."

No one's laughing—especially none of the other sleep-deprived new parents out there. And no one's really wondering why you're so exhausted, either. After all, you're juggling endless feeding, burping, changing, rocking, and pacing. You're trying to tackle the mountain of laundry that seems to grow larger and more daunting each day and the pile of thank-you notes that never seem to get written. You're shopping (out of diapers—again?), and you're schlepping (who knew how much baby stuff you'd need to lug just to pick up milk at the supermarket?). And you're doing it all on an average of about three hours' sleep (if you're lucky) a night, with a body that's still recovering from childbirth. In other words, you have multiple good reasons to be calling yourself Our Lady of Perpetual Exhaustion.

Is there a cure for this maternal fatigue syndrome? Not really—at least not until your baby starts sleeping through the night. But in the meantime, there are many ways of regaining some of your get-up-and-go—or at least enough so you can keep getting up and going:

Get some help. Hire help if you can afford to. If you can't, rely on volunteers. Now's a good time to let your mom, your mother-in-law, or your best friends lend their helping hands. Suggest they take baby out for a stroll while you grab a power nap or they pick up your groceries, dry cleaning, or that bag of diapers you desperately need.

Share the load. Parenting—when there are two parents—is a two-person job. Even if your partner-in-parenting is holding down a 9 to 5, he should be sharing the baby load when he's home. Ditto the cleaning, laundry, cooking, and shopping. Together, divide and conquer the responsibilities, then write down who's on for what and when so there's no confusion. (If you're a single parent, enlist a close friend to help out as much as possible.)

Don't sweat the small stuff. The only small stuff that matters right now is your baby. Everything else should take a distant backseat until you're feeling more energetic. So let the dust bunnies breed where they may (even if it's on top of those thank-you notes you don't have time to get to). And while you're ignoring those thank-you notes, buy some time by sending out a bulk e-mail with baby's picture attached.

Find deliverance. Now that you've delivered, it's time to find stores and restaurants that will deliver, too—whether it's the hot meal you'd never have time to cook, or the rectal thermometer you forgot to buy. Even groceries can find their way to your home via the Internet. Ditto all those baby essentials. Order in bulk so you don't run out of diapers so quickly (but don't buy so far in advance that baby outgrows the diapers before you get a chance to use them).

Sleep when the baby sleeps. Yes, you've heard it before, and probably snorted at the thought. After all, baby's nap time is the only time you can tackle the 300 other things that never seem to get done. But stop snorting and start snoring. Lie down for even 15 minutes during one of the baby's daytime naps, and you'll feel better able to handle the crying when it starts again (in 15 minutes).

Feed your baby, feed yourself. Yes, you're busy feeding baby—but don't forget to feed yourself, too. Fight fatigue by grazing on snacks and mini meals that combine protein and complex carbs to serve up long-term energy instead of the momentary rush: string cheese and crackers; trail mix; precut veggies with bean dip; a smoothie; a yogurt, banana, and a granola bar. Keep your fridge, your glove compartment, and your diaper bag stocked with such grab-and-go snacks so you're never running on empty. While sugar and caffeine (that king-size candy bar and that five-shot latte, taken in quick succession) may seem the obvious solution for the energy-challenged, remember this: Though they may give you the boost you crave in the short term, they'll quickly lead to an energy crash and burn. And don't just eat; drink plenty of water, too—not only because you've lost a lot of fluid during delivery, but because dehydration can lead to exhaustion. All of these tips apply to all new moms, but are especially important for nursing moms who are still eating for two.

If you're really beat, check with your practitioner to rule out any other physical cause responsible for your exhaustion (such as postpartum thyroiditis; see page 460). If you're feeling a little blue or depressed (see page 456), take steps to get that under control, too, because baby blues are tied to fatigue as well (and also to thyroiditis). If you get a clean bill of health, rest assured—that is, when you can rest at all—your zombie days are numbered. You will live to sleep again.

Hair Loss

"My hair seems to be falling out suddenly. Am I going bald?"

You're not going bald—you're just going back to normal. Ordinarily, the average head sheds 100 hairs a day (just not all at once, so you don't usually notice them), and those hairs are being continually replaced. During pregnancy, however, the hormonal changes keep those hairs from falling out, which means your head hangs on to them (remember how thick your hair felt back in the pregnant days?). But all good things must come to an end, including your reprieve on hair fall. All those hairs that were slated to go during pregnancy will be shed sometime after delivery, usually in the first six months postpartum—and often in unsettling clumps. Some women who are breastfeeding exclusively report that hair fall doesn't begin until they wean their baby or supplement the nursing with formula or solids. You'll take comfort knowing that by the time your baby is ready to blow out the candles on that first birthday cake (and has a full head of hair of his or her own), your hair should be back to normal—and business as usual—too.

To keep your hair healthy, continue taking a vitamin supplement, eat well, and treat your mane humanely. That means shampooing only when necessary (as if you had time for any shampoos now), using a conditioner and/or a detangling leave-on spray to reduce the need to tug at tangles, using a wide-toothed comb if you do have to untangle wet, and avoiding frying your hair with curling or flat irons (as if you have the time to style it, anyway).

Talk to your practitioner if your hair loss seems really excessive.

Postpartum Urinary Incontinence

"I thought I'd have more control over my bladder once my baby was born, but I gave birth nearly two months ago and I'm still peeing when I cough or laugh. Is it going to be like this forever?"

So your new-mom bladder is letting you—and your panties—down? It's completely normal to occasionally leak some urine involuntarily in the months (yes, months) following delivery, usually while laughing, sneezing, coughing, or performing any strenuous activity—and it's pretty common (more than a third of moms spring this particular leak postpartum). That's because pregnancy, labor, and delivery weakened the muscles around your bladder and pelvis, making it harder for you to control the flow of urine (it took a licking and therefore keeps on dripping). Plus, as your uterus shrinks in the weeks following delivery, it sits directly on the bladder, compressing it and making it more difficult to stem the tide. Hormonal changes after pregnancy can also batter your bladder.

It can take between three and six months, or even longer, to regain complete bladder control. Until then, use panty liners or pads to absorb leaking urine (no tampons, please—they don't block the flow of urine, because it's a different outlet, and they're off-limits postpartum period anyway), and take these steps to help regain control faster:

Keep your Kegels up. Thought you were done with your Kegels now that your baby's delivered? Not so fast. Continuing those pelvic floor–strengthening exercises will help you recover bladder control now and preserve it later on in life.

Keep your weight down. Start shedding those pregnancy pounds sensibly, because all those extra pounds are still applying pressure on your bladder.

Train your bladder to behave. Urinate every 30 minutes—before you have the urge—and then try to extend the time between pees, going (without going) a few more minutes each day.

Stay regular. Try to avoid constipation, so full bowels don't put added pressure on your bladder.

Drink up. Keep drinking at least eight glasses of fluid every day. It might seem that cutting back on water might cut down on the leak, but dehydration makes you vulnerable to UTIs. An infected bladder is more likely to leak, and a leaking bladder is more likely to become infected.

Fecal Incontinence

"I'm so embarrassed because I've been passing gas involuntarily lately and even leaking a little feces. What can I do about it?"

As a new mother, you definitely expected to be cleaning up after your baby—but you probably didn't count on cleaning up after yourself. Yet some newly delivered moms do add fecal incontinence and the involuntary passing of gas to that long list of unpleasant postpartum symptoms. That's because during labor and childbirth, the muscles and nerves in the pelvic area are stretched and sometimes damaged, which can make it difficult for you to control how and when waste (and wind) leaves your body. In most cases, the problem takes care of itself as the muscles and nerves recover, usually within a few weeks.

Until then, skip hard-to-digest foods (nothing fried, no beans, no cabbage), and avoid overeating or eating on the run (the more air you gulp, the more you

are likely to pass it as gas). Keeping up with your Kegels can also help tighten up those slack muscles as well as the ones that control urine (which also may be leaking these days).

Postpartum Backache

"I thought all my back pain would go away after delivery, but It hasn't. Why?"

Welcome back, backache. If you're like nearly half of all newly delivered moms, your old pal from pregnancy has returned for an unwelcome visit. Some of the pain still has the same cause—hormonally loosened ligaments that haven't yet tightened up. It may take time, and several weeks of soreness, before these ligaments regain their strength. Ditto for the stretched-out and weakened abdominal muscles that altered your posture during pregnancy, putting strain on your back. And of course, now that you've got a baby around, there's another reason for that pain in your back: all that lifting, bending, rocking, feeding, and toting you're doing. Especially as that cute little load you're carrying around gets bigger and heavier, your back will be up against growing stress and strain.

While time heals most things, including those postpartum aches and pains, there are other ways to get your back back on track:

- Tone that tummy. Ease into some undemanding exercises, like pelvic tilts, that will strengthen the muscles that support your back.

- Mend when you bend. And lift. Give your back a break by bending from your knees to pick up that dropped diaper or lift that baby.

- Don't be a slouch on the couch. When feeding your baby, don't slump over

---

Help for Leaks That Won't Let Up

Tried every do-it-yourself trick for dealing with postpartum urinary or fecal incontinence—including Kegel-ing until you're blue in the face—but you're still left with a leak? Don't let embarrassment keep you from talking to your practitioner. He or she might suggest biofeedback (a mind-body technique that can be surprisingly effective in relieving incontinence), other treatments, or in a particularly tough case, surgery. Fortunately, the situation most often resolves itself without that kind of intervention.

(as tempting as that might be, given your state of exhaustion). Your back will thank you if it's well supported (using pillows, armrests, or whatever else lets you sit pretty).

■ Get off your feet. Sure, you're running (and rocking) all the time, but whenever you don't have to, take a seat. When you have to stand, placing one foot on a low stool will take some pressure off your lower back.

■ Watch your posture. Listen to your mom, Mom—and stand up straight, even when you're swaying from side to side. Slouched shoulders result in an aching back. As your baby gets bigger, avoid resting that growing weight on one hip, which will throw your back off further, plus lead to hip pain.

■ Put your feet up. Who deserves to put their feet up more than you? Plus, elevating your feet slightly when sitting—and baby feeding—will ease the strain on your back.

■ Wear your baby. Instead of always holding your baby, wear him or her in a baby carrier or a sling. Not only will it be soothing to baby, it'll be soothing to your achy back and arms.

■ Pull a switch. Many moms play favorites with their arms, always carrying (or bottle feeding) their baby in one arm or the other. Instead, alternate arms so they each get a workout (and your body doesn't get a lopsided ache).

■ Rub it. A professional massage, if you can spare the time and the change, is definitely what your muscles are aching for. But in a pinch, ask your spouse to step in and rub.

■ Turn up the heat. A heating pad can spell relief from back pain and muscle aches. Apply it often, especially during those marathon feeding sessions.

As your body adjusts to pumping baby, you'll probably find that pain in your back (and arms, and hips, and neck) diminishing, and you may even find yourself sporting some brand-new triceps. In the meantime, here's something else that might help ease your aches by easing your load: Empty that diaper bag. Lug around only what you absolutely need, which is plenty heavy anyway.

Baby Blues

"I was sure I'd be thrilled once my baby was born. But I'm feeling down instead. What's going on?"

It's the best of times; it's the worst of times. And it's how an estimated 60 to 80 percent of new moms feel after childbirth. So-called baby blues appear (appropriately) out of the blue—usually three to five days after delivery, but sometimes a little earlier or a little later—bringing on unexpected sadness and irritability, bouts of crying, restlessness, and anxiety. Unexpected because—well, for one thing, isn't having a baby supposed to make you happy, not miserable?

It's actually easy to understand why you're feeling this way if you step back for a moment and take an objective look at what's been going on in your life, your body, and your psyche: rapid changes in hormone levels (which drop precipitously after childbirth); a draining delivery, followed by an exhausting homecoming, and all compounded by the round-the-clock demands of newborn care; sleep deprivation; possible feelings of letdown (you were expecting motherhood to come naturally—it hasn't; you were expecting cute and round—you got puffy and cone-headed); breastfeeding stumbling blocks (sore nipples, painful engorgement); unhappiness over your looks (the bags under your eyes, the pooch around your belly, the fact that there are more dimples on your thighs than on your baby's); and stress in your relationship with your partner (what relationship?). With such an overwhelming laundry list of challenges to confront (and don't even get you started on the laundry that's on that list), it's no wonder you're feeling down.

The baby blues will likely fade over the next couple of weeks as you adjust to your new life and start getting a little more rest—or, more realistically, begin functioning more effectively on less rest. In the meantime, try the following tips to help lift yourself out of that postpartum slump:

Lower the bar. Feeling overwhelmed and inadequate in your role as a newbie mom? It may help to remember that you won't be for long. After just a few weeks on the job, you're likely to feel much more comfortable in those maternal shoes. In the meantime, lower your expectations for yourself—and for your baby. Then lower them some more. Make this your mantra, even after you've become a parenting pro: There's no such thing as a perfect parent, or a perfect baby. Expecting too much means you'll be letting yourself down—and bringing your mood down, too. Instead, just do the best you can (which at this point may not be as well as you'd like, but that's okay).

Don't go it alone. Nothing is more depressing than being left alone with a crying newborn, that mountain of spit-up-stained laundry, a leaning tower of dirty dishes, and the promise (make that guarantee) of another sleep-deprived night ahead. So ask for help—from your spouse, your mother, your sister, your friends, a doula, or a cleaning service.

Get dressed. Sounds trite, but it's surprisingly true. Spending a little time making yourself look good will actually help you feel good. So hit the shower and maybe even the blow-dryer before your spouse hits the commuter train, trade in the stained sweats for a clean pair, and consider applying a little makeup (and a lot of concealer).

Get out of the house. It's amazing what a change of scenery can do for your state of mind—especially when the scenery suddenly doesn't include that pile of unopened mail (and unpaid bills). Try to get out of the house at least once a day: Take your baby for a walk in the park, visit with friends (and, if your friends are also moms, you can swap sob stories—and then laugh about them), stroll the mall. Anything that will keep you from hosting another self-pity party.

Treat yourself. Try a movie, a dinner date with your spouse, a 30-minute manicure (someone's bound to agree to watch the baby for that long), or even a long shower. Occasionally, make yourself a priority. You deserve it.

Get moving. Exercise boosts those feel-good endorphins, giving you an all-natural (and surprisingly lasting) high. So join a postpartum exercise class (preferably one that includes babies in the fun or at a club that offers child care), work out to an exercise DVD, step out for some stroller exercise (exercises that tone with the help of a stroller full of baby), or just simply step out for a walk.

Be a happy snacker. Too often, new moms are too busy filling their babies' tummies to worry about filling their own. A mistake—low blood sugar sends not only energy levels plummeting but moods, too. To keep yourself on a more even keel, physically and emotionally, stash sustaining, easy-to-munch snacks within quick reach. Tempted to reach for a chocolate bar instead? Reach away—

especially if chocolate really makes you happy—just not too often, because sugar-induced blood sugar highs have a way of crashing quickly.

Cry—and laugh. If you need a good cry, go for it. But when you're done, turn on a silly sitcom and laugh. Laugh, too, at all the mishaps you're likely having (instead of crying over them)—you know, the diaper blowout, the breasts that leaked in line at the market, the spit-up that spewed only after you realized you left home without wipes. You know what they say: Laughter is the best medicine. Plus, a good sense of humor is a parent's best friend.

Still blue, no matter what you do? Keep on reminding yourself that you'll outgrow the baby blues within a week or two—most moms do—and you'll be enjoying the best of times, most of the time, in no time.

If feelings of depression persist (lasting more than two weeks) or worsen, and start interfering with your functioning, call your practitioner right away and see the next column.

"I feel amazing and have since the moment I delivered three weeks ago. Is all this good feeling building up to one amazing case of letdown?"

Baby blues are common, but they're by no means on every newly delivered mom's to-do list. In fact, there's no reason to believe you're in for an emotional crash just because you've been feeling upbeat. Since baby blues usually occur within the first or second postpartum week, it's pretty safe to assume you've escaped them.

The fact that you're not feeling down, however, doesn't necessarily mean that everybody in your house has escaped the blues. Studies show that while new fathers (who, believe it or not,

also go through hormonal changes postpartum) are unlikely to be depressed when their wives are, their risk of falling into a postpartum slump increases dramatically when the new mother is feeling great. So be sure your spouse isn't down with the baby blues; some new dads try to hide such feelings to avoid dumping on their spouses.

Postpartum Depression

"My baby is over a month old, and I still can't stop feeling depressed. Shouldn't I be feeling better by now?"

When the blues just won't fade, chances are postpartum depression is the reason why. Though "baby blues" and "postpartum depression" are often used interchangeably, they're actually two very different conditions. True postpartum depression (PPD) is less common (affecting about 15 percent of women) and much more enduring (lasting anywhere from a few weeks to a year or more). It may begin at delivery, but more often not until a month or two later. Sometimes PPD is late onset; it doesn't start until a woman gets her first postpartum period or until she weans her nursing baby (possibly because of fluctuating hormones). More susceptible to PPD are women who have had it before, have a personal or family history of depression or severe PMS, spent a lot of time feeling down during pregnancy, had a complicated pregnancy or delivery, or have a sick baby.

The symptoms of PPD are similar to those of baby blues, though much more pronounced. They include crying and irritability; sleep problems (not being able to sleep or wanting to sleep the day away); eating problems (having no appetite or an excessive one); persistent feelings of sadness, hopelessness,

Getting Help for Postpartum Depression

No new mother should have to suffer from postpartum depression (PPD). Sadly, too many do, either because they believe it's normal and inevitable after delivery (it isn't) or because they're ashamed to ask for help (they shouldn't be).

Public education campaigns are under way to spread the word about PPD, to make sure that a woman who needs help gets it as quickly as she can—so she can start enjoying her new baby as soon as possible. Hospitals are, or will be, required to send new mothers home with educational materials about PPD, so that they (and their spouses) will be more likely to spot the symptoms early and seek treatment. Practitioners are becoming better educated, too—learning how to look for risk factors during pregnancy that might predispose a woman to PPD, to screen routinely for the illness postpartum, and to treat it quickly, safely, and successfully. Several standardized tests (Edinburgh Postnatal Depression Scale and Cheryl Beck's Postpartum Depression Screening Scale) are effective in screening for PPD.

PPD is one of the most treatable forms of depression. So if it strikes you, don't suffer with it any longer than you have to. Speak up—and get the help you need now. For more help, contact Postpartum Support International, (800) 944-4PPD (4773); postpartum.net.

and helplessness; an inability (or lack of desire) to take care of yourself or your newborn; social withdrawal; excessive worry; aversion to your newborn; feeling all alone; and memory loss.

If you haven't already tried the tips for fading the baby blues (see page 456), do try them now. Some of them may be helpful in easing postpartum depression, too. But if your symptoms have persisted for more than two weeks without any noticeable improvement or if you're having more serious symptoms for more than a few days, chances are your PPD won't go away without professional attention. Don't wait to see if it does. First, call your practitioner and be up-front about how you're feeling. He or she may run a thyroid test; because irregularities in thyroid hormone levels can lead to emotional instability, this is often one of the first steps taken when evaluating postpartum depression (see next page). If your thyroid levels check out normally, ask for a referral to a therapist who has a clinical background in the treatment of postpartum depression and make an appointment promptly. Antidepressants (several are safe even if you're breastfeeding), combined with counseling, can help you feel better fast. Some physicians prescribe low doses of antidepressants during the last trimester of pregnancy to women with a history of depression; others recommend that women who are at high risk take antidepressants right after delivery to prevent postpartum depression. Bright light therapy may also bring relief from the symptoms of PPD. (In light therapy, you sit with your eyes open in front of a box that emits a type of light that mimics daylight, causing a positive biochemical change in your brain that can cheer you up.) Whichever treatment (or combination of treatments) you and your therapist decide is right for you, keep in mind that swift intervention is

Thyroiditis Got You Down?

Nearly all new mothers feel run-down and tired. Most have trouble losing weight. Many suffer from some degree of depression and a certain amount of hair loss. It may not be a pretty picture, but for the majority of moms, it's a completely normal one in the postpartum period—and one that gradually begins to look better as the weeks pass. For the estimated 5 to 9 percent of women who suffer from postpartum thyroiditis (PPT), however, this picture may not improve with time. And, because the symptoms of PPT are so similar to those weathered by all new mothers, the condition may go undiagnosed and untreated.

PPT may start anywhere from one to three months after delivery with a brief episode of hyperthyroidism (too much thyroid hormone). This period of excess thyroid hormone circulating in the bloodstream may last a few weeks or longer. During this hyperthyroid period, a woman may be tired, irritable, and nervous; feel very warm; and experience increased sweating and insomnia—all of which are common in the immediate postpartum period anyway, making an easy diagnosis more elusive. Treatment isn't usually needed for this phase.

This period will typically (but not always) be followed by one of hypothyroidism (too little thyroid hormone). With hypothyroidism, fatigue continues, along with depression (longer lasting and often more severe than typical baby blues), muscle aches, excessive hair loss, dry skin, cold intolerance, poor memory, and an inability to lose weight.

If your postpartum symptoms seem to be more pronounced and persistent than you would have expected, and especially if they are preventing you from eating, sleeping, and enjoying your new baby, check with your practitioner. Tests can determine whether PPT is the cause of your troubles. Be sure to mention any history of thyroid problems in your family, since there is a very strong genetic link.

Most women recover from PPT within a year after delivery. In the meantime, treatment with supplementary thyroid hormone can help them feel much better much faster. About 25 percent of women who have the condition, however, remain hypothyroid, requiring lifetime treatment (which is as easy as taking a pill every day and having a yearly blood test). Even in those who recover spontaneously, thyroiditis is likely to recur during or after subsequent pregnancies. Some may develop hypothyroidism or Graves disease (hyperthyroidism) later in life. For this reason, it makes sense for women who have had PPT to have a yearly thyroid screening and, if they are planning another pregnancy, to be screened in the preconception period and during pregnancy (because an untreated thyroid condition can interfere with conception and cause problems during pregnancy).

critical. Without it, depression can prevent you from bonding with, caring for, and enjoying your baby. It can also have a devastating effect on the other relationships in your life (with your spouse, with other children), as well as on your own health and well-being.

Some women, instead of (or in addition to) feeling depressed postpartum, feel extremely anxious or fearful, sometimes experiencing panic attacks that include rapid heartbeat and breathing, hot or cold flashes, chest pain, dizziness, and shaking. These symptoms also require prompt treatment by a qualified therapist, which may include medication.

About 30 percent of women suffering from PPD also exhibit signs of postpartum obsessive-compulsive disorder (PPOCD), though PPOCD can also occur by itself. Symptoms of PPOCD include obsessive-compulsive behaviors, such as waking up every 15 minutes to make sure the baby is still breathing, furious housecleaning, or having obsessive thoughts about harming the newborn (such as throwing the baby out the window or dropping him or her down the stairs). Women suffering from PPOCD are appalled by their gruesome and violent thoughts, though they won't act on them (only those suffering from postpartum psychosis might; see below). Still, they can be so afraid of losing control and following through with these impulses that they may end up neglecting their babies. Like PPD, treatment for PPOCD includes a combination of antidepressants and therapy. If you're having obsessive thoughts and/or behaviors, be sure to get help by telling your practitioner about your symptoms.

Much more rare and much more serious than PPD is postpartum psychosis. Its symptoms include loss of reality, hallucinations, and/or delusions. If you're experiencing suicidal, violent, or aggressive feelings, are hearing voices or seeing things, or have other signs of psychosis, call your doctor and go to the emergency room immediately. Don't underplay what you're feeling, and don't be put off by reassurances that such feelings are normal during the postpartum period—they're not. To be sure you don't act out any dangerous feelings while you're waiting for help, try to get a neighbor, relative, or friend to stay with you or put your baby in a safe place (such as the crib).

Losing Weight Postpartum

"I knew I wouldn't be ready for a bikini right after delivery, but I still look six months pregnant two weeks later."

Though childbirth produces more rapid weight loss than any diet you'll find on the bestseller lists (an average of 12 pounds overnight), most women don't find it quite rapid enough. Particularly after they catch a glimpse of their paunchy postpartum profiles in the mirror.

The fact is, no one comes out of the delivery room looking much slimmer than when they went in. Part of the reason for that protruding postpartum abdomen is your still-enlarged uterus, which will be reduced to prepregnancy size by the end of six weeks, reducing your girth in the process. Another reason for your belly bloat might be leftover fluids, which should be flushing out soon. But the rest of the problem lies in those stretched-out abdominal muscles and skin, which will likely take some effort to tone up. (See Getting Back into Shape, page 465.)

As hard as it might be to put it out of your mind, don't even think about the shape your body's in during the first six weeks postpartum, especially if you're breastfeeding. This is a recovery period, during which ample nutrition (and rest) is important for both energy and resistance to infection. Sticking to a healthy postpartum diet should start you on the way to slow, steady weight loss. If, after six weeks, you aren't losing any weight, you can start cutting back somewhat on calories. If you're nursing, don't go overboard. Eating too few calories can reduce milk production, and burning fat too quickly can release toxins into the blood, which can end up in your breast milk. If you're not nursing, you can go on a sensible, well-balanced weight-loss diet six weeks postpartum.

Some women find that the extra pounds melt off while they're breastfeeding; others are dismayed to find the scale doesn't budge. If the latter turns out to be the case with you, don't despair; you'll be able to shed any remaining excess poundage once you've weaned your baby.

How quickly you return to your prepregnant weight will also depend on how many pounds you put on during pregnancy. If you didn't gain much more than 25 to 35 pounds, you'll likely be able to pack away those pregnancy jeans in a few months, without strenuous dieting. If you gained 35 or more pounds, you may find it takes more effort and more time—anywhere from 10 months to 2 years—to return to prepregnancy weight and your skinny jeans.

Either way, give yourself a break—and give yourself some time. Remember, it took you nine months to gain that pregnancy weight, and it may take at least that long to take it off.

Long-Term C-Section Recovery

"It's been a week since my C-section. What can I expect now?"

While you've definitely come a long way since you were wheeled into recovery, like every new mom you still have some recuperation ahead of you in the next few weeks. Keep in mind that the more conscientious you are about getting the rest you need now—as well as about following your practitioner's instructions—the shorter that recuperation time will ultimately be. In the meantime, you can expect:

Little or no pain. Most of it should have dissipated by now. But if you do hurt, some acetaminophen (Tylenol) should do the trick.

Progressive improvement. Your scar will be sore and sensitive for a few weeks, but it will improve steadily. A light dressing may protect it from irritation, and you will probably be more comfortable wearing loose clothing that doesn't rub. Occasional sensations of pulling or twitching and other brief pains around the incision site are a normal part of healing and eventually subside. Itchiness may follow—ask your practitioner to recommend an anti-itch ointment that you can apply. The numbness surrounding the scar will last longer, possibly several months. Lumpiness in the scar tissue will probably diminish, and the scar may turn pink or purple before it finally fades.

If pain becomes persistent, if the area around the incision turns an angry red, or if a brown, gray, green, or yellow discharge oozes from the wound, call your doctor. The incision may have become infected. (A small amount of clear fluid discharge is usually normal, but report it to your physician anyway.)

A four-week wait (at least) for sex. The guidelines are pretty much the same as they are for those who've delivered vaginally, though how well your incision is healing may also be factored into how long you'll need to wait. See the next question for more.

To get moving. Once you're free of pain, you'll be able to begin exercising. Kegel exercises are still important even if you delivered with your perineum intact, because pregnancy took its toll on those pelvic floor muscles. Concentrate, too, on exercises that tighten the abdominal muscles. (See Getting Back into Shape, page 465.) Make "slow and steady" your motto; get into a program gradually and continue it daily. Expect it to take several months before you're back to your old self.

Resuming Sex

"When can we start having sex again?"

That's at least partly up to you, though you'll also want to include your practitioner in the decision (probably not in the heat of the moment). Couples are typically advised to pick up where they left off whenever the woman feels physically ready—usually around four weeks postpartum, though some practitioners give the green light to sex as early as two weeks postpartum, and others still follow the old six-week rule routinely. In certain circumstances (for instance, if healing has been slow or you had an infection), your practitioner may recommend waiting longer. If your practitioner still has you in a holding pattern, but you think you're ready to move forward, ask if there's a reason why you shouldn't. If there isn't, ask your practitioner if you can get busy earlier. If it turns out there is a reason why sex might not be safe yet, hit the cold shower—though maybe together—and wait for clearance. Keep in mind that time will fly when you're caring for a newborn. In the meantime, satisfy each other with lovemaking that doesn't involve penetration.

"My midwife told me I can start having sex, but I'm afraid it's going to hurt. Plus, to be honest, I'm really not in the mood."

Doing "it" isn't topping your to-do list these days—or, more likely, isn't even making the top 20? No surprise there (or down there). Most women lose that loving feeling during the postpartum period—and beyond—for a variety of reasons. First, as you already suspect, postpartum sex can be more pain than pleasure—especially if you delivered vaginally, but, surprisingly, even if you labored and then had a C-section. After all, your vagina has just been stretched to its earthly limits, and possibly torn or surgically cut and sutured to boot—leaving you too sore to sit, never mind contemplate sex. Your natural lubrications haven't turned on yet, making you feel uncomfortably dry where you'd rather be moist—especially if you're breastfeeding. Adding to the pain potential: Low levels of estrogen cause the vaginal tissue to remain thin, and thin is not in as far as vaginas are concerned.

But your libido has other problems to contend with postpartum besides the physical ones: Your understandable preoccupation with a very little and very needy person, who is given to waking up with a full diaper and an empty tummy at the least opportune times. Not to mention a number of other very effective mood killers (the pungent smell of day-old spit-up on your sheets, the pile of dirty baby clothes at the foot of your bed, the baby oil on your nightstand where there used to be massage oil, the fact that you can't remember when you had your last shower). It's no wonder sex isn't on the schedule.

Will you ever live to make love again? Absolutely. Like everything else in your new and often overwhelming life, it'll just take time and patience (especially from your partner, who's almost certainly ready for this dry spell to end). So wait until you're feeling ready, or help yourself get ready with the following tips:

Lubricate. Using K-Y jelly, Astroglide, or another lubricant until your own natural secretions return can reduce pain and, ideally, increase pleasure. Buy them in economy sizes, so you'll be more likely to use them liberally—on both of you.

Loosen up. Speaking of lubrication, drinking a small glass of wine can also help you unwind—and keep you from

Craving More?

For much more information on easing back into sex, birth control, and enjoying the first year, see *What to Expect the First Year.*

tensing up and experiencing pain during intercourse (just make sure you drink it right after a feeding if you're nursing). Another great way to loosen up is massage, so request one prior to closing the deal.

Warm up. Of course, your partner's probably as eager as he's ever been to get down to business. But though he may not need much—if any—foreplay, you definitely do. So ask for it. And then ask for some more. The greater the effort he puts into warming you up (time permitting before baby wakes up again, of course), the better the main event will be for both of you.

Tell it like it is. You know what hurts and what feels good, but your partner doesn't unless you provide him a clearly marked map ("Turn left . . . no, right . . . no, down . . . up just a smidge—there, perfect!"). So speak up when you'd like things to heat up.

Position properly. Experiment and find a position that puts less pressure on any tender areas and gives you control over the depth of penetration (this is one time when deeper will definitely not be better). Woman-on-top (if you have the energy) or side-to-side positions are both great postpartum picks for those reasons. Whoever's in charge of the strides, make sure they're performed at a comfortably slow speed.

Pump it up. No, not that kind of pumping. Pump blood and restore muscle

tone to your vagina by doing the exercise you're probably sick of hearing about (but should keep doing anyway): Kegels. Do them day and night (and don't forget to do them when you're doing "it," too, since that squeeze will please you both).

Find alternative means of gratification. If you're not having fun yet through intercourse, seek sexual satisfaction through mutual masturbation or oral sex. Or if you're both too pooped to pop, find pleasure in just being together. There's absolutely nothing wrong (and everything right) about lying in bed together, cuddling, kissing, and swapping baby stories.

Bottom line on your bottom line: Even if sex does hurt a bit the first time (and second and third time), don't write it off—or give it up. It won't be long (though it may seem that way) before the pleasure will be all yours—and your partner's—again.

Becoming Pregnant Again

"I thought that breastfeeding was a form of birth control. Now I hear you can get pregnant while nursing, even before you get your period."

Unless you don't mind becoming pregnant again soon, don't even think about relying on breastfeeding for contraception.

It's true that, on average, women who nurse resume normal cycles later than those who don't. In mothers who aren't nursing, periods usually kick in again somewhere between 6 and 12 weeks after delivery, whereas in nursing mothers the average is somewhere between 4 and 6 months. As usual, however, averages are deceptive. Nursing moms have been known to begin their periods as early as 6 weeks and later than 18 months postpartum. The problem is, there's no sure way to predict when you will get your first postbaby period, though several variables can influence the timing: for example, frequency of nursing (more than three times a day seems to suppress ovulation better), duration of nursing (the longer you nurse, the greater the delay in ovulation), and whether or not feedings are being supplemented (your baby's taking formula, solids, even water can interfere with the ovulation-suppressing effect of nursing).

Why worry about birth control before that first postpartum visit from Aunt Flo? Because the point at which you ovulate for the first time after delivery is as unpredictable as when you menstruate. Some women have a sterile first period; that is, they don't ovulate during that initial cycle. Others ovulate before the period, and therefore they can go from pregnancy to pregnancy without ever having had a period. Since you don't know which will come first, the period or the egg, contraceptive caution is highly advisable.

Of course, accidents can happen. So even if you've been using contraception—and especially if you haven't been—pregnancy is still a possibility. If you do have any suspicion that you might be expecting again, the best thing to do is take a pregnancy test. See page 42 for information on back-to-back pregnancies.

See page 42 for information on back-to-back pregnancies.

Getting Back into Shape

It's one thing to look six months pregnant when, in fact, you are six months pregnant, and quite another to look it when you've already delivered. Yet most women can expect to come out of the birthing room not much trimmer than when they went in—with a little bundle in their arms and a sizable one still around their middles. As for the zip-up jeans optimistically packed for the going-home trip, they're likely to stay packed, with baggy sweats the comfortable substitute.

How soon after you become a new mother will you stop looking like a mother-to-be? The answer will depend primarily on four factors: how much weight you gained during pregnancy, how well you control your intake of calories, how much exercise you get, and your metabolism and your genes.

"Who needs exercise?" you may wonder. "I haven't stopped moving since I got home from the hospital. Doesn't that count?" Unfortunately, not much. Exhausting as it is caring for a newborn, that kind of activity won't tighten up the perineal and abdominal muscles that have been stretched and left saggy by pregnancy and childbirth—only an exercise program will. And the right kind of postpartum exercise will do more than tone you up. It will help keep baby-toting backaches at bay, promote healing and hasten recovery from labor and delivery, help pregnancy-loosened joints tighten up, improve circulation, and reduce the risk of a variety of other unpleasant postpartum symptoms, from varicose veins to leg cramps. Kegel exercises, which target the perineal

Basic Position

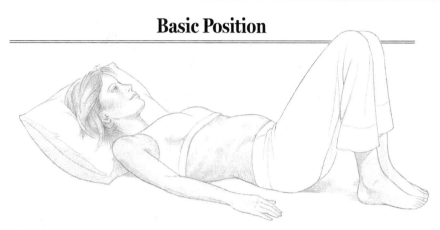

Lie on your back, knees bent, soles flat on the floor. Support your head and shoulders with cushions, and rest your arms flat at your sides.

Pelvic Tilt

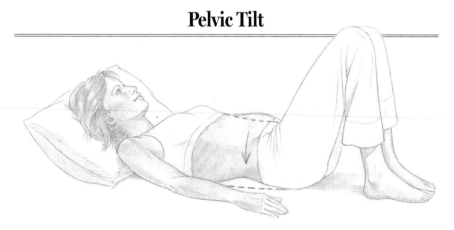

Lie on your back in the basic position. Take a breath. Then exhale as you press the small of your back against the floor for 10 seconds. Then relax. Repeat three or four times to start, increasing gradually to 12, and then 24.

muscles, will help you avoid stress and urinary incontinence and postpartum sexual problems. Finally, exercise can make you happier. As exercise-released endorphins circulate in your system, boosting your mood and your ability to cope, you'll find yourself much better equipped to handle the stresses of new parenthood. In fact, research shows that moms who resume exercising within six weeks of delivery feel better about themselves—and just plain feel better.

And you can probably start sooner than you think. If your delivery was vaginal and uncomplicated and you don't have any other major health issue that

Leg Slides

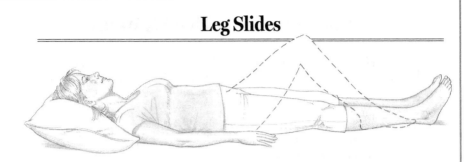

Assume the Basic Position. Slowly extend both legs until they are flat on the floor. Slide your right foot, flat on the floor, back toward your buttocks, inhaling as you go. Keep the small of your back against the floor. Exhale as you slide your leg back down. Repeat with your left foot. Start with three or four slides per side, and increase gradually until you can do a dozen or more comfortably. After three weeks, move to a modified leg lift (lifting one leg at a time slightly off the floor and lowering it again very slowly), if it is comfortable.

Head/Shoulder Lift

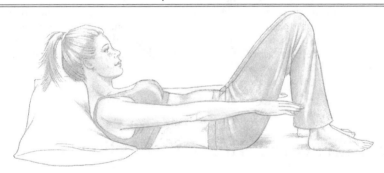

Assume the Basic Position. Take a deep relaxing breath; then raise your head very slightly and stretch your arms out, exhaling as you do. Lower your head slowly and inhale. Raise your head a little more each day, gradually working up to lifting your shoulders slightly off the floor. Don't try full sit-ups during the first six weeks—and then only if you have always had very good abdominal muscle tone. Check first, too, for an abdominal separation (see page 469).

might slow you down, you can begin your postpartum exercise program as early as 24 hours after delivery. (If you've had a surgical or a traumatic delivery, check with your doctor first.)

Don't even think about starting off with a bang, however; your recovering body needs to take it slowly and care-fully. The following three-phase program will help guide you. You can supplement it by using a postpartum exercise book or DVD, joining a class for new mothers (the camaraderie helps with motivation, and many include infants in the routines), and making daily strolls with baby a part of your routine.

Workout Rules for the First Six Weeks

- Wear a supportive bra and comfortable clothing.

- Try to divide your exercise schedule into two or three brief sessions rather than doing one long session a day (this tones muscles better and will be easier on your recovering body—plus you're more likely to be able to fit it in).

- Start each session with the exercise you find least strenuous.

- Do exercises slowly, and don't do a rapid series of repetitions. Instead, rest briefly between movements (the muscle buildup occurs then, not while you are in motion).

- As during pregnancy, avoid jerky, bouncy, erratic motions during the first six weeks postpartum, while your ligaments are still loose. Also avoid knee-to-chest exercises, full sit-ups, and double leg lifts during this period.

- Be sure to replenish fluids lost during exercise. Keep a water bottle next to you during your workouts and sip often. Aim for an extra cup or two of fluids for short bouts of exercise (more if your workouts are longer or more strenuous).

- Take it slowly and sensibly. "No pain, no gain" wasn't a motto created with new moms in mind. Don't do more than recommended, even if you feel you can, and stop before you feel tired. If you overdo it, you probably won't feel it until the next day, by which time you may be so exhausted and achy that you won't be able to exercise at all.

- Don't let taking care of your baby stop you from taking care of yourself. Your baby will love lying on your chest as you go through your exercise routine.

Phase 1: Twenty-Four Hours After Delivery

Can't wait to get back on the workout wagon? Easy does it, starting with:

Kegels. You can really start your Kegels as soon as you've delivered (see page 295 for directions if you haven't done them before), though you probably won't be able to feel yourself doing them at first, thanks to perineal numbness. Kegels can be done in any comfortable position, and comfort is key when you've just delivered a baby. Any time is a good time for Kegels, but try to get in the habit of doing them while you're feeding your baby—which you'll be doing a lot in the months to come. Work up to 25 repetitions four to six times a day, and continue for the rest of your life for good pelvic health (and increased sexual pleasure).

Deep diaphragmatic breathing. In the Basic Position (see box, page 466), place your hands on your abdomen so you can feel it rise as you inhale slowly through your nose; tighten the abdominal muscles as you exhale slowly through your mouth. Start with just two or three deep breaths at a time, to prevent hyperventilating, and work up gradually. (Signs that you've overdone it are dizziness or faintness, tingling, or blurred vision.)

Phase 2: Three Days After Delivery

Anxious to get that pre-baby body back? Then you'll be happy to hear that it's time to move up another rung on the exercise ladder. But before you take that step, make sure the pair of vertical muscles that form your abdominal wall have not separated during pregnancy. If they have, you'll have to close them up before the workouts start heating up (see box below). Once the separation has closed, or if you've never had one, move on to Head/Shoulder Lifts, Leg Slides, and Pelvic Tilts (see illustrations on pages 466 and 467).

All these exercises should be done in the Basic Position. At first, do them in bed, then move on to a well-cushioned floor. (An exercise mat is a good investment, not only because it makes these exercises easier and more comfortable to do now, but because your baby can practice rolling over and try his or her first tentative crawls on it later on in the year.)

Close the Gap

Don't look now, but there's probably a hole in the middle of your belly (and it's not your navel). A very common pregnancy condition known in obstetrical circles as diastasis, it's a gap in your abdominal muscles that can develop as the abdomen expands. It can take a month or two after delivery for this gap to close, and you'll have to wait until it does before you start those crunches and other abdominal exercises or you'll risk an injury. To determine if you have a separation, examine yourself this way: As you lie in the Basic Position, raise your head slightly with your arms extended forward; then feel for a soft lump above your navel. Such a lump indicates a separation.

If you do have a separation, you may be able to help correct it more quickly with this exercise: Assume the Basic Position and inhale. Now cross your hands over your abdomen, using your fingers to draw the sides of your abdominal muscles together as you breathe out, pulling your belly button inward toward the spine while raising your head slowly. Exhale as you lower your head slowly. Repeat three or four times, twice a day.

Phase 3: After Your Postpartum Checkup

Now, with your practitioner's go-ahead, you can gradually graduate to a more active workout program that includes walking, running, bicycling, swimming, water workouts, aerobics, yoga, Pilates, weight training, or similar routines. Or sign up for a postpartum exercise class. But don't try to do too much too soon. As always, let your body be your guide.

Milk It

Good news for nursing moms who want to exercise their right to work out. Exercise—even the high-intensity type—doesn't turn your breast milk sour, as you might have heard. Salty, maybe, from the sweat on your nipples—but your baby might actually enjoy that added tang. So go ahead (when your practitioner's given the go-ahead) and exercise to your body's content. Feeding your baby before a workout (or pumping) might make you more comfortable (since your breasts won't be as full), but it isn't necessary. And don't forget to wear a bra that offers you plenty of support—you need it more than ever.

PART 5

For Dads

Fathers Are Expectant, Too

THOUGH IT'S CERTAINLY TRUE—future medical breakthroughs and Hollywood movies notwithstanding—that only women can become pregnant, it's just as true that fathers are expectant, too. As a dad, you're not only an essential member of your baby-making team, but an invaluable nurturer of both your pregnant spouse and your unborn offspring. In the months to come, you'll participate fully in the amazing process of pregnancy—in the excitement, in the responsibility, and, of course, in the worry. Some of your concerns will overlap those of mom-to-be; others will be uniquely yours. And just like your mate, you're entitled to your share of reassurance, not just during the pregnancy and the birth, but during the postpartum period as well.

And so this chapter is dedicated to the equal, but sometimes neglected, partner-in-reproduction. Keep in mind, however, that the pages that follow aren't intended for your eyes only, any more than the rest of the book is intended only for the mother-to-be. Your spouse can gain some valuable insights into what you're feeling, won-

Get Ready, Get Set . . . Then Go

Giving your baby the best start in life can start even before sperm meets egg. If your partner isn't yet pregnant, you both have time to get yourselves into tip-top baby-making shape first. Read Chapter 1, and follow the suggestions for the preconception period. If you're already expecting, no problem. Just start taking good care of yourselves and each other now.

dering about, and hoping by reading this chapter; you can better understand the physical and emotional challenges she'll be facing during pregnancy, childbirth, and postpartum—and at the same time better prepare yourself for your own role in this adventure—by reading the rest of this book.

What You May Be Wondering About

Dealing with Her Symptoms

"My wife is having every symptom in the book, literally: nausea and cravings and peeing all the time. I'm not sure what to do—I feel so helpless."

Seem like the woman in your life has been taken over by aliens? Close—she's been taken over by pregnancy hormones (which can sometimes make an alien invasion seem like a walk in the park). These hormones, vital to baby production, can also produce a wide variety of uncomfortable (and sometimes bewildering) symptoms: hard for her to cope with and hard for you to stand by helplessly and watch.

Fortunately, you don't have to just stand there—you can actually do something. To help your pregnant partner feel better while helping yourself feel less helpless, read about the symptoms individually in this book, plus try some of the following father-focused symptom-fighting strategies:

Morning sickness. Morning sickness is one pregnancy symptom that definitely doesn't live up to its name. It's a 24/7 experience that can send your spouse running to the bathroom morning, noon, and night—and hugging the toilet far more than she'll be hugging you. So take steps to help her feel better—or at least not worse. Lose the aftershave that she suddenly finds repulsive and get your onion ring fix out of her sniffing range (her sense of smell is in overdrive). Fill her gas tank so she doesn't have to come nose-to-nozzle with the fumes at the pump. Fetch her foods that quell her queasies and don't provoke another run to the toilet—ginger ale, soothing smoothies, crackers (but ask first—what spells r-e-l-i-e-f for one queasy woman spells v-o-m-i-t to another). Be there for support when she's throwing up—hold back her hair, bring her some ice water, rub her back. Encourage her to eat small meals throughout the day instead of three large ones (spreading out the load and keeping her tummy filled may ease her nausea). And remember, no jokes. If you'd been throwing up for 10 straight weeks, you wouldn't find it amusing. Neither does she.

Cravings and aversions. Have you noticed that she's gagging over foods she used to love—or going gaga over foods she's never eaten before (or eaten in such peculiar combinations)? Don't tease her about these cravings and aversions—she's as powerless to control them as you are to understand them. Instead, indulge her by keeping the offending foods out of smelling distance. (Love chicken wings? Love them somewhere else.) Surprise her with the pickle-melon-and-Swiss sandwich she suddenly can't live without. Go the extra mile—or two miles—to the all-night mart for that midnight pint of triple fudge brownie, and you'll both feel better.

A Partner in Parenting by Any Name

Most of the tips in this chapter also apply to the partner in a nontraditional family. Pick and choose questions and answers that fit your situation or can be applied to it.

Exhaustion. If you think *you're* tired at the end of the day, think about this: Your spouse expends more energy lying down on the sofa building a baby than you do bodybuilding at the gym. Which makes her a lot more tired than you've ever known her to be—and a lot more tired than you can even imagine. So pick up the slack. And your slacks. And the trail of socks and sneakers in the hallway. Beat her to the vacuuming and the dusting and the laundry and the toilet cleaning. (The fumes from the cleaning products will make her feel sicker anyway.) Encourage her to watch your cleanup routine from a fully reclining position on the sofa (even if that's always been your favorite position).

Trouble sleeping. She's making a baby, but chances are she isn't sleeping like one. So instead of snoring up a storm next time her pregnancy insomnia strikes, keep your spouse company while she waits for the sandman to show up. Buy her a body pillow to help get her comfy or build her a cozy fort of support with your extra pillows. Relax her with a backrub, run her a bath, bring her a warm cup of milk and a muffin. Do a little pillow talking. Cuddle as needed and as wanted. And if one thing leads to another, you might both sleep better. (Don't expect a sexual nightcap for your

efforts, though—there are plenty of reasons why she might not be in the mood these days.)

Frequent urination. There she goes—again. Urinary frequency will be your spouse's constant companion in her first trimester, and it'll come back with a vengeance in the last trimester, too. So try not to hog the bathroom, and always leave it ready for her use. Remember to put the seat down after every use (especially at night), and keep the hallway free of obstacles (your briefcase, your sneakers, that magazine) and lit by a nightlight so she won't trip on her way to the toilet. And be as understanding as you can when she has to get up three times during the movie or stop six times on the way to your parents' house.

Sympathy Symptoms

"It's my wife who's pregnant, so why am I having morning sickness?"

Feeling curiously . . . pregnant? Women may have a corner on the pregnancy market but not on pregnancy symptoms. As many as half, or even more (depending on the study), of expectant fathers suffer from some degree of couvade syndrome, or "sympathetic pregnancy," during their wives' gestation. The symptoms of couvade can mimic virtually all the normal symptoms of pregnancy, including nausea and vomiting, abdominal pain, appetite changes, weight gain, food cravings, constipation, leg cramps, dizziness, fatigue, and mood swings.

Any number of emotions that have settled down in your psyche these days could trigger these symptoms, from sympathy (you wish you could feel her pain, and so you do), to anxiety (you're stressed about the pregnancy or about becoming a father), to jealousy (she's getting center stage; you'd like to share it). But there's more to sympathy symptoms than just sympathy (and other normal father-to-be feelings). In fact, there are actually physical factors in play. Believe it or not, your wife's female hormones aren't the only ones surging these days. Research shows that pregnancy and the postpartum period step up dad's supply, too. Though you (and your fellow fathers-to-be) won't be churning out enough female hormones to grow breasts, you might produce enough to grow a little belly, or send you heaving at the sight of your favorite burger, or running to the fridge for a midnight pickle fest (or all three). And these hormonal fluctuations aren't random or a sign of Mother Nature's twisted sense of humor. They're designed to get you in touch with your nurturing side—nature's way of bringing out the parent in you. Which doesn't only prepare you for the diaper-changing ahead, but helps you cope with the changes you're both facing now. These hormone shifts also make it easier for you to channel those sometimes uncomfortable feelings into productive pursuits. Apply your sympathy to cooking dinner and scrubbing the toilet; work through those anxieties by talking them out with your spouse and with friends who are already dads; feel less left out by becoming more involved in the pregnancy and baby prep.

Rest assured, all symptoms that don't go away during pregnancy will disappear soon after delivery, though you may find that others crop up postpartum. And don't stress out if you don't have a single sick—or queasy or achy—day during your wife's pregnancy. Not suffering from morning sickness or putting on weight doesn't mean you don't empathize and identify with your spouse or that you're not destined for nurturing—just that you've found other ways to express your feelings. Every expectant father, like every expectant mother, is different.

Feeling Left Out

"I hardly feel I have anything to do with the pregnancy, now that conception's out of the way."

Many fathers-to-be feel like they're on the outside looking in, and that's not surprising. After all, mom's the one getting all the attention (from friends, from family, from the practitioner). She's the one with the physical connection to the baby (and the belly to back it up). You know you're about to become a father, but you don't have much to show for it now.

Not to worry. Just because the pregnancy's not taking place in your body doesn't mean you can't share it. Don't wait for an invitation to get you off the bench. Your spouse has a lot on her mind (and a lot to get off her chest), and it's up to you to get into the game. Open up to her about feeling shut out, and ask her to let you in. She might not even realize she's excluding you from the pregnancy, or she may think you're not particularly interested in it.

But also remember, the best way to keep from feeling left out is to step up to the plate and get involved. Here's how:

- Be a prenatal regular. Whenever you can (and if you're not already), join her at her practitioner checkups. She'll appreciate the moral support, but you'll appreciate the chance to hear the practitioner's instructions for yourself (so you can help her follow them better—and help her remember them if pregnancy forgetfulness leaves her in a fog). Plus you'll get to ask all those questions you have. The visits will also give you much-needed insight into the miraculous changes going on in your spouse's body. Best of all, you'll get to experience those momentous milestones with her

Resources for Dads

Expectant fathers are just as hungry for reassurance, support, information, and empathy as expectant mothers. Here are some places you can turn to, both during pregnancy and once you're a full-fledged dad: whattoexpect.com; fathermag.com; fathersforum.com; fatherville.com; bcnd.org.

(hearing the heartbeat, seeing those tiny limbs on ultrasound).

- Act pregnant. You don't have to show up for work in a baby-on-board T-shirt or start sporting a milk mustache. But you can be a true partner in pregnancy: Exercise with her (it'll tone you up, too); take a pass on the alcohol (it's much easier for her to toe the teetotaling line when she has a comrade-in-club-soda); eat well (at least when you're around her); and if you smoke, quit (permanently, since secondhand smoke isn't good for anyone—especially your baby).

- Get an education. Even dads with advanced degrees (including those with MDs) have a lot to learn when it comes to pregnancy, childbirth, and baby care, just as moms do the first time. Read books and magazines; visit websites. Attend childbirth classes together; attend classes for fathers, if they're available locally. Chat up friends and colleagues who've become new fathers recently or chat with other pregnant dads online.

- Make contact with your baby. A pregnant woman may have the edge in bonding with the unborn baby because it's comfortably ensconced in

her uterus, but that doesn't mean you can't start getting to know the new family member, too.

Talk, read, sing to your baby frequently; a fetus can hear from about the end of the sixth month on, and hearing your voice often now will help your newborn recognize it after delivery. Enjoy baby's kicks and squirms by resting your hand or your cheek on your wife's bare belly for a few minutes each night. It's a nice way to get close to her, too.

- Shop for a layette, and a crib, and a stroller with your partner. Decorate the nursery together. Pore over baby-name books. Attend consultations with prospective baby doctors. In general, become active in every aspect of planning and preparing for the baby's arrival.

- Consider taking off. Start looking into your company's paternity-leave policy. This way, you'll be sure not to be left out of all the fun after the baby is born.

Sex

"Ever since my wife's became pregnant, she's been really oversexed. Is that normal (not that I'm complaining)? Is it safe to have sex so often?"

The rumors are true: Some women really can't get enough when they're expecting. And for good reason. Your wife's genitals are swollen with hormones and blood now that she's pregnant, leaving the nerves down below set on tingle mode. Other parts are swollen, too (you might have noticed), including places (such as those breasts and hips) that can make a woman feel more womanly than ever—and more sensually charged. All of which is normal (as is feeling less in the mood, which many women feel,

Expectant Sex Explained

Sure, you've done it before. But have you done it pregnancy-style? Though the basic rules of the game apply when you're expecting, you'll find that pregnant sex requires a few adjustments, a little finessing, and a lot of flexibility—literally. Here are some suggestions to get you going in the right direction:

- Wait for the green light. She was hot to trot yesterday, but today she's cold as ice to your advances? As a pregnant woman's moods swing, so does her sex drive. You'll have to learn to swing along (and to hold on tight).

- Warm her up before you start your own engine. This may go without saying (always), but it's a must when she's expecting. Go as slowly as she needs you to, making sure she's fully charged on foreplay before you hit the road.

- Stop for directions. The road map of what feels good and what doesn't may have changed (even since last week), so don't rely on possibly outdated directions. Always ask before going in. You may need to tread especially lightly when it comes to those super-size breasts. Though they may have swelled to heart-quickening proportions, they can be tender to even the gentlest touch, especially in the first trimester. Which means you may have to look but not touch for a while.

- Put her in the driver's seat. Choose positions with her comfort in mind. A top pregnancy favorite is her on top, since she can control penetration best this way. Another is her facing away on her side (spooning each other). And when her belly starts getting between you, get around it creatively: Try it from behind with her on her knees or sitting on your lap while you lie down.

- Be prepared for rerouting. All roads aren't leading to intercourse? Find alternate paths to pleasure that you both can enjoy—masturbation, oral sex, two-way massage.

too)—safe, also, as long as the practitioner has given the sex go-ahead.

So be there for the taking whenever she's in the mood to grab you. Feel lucky that you're getting lucky so often. But always take your cues from her, especially now. Proceed with seduction if she's up for it and into it, but don't go without the green light.

Though some women are in the mood throughout their nine months, others find that the party doesn't get started until the second trimester; still others find desire spikes in the second, only to dip in the third. So be ready to roll with her changing sexual agenda when she goes from turned on to turned off in 60 seconds (frustrating, possibly, but completely normal). Keep in mind, too, that there will be some logistical challenges in mid- to late pregnancy as her body goes from two-seater to semi.

"I find my wife incredibly sexy now. But she hasn't been in the mood since the day we found out we were pregnant."

Even couples who have always been in sexual sync can find themselves suddenly out of step in the sack once they're expecting. That's because so many factors, both physical and emotional, can affect sexual desire, pleasure, and performance during pregnancy.

Your libido may be getting a lift just from liking what you see; many men find the roundness, fullness, and ripeness of the pregnant form surprisingly sensual, even extra erotic. Or your lust may be fueled by affection; the fact that you're expecting a baby together may have deepened your already strong feelings for your wife, arousing even greater passions.

But just as your sexual overdrive is both understandable and normal, so is her decreased drive. It could be that pregnancy symptoms have leveled her libido (it's not so easy to lose yourself in the moment when you're busy losing your lunch, or to get hot when you're bothered by backache and swollen ankles, or to get it on when you barely have the energy to get up), particularly in those uncomfortable first and third trimesters. Or that she's as turned off by her new roundness as you are turned on by it (what you see as a sexy round bottom, she may see as a big fat ass). Or that she's preoccupied with all things baby and/or having a hard time blending the roles of mother and lover.

When she's not in the mood (even if she's *never* in the mood), don't take it personally. Try, try, again another time, but always be a good sport while you're waiting for your ship to come in. Accept those "not now's" and those "don't touch there's" with an understanding smile and a hug that lets her know you love her even when you can't show it the way you'd like to. Remember, she's got a lot going on in her mind (and in her body) right now, and it's a safe bet that your sexual needs aren't front and center on her plate.

There's definitely a possibility that your patience will pay off, most likely in the second trimester, when some women get their sexual groove back. Even if your sex life doesn't perk up then or if it drops off again in the third trimester

(because of an increase in her fatigue or back pain or because of that growing basketball belly) or in the postpartum period (when neither one of you is likely to be much in the mood), don't worry. Nurturing the other aspects of your relationship (making that love connection without actually making love) will ensure that you'll eventually be able to pick up where you left off sexually.

In the meantime, don't push your sexual agenda, but do step up the romance, communication, and cuddling. Not only will these bring you closer together, but because they're powerful aphrodisiacs for many women, they may just bring you what you're craving. When one thing does lead to another, make sure you proceed with care and caution (see box, page 477)

And don't forget to tell your partner—often—how sexy and attractive you find the pregnant her. Women may be intuitive, but they're not mind readers.

"Now that we're expecting, I just don't seem very interested in sex. Is this normal?"

Expectant fathers, like expectant mothers, can experience a wide range of reactions when it comes to their pregnancy libidos—some of them bewildering, and all of them normal. And there are plenty of good reasons why your sex drive may be in a slump now. Perhaps you and your spouse worked so conscientiously at conception that sex suddenly feels too much like hard work. Maybe you're so focused on the baby and on becoming a dad that your sexual side is taking a backseat. Or the changes in your spouse's body are taking some getting used to (especially because they're an in-your-face reminder of how your life and relationship are also changing). Or fear that you'll hurt her or your baby during sex (you won't) has sent your mojo into hiding. Or it could be a hang-up thing—the hang-up being that you've never made love to a mother before (even though that mother happens to be a woman you've always enjoyed making love to). Or it could be the weirdness factor that's keeping you down: Getting close to your pregnant spouse might mean getting too close for comfort to your baby during a decidedly adult activity (even though baby's completely oblivious). The normal hormonal changes that expectant fathers experience can also slow them sexually.

Confusing these conflicted feelings even more could be miscommunication: You think she's not interested, so you subconsciously put your urges on ice. She thinks you're not interested, so she gives desire a cold shower.

Try to focus less on the quantity of sex in your relationship and more on the quality of the intimacy you're sharing. Less may not be more, but it can still be fulfilling. You might even find that stepping up the other kinds of intimacy—the hand-holding, the unexpected hugs, the confiding of your feelings—might put you both more in the mood for lovemaking. Don't be surprised, too, if your libido gets a boost once both of you have adjusted to the emotional and physical changes of pregnancy.

It's also possible that your sexual slowdown will continue throughout the nine months—and beyond, too. After all, even couples who can't get enough while they're expecting find that their sex lives can come to a screeching halt once there's a baby in the house, at least for the first couple of months. All of this is fine—and all of it is temporary. Meanwhile, make sure the nurturing of your baby doesn't interfere with the care and feeding of your relationship. Put romance on the table regularly (and while you're at it, put some candles

there, too, plus a dinner you cooked up while she was napping). Surprise her with flowers or a sexy negligee (they make them for expectant moms, too). Suggest a moonlit stroll or hot cocoa and cuddles on the couch. Share your feelings and fears, and encourage her to share hers. Keep the hugs and kisses coming (and coming . . . and coming). You'll both stay warm while you're waiting for things to heat up again.

Also be sure that your wife knows that your lack of libido has nothing to do with her physically or emotionally. Expectant moms can suffer a crumbling of confidence when it comes to their pregnant body image, particularly as those pounds start piling on. Letting her know (often, through words and touch) that she's more attractive to you than ever will help keep her from taking your drop in sexual interest personally.

For more tips on enjoying sex more when you're doing it less, see page 260.

"Even though the doctor told us that sex is safe during pregnancy, I have trouble following through because I'm afraid of hurting my wife or the baby."

Plenty of fathers-to-be confront that very same fear factor when it comes to expectant lovemaking. And that's not surprising. It's only natural to put your expectant wife and baby-to-be first and to try to protect them at all costs (including at the cost of your pleasure).

But fear not, and take it from the practitioner. If he or she has greenlighted sexual intercourse during pregnancy (and most of the time, that's exactly what'll happen), sex is completely safe up to delivery. Your baby is way out of your reach (even for the particularly gifted), well secured and sealed off in its uterine home, impervious to harm, unable to view or be aware of the proceedings, and perfectly oblivious to what's going on when you're getting it on. Even those mild contractions your spouse might feel after orgasm are nothing to worry about, since they're not the kind that triggers premature labor in a normal pregnancy. In fact, research shows that low-risk women who stay sexually active during pregnancy are actually less likely to deliver early. And not only will making love to your wife do her no harm, but it can do her a world of good by filling her increased needs for physical and emotional closeness, and by letting her know that she's desired at a time when she may be feeling her least desirable. Though you should proceed with care (take your cues from her and keep her needs top priority), you can certainly proceed—and feel good about it.

Still concerned? Let her know. Remember, open and honest communication about everything, including sex, is the best policy.

Pregnancy Dreams

"I've been having the strangest dreams lately—and I'm not sure what to make of them."

So your dream life has been more interesting than your real life these days? You've got lots of company. For just about all expectant mothers and fathers, pregnancy is a time of intense feelings, feelings that run the roller coaster from joyful anticipation to panic-stricken anxiety and back again. It's not surprising that many of these feelings find their way into dreams, where the subconscious can act them out and work them through safely. Dreams about sex, for instance, might be your subconscious telling you what you probably already know: You're worried about how pregnancy and having a baby is affecting and will con-

tinue to affect your sex life. Not only are such fears normal, they're valid. Acknowledging that your relationship is in for some changes now that baby's making three is the first step in making sure your twosome stays cozy.

R-rated dreams are most common in early pregnancy. Later on, you may notice a family theme in your dreams. You may dream about your parents or grandparents as your subconscious attempts to link past generations to the future one. You may dream about being a child again, which may express an understandable fear of the responsibilities to come and a longing for the carefree years of the past. You may even dream about being pregnant yourself, which may express sympathy for the load your spouse is carrying, jealousy of the attention she's getting, or just a desire to connect with your unborn baby. Dreams about dropping the baby or forgetting to strap your newborn into the car seat can express your insecurities about becoming a father (the same insecurities every expectant parent shares). Uncharacteristically macho dreams— scoring a touchdown or driving a race car—can communicate the subconscious fear that becoming a nurturer will chip away at your manliness. The flip side of your subconscious may also get equal time (sometimes even in the same night); dreaming about taking care of your baby helps prepare you for your new role as doting dad. Dreams about loneliness and being left out are extremely common; these speak to those feelings of exclusion that so many expectant fathers experience.

Not all of your dreams will express anxiety, of course. Some dreams—of being handed or finding a baby, of baby showers or family strolls through the park—show how excited you are about the imminent arrival. (You'll find more dream themes on page 291.)

It's Your Hormones (Really)

Think just because you're a guy you're immune to the hormonal swings usually reserved for females? Think again. Research has revealed that expectant and new dads experience a drop in their testosterone levels and an increase in the hormone estradiol—a female sex hormone. It's speculated that this shift in hormones, which is actually common across the animal kingdom, turns up the tenderness in males. It may also contribute to some pretty strange and surprising pregnancy-like symptoms in fathers-to-be, including food cravings, queasiness, weight gain, and mood swings. What's more, it may keep dad's libido in check (often a good thing, since a raging sex drive can sometimes be inconvenient during pregnancy—and definitely when there's a new baby in the house). Hormone levels typically return to normal within three to six months, bringing with them an end to those pseudo pregnancy symptoms—and a return to libido business as usual (though not necessarily to sex life as usual until baby's sleeping through the night).

One thing is for sure: You're not dreaming alone. Expectant mothers (for the same reasons) are subject to strange dreams, too—plus the hormones make them even more vivid. Sharing dreams with each other in the morning can be an intimate, enlightening, and therapeutic ritual, as long as you don't take them too seriously. After all, they're just dreams.

Surviving Her Mood Swings

"I've heard about mood swings during pregnancy, but I wasn't prepared for this. One day she's up, the next day she's down, and I can't seem to do anything right."

Welcome to the wonderful—and sometimes wacky—world of pregnancy hormones. Wonderful because they're working hard to nurture the tiny life that's taken up residence inside your spouse's belly (and that you'll soon be cuddling in your arms). Wacky because, in addition to taking control of her body (and often making her miserable), they're also taking control of her mind—making her weepy, over-the-top excited, disproportionately pissed, deliriously happy, and stressed out . . . and that's all before lunch.

Not surprisingly, an expectant mom's mood swings are usually the most pronounced during the first trimester when those pregnancy hormones are in their greatest state of flux (and when she's just getting used to them). But even once the hormones have settled down in the second and third trimesters, you can still expect to be riding the emotional roller coaster with your spouse, which will continue to take her to emotional highs and lows (and fuel those occasional outbursts) right up until delivery, and beyond.

So what's an expectant dad to do? Here are some suggestions:

Be patient. Pregnancy won't last forever (though there will be times in the ninth month where you both may wonder if it will). This, too, shall pass, and it'll pass a lot more pleasantly if you're patient. In the meantime, try to keep your perspective—and do whatever you can to channel your inner saint.

Don't take her outbursts personally. And don't hold them against her. They are, after all, completely out of her control. Remember, it's the hormones talking—and crying for no apparent reason. Avoid pointing out her moods, too. Though she's powerless to control them, she's also probably all too aware of them. And chances are, she's no happier about them than you are. It's no picnic being pregnant.

Help slow down the swings. Since low blood sugar can send her mood swinging, offer her snacks when she's starting to droop (a plate of crackers and cheese, a fruit-and-yogurt smoothie). Exercise can release those feel-good endorphins she's in need of now, so suggest a before- or after-dinner walk (also a good time to let her vent fears and anxieties that might be dragging her down).

Go the extra yard. That is, go to the laundry room, to her favorite takeout on the way home from work, to the supermarket on Saturday, to the dishwasher to unload . . . you get the picture. Not only will she appreciate the efforts you make—without being asked—but you'll appreciate her happier mood.

Your Pregnancy Mood Swings

"Ever since we got the positive pregnancy test, I seem to be feeling really down. I didn't think fathers were supposed to get depressed during pregnancy."

Fathers share a lot more than the expected bundle of joy with their partners. Long before that bundle arrives, they can share in many of the symptoms, including pregnancy mood slumps—which are surprisingly common in expectant dads. While you can't be as quick to blame your hormones as your spouse can (though men's hormones do fluctuate somewhat during pregnancy, too), it's likely that your emotional low can be linked to the host of normal but conflicted feelings—from anxiety to fear to ambivalence—that most dads-to-be (and moms-to-be) find themselves trying to work out in the months leading up to this major life change.

But you can help boost your pregnancy mood—and perhaps prevent the postpartum blues, which about 10 percent of new fathers suffer from—by:

- Talking. Let your feelings out so they don't bring you down. Share them with your wife (and don't forget to let her share hers, too), making communication a daily ritual. Talk them over with a friend who recently became a father (no one will get it like he will) or even with your own father. Or find an outlet online—a message board for new or expectant dads.

- Moving. Nothing gets your mood up like getting your pulse up. Not only will a workout help you work out your feelings—or pound them out, or pump them out—but it can give your feel-good endorphins a long-lasting boost.

- Getting baby-busy. Gear up for the anticipated arrival by pitching in with all the baby prep that's likely going on. You may find that getting in the baby spirit helps give your spirits a boost.

- Cutting out (or cutting down). Drinking a lot can swing your moods even lower. Though alcohol has a reputation for being a mood booster, it's technically a depressant, so there's a reason why the morning after is never as happy as the night before. Plus, it's a coping mechanism that covers up the feelings you're trying to cope with. Ditto with other drugs.

If these suggestions don't help lift your mood, or if your depression deepens or begins to interfere with your relationship with your spouse, your work, and other aspects of your life, don't wait it out. Seek professional help (from your physician or a therapist) so you can start enjoying what should be a happy and exciting life change.

Labor and Delivery Worries

"I'm excited about our baby's birth, but I'm stressed out about handling it all. What if I can't keep it together?"

Few fathers enter the birthing room without a little trepidation—or a lot. Even obstetricians who've assisted at the births of thousands of other people's babies can experience a sudden loss of self-confidence when confronted with their own baby's delivery.

Yet very few of those father-to-be fears—of freezing, falling apart, fainting, getting sick, and otherwise humiliating themselves or their spouses or falling short of their expectations—are ever realized. In fact, most dads handle childbirth with surprising ease, keeping their composure, their cool, and their lunch. And though being prepared for the birth—by taking childbirth education classes, for instance—generally makes the experience more satisfying for all involved, even most unprepared fathers come through labor and delivery better than they ever would have imagined.

But, like anything new and unknown, childbirth becomes less scary and intimidating if you know what to expect. So become an expert on the subject. Read the section on labor and delivery, beginning on page 380. Check out the Internet. Attend childbirth education classes, watching the labor and delivery DVDs with your eyes wide open. Visit the hospital or birthing center ahead of time so it'll be familiar ground on labor day. Talk to friends who've attended the births of their children—you'll probably find that they were stressed out about the birth beforehand, too, but that they came through it like pros.

Though it's important to get an education, remember that childbirth isn't the final exam. Don't feel you're under any pressure to perform. Midwives and doctors won't be evaluating your every move or comparing you to the coach next door. More important, neither will your spouse. She won't care if you forget every coaching technique you learned in class. Your being beside her, holding her hand, urging her on, and providing the comfort of a familiar face and touch is what she'll need—and appreciate—most of all.

Still having performance anxiety? Some couples find that having a doula present during birth helps them both to get through labor and delivery with less stress and more comfort (see page 298).

"The sight of blood makes me sick, so I'm worried about being at the delivery."

Most expectant fathers—and mothers—worry about how they'll handle seeing blood at delivery. But chances are you won't even notice it, never mind be bothered by it—for a couple of reasons. First of all, there typically isn't very much blood to see. Second, the excitement and wonder of watching your baby arrive is likely to keep you both pretty preoccupied (that, and the efforts of birthing, of course).

If at first glance the blood does bother you (and it's really likely it won't), keep your eyes focused on your spouse's face as you coach her through those last pushes. You'll probably want to turn back to the main event for that momentous moment; at that point, blood is going to be the last thing you'll notice.

"My wife is having a scheduled C-section. Is there anything I need to know ahead of time?"

The more you learn about C-sections now, the better the experience will be for both of you. Even though you won't be helping out as much as you would if you were coaching your partner through a vaginal birth, your participation will be more valuable than you might think. A dad's reaction at a cesarean delivery can actually affect the level of fear and anxiety his partner experiences—and a less-stressed father contributes greatly to a less-stressed mother. And there's no better way to reduce your stress than knowing what to expect. So sign up together for a childbirth education class that includes C-sections in the curriculum, read up on surgical deliveries and recoveries (see pages 398 and 432), and get as prepped as you can.

Remember that any kind of surgery can seem like a scary proposition, but C-sections are extremely safe for both mom and baby. Plus, most hospitals now strive to make them as family friendly as possible, allowing you to watch (if you want to), sit by your spouse's side, hold her hand, and hold the baby right after birth—just like the couples delivering vaginally down the hall.

Anxiety Over Life Changes

"Ever since I saw him on ultrasound, I've been excited about our son's birth. But I've also been worrying about how different our lives will be once we become parents."

Little babies do bring some large life changes, no doubt about it—and all expectant parents worry about them. Moms-to-be stress about these upcoming changes, too, but being so physically invested in the pregnancy process gives them a head start on working them through (their lives are already different, big time). For dads, the changes can seem less gradual, more jolting. But thinking about them—and even stressing about them—now is actually a really good thing, since it gives you a chance to prepare realistically for the impact parenthood will have on your life. The most common dad-to-be worries include:

Will I be a good father? There isn't a dad-to-be (or mom-to-be) who doesn't have this one on his top-10 worry list. To help you cross it off yours, see page 486.

Will our relationship change? Just about every set of new parents finds that their relationship undergoes some change when baby makes three. Anticipating this change realistically during pregnancy is an important first step in dealing with it effectively postpartum. No longer will being alone together be as simple as closing the blinds and letting voice mail pick up calls; from the moment baby comes home from the hospital, spontaneous intimacy and complete privacy will be precious, and often unattainable, commodities. Romance may have to be planned (a quickie grabbed during baby's nap) rather than spur of the moment, and interruptions may be the rule (you can't let voice mail pick up the baby, after all). But as long as you both make the effort to make time for each other—whether that means catching up with each other over a late dinner once baby's in bed, or giving up a game with the guys so you can play games of an entirely different kind with your spouse, or starting a weekly date night—your relationship will weather

Being There

The very best way to start off your new life as a father is at home with your new family. So if it's possible and financially feasible, consider taking off as much time as you can right after delivery—through the Family and Medical Leave Act (which allows for 12 weeks of unpaid leave for mothers and fathers; see page 187), the policy at your company (ask ahead of time what it is), or by taking a chunk of vacation time (the beach will be there next year, but your baby will be a newborn only once). Or if that's impossible (or not your preference), consider working part-time for a few weeks or doing some work from home.

Should none of these possibilities prove practical, and job responsibilities call, maximize the time you have off from work. Make sure you're home as much as you can be; learn to say no to overtime, early or late meetings, and business trips that can be put off or passed off. Especially in the postpartum period, when your spouse is still recovering from labor and delivery, try to do more than your share of household chores and baby care whenever you're home. Keep in mind that no matter how physically or emotionally stressful your occupation, there is no more demanding job than caring for a newborn.

Make bonding with your new baby a priority, but don't forget to devote some time to nurturing your spouse as well. Pamper her when you're home, and let her know you're thinking of her when you're at work. Call her often to offer support and empathy (and so she can unload as much as she needs to); surprise her with flowers or takeout from a favorite restaurant.

---

the changes well. Many couples, in fact, find that becoming a threesome deepens, strengthens, and improves their twosome—bringing them closer together than they've ever been before.

How will we divide the child care? Parenting is a two-person job (at least when there are two parents), but that doesn't mean it's clear just how the division of labor will play out once baby makes three. Don't wait until baby needs his first midnight diaper change or his first bath to decide this question. Start divvying up duties now—fairly. Some details of your plan may change once you really start operating as parents (she had signed up for baths, but you turn out to be the better bather), but exploring the options in theory now will make you feel more confident about how baby care is going to work in practice later.

Plus, it'll encourage you to communicate about it openly—something every team needs to do to be effective.

How will work be affected? That depends on your work schedule. If you currently work long hours with little time off, you may need (and want) to make some changes to make fatherhood the priority in your life that you'll want it to be. And don't wait until you officially become a father. Think about taking time off now for doctor's visits, as well as to help your exhausted spouse with baby preparations. Start weaning yourself off those 12-hour days, and resist the temptation to continue your day at the office at home. Avoid trips and a heavy workload during the two months before and after your baby's ETA, if you can. And if it's at all possible, consider taking paternity leave in the early weeks of baby's life.

Will we have to give up our lifestyle? You probably won't have to say good-bye to accustomed activities or your social life as you knew it, but you should expect to make some adjustments, at least up front. A new baby does, and should, take center stage, pushing some old lifestyle habits temporarily aside. Parties, movies, and sports may be tricky to fit in between feedings; cozy dinners for two at your favorite bistro may become noisy meals for three at family restaurants that tolerate squirming infants. Your circle of friends may change somewhat, too; you may suddenly find yourself gravitating toward fellow stroller-pushers for empathetic companionship. Not to say that there won't be a place for old friends—and pastimes from your past—in your new life with baby; just that your priorities will likely do some necessary shifting.

Can I afford a larger family? With child-rearing costs going through the roof, many expectant parents lose sleep over this very legitimate question. But there are plenty of ways to cut those costs, including opting for breastfeeding (no bottles or formula to buy), accepting all the hand-me-downs that are offered (new clothes start to look like hand-me-downs after a few spitting-up episodes anyway), and letting friends and family know which gifts you really need rather than allowing them to fill baby's shelves with stuff you'll never use. If either of you is planning to take extra time off from work (or to put career plans on hold for a while) and this concerns you from a financial standpoint, weigh it against the costs of quality child care and commuting. The income lost may not be so great after all.

Most important: Instead of thinking of what you won't have in your life anymore (or won't have as much opportunity for), try to start thinking of what

you will have in your life: a very special little person to share it with. Will your life be different? Absolutely. Will it be better? Immeasurably.

Fathering Fears

"I want to be a good father, but the thought is terrifying. I've never even seen or held a newborn, much less taken care of one."

Few men are born fathers, any more than women are born mothers. Though parental love may come naturally, parental skills (the stuff you're nervous about) have to be learned. Like every other new dad and mom, you'll grow into parenthood one challenge, one bath, one all-night rocking session, one cuddle and coo at a time. Gradually, with persistence, hard work, and a lot of love (that'll be the easy part, once you gaze into that little face), the role that seems daunting—yes, terrifying—now will become second nature. Though you'll learn plenty on the job—and from your mistakes, which every new parent makes plenty of—you might feel a little more comfortable with some formal preparation.

Fortunately, classes that teach all the baby basics—from diapering to bathing, feeding to playing—are finding their way into communities across the country. There are boot camps for new dads and other preparatory classes in many hospitals and community centers. Ask about those or classes you can take together as a couple at the next prenatal appointment, check into them at the hospital or birthing center you'll be delivering at, or do some research online. Put an infant CPR class on your to-do list, too. You can also learn the ropes by reading *What to Expect the First Year* or online at whattoexpect.com. If you have friends who have recently arrived infants, turn to them for some hands-on instruction. Ask them to let you hold, diaper, and play with their babies.

And remember, too, as you learn, that just as mothers have different parenting techniques, so do dads. Relax, trust your instincts (surprise . . . fathers have them, too), and feel free to find the style that works for both you and your baby. Before you know it, you'll be fathering with the best of them.

Breastfeeding

"My wife is thinking about breastfeeding our new baby, and I know it would be good for him—but I feel a little weird about it."

Up until now, you've thought of your wife's breasts sexually. And that's natural. But here's something that's also natural. Breasts are built the way they are for another good reason and to serve another really important purpose: baby feeding. There is no more perfect food for an infant than breast milk, and no more perfect food delivery system than a breast (make that two breasts). Breastfeeding offers an overwhelming number of health benefits for a baby (from preventing allergies, obesity, and illness to promoting brain development) and for its mother (nursing is linked to a speedier recovery postpartum and possibly a reduced risk of breast cancer later on in life). You can read more about those amazing benefits starting on page 331.

Without a doubt, your wife's decision to choose breast over bottle can make a dramatic difference in your child's life—and in hers. So try to put your feelings aside, and give her your vote of breastfeeding confidence—which counts a lot more than you'd think. Even though you don't know letdown from latch-on, you'll have a tremendous influence on whether your wife sticks with breastfeeding (and the longer she sticks with it, the

more health benefits for both her and baby). In fact, research shows that moms are far more likely to try and succeed at nursing when fathers are supportive than if they're ambivalent. So take your influence seriously. Read up on nursing, watch a DVD, talk to other dads whose wives have breastfed, and ask whether a lactation consultant (basically, a nursing coach) will be available at the hospital or birthing center when the baby's ready to chow down for the first time. (Lesson one: It's a natural process, but it doesn't come naturally.) If your wife is too embarrassed to ask for help—or she's just too tired after delivery—be her breastfeeding advocate and make sure she gets it.

Sure, seeing your wife breastfeeding might seem weird at first—almost as weird as breastfeeding might feel to her initially—but before long, it will seem natural, normal, and incredibly special.

"My wife is breastfeeding our son. There's a closeness between them that I can't seem to share, and I feel left out."

Certain biological aspects of parenting naturally exclude you: You can't be pregnant, you can't give birth, and you can't breastfeed. But, as millions of new fathers discover each year, those natural physical limitations don't have to relegate you to spectator status. You can share in nearly all the joys, expectations, trials, and tribulations of your wife's pregnancy, labor, and delivery—from the first kick to the last push—as an active, supportive participant. And though you'll never be able to put your baby to the breast (at least not with the kind of results baby's looking for), you can share in the feeding process:

Be your baby's supplementary feeder. Once breastfeeding is established, there's more than one way to feed a baby. And though you can't nurse, you can be the one to give supplementary bottles

Your Baby Blues

You're overjoyed to be a father, and that's putting it mildly. So why are you also feeling emotionally spent? After all that buildup, all the planning and spending and drama, your child has been born, and you feel not only run-down (that's the sleep deprivation talking) but also a tiny bit let down. Welcome to the Postpartum Club, when you suddenly realize why the word *baby* is so often followed by the word *blues*. Not every new parent experiences the so-called baby blues, but you can expect a profusion of emotions in both of you (fortunately, usually only one of you at a time). Be ready. And be strong. You'll need the patience of a saint, the endurance of a triathlete, a temper with a mile-long fuse, and a sense of humor (big time) to work through this period of adjustment. Adapt the tips for her baby blues (page 456) to your needs during this rough patch. If those don't help, and baby blues progress to depression, ask your doctor for help so you can start enjoying life with your new baby.

(if those will be on the menu for baby). Not only will your being the supplementary feeder give mom a break (whether in the middle of the night or in the middle of dinner), it will give you extra opportunities for closeness with your baby. Make the most of the moment—instead of propping the bottle up to the baby's mouth, strike a nursing position, with the bottle where that breast would be and your baby snuggled close. Opening up your shirt, which allows for skin-to-skin contact, will enhance the experience for both of you.

Don't sleep through the night until your baby does. Sharing in the joys of feeding also means sharing in the sleepless nights. Even if you're not giving supplementary bottles, you can become a part of nighttime feeding rituals. You can be the one to pick baby up, do any necessary diaper changing, deliver him to his mom for his feeding, and return him to bed once he has fallen asleep again.

Participate in all other baby rituals. Nursing is the only baby-care activity limited to mothers. Dads can bathe, diaper, and rock with the best of moms, given the chance.

Bonding

"I'm so excited about our new baby that I'm afraid I'm almost overdoing the attention I'm giving her."

Some things in life you can overdo—but not loving and caring for your baby. Not only do infants thrive on attention from their fathers, there is no better way to cement your relationship with your new offspring. All the time you're spending with the baby will also help your spouse bond better with the baby (a mother who carries the load of baby care alone may find herself too exhausted and resentful to bond well).

And if you're surprised by your enthusiasm for your daughter, don't be. Studies have found that males in both the human and animal kingdoms experience a surge in female hormones when their babies arrive. Nurturing, long thought the province of mothers, apparently comes naturally to dads, too.

As you're busy nurturing your newborn, however, don't forget another relationship that needs looking after: the one with your spouse. Make sure she knows how much you love her, too. And make sure she gets her share of attention.

"I've heard about bonding, and we both got a chance to hold our baby when he arrived. But four days later, I feel love, but I still don't feel all that connected."

Bonding begins with that first cuddle, but it's just the very start of your relationship with your baby. That brand-new connection between you will deepen and strengthen, not just over the next weeks, but over the many years you'll be sharing as father and son.

In other words, don't expect instant results—and don't worry because you feel you haven't had them. Look at every moment with your new son as a new opportunity to build the bond you've started. Every diaper change, every bath, every kiss, every caress, every look into that tiny little face, you'll be bonding.

Keep an Eye on Her Mood

Baby blues are one thing (they're normal and self-limiting), but true postpartum depression is another. It's a serious medical condition that requires prompt, professional treatment. If the mom in your life still seems truly overwhelmed several weeks after the baby comes home or experiences bouts of crying, irritability, or sleep disruptions (other than those caused by the baby), or if she's not eating or otherwise functioning normally—as normally as can be expected given her new responsibilities—encourage her to talk to her practitioner about it. Don't leave it up to her if she says no. She may not recognize the signs of depression. Make sure she gets the treatment she needs to feel better. See page 458 for signs of postpartum depression.

Making eye contact and skin contact (open your shirt and hold him against your chest as you sing him to sleep) can enhance the closeness and tighten the bond. (This kind of contact will also, according to research, speed his brain development, so it's good for both of you.) Keep in mind that the relationship may seem a little one-sided at first (until your newborn is alert enough to be responsive, you'll be doing all the smiling and cooing), but every moment of your attention is contributing to your baby's fledgling sense of well-being and letting him know he's loved. The feedback you'll get once the smiles start coming will confirm your time was well spent—and the connection with your baby was there all along.

If you find your spouse is monopolizing the baby care (she may do this without even being aware of it), let her know you'd like to take on at least your share. Volunteering to spend time alone with the baby whenever possible—while your spouse takes an exercise class, meets a friend for coffee, or just soaks in a tub with a good book—will guarantee that maternal good intentions won't interfere with you and your son getting to know each other. And don't feel you have to spend your quality time with your son at home. Newborns are highly portable, so feel free to pack a diaper bag, strap him into a stroller, car seat, or baby carrier, and take a stroll or run an errand with baby in tow.

Feeling Unsexy After Delivery

"The delivery of our baby was absolutely awesome. But seeing her born seems to have turned me off sexually."

Human sexual response, compared to that of other animals, is

Postpartum Sex?

Are you experiencing the longest sexual dry spell you've had since freshman year? Think you're exhibiting the symptoms of dreaded DSB (deadly sperm backup)? Be patient: Their time will come, and so will yours. Your spouse is still recovering from a significant shock to her system—not just the birthing, but the nine months preceding. She's been through the wringer physically. The doctor or midwife may have already said that sex is technically okay to start up again, but your partner will be the ultimate decision maker on this one. Once she agrees to give it a try, you'll need to proceed very slowly and extremely gently. Ask her what feels good, what hurts, what you can do to help. And don't even consider laying into the entree until you've served up at least a few foreplay appetizers (she'll need lots of massage, and lubrication will help get her juices going because hormonal changes have left her extra dry). Don't be surprised if you get an accidental eyeful of milk right in the middle of the action (milk happens, especially early on). Share a laugh, and get back to business.

extremely delicate. It's at the mercy not only of the body but of the mind as well (dogs don't think about it—they just do it). And the mind can, at times, play plenty of tricks. One of those times, as you probably already know, is during pregnancy. Another, as you're discovering, is during the postpartum period.

It's very possible that the cause of your sudden sexual ambivalence has nothing to do with having seen your baby delivered. Most brand-new fathers find both the spirit and the flesh somewhat less willing after delivery (although there's nothing abnormal about those who don't) for many very understandable reasons: fatigue; fear that your baby will wake up crying at that first kiss (particularly if she is sharing your room); concern that you may hurt your spouse by having sex before her body is completely healed; and, finally, a general physical and mental preoccupation with your newborn, which sensibly concentrates your energies where they are most needed at this stage of your lives. Your feelings may also be influenced by the temporary increase in female hormones and drop in testosterone that many new fathers experience, because it's the male hormones, in both women and men, that fuel libido. That's probably nature's way of helping you nurture—and nature's way of keeping sex off your mind when there's a new baby in the house.

In other words, it's probably just as well that you aren't feeling sexually motivated, particularly if your wife—like most women in the immediate postpartum period—isn't feeling emotionally or physically up to it, either. Just how long it will take for your interest, and hers, to return is impossible to predict. As with all matters sexual, there is a wide range of normal. For some couples, desire precedes even the practitioner's go-ahead—which, depending on the circumstances, may be anywhere from two to six weeks. For others, six months can pass before sex makes a postpartum comeback. Some women find their libidos lacking until they stop breastfeeding, but that doesn't mean they can't enjoy the closeness of lovemaking.

Some fathers, even if they've been prepared for the childbirth experience, do come out of it feeling as if the special place that's always been meant for pleasure has suddenly taken on a practical purpose. But as the weeks pass, that feeling usually does, too. The vagina, after all, has two really important functions: practical and sexual. Neither excludes the other, and, if you think about it, they're very much interconnected. The vagina is used for childbirth only briefly, but it's a source of pleasure for you and your wife for a lifetime.

While you're waiting for your libido to make its inevitable return (and it will!), make sure you're paying your partner plenty of the attention she's undoubtedly in need of. Women who've just delivered typically don't feel their most desirable, and even if she's not in the mood for love—she's definitely in the mood to hear that you love her (and think she's beautiful and sexy). It can't hurt, either, to try some romantic moves to get you both back into the mood—as hard as that might be to accomplish when you've got a newborn in the house. Light some scented candles once baby's finally asleep to mask that pervasive aroma of dirty diapers; offer her a sensuous no-strings-attached massage; bring on the cuddles while you're both collapsed on the coach. Who knows—you might feel that libido return sooner than you'd think.

"Now that my wife's breastfeeding, I can't help feeling differently about her breasts. They seem too functional to be sexy."

Like the vagina, breasts were designed to serve both a practical and a sexual purpose (which, from a procreative perspective, is also practical). And though these purposes aren't mutually exclusive in the long run, they can conflict temporarily during lactation.

Some couples find breastfeeding a sexual turn-on, especially if breasts are full for the first time. Others, for aesthetic reasons (leaking milk, for instance) or because they feel uncomfortable about using the baby's source of nourishment for their sexual pleasure, find it a very definite turn-off. They may find this effect wears off, however, as breastfeeding becomes more second nature for all concerned.

Whatever turns you on—or off—is what is normal for you. If you feel your wife's breasts are too functional to be sexy now, focus foreplay elsewhere until you've become more comfortable sharing them with baby (or until baby has been weaned). Be sure, however, to be open and honest with your wife. Taking a sudden, unexplained hands-off approach to her breasts could leave her feeling unappealing. Be careful, also, not to harbor any resentment against the baby for sharing the breasts you love so much; try to think of nursing as a temporary "loan" instead. And enjoy the "interest" that comes with the loan—a healthy, well-fed newborn.

PART 6

Staying Healthy When You're Expecting

CHAPTER 20

If You Get Sick

So you probably expect to deal with at least a few of the less pleasant pregnancy symptoms during your nine-month stint (a little morning sickness, a few leg cramps, some indigestion and exhaustion), but maybe you weren't planning on coming down with a nasty cold or an ugly (and itchy) infection. The truth is, pregnant women can get sick with the best of them—and even better than the best of them, since suppression of the normal immune system makes expectant moms easier targets for germs of every variety. What's more, being sick for two can make you at least twice as uncomfortable—especially since so many of the remedies you're used to reaching for may need to stay behind medicine cabinet doors for a while.

Fortunately, such pregnancy-unrelated illnesses won't affect your pregnancy (though they may affect the way you feel). Prevention is, of course, the best way to avoid getting sick in the first place and to keep that healthy glow of pregnancy going strong. But when it fails (as when a coworker brings the flu to the office, your nephew's wet kisses are loaded with cold germs, or you pick up some bacteria with those fresh-picked blueberries), quick treatment, in most cases under the supervision of your practitioner, can help you feel better fast.

What You May Be Wondering About

The Common Cold

"I'm sneezing, coughing, and my head is killing me. Can this nasty cold affect my baby?"

Common colds are even more common when you're pregnant because your normal immune system is suppressed. The good news is that you're the only one those nasty bugs will be bugging. Your baby can't catch your cold or be affected by it in any way. The not-so-good news: The medications and supplements that you might be used to reaching for to find relief (or to prevent a cold), including aspirin and ibuprofen, megadoses of vitamins, and most herbs, are usually off limits when you're expecting (see page 509 for information on taking medications during pregnancy). So before you pick the shelves of the drugstore clean, pick up the phone and call your practitioner to ask which remedies are considered safe in pregnancy, as well as those that will work best in your case—there will probably be several you can choose from. (If you've already taken a few doses of a medication that isn't recommended for use during pregnancy, don't worry. But do check with your practitioner for extra reassurance.)

Even if your standard cold medication is shelved for now, you don't have to suffer (or play mother-to-be martyr) when you're laid up in bed with a runny nose and hacking cough—or even if you just feel a cold coming on. Some of the most effective cold remedies don't come in a bottle and are also the safest for both you and your baby. These tips can help nip a cold in the bud, before it blossoms into a nasty case of sinusitis or another secondary infection, while helping you to feel better faster. At the very first sneeze or tickle in the throat:

- Rest, if you feel the need. Taking a cold to bed doesn't necessarily shorten its duration, but if your body is begging for some rest, be sure to listen. On the other hand, if you feel up to it (and you're not running a fever or coughing), light to moderate exercise can actually help you feel better faster.

- Don't starve your cold, fever—or baby. Eat as nutritiously as you can, given how crummy you feel and how little appetite you probably have. Choose foods that appeal to you or at least don't turn you off completely. Try to have some citrus fruit or juice (oranges, tangerines, grapefruit) as well as plenty of other fruits and vegetables rich in vitamin C every day, but don't take extra vitamin C supplements (beyond what comes in your pregnancy vitamin supplement) without medical approval. The same holds true for zinc and echinacea.

- Flood yourself with fluids. Fever, sneezes, and a runny nose will cause your body to lose fluids that you and your baby need. Warm beverages will be particularly soothing, so keep a thermos of a hot drink or hot soup next to your bed and try to drink at least a cupful an hour. Water and cold juices work fine, too, if that's what you're thirsting for.

- When you're lying down or sleeping, use a couple of pillows to keep your head elevated. This will make it easier for you to breathe through a stuffy nose. Nasal strips (which gently pull your nasal passages open, making breathing easier) may help, too. They're sold over the counter and are completely drug free.

- Keep your nasal passages moist with a humidifier and by squirting the inside of your nose with saline nose drops (which are also drug free and completely safe).

- If your throat is sore or scratchy, or if you're coughing, gargle with salt water (¼ teaspoon of salt to 8 ounces of warm water).

- Try to bring down a fever promptly. For more on fever treatment, see page 497.

- Don't put off calling the doctor or refuse to take a medication he or she prescribes because you think all drugs are harmful in pregnancy. Many are not. But do be sure the prescribing doctor knows you're expecting.

Is It the Flu or a Cold?

Here's how to tell which bug has you down:

The cold. A cold, even a bad one, is milder than the flu. It often starts with a sore or scratchy throat (which typically lasts only a day or two) followed by the gradual appearance of cold symptoms. These include a runny, and later stuffy, nose; lots of sneezing; and possibly slight achiness and mild fatigue. There is little or no fever (usually less than 100°F). Coughing may develop, particularly near the cold's end, and may continue for a week or more after other symptoms have subsided.

The flu. Influenza (or the flu) is more severe and comes on more suddenly. Symptoms include fever (usually 102°F to 104°F), headache, sore throat (which generally worsens by the second or third day), often intense muscle soreness, and general weakness and fatigue (which can last a couple of weeks or longer). There may also be occasional sneezing and often a cough that can become severe. In some cases, nausea or vomiting may occur, but don't confuse this with what is often called the "stomach flu" (see page 501). You can easily avoid coming down with the flu by getting a flu shot.

If your cold is severe enough to interfere with eating or sleeping, if you're coughing up greenish or yellowish mucus, if you have a cough with chest pain or wheezing, if your sinuses are throbbing (see the next question), or if symptoms last more than a week, call your doctor. It's possible that your cold has settled into a secondary infection and prescribed medication may be needed for your safety and your baby's.

Sinusitis

"I've had a cold for about a week. Now my forehead and cheeks are starting to really hurt. What should I do?"

Sounds as though your cold has turned into sinusitis. Signs of sinusitis include pain and often tenderness in the forehead and/or one or both cheeks (beneath the eye), and possibly around the teeth (pain usually worsens when you bend over or shake your head), as well as thickened and darkened (greenish or yellowish) mucus.

Sinusitis following a cold is fairly common, but it is far more common among pregnant women. That's because your hormones tend to swell mucous membranes (including those in and leading to the sinuses), causing blockages that allow germs to build up and multiply in the sinuses. These germs tend to linger longer there, because immune cells, which destroy invading germs, have difficulty reaching the sinuses' deep recesses. As a result, sinus infections that aren't treated can persist for weeks—or even become chronic. Treatment with antibiotics (your practitioner will be able to prescribe one that is safe during pregnancy) can bring relief quickly.

Flu Season

"It's fall, and I'm wondering if I should get a flu shot. Is it safe during pregnancy?"

A flu shot is definitely your best line of defense during flu season. Not only is it safe to receive while you're pregnant, it's considered a good move. In fact, the Centers for Disease Control and Prevention (CDC) recommends that any woman who will be pregnant during flu season (generally October through March) be given the flu shot. And since the CDC puts pregnant women at the top of the priority list for getting vaccinated (along with the elderly and children between the ages of 6 months and 5 years), moms-to-be can waddle to the front of the flu-shot line, even if the vaccine is in short supply. Talk to your ob-gyn or midwife about getting a flu shot. If he or she doesn't offer it, make an appointment with your general practitioner to get one. You can also look for flu-shot clinics that are sometimes set up at local drug and grocery stores during flu season.

The flu vaccine must be taken prior to each flu season—or at least early in the season—for best protection. It's not 100 percent effective because it protects only against the flu viruses that are expected to cause the most problems in a particular year. Still, it greatly increases the chance that you will escape the season flu free. And even when it doesn't prevent infection, it usually reduces the severity of symptoms. Side effects occur infrequently and are generally mild.

When going for your flu shot, ask if you can receive thimerosal-free (or -reduced) vaccine. And stick with the needle, not the nasal spray vaccine (FluMist). That vaccine, unlike the flu shot, is made from live flu virus (which means it could actually give you a mild case of the flu) and is not recommended for pregnant women.

If you suspect you might have the flu (see symptoms in box, facing page), call your doctor so that you can be treated (and so that the flu doesn't progress to pneumonia). Treatment is typically symptomatic—aimed at reducing fever (take steps right away to bring down any fever; see next question), aches and pains, and nasal stuffiness. Most important if you've got the flu (or any virus) when you're expecting: Rest and drink plenty of fluids, essential for preventing dehydration.

Flu Shot for Two

Getting a flu shot is good for you when you're expecting, but did you know that its benefits carry over to your newborn as well? Researchers have found that babies born to mothers who were given the flu shot during the last trimester of pregnancy appear to be protected against the virus for the first six months of life. Which means that by getting a flu shot now, you'll be keeping your baby protected until it's time for his or her first flu shot.

Fever

"I'm running a little fever. What should I do?"

During pregnancy, a low-grade fever (one that's under 100.4°F) isn't usually something to be concerned about. But it's also not something to be ignored, which means you should take steps to bring any fever down promptly. Keep a close eye on your temperature, too, to make sure it doesn't start rising.

Any fever over 100.4°F while you're expecting is more of a concern and should be reported to your practitioner right away. That's because the cause (such as an infection that should be treated with antibiotics) can pose a pregnancy problem even when the fever doesn't. While you're waiting to speak to your practitioner, take two acetaminophen (Tylenol) to start reducing the fever. Taking a tepid bath or shower, drinking cool beverages, and keeping clothing and covers light will also help bring your temperature down. Aspirin or ibuprofen (Advil or Motrin) should *not* be taken when you're expecting unless they've been specifically recommended by your practitioner.

If you had a high fever earlier in pregnancy and did not report it to your practitioner, mention it now.

Strep Throat

"My three-year-old came down with strep throat. If I catch it, is there a risk to the baby?"

If there's one thing kids are good at sharing, it's their germs. And the more kids you have at home (particularly of the child-care-attending or school-going variety), the greater your chances of coming down with colds and other infections while you're expecting.

So step up preventive measures (don't share drinks, resist the temptation to finish that peanut-butter-and-germ sandwich, wash your hands frequently) and boost your immune system—which is lowered during pregnancy anyway—by eating well and getting enough rest.

If you do suspect that you've succumbed to strep, go to your practitioner for a throat culture right away. The infection will not harm the baby, as long as it is treated promptly with the right type of antibiotic. Your practitioner will prescribe one that is effective against strep and perfectly safe for use during pregnancy. Don't take medication prescribed for your children or someone else in the family.

Urinary Tract Infection

"I'm afraid I have a urinary tract infection."

Your poor battered bladder, which spends months on end being pummeled by your growing uterus and its adorable occupant, is the perfect breeding ground for less welcome visitors: bacteria. These little bugs multiply fast in areas where urine pools or is prevented from moving along, meaning anywhere along a urinary tract that's being squished by the expanding uterus. (It's that same compression that makes you unable to sleep through the night without getting up several times to pee.) That here-and-there compression, added to the muscle-relaxing properties of the hormones flooding your body, makes it much easier for the intestinal bacteria that live quietly on your skin and in your feces to enter your urinary tract and make you miserable. In fact, urinary tract infections (UTIs) are so common in pregnancy that at least 5 percent of pregnant women can expect to develop at least one, and those who have already had one have a 1 in 3 chance of an encore. In some women, a UTI is "silent" (without symptoms) and diagnosed only after a routine urine culture. In others, symptoms can range from mild to quite uncomfortable (an urge to urinate frequently, pain or a burning sensation when urine—sometimes only a drop or two—is passed, pressure or sharp pain in the lower abdominal area). The urine may also be foul smelling and cloudy.

Diagnosing a UTI is as simple as dipping an indicator stick into a urine sample at your practitioner's office; the stick will react to red or white blood cells in the sample. Red blood cells indicate bleeding in the urinary tract; white cells indicate a likely infection. Treating a UTI is as simple as taking a full course of prescribed antibiotics specifically aimed at the type of bacteria found when a lab analyzed that urine sample. (Don't hesitate to take them—your practitioner will prescribe one of the many antibiotics that are safe for use during pregnancy.)

Of course, your best bet is to prevent a UTI in the first place. There are a number of steps you can take to reduce your chances of developing one during your pregnancy (or, in conjunction with medical treatment, help speed recovery when infection occurs):

- Drink plenty of fluids, especially water, which can help flush out any bacteria. Cranberry juice may also be beneficial, possibly because the tannins it contains keep bacteria from sticking to the walls of the urinary tract. Avoid coffee and tea (even decaffeinated varieties) and alcohol, which may increase risk of irritation.

- Wash your vaginal area well and empty your bladder just before and after sex.

- Every time you urinate, take the time to empty your bladder thoroughly. Leaning forward on the toilet will help accomplish this. It sometimes also helps to "double void": After you pee, wait five minutes, then try to pee again. And don't put off the urge when you have it; regularly "holding it in" increases susceptibility to infection.

- To give your perineal area breathing room, wear cotton-crotch underwear and panty hose, avoid wearing tight pants, don't wear panty hose under pants, and sleep without panties or pajama bottoms on if possible (and comfortable).

- Keep your vaginal and perineal areas meticulously clean and irritation free. Wipe front to back after using the toilet to keep fecal bacteria from entering your vagina or urethra (the short tube through which urine is excreted from the bladder). Wash daily (showers are better than baths), and avoid bubble bath and perfumed products—powders, shower gels, soaps, sprays, detergents, and toilet paper. Also, stay out of pools that aren't properly chlorinated.

- Some practitioners recommend eating yogurt that contains active cultures or taking probiotics while you're on antibiotics to help restore the balance of beneficial bacteria. Ask your practitioner; some probiotics are definitely more potent than others.

- Keep your resistance high by eating a nutritious diet, getting enough rest and exercise, and not letting your life get too stressful.

UTIs in the lower part of the urinary tract are no fun, but a more serious potential threat is that bacteria from an untreated UTI will travel up to your kidneys. Kidney infections that aren't treated can be quite dangerous and may lead to premature labor, low-birthweight babies, and more problems. The symptoms are the same as those of UTIs but are frequently accompanied by fever (often as high as 103°F), chills, blood in the urine, backache (in the midback on one or both sides), nausea, and vomiting. Should you experience these symptoms, notify your practitioner immediately so you can be treated promptly.

Yeast Infection

"I think I have a yeast infection. Should I go get some of the medication I usually use, or do I need to see the doctor?"

Pregnancy is never a time for self-diagnosis or treatment—not even when it comes to something as seemingly simple as a yeast infection. Even if you've had yeast infections a hundred

Bacterial Vaginosis

Bacterial vaginosis (BV) is the most common vaginal condition in women of childbearing age, affecting up to 16 percent of pregnant women. A BV condition, which occurs when certain types of bacteria normally found in the vagina begin to multiply in large numbers, is often accompanied by an abnormal gray or white vaginal discharge with a strong fishlike odor, pain, itching, or burning (though some women with BV report no signs or symptoms at all). Doctors are not exactly sure what causes the normal balance of bacteria in the vagina to be disrupted, though some risk factors have been identified, including having multiple sex partners, douching, or using an IUD. BV is not transmitted during sexual contact but is associated with sexual activity (women who have never had sexual intercourse are rarely affected).

During pregnancy, BV is associated with a slight increase in such complications as premature rupture of the membranes and amniotic fluid infection, which may lead to premature labor. It may also be associated with miscarriage and low birthweight. Some doctors test for BV in women who are at high risk for preterm delivery, but no clear evidence indicates that treating such high-risk women reduces the incidence of prematurity. That said, treating symptomatic BV with antibiotics is effective at relieving symptoms. Some research has also suggested that treatment may reduce the complications associated with preterm births triggered by BV and may decrease the number of days these babies spend in the NICU.

times before, even if you know the symptoms backward and forward (a yellowish, greenish, or thick and cheesy discharge that has a foul odor, accompanied by burning, itching, redness, or soreness), even if you've treated yourself successfully with over-the-counter preparations in the past—this time around, call your practitioner.

How you will be treated will depend on what kind of infection you have, something only your practitioner can determine via lab tests. If it does turn out to be a yeast infection, which is very common in pregnancy, your practitioner may prescribe vaginal suppositories, gels, ointments, or creams. The oral anti-yeast agent fluconazole (Diflucan) may also be prescribed during pregnancy, but only in low doses and for no longer than two days.

Unfortunately, medication may banish a yeast infection only temporarily; the infection often returns off and on until after delivery and may require repeated treatment.

You may be able to speed your recovery and prevent reinfection by keeping your genital area clean and dry. Do this by practicing meticulous hygiene, especially after going to the bathroom (always wipe from front to back); rinsing your vaginal area thoroughly after soaping during a bath or shower; skipping irritating or perfumed soaps, and bubble baths; wearing cotton underwear; and avoiding tight pants or leggings (especially those that aren't cotton). In general, let the area breathe whenever you can (sleeping without underwear, if possible).

Eating yogurt containing live probiotic cultures may help keep those yeast bugs at bay. You can also ask your practitioner about using an effective probiotic supplement (many on the market aren't effective). Some chronic yeast infection sufferers find that cutting down on the sugar and baked goods made with refined flour helps, too. Do not douche, because it upsets the normal balance of bacteria in the vagina.

Stomach Bugs

"I've got a stomach bug, and I can't keep anything down. Will this hurt my baby?"

Just when you thought it was safe to come out of the bathroom, you're back with a bug (good-bye morning sickness, hello stomach flu). And if you're still in your first trimester when the bug hits, it could be hard to differentiate the symptoms from those of morning sickness.

Luckily, having a stomach virus won't hurt your fetus, even while it's hurting your stomach. But just because the virus isn't bugging baby doesn't mean it shouldn't be treated. And whether your tummy is turning from hormones, a virus, or from egg salad that sat on the lunch cart too long, the treatment is the same: Get the rest your body's aching for, and focus on fluids, especially if you're losing them through vomiting or diarrhea. They're much more important in the short term than solids.

If you're not urinating frequently enough or your urine is dark (it should be straw-colored), you may be dehydrated. Fluid needs to be your best buddy now: Try taking frequent small sips of water, diluted juice (white grape is easiest on the tummy), clear broth, weak decaffeinated tea, or hot water with lemon. If you can't manage to sip, suck on ice chips or a Popsicle. Follow your stomach's lead when it comes to adding solids—and when you do, keep it bland, simple, and fat-free (white rice or dry toast, low-fiber cereal, applesauce, bananas). And don't

forget that ginger's good for what ails any sick stomach. Take it in tea or in flat ginger ale (best if there's actually ginger in it) or another ginger beverage, or suck or chew on some ginger candies. Remember, too, to supplement when you can. Getting your vitamin insurance is an especially good idea now, so try to take your supplement when it's least likely to come back up. Don't worry, however, if you can't manage to keep it down for a few days or so; no harm done.

If you can't get anything down, talk to your practitioner. Dehydration is a problem for anyone suffering with a stomach bug, but it's especially problematic when you need to stay hydrated for two. You might be advised to take some rehydration fluid (like Pedialyte, which also comes in a soothing freezable form).

Check with your practitioner before you open up your medicine cabinet looking for relief. Antacids like Tums and Rolaids are considered safe to take during pregnancy, and some practitioners may okay gas relievers, but be sure to ask first. Your practitioner may also say you can take certain antidiarrheal medicines, but probably only after your first trimester is safely behind you (see page 511). As always, check with your practitioner before taking anything, just to play it safe.

And sick tummies, take heart: Most stomach bugs clear up by themselves within a day or so.

Listeriosis

"A friend who is pregnant said to stay away from certain dairy products because they can make you sick when you're expecting. Is this true?"

More bad news for adventurous eaters. Unpasteurized milk and cheeses made from unpasteurized milk (including some mozzarella, blue cheese,

Mexican cheeses, Brie, Camembert, and feta) can sometimes make you sick, and that extremely unlikely possibility becomes slightly more likely when you're expecting. These foods, along with unpasteurized juices, raw or undercooked meat, fish and shellfish, poultry, eggs, unwashed raw vegetables, and hot dogs and deli meats, can very occasionally contain Listeria. These bacteria can cause serious illness (listeriosis), especially in high-risk individuals, including young children, the elderly, those with compromised immune systems, and pregnant women, whose immune systems are also somewhat suppressed. Though the overall risk of contracting listeriosis is extremely low—even in pregnancy—the potential of its causing problems in pregnancy is higher. Listeria, unlike many other germs, enters the bloodstream directly and therefore can get to the baby quickly through the placenta (other food contaminants generally stay in the digestive tract and may only pose a threat if they get into the amniotic fluid).

Listeriosis is hard to detect—partly because symptoms can appear anytime between 12 hours and 30 days after contaminated food is eaten, and partly because the symptoms (headache, fever, fatigue, muscle aches, and occasionally nausea and diarrhea) are similar to those of flu, and some can even be mistaken for pregnancy side effects. Antibiotics are needed to treat and cure listeriosis. Untreated, the illness can cause serious complications for mom and baby.

So, clearly, it's important to prevent infection in the first place by staying away from the risky foods that might possibly carry Listeria, especially now, even if it means that your taco salad comes without the fresh queso. See page 116 for more tips on food safety and the prevention of food-borne diseases. Keep in mind, though, that the risk of contracting the infection from day-to-day eating is extremely low, even among expectant diners, so don't stress about the queso you've sprinkled or the smoked turkey you've gobbled up until now.

Toxoplasmosis

"Though I've given all the cat-care chores over to my husband, just the very fact that I live with cats makes me nervous about toxoplasmosis. How would I know if I came down with it?"

Chances are you wouldn't. Most people who are infected show no symptoms at all, though some do notice mild malaise, slight fever, and swollen glands two or three weeks after exposure, followed by a rash a day or two later.

But chances are, too, that you wouldn't come down with the disease in the first place. If you've lived with cats for a long time, it's very likely that you've already become infected and have developed antibodies to the virus that causes toxoplasmosis.

If you turn out not to be immune, and you do experience the symptoms of toxoplasmosis, you'll probably be tested. (Don't try to test yourself, however, since home tests for toxoplasmosis are highly unreliable.) In the unlikely event that the test comes back positive, you'll probably be treated with antibiotics to reduce the risk of transmitting the infection to your baby.

There is little risk to an expectant mother from toxoplasmosis, and the risk of a fetus becoming infected if mom has contracted the infection and is untreated is only about 15 percent. The earlier in pregnancy a mother is infected, the less likely the illness will be transmitted to her baby but the more serious the consequences will be. The later in the pregnancy, the greater the transmission rate but the less severe the potential consequences. Fortunately, the number of pregnant women who contract toxoplasmosis is small to begin with, and only 1 in 10,000 babies is born with severe congenital toxoplasmosis.

Recent advances have made it possible to test fetal blood and/or amniotic fluid and the fetus's liver via ultrasound to learn whether or not the fetus has actually become infected, though not usually before 20 to 22 weeks. If no infection is detected, the fetus is most likely fine.

The best "treatment" of toxoplasmosis, however, is prevention. See page 79 for tips on how to avoid infection.

Cytomegalovirus

"My son came home from preschool with a note saying that there's an outbreak of CMV at his school. Is this something I should worry about catching during pregnancy?"

Luckily, the chances of picking up cytomegalovirus (CMV) from your son and passing it on to your baby are remote. Why's that? A majority of adults were infected in childhood, and if you're among that majority, you can't "catch" CMV now (though it could become "reactivated"). Even if you did come down with a new CMV infection during pregnancy, the risks to your baby are low. Though half of infected moms give birth to infected infants, only a tiny percentage of them ever show any ill effects. The risks are lower still in a baby whose mom had a reactivated infection during pregnancy.

Still, unless you know for sure that you're immune to CMV because you had the infection before, your best defense is a good offense. Take preventative measures such as washing up carefully after changing your son's diapers or helping him out at the potty, and resist nibbling on your preschooler's leftovers. (And if you work in a child-care or preschool setting, always practice good hygiene protocol.)

Though CMV often comes and goes without any obvious symptoms, it's occasionally marked by fever, fatigue, swollen glands, and sore throat. If you notice any of these symptoms, check with your doctor. Whether these symptoms signal CMV or another illness (such as flu or strep throat), you'll need some sort of treatment.

Fifth Disease

"I was told that a disease I had never even heard of before—fifth disease—could cause problems in pregnancy."

Fifth disease is the fifth of a group of six diseases that cause fever and rash in children. But unlike its sister diseases (such as measles and chicken pox, the ones that get all the attention), fifth disease isn't widely known because its symptoms are mild and can go unnoticed—or may even be totally absent. Fever is present in only 15 to 30 percent of cases. For the first few days, the rash gives the cheeks the appearance of having been slapped, then spreads in a lacy pattern to trunk, buttocks, and thighs, recurring on and off (usually in response to heat from the sun or a warm bath) for one to three weeks. It is often confused with the rash of rubella and other childhood illnesses or even a sun- or windburn.

Concentrated exposure from caring for a child sick with fifth disease or from teaching at a school where it is epidemic somewhat increases that very small risk of contracting the illness. But half of all women of childbearing age had fifth disease during childhood and are already immune, so infection, happily, isn't common among pregnant women. In the unlikely event that a mom catches fifth disease and her fetus does become infected, the virus can disrupt the developing baby's ability to produce red blood cells, leading to a form of anemia or other complications. If you do contract fifth disease, your practitioner will follow you for signs of fetal anemia with weekly ultrasounds for eight to ten weeks. If the baby is infected during the first half of pregnancy, the risk of miscarriage increases.

Again, the odds that fifth disease will affect you, your pregnancy, or your baby are very remote. Still, as always, it makes sense to take the appropriate steps to avoid any infection while you're expecting (see opposite page).

Measles

"I can't remember if I was vaccinated against measles when I was a child. Should I be immunized now?"

No. Measles vaccine (a component of the MMR vaccine) isn't given during pregnancy because of the theoretical risk to the fetus from the vaccine, though there have been no reports of problems among newborns whose mothers were inadvertently vaccinated. Besides, the chances are good that you are already immune to measles, since most women of childbearing age either had the disease or were vaccinated against it as children. If your medical history doesn't include this information and your parents can't recall it, your doctor can run a test to determine whether you are immune. Even if you're not immune, the risk that you might contract measles is extremely remote because the disease has been practically wiped out in the United States (which means it would be highly unlikely that you'd be able to catch it here).

In the exceedingly unlikely event that you are exposed directly to someone with measles and are not immune, your doctor may administer gamma globulin (antibodies) during the incubation period—between exposure and the start of symptoms—to decrease the severity of the illness should you come down with it. Measles, unlike rubella, does not appear to cause birth defects, though it may be linked to an increased risk of miscarriage or premature labor. If you were to contract measles near your due date, there is a risk that your newborn might catch the infection from you. Again, gamma globulin may be administered to reduce the severity of such an infection. Keep in mind that all this is pretty much theoretical, given how rare measles are these days.

Mumps

"A coworker of mine came down with a bad case of the mumps. Should I get immunized so I don't get it myself?"

It's not that easy to get mumps these days—in fact, it's pretty close to impossible. Fewer than 250 Americans contract mumps each year, thanks to routine childhood immunization with MMR (measles, mumps, rubella). And chances are you were vaccinated, too, when you were a child (or, less likely, that you actually had the disease), which means you can't catch it now. If you're not sure whether you were immunized against or had mumps, check with your parents or the doctor who cared for you as a child, if that's possible.

If it turns out you're not immune, you can't be immunized now because the vaccine might be harmful to your fetus. Even without immunity, though, the risk of contracting mumps is very low. It isn't highly contagious through casual contact. However, because the disease appears to

Staying Well

In pregnancy, when you need to stay well for two, the proverbial ounce of prevention is worth far more than a pound of cure. The following suggestions will increase your chances of staying well when you're expecting (and when you're not):

Keep your resistance up. Eat the best diet possible, get enough sleep and exercise, and don't run yourself down by running yourself ragged. Reducing stress in your life as much as you can also helps keep your immune system in tip-top shape.

Avoid sick people like the plague. As best as you can, try to stay away from anyone who has a cold, flu, stomach virus, or anything else noticeably contagious. Keep your distance from coughers on the bus, avoid lunching with a colleague who's complaining of a sore throat, and evade the handshake of a friend with a runny nose (germs as well as greetings can be exchanged in a handshake). Also avoid crowded or cramped indoor spaces when you can.

Wash your hands. Hands are the major spreader of infections, so wash them often and thoroughly with soap and warm water (about 20 seconds does the trick), particularly after exposure to someone you know is sick and after spending time in public places or riding on public transportation. Hand washing is especially important before eating. Keep a hand sanitizer in your glove compartment, in your desk drawer, and in your handbag or briefcase so you can wash up when there's no sink in sight.

Don't share the germs. At home, try to limit germ-spreading contact with sick children or a sick spouse as much as possible. Avoiding finishing up their sandwich scraps and drinking from their cups. And while every sick child needs a dose of kiss-and-hug therapy from mom now and then, be sure to wash your hands and face after those comforting cuddles. Wash your hands, too, after touching their germy sheets, towels, and used tissues, especially before touching your own eyes, nose, and mouth. See that the little patients wash their hands frequently, too, and try to get them to cough and sneeze into their elbows instead of their hands (a good tip for adults, too). Use disinfectant spray or wipes on telephones, computer keyboards, remotes, and other surfaces they handle.

If your own child or a child you regularly spend time with develops a rash of any kind, avoid close contact and call your doctor as soon as you can unless you already know that you are immune to chicken pox, fifth disease, and CMV.

Be pet smart. Keep pets in good health, updating their immunizations as necessary. If you have a cat, take the precautions to avoid toxoplasmosis (page 79).

Look out for Lyme. Avoid outdoor areas where Lyme disease is prevalent, or be sure to protect yourself adequately (see page 507).

To each his or her own. Maintain a no-sharing policy when it comes to toothbrushes and other personal items (and don't let those toothbrushes mingle bristle-to-bristle). Use disposable cups for rinsing in the bathroom.

Eat safe. To avoid food-borne illnesses, practice safe food preparation and storage habits (see page 116).

trigger uterine contractions and is associated with an increased risk of miscarriage in the first trimester or preterm labor later, be alert for the first symptoms of the disease (possibly vague pain, fever, and loss of appetite before the salivary glands become swollen; then ear pain and pain on chewing or on taking acidic or sour food or drink). Notify your practitioner of such symptoms immediately because prompt treatment can reduce the chance of problems developing. You might also want to consider the MMR vaccine before deciding to get pregnant again, just to be on the safe side.

Rubella

"I might have been exposed to rubella on a trip out of the country. Should I be worried?"

Happily, the vast majority of pregnant women in the United States are immune to rubella (German measles), either because they were immunized against it as a child (it's the "R" in the MMR vaccine) or contracted it at some other time in their lives (usually during childhood). In fact, the CDC considers rubella to be eradicated here, so the odds are good that you can't catch it and, consequently, have nothing to worry about. If you're not sure whether or not you are immune (around 25 percent of women may not be immune because they were born outside the United States), you can find out with a simple test—a rubella antibody titer—that measures the level of antibodies to the virus in your blood and is performed routinely at the first prenatal visit by most practitioners. If this test was not performed earlier, it should be now.

In the unlikely event you turn out not to be immune (or if the antibody levels in your blood are low), you still don't have to consider drastic measures imme-

diately. For the virus to do its damage, you have to actually come down with the illness. The symptoms, which show up two or three weeks after exposure, are usually mild (malaise, slight fever, and swollen glands, followed by a slight rash a day or two later) and may sometimes pass unnoticed. If you did come down with rubella during pregnancy (and, again, the odds are extremely remote), whether your baby would be at risk would depend on when you contracted it. During the first month, the chance of a baby developing a serious birth defect from in utero exposure is pretty high. By the third month, the risk is significantly lower. After that, the risk is lower still.

There is no way of absolutely preventing an exposed woman with no immunity from coming down with rubella—but because the chance of being exposed to rubella in the United States is almost nil, that scenario is just about never encountered. Still, if you aren't immune and don't contract the disease this time around, avoid the concern entirely in subsequent pregnancies by being vaccinated after this delivery. As a precaution, you will be advised not to become pregnant for one month following vaccination. But should you conceive accidentally during this time, or if you were vaccinated early in this pregnancy, before you knew you had conceived, don't worry. Apparently, there is no risk when an expectant woman is inadvertently vaccinated early in pregnancy or if she conceives soon after vaccination.

Chicken Pox (Varicella)

"My toddler was exposed to chicken pox at her child-care center—by a child who wasn't immunized. If she comes down with it, could the baby I'm now carrying be hurt?"

Not likely. Well insulated from the rest of the world, a fetus can't catch chicken pox from a third party—only from its mother. Which means you would have to catch it first, something that's unlikely. First of all, your child probably won't catch it and bring it home if she was immunized with the varicella vaccine. Second of all, it's very likely you had the infection as a child (85 to 95 percent of the U.S. adult population has had it) and are already immune. Ask your parents or check your health records to find out whether you have had chicken pox. If you can't find out for sure, ask your practitioner to run a test now to see if you are immune.

Though the chances of your becoming infected are slim if you aren't immune, an injection of varicella-zoster immune globulin (VZIG) within 96 hours of a documented personal exposure (in other words, direct contact with someone who has been diagnosed with chicken pox) may be recommended. It isn't clear whether or not this will protect the baby should you come down with chicken pox anyway, but it should minimize complications for you—a significant plus, since this mild childhood disease can be quite severe in adults. If you should be hit with a severe case, you may be given an antiviral drug to further reduce the risk of complications.

If you become infected during the first half of your pregnancy, the chances are very low (around 2 percent) that your baby could develop a condition called congenital varicella syndrome, which can cause some birth defects. If you come down with chicken pox later in your pregnancy, there's almost zero danger to the baby. The exception is if you get chicken pox just before (within a week of) giving birth or just after delivery. In that extremely unlikely scenario, there's a small chance your newborn will arrive infected and will develop the characteristic rash within a week or so. To prevent neonatal infection, your baby will be given an infusion of chicken pox antibodies immediately after delivery (or as soon as it becomes apparent that you've been infected postpartum).

Incidentally, shingles, or herpes zoster, which is a reactivation of the chicken pox virus in someone who had the disease earlier, does not appear to be harmful to a developing fetus, probably because the mother and thus the baby already have antibodies to the virus.

If you are not immune and escape infection this time, ask your doctor about getting immunized after delivery, to protect any future pregnancies. Immunization should take place at least a month before any new conception.

Lyme Disease

"I live in an area that's high risk for Lyme disease. Is Lyme dangerous when you're pregnant?"

Lyme disease is most common among those who spend time in woods frequented by deer, mice, or other animals carrying deer ticks, but it can also be picked up in forest-free cities via greenery brought from the country or purchased at a farmers' market.

The best way to protect your baby—as well as yourself—is by taking preventive measures. If you are out in woodsy or grassy areas, or if you are handling greenery grown in such areas, wear long pants, tucked into boots or socks, and long sleeves; use an insect repellent effective for deer ticks on your clothing. When you return home, check your skin carefully for ticks. If you find one, remove it right away by pulling straight up on it with tweezers; then drop it into a small bottle and have it tested by your doctor (removing a tick within 24 hours almost entirely eliminates the possibility of infection).

If you've been bitten by a tick, see your doctor immediately; a blood test may be able to determine whether you are infected with Lyme. (Early symptoms may include a blotchy bull's-eye rash at the bite site, fatigue, headache, stiff neck, fever and chills, generalized achiness, swollen glands near the site of the bite; later symptoms may include arthritis-like pain and memory loss.)

Fortunately, studies have shown that prompt treatment with antibiotics completely protects a baby whose mother is infected with Lyme—and keeps mom from becoming seriously ill.

Hepatitis A

"One of the toddlers in the child-care center where I work was just diagnosed as having hepatitis A. If I get it, could it affect my pregnancy?"

Hepatitis A is very common, almost always a mild disease (often with no noticeable symptoms), and rarely passed on to a fetus or newborn. So even if you did catch it, it shouldn't affect your pregnancy. Still, you're better off not contracting an infection of any kind in the first place. So take precautions: Be sure to wash your hands after changing diapers or taking your young charges to the bathroom (hepatitis A is passed by the fecal-oral route), and be sure to wash up well before eating. You might also want to ask your physician about immunization against hepatitis A.

Hepatitis B

"I'm a carrier of hepatitis B and just found out that I'm pregnant. Will my being a carrier hurt my baby?"

Knowing that you're a carrier for hepatitis B is the first step in making sure your condition won't hurt your baby. Because this liver infection can be passed on from mother to baby during delivery, prompt steps will be taken at your baby's birth to make sure that doesn't happen. Your newborn will be treated within 12 hours with both hepatitis B immune globulin (HBIG) and the hepatitis B vaccine (which is routine at birth anyway). This treatment can almost always prevent the infection from developing. Your baby will also be vaccinated at one or two months and then again at six months (this, too, is a routine part of the hepatitis B series), and may be tested at 12 to 15 months to be sure the therapy has been effective.

Hepatitis C

"Should I be worried about hepatitis C during pregnancy?"

Hepatitis C can be transmitted from infected mother to child during delivery, with a transmission rate of about 7 to 8 percent. But because hep C is usually transmitted via blood (for instance, through past transfusions or illegal drug injections), unless you've had a transfusion or are in a high-risk category, it's unlikely you'd be infected. The infection, if diagnosed, can potentially be treated, but not during pregnancy.

Bell's Palsy

"I woke up this morning with pain behind my ear, and my tongue felt numb. When I looked in the mirror, the whole side of my face looked droopy. What's going on?"

It sounds like you've got Bell's palsy, a temporary condition caused by damage to the facial nerve, resulting in weakness or paralysis on one side of the face. Bell's palsy strikes pregnant women three times more often than it does women who are not pregnant (though it's quite uncommon in general) and most often occurs in the third trimester or in the early postpartum period. Its onset is sudden, and most people with the condition—like you— wake up without warning to find their face drooping.

The cause of this temporary facial paralysis is unknown, though experts suspect that certain viral or bacterial infections may cause swelling and inflammation of the facial nerve, triggering the condition. Other symptoms sometimes accompanying the paralysis include pain behind the ear or in the back of the head, dizziness, drooling (because of the weak muscles), dry mouth, inability to blink, impaired sense of taste and tongue numbness, even impaired speaking in some cases.

The good news is that Bell's palsy will not spread beyond your face and won't get worse. More good news: Most cases completely resolve within three weeks to three months without treatment (though for some it can take as long as six months to completely go away). And the best news of all: The condition poses no threat to to your pregnancy or your baby. Though you should definitely put a call in to your practitioner, chances are treatment won't be necessary.

Medications During Pregnancy

Open any prescription or over-the-counter drug insert and read the fine print. Virtually all will warn against pregnant women using medications without a doctor's advice. Still, if you're like the average expectant mom, you'll wind up taking at least one prescription drug during your pregnancy and even more over-the-counter medications. How will you know which are safe and which aren't?

No drug—prescription or over-the-counter, traditional or herbal—is 100 percent safe for 100 percent of the people, 100 percent of the time. And when you're pregnant, there's the health and well-being of two people, one very small and vulnerable, to consider every time you take a drug. Happily, only a few drugs are known to be harmful to a developing fetus, and many drugs can be used safely during pregnancy. In fact, in certain situations, using a medication during pregnancy is absolutely necessary.

It's always wise to weigh the potential risks of taking a medication against the potential benefits it will provide, but never more so than during pregnancy. Involving your practitioner in the decision of whether or not to take a drug is a good idea in general, but when you're pregnant, it's essential. So check with your practitioner before taking any medication while you're expecting, even an over-the-counter drug you've used routinely in the past.

One of the tools your practitioner will use to determine the safety of a particular medication is the five-letter rating (A, B, C, D, or X) set up by the Food and Drug Administration to determine whether a drug poses a risk to a fetus. Categories A and B drugs are thought to be generally safe, with those in the A category having undergone controlled studies that showed no risk to the fetus, and those in the B category shown to have no risk to animals or no risk to humans even if animal studies showed an adverse effect. Category C means that the data is inconclusive. The other categories (D and X) are given to drugs that have a demonstrated risk to the fetus (though in some rare life-threatening cases, doctors may prescribe a Category D drug because the risk to the mother—if she doesn't take the drug—is too great). Still, this system is far from perfect since the FDA doesn't require drug manufacturers to conduct long-term studies on pregnant women, for obvious reasons.

Still confused about the ABCs of medications during pregnancy? Here's the bottom line: Never take any drug—prescription, over-the-counter, or herbal—without talking to your doctor or midwife first.

Common Medications

A number of medications are considered safe for pregnant women to take, and these medications can be a welcome relief if you're down and out with a stuffy nose or a pounding headache. Other medications are not recommended in most cases—though in certain cases they may be okayed, such as after the first trimester or for a specific problem. And many medications are completely off-limits when you're expecting. Here's the lowdown on some of the more common medications you may come across during pregnancy:

Tylenol. Acetaminophen is usually given the green light for short-term use during pregnancy, but be sure to ask your practitioner for the proper dosage before taking it for the first time.

Aspirin. Your practitioner will probably advise that you not take aspirin—especially during the third trimester, since it increases the risk for potential problems for the newborn, as well as complications before and during delivery, such as excessive bleeding. Some studies suggest that very low dosages of aspirin may help to prevent preeclampsia in certain circumstances, but only your practitioner will be able to tell you whether it should be prescribed in your case. Other studies suggest that low-dose aspirin, in combination with the blood-thinning medication heparin, may reduce the incidence of recurrent miscarriage in some women with a condition known as antiphospholipid antibody syndrome. Again, only your practitioner can let you know if these medications are safe for you and under what circumstances.

Advil or Motrin. Ibuprofen should be used with caution in pregnancy, especially during the first and third trimesters, when it can have the same negative effects as aspirin. Use it only if it's specifically recommended by a physician who knows you are pregnant.

Aleve. Naproxen, a nonsteroidal anti-inflammatory drug (NSAID), is not recommended for use in pregnancy at all.

Nasal sprays. For short-term relief from a stuffy nose, most nasal sprays are fine to use. Check with your practitioner for his or her preferred brand and dosing suggestions. Saline sprays are always safe to use, as are nasal strips.

Antacids. Heartburn that won't quit (you'll have plenty of that) often responds to Tums or Rolaids (plus you'll get a dose of calcium to boot). But check with your practitioner for the right dosage.

Gas aids. Many practitioners will okay gas aids, such as Gas-X, for the occasional relief of pregnancy bloat, but check with yours first.

Antihistamines. Not all antihistamines are safe during pregnancy, but several will probably get the green light from your practitioner. Benadryl is the most commonly recommended antihistamine during pregnancy. Claritin is also considered safe, but check with your practitioner, because not all will give it the okay, particularly in the first trimester. Many practitioners allow the use of chlorpheniramine (Chlor-Trimeton) and triprolidine on a limited basis.

Sleep aids. Unisom, Tylenol PM, Sominex, Nytol, Ambien, and Lunesta are generally considered safe during pregnancy, and they are okayed by many practitioners for occasional use. Always check with your practitioner before taking these or any sleep aids.

Decongestants. Sudafed is considered the safest oral decongestant if you must use one during pregnancy, as long as it's used in a limited amount. Be sure to check with your practitioner first and to get the right dosage information.

Antidiarrheals. Kaopectate is considered safe for use during pregnancy in limited amounts and for a limited time period, but ask your practitioner first to be sure (most will advise waiting until after the first trimester). Pepto-Bismol (and other salicylates) should probably not be used during pregnancy.

Antibiotics. If your doctor has prescribed antibiotics for you during pregnancy, it's because the bacterial infection you have is more dangerous than taking the antibiotics to fight it off (many are considered completely safe). You'll usually be put on antibiotics that fall into the penicillin or erythromycin families. Certain antibiotics are not recommended (such as tetracyclines), so be

> ## Keeping Current
>
> The many lists of safe, possibly safe, possibly unsafe, and definitely unsafe drugs and medication during pregnancy change all the time, especially as new medications are introduced, others change from being prescription-only to over-the-counter, and still others are being studied to determine their safety during pregnancy. To stay current on what is or isn't safe, always ask your practitioner first. You can also turn to the U.S. Food and Drug Administration (contact your regional office, or visit fda.gov) for information. Or try the local office of the March of Dimes, or contact the March of Dimes Resource Center at (888) MODIMES (663-4637); marchofdimes.com. You can also go to safefetus.com to check on the safety of a certain medication during pregnancy.

sure that any doctor prescribing antibiotics while you're expecting knows that you're pregnant.

Antidepressants. Untreated depression in an expectant mom can have many adverse effects on her baby. Though the research on the effects of antidepressants on pregnancy and on the fetus is ever changing, it does appear that there are several medications that are safe to use, others that should be completely avoided, and still others that can be considered on a case-by-case basis, their use weighed against the risk of untreated (or undertreated) depression. See page 518 for more on antidepressants.

Antinausea. Unisom Sleep Tabs (which contain the antihistamine doxylamine), taken in combination with vitamin B$_6$, decrease the symptoms of morning sickness but should only be used when recommended by your practitioner. The downside of taking this remedy during the day: sleepiness.

Topical antibiotics. Small amounts of topical antibiotics, such as bacitracin or Neosporin, are safe during pregnancy.

Topical steroids. Small amounts of topical hydrocortisones (such as Cortaid) are safe during pregnancy.

If You Need Medication During Pregnancy

If your practitioner recommends that you take a certain medication while you're expecting, follow these steps for increased benefit and reduced risk:

- Discuss with your practitioner the possibility of taking the medication in the smallest effective doses for the shortest possible time.

Herbal Cures

Herbal supplements and remedies make the most tempting of promises (better memory! sounder sleep! improved immunity!), especially when pregnancy leaves you with fewer self-medicating options open and your medicine cabinet at least partially closed. Would it really hurt to pop a couple of ginkgo biloba pills to give your brain cells a fighting chance of remembering to pay this month's electric bill? Or melatonin to guarantee that you'll sleep like a baby (even when it's a baby-to-be who's keeping you awake)? And what about an echinacea or two to fend off the germs after you were sneezed on (twice) at that afternoon meeting? After all, the bottles say "all-natural," and you did buy them at the health-food store (what could be healthier than that?).

Actually, it could hurt—particularly now that you're sharing those pills with a little someone else. "All-natural" doesn't make herbal preparations "all safe," and neither does a health-food-store pedigree. Herbal preparations are not tested or approved by the FDA and are not required to undergo clini-

cal trials, which means that their safety (or lack of) is unknown. Even herbs that you've heard could be helpful during pregnancy could be dangerous at different points during those nine months. For example, some herbs purported to help bring on labor can cause premature labor if taken before full term. And many herbs are downright dangerous if taken at any time during pregnancy (such as basil oil, black or blue cohosh, clove oil, comfrey, juniper, mistletoe, pennyroyal, sassafras, wild yam, and many others).

It's always smart to proceed with caution when you're self-medicating with herbals, but twice as smart when you're self-medicating for two. To play it safe, don't take any herbal preparation—even ones you used freely preconception—unless it's prescribed by your practitioner for use during pregnancy.

If you'd like to feel like a natural woman during your pregnancy, look into other natural therapies that do not include ingesting anything (such as CAM treatments like acupuncture, massage, and meditation).

- Take the medication when it's going to benefit you the most—a cold medication at night, for instance, so it will help you sleep.

- Follow directions carefully. Some medications must be taken on an empty stomach; some should be taken with food or milk. If your physician hasn't given you any instructions, ask your pharmacist for particulars—most provide handouts with full directions and information (including possible side effects) on each prescription drug they sell. Don't panic if you see that the drug isn't recommended during pregnancy—the vast majority of drugs carry that warning, even if they're considered safe. As long as a practitioner who knows that you're expecting and is familiar with pregnancy drug safety has prescribed or recommended it, it's okay to take it.

- Explore nondrug remedies, and use them, as appropriate, to supplement the drug therapy. For instance, eliminate as many offending allergens from your home as you can, so your physician can reduce the amount of prescribed antihistamines you take. Keep in mind that herbal remedies are still considered drugs and shouldn't be taken without a practitioner's approval.

- Make sure the medication gets where it's supposed to by taking a sip of water before you swallow a capsule or tablet, to make it go down more easily, and by drinking a full glass afterward, to ensure that it is washed speedily down to where it will be absorbed.

- For additional safety, try to get all your prescriptions at the same pharmacy. The pharmacist will have you and all your prescriptions on the computer and should be able to warn you of potential drug interactions. Also, be sure you've gotten the right prescription (or over-the-counter medication). Check the name and dosage on the bottle to be sure it's the one specified by your doctor (many drug names and patient names are similar, and pharmacies do occasionally make mistakes). For additional reassurance, ask the pharmacist what the drug is meant to treat or check out the printed material that comes with the drug. If you know you were supposed to get an antihistamine for your allergies and the drug you are handed is for hypertension, you've obviously got the wrong medication.

- Ask about possible side effects and which ones should be reported to your doctor.

Once you've made certain that a prescribed drug is considered safe for use during pregnancy, don't hesitate to take it because you're still afraid it might somehow harm your baby. It won't, but delaying treatment might.

CHAPTER 21

If You Have a Chronic Condition

ANYONE WHO'S LIVED WITH A chronic condition knows that life can get pretty complicated, what with special diets, medications, and/or monitoring. Add pregnancy into the mix, and you've got your hands even fuller, with the special diet needing to be tweaked, medications modified, and monitoring stepped up. Happily, with some extra precautions and extra effort, most chronic conditions are now completely compatible with pregnancy.

Just how your chronic condition will be affected by pregnancy and how pregnancy will affect your chronic condition will depend on plenty of factors, many of them uniquely yours. This chapter outlines general recommendations for pregnant women with common chronic conditions. Use this alphabetized list as a guide, but be sure to follow your doctor's orders, since they've probably been tailored to your specific needs.

What You May Be Wondering About

Asthma

"I've had asthma since I was a child. I'm concerned that the attacks and the medication I take for them might be harmful now that I'm expecting."

Finding out you're pregnant can take any woman's breath away—but when you're asthmatic, being breathless and pregnant can understandably bring up some extra concerns. While it's true that a severe asthmatic condition does put a pregnancy at somewhat higher risk, fortunately, this risk can be almost completely eliminated. In fact, if you're under close, expert medical supervision—by a team that includes your obstetrician, your internist, and/or your asthma doctor—your chances of having a normal pregnancy and a healthy baby are about as good as a nonasthmatic's (which means you can breathe a little easier now).

Though well-controlled asthma has only a minimal effect on pregnancy, pregnancy can have an effect on asthma, but the effect varies from expectant mom to expectant mom. For about a third of pregnant asthmatics, the effect is positive: Their asthma improves. For another third, their condition stays about the same. For the remaining third (usually those with the most severe disease), the asthma worsens. If you've been pregnant before, you're likely to find that your asthma behaves pretty much the same way in this pregnancy as it did in earlier ones.

It's not surprising that getting your asthma under control before you conceive or as early in pregnancy as possible is the best strategy for you and your baby. The following steps will help you do that, if you haven't yet:

- Identify environmental triggers. Allergies are a major cause of asthma, and you probably already know which ones trigger problems for you. Avoid them, and you'll find the breathing a lot easier during your pregnancy (see page 205 for tips on avoiding allergens). Common offenders are pollen, animal dander, dust, and mold. Such irritants as tobacco smoke, household cleaning products, and perfumes can also provoke a reaction, so it's a good idea to steer clear of them (and, of course, you should quit smoking if you're a smoker—ditto for your

spouse). If you were started on allergy shots before pregnancy, you'll be able to continue.

- Exercise with care. If your asthma is exercise-induced, prescribed medication taken before your workout or any other kind of exertion can usually prevent an attack. Talk to your practitioner about other exercise guidelines.

- Stay healthy. Try to avoid colds, flu, and other respiratory infections, which are also asthma triggers (for tips on staying well, see box, page 505). Your doctor may give you medication to ward off an asthma attack at the beginning of a cold, and will probably want to treat any but the most minor bacterial respiratory infections with antibiotics. A flu shot—recommended for every expectant mom—is especially important for you, as is a vaccine for pneumococcal infection, if you're considered high risk (ask your doctor). If you suffer from chronic sinusitis or reflux—both of which are more common in pregnancy anyway—be sure to ask your doctor for a treatment plan, because both conditions can interfere with the management of your asthma.

- Keep a close eye on your peak flow. Follow your doctor's directions to make sure you're getting the oxygen you and your baby need. Monitor your breathing with a peak-flow meter, according to your physician's directions.

- Take a fresh look at your meds. All the medication rules change when you're expecting, so be sure you use only those that your physician has prescribed during your pregnancy. If your symptoms are mild, you may be able to get away without any medication. If they're moderate to severe, you'll be given one of the several medications that are considered safe during pregnancy (in general, inhaled medications appear to be safer than oral medication). Don't hesitate to take medication that you need—remember, you're breathing for two now.

If you do have an asthma attack, treating it promptly with your prescribed medication will help ensure that your baby isn't shortchanged of oxygen. But if the medication doesn't help, call your doctor or head for the nearest emergency room immediately. Asthma attacks may trigger early uterine contractions, but the contractions usually stop when the attack does (which is why it's so important to stop it quickly).

Because of your breathing problems history, you may find the breathlessness that typically comes with late pregnancy especially concerning. But don't worry—it's normal, and it isn't dangerous. Keep in mind, though, that as your growing uterus begins to crowd your lungs, you may notice that your asthmatic flare-ups worsen. Just be sure you treat these attacks quickly.

How will asthma affect your labor and delivery? If you're considering going without medication, you'll be happy to hear that asthma usually doesn't interfere with the breathing techniques of Lamaze and other childbirth education methods. If it's an epidural you have your heart set on, that shouldn't be a problem either (but narcotic analgesics, such as Demerol, will probably be avoided because they may trigger an asthma attack). Though asthma flare-ups during childbirth are rare, your doctor will probably recommend that you continue your regular medications when you're in labor; if

Cancer in Pregnancy

Cancer isn't common during pregnancy, but it happens, just as it can happen during any other time of life. Pregnancy doesn't cause cancer or increase your chances of developing cancer. They're just two life events, one joyous and one challenging, that sometimes take place at the same time.

Treatment for cancer during pregnancy is a delicate balancing act between providing the best treatment for the mother and limiting any possible risk to the fetus. The type of treatment you'll get will depend on many factors: how far the pregnancy has progressed; the type of cancer; the stage of the cancer; and, of course, on your wishes. The decisions you may face in balancing your well-being against your baby's may be emotionally wrenching,

and you'll need plenty of support in making them.

Because some cancer treatments can harm the fetus, especially during the first trimester, doctors usually delay any treatment until the second or third trimesters. When cancer is diagnosed later in pregnancy, doctors may wait until after the baby is born to begin treatment, or they may consider inducing labor early. The reassuring news is that women diagnosed during pregnancy respond just as well to cancer treatment as women who are not pregnant, all other factors being equal.

For more help, contact the National Cancer Institute: cancer.gov, as well as pregnantwithcancer.org or (800) 743-4471, a support system for expectant women with cancer.

your asthma has been serious enough to require oral steroids or cortisone-type medications, you may also require IV steroids to help you handle the stress of labor and delivery. Your oxygenation will be checked when you are admitted to the hospital, and if it is low, preventive medications may be given. Though some babies of moms with asthma experience rapid breathing after delivery, that's usually only temporary.

As for your asthma postpartum, chances are you'll find your symptoms will return to the way they were pre-pregnancy within three months after delivery.

Cystic Fibrosis

"I have cystic fibrosis, and I know that makes pregnancy complicated—but how complicated?"

As someone who's lived with cystic fibrosis (CF) for her whole life, you're already used to the challenges that the condition comes with—but you're also used to working hard at overcoming them. And though the challenges do increase somewhat with pregnancy, there are plenty of things that you and your doctors can do to help make your pregnancy safe and successful.

The first challenge may be gaining enough weight, so working closely with your doctors to ensure that the numbers on the scale keep climbing will be important (a nutritionist may be a helpful addition to your pregnancy team). To keep a closer eye on your weight and your baby's growth—as well as on all aspects of your pregnancy—you'll have more frequent prenatal visits than the average mom-to-be (on the plus side, that means more chances to hear your baby's heartbeat—and more opportunities to ask questions). Your activity

may be limited, and because you'll be at higher risk for premature delivery, additional precautions will be taken to reduce the risk and help ensure that your baby stays safely put until term. It's also possible that periodic hospitalization may be necessary.

Genetic counseling (if you haven't had it already) will be able to determine whether your baby is at risk for being born with CF or not ("not" being the much more likely scenario). If your spouse isn't a carrier for CF, there's very little chance that your baby will be affected by it (though he or she will be a carrier). If your spouse is a carrier, there's a 1 in 2 chance that your baby will be affected; prenatal testing can let you know for sure.

Since you're breathing for two now, your doctors will be keeping a close watch on your pulmonary care—especially as your growing uterus leaves less room for your lungs to expand. You'll also be monitored for pulmonary infection. Some women with severe lung disease may find that their condition can get a little worse while they're pregnant, but only temporarily. In general, pregnancy doesn't seem to have any negative long-term effect on CF at all.

Pregnancy isn't easy no matter what, and it's certainly more challenging for women with CF. But that cuddly reward—the beautiful baby you're working so hard for—can make all those challenges more than worthwhile.

Depression

"I was diagnosed with chronic depression a few years ago, and I've been on low-dose antidepressants ever since. Now that I'm pregnant, should I stop taking the meds?"

More than one out of ten women of childbearing age battles with bouts of depression, so you're far from alone. Luckily for you and all the other expectant moms who share your condition, there's a happy outlook: With the right treatment, women with depression can have perfectly normal pregnancies. Deciding what that treatment should consist of during pregnancy is a delicate balancing act, however, especially when it comes to the use of medications. Together with your psychiatrist and prenatal practitioner, you'll need to weigh the risks and benefits of taking such meds—and not taking them—while you're growing a baby.

Maybe it seems like a simple decision to make, at least at first glance. After all, could there ever be a good reason to put your emotional well-being over your baby's physical well-being? But the decision is actually a lot more complicated than that. For starters, pregnancy hormones can do a number on your emotional state. Even women who've never had an encounter with mood disorders, depression, or any other psychological condition may experience wild emotional swings when they're expecting—but women with a history of depression are at greater risk of having depressive bouts during pregnancy and are more likely to suffer from postpartum depression. And this is especially true for women who stop taking their antidepressants during pregnancy.

What's more, untreated depression isn't likely to affect only you (and those you're close to), it's also likely to affect your baby's health. Depressed mothers-to-be may not eat or sleep as well or pay as much attention to their prenatal care, and they may be more likely to drink and smoke. Any or all of those factors, combined with the debilitating effects of excessive anxiety and stress, have been linked in some studies to an increased risk of preterm birth, low birthweight, and a lower Apgar score for babies. Treating depression effectively, however—and keeping it under control during pregnancy—allows a mother-to-be to nurture her body and her developing baby.

So what does all this mean for you? It means you might want to think twice (and consult with your physician, of course) before you consider tossing your antidepressants. And in doing your thinking—and your consulting—you and your doctor will also want to consider which antidepressant best suits your needs now that you're expecting, which may or may not be the same one (or ones) you were using preconception. Certain meds are safer than others, and some aren't recommended for pregnancy use at all. Your doctor can give you the most up-to-date information, because it's ever-changing. What is known right now is that Wellbutrin is often a good choice during pregnancy. Prozac, Paxil, Zoloft, and other selective serotonin reuptake inhibitors (SSRIs) carry very little risk to the baby and can therefore also be good choices. Studies do show that pregnant women on Prozac might be somewhat more likely to deliver prematurely, and newborns exposed to Prozac and other SSRIs in the womb may experience short-term withdrawal symptoms (lasting no more than 48 hours), including excessive crying, tremors, sleep problems, and gastrointestinal upset immediately after birth. Still, researchers caution that these risks shouldn't keep pregnant women from taking Prozac (or other SSRIs) if their depression can't be treated effectively in other ways, because untreated depression carries its own risks, many with long-term effects.

Your prenatal practitioner—along with your mental health care provider—will be able to steer you toward the best medications for you during pregnancy, so discuss the options with both of them.

Remember, too, that nonmedicinal approaches can also sometimes help manage depression. Psychotherapy may be effective on its own or in conjunction with medication. Other therapies that can sometimes be helpful when used along with medication include bright light therapy and CAM approaches. Exercise (for its release of feel-good endorphins), meditation (which can help you manage stress), and diet (keeping blood sugar up with regular meals and snacks and getting plenty of omega-3 fatty acids may help give your mood a boost) can also be beneficial additions to a treatment program. Talk to your practitioner and mental health care provider to see if these options have a place in yours.

Diabetes

"I'm a diabetic. How will that affect my baby?"

There's lots of good news for pregnant diabetics these days. In fact, with expert medical care and diligent self-care, you have about the same excellent chances of having a successful pregnancy and a healthy baby as any other expectant mom.

Research has proven that the key to managing a diabetic pregnancy successfully—whether the diabetes is type 1 (juvenile-onset diabetes, in which the body doesn't produce insulin) or type 2 (adult-onset diabetes, in which the body doesn't respond as it should to insulin)—is achieving normal blood glucose levels before conception and maintaining them throughout the nine months following it.

Whether you came into pregnancy as a diabetic or you developed gestational diabetes along the way, all of the following will help you have a safe pregnancy and a healthy baby:

The right doctor. The OB who supervises your pregnancy should have plenty of experience caring for diabetic mothers-to-be, and he or she should work together with the doctor who has been in charge of your diabetes. You'll have more prenatal visits than other expectant moms and will probably be given more doctor's orders to follow (but all for a very good cause).

Good food planning. A diet geared to your personal requirements should be carefully planned with your physician, a nutritionist, and/or a nurse-practitioner with expertise in diabetes. The diet will probably be high in complex carbohydrates, moderate in protein, low in cholesterol and fat, and contain few or no sugary sweets. Plenty of dietary fiber will be important, since some studies show that fiber may reduce insulin requirements in diabetic pregnancies.

Carbohydrate regulation is typically not as strict as it used to be because fast-acting insulin can be adjusted if you go over your limit at one meal or another. Still, the extent of your carbohydrate restriction will depend on the way your body reacts to particular foods. Most diabetics do best getting their carbohydrates from vegetable, grain (whole is best), and legume sources rather than from fruits. To maintain normal blood sugar levels, you'll have to be particularly careful to get enough carbohydrates in the morning. Snacks will also be important (even more important than they are for the average mom-to-be), and, ideally, they should include both a complex carbohydrate (such as whole-grain bread) and a protein (such as beans or cheese or chicken). Skipping meals or snacks can dangerously lower blood sugar, so try to eat on schedule, even if morning sickness or indigestion are putting a damper on your appetite. Eating six mini meals a day, regularly spaced, carefully planned, and supplemented as needed by healthy snacks, is your smartest strategy.

Sensible weight gain. It's best to try to reach your ideal weight before conception (something to remember if you plan another pregnancy). But if you start your pregnancy overweight, don't plan on using your nine-month stint for slimming down. Getting enough calories is vital to your baby's well-being. Aim to gain weight according to the guidelines set by your physician (slow and steady does it best). Your baby's growth will be monitored using ultrasound, because babies of diabetics sometimes grow very large, even if mom's weight is on target.

Exercise. A moderate exercise program, especially if you have type 2 diabetes, will give you more energy, help to regulate your blood sugar, and help you get in shape for delivery. But it must be planned in conjunction with your medication schedule and diet, with the help of your medical team. If you experience no other medical or pregnancy complications and are physically fit, moderate exercise—such as brisk walking, swimming, and stationary biking (but not jogging)—will likely be on the workout menu. Chances are that only very light exercise (leisurely walking, for instance) will get the green light if you were out of shape prior to pregnancy or if there are any signs of problems with your diabetes, your pregnancy, or your baby's growth.

Precautions you may be asked to take when exercising probably won't differ much from safe exercise tips for any pregnant woman: Have a snack before your workout; don't exercise to the point of exhaustion; and never exercise in a very warm environment (80°F or higher). If you're on insulin, you'll probably be advised to avoid injecting

it into the parts of the body being exercised (your legs, for example, if you're walking) and not to reduce your insulin intake before you exercise.

Rest. Getting enough rest is very important, especially in the third trimester. Avoid overdoing it, and try to take some time off during the middle of the day for putting your feet up or napping. If you have a demanding job, your doctor may recommend that you begin your maternity leave early.

Medication regulation. If diet and exercise alone don't control your blood sugar, you'll likely be put on insulin. If you end up needing insulin for the first time, your blood sugar can be stabilized under close medical supervision. If you were taking oral medication before you conceived, you might be switched to injected insulin or an under-the-skin insulin pump during pregnancy. Since levels of the pregnancy hormones that work against insulin increase as pregnancy progresses, your insulin dose may have to be adjusted upward periodically. The dose may also have to be recalculated as you and your baby gain weight, if you get sick or are under emotional strain, or if you overdo your carbs. Studies show that the oral drug glyburide may be an effective alternative to insulin therapy during pregnancy for some mild cases.

In addition to being sure your diabetes medication is on target, you'll need to be extremely careful about any other medications you take. Many over-the-counter drugs can affect your insulin levels—and some may not be safe in pregnancy—so don't take any until you check with both the physician who is overseeing your diabetes and the one taking care of your pregnancy.

Blood sugar regulation. You may have to test your blood sugar (with a simple finger-prick method) at least four or as often as ten times a day (possibly before and after meals) to be sure it's staying at safe levels. If you have type 1 diabetes, your blood may also be tested for glycosylated hemoglobin (hemoglobin A1c), because high levels of this substance may be a sign that sugar levels aren't being well controlled. To maintain normal blood glucose levels, you'll have to eat regularly, adjust your diet and exercise as needed, and, if necessary, take medication. If you were insulin-dependent before pregnancy, you may be more subject to low blood sugar episodes (hypoglycemia) than when you weren't pregnant, especially in the first trimester—so careful monitoring is a must. And don't leave home (or go anywhere) without packing the right snacks.

Urine monitoring. Since your body may produce ketones—acidic substances that can result when the body breaks down fat—during this close regulation of your diabetes, your urine may be checked for these regularly.

Careful monitoring. Don't be concerned if your physician orders a lot of tests for you, especially during the third trimester, or even suggests hospitalization for the final weeks of your pregnancy. This doesn't mean something is wrong, only that he or she wants to be sure everything stays right. The tests will primarily be directed toward regular evaluation of your condition and of your baby to determine the optimal time for delivery and whether any other intervention is needed.

You will probably have regular eye exams to check the condition of your retinas and blood tests and urine collections every 24 hours to evaluate your kidneys (retinal and kidney problems tend to worsen during pregnancy but usually return to prepregnancy status

after delivery if you've been taking care of yourself throughout pregnancy). The condition of your baby and the placenta will likely be evaluated throughout pregnancy with stress and/ or nonstress tests (see page 348), biophysical profiles, and ultrasound (to size up your baby to be sure it's growing as it should be and so that delivery can be accomplished before the baby gets too big for a vaginal delivery). And because there's a slightly higher risk of heart problems in the babies of diabetics, you'll get a detailed ultrasound of the fetal anatomy at 16 weeks and a special ultrasound of the fetal heart (fetal electrocardiogram) at about 22 weeks to make sure everything's going well.

After the 28th week, you may be asked to monitor fetal movements yourself three times a day (see page 289 for one way to do this, or follow your doctor's recommendation).

Because diabetics are at somewhat higher risk for preeclampsia, your doctor will watch you closely for early signs of that condition, too.

Elective early delivery. Women who develop gestational diabetes, as well as women with preexisting mild diabetes that is well controlled, can carry to their due date safely. But when mom's normal blood sugar levels have not been well maintained throughout pregnancy, or if the placenta deteriorates early, or if other problems develop late in pregnancy, her baby may be delivered a week or two before term. The various tests mentioned above help the physician decide when to induce labor or perform a C-section—late enough so the fetal lungs are sufficiently mature to function outside the womb, but not so late that the baby's safety is compromised.

Don't worry if your baby is placed in a neonatal intensive care unit immediately after delivery. This is routine procedure in most hospitals for infants of diabetic mothers. Your baby will be observed for respiratory problems (which are unlikely if the lungs were tested and found to be mature enough for delivery) and for hypoglycemia (which, though more common in babies of diabetics, is easily treated). You should be able to get your baby back soon so you can start nursing, if that's your plan.

Epilepsy

"I have epilepsy, and I desperately want to have a baby. Can I have a safe pregnancy?"

With the right precautions, there could definitely be a healthy baby in your future. Your first step—preferably before you take care of the conception part—is to get your condition under the best possible control, with the help of your neurologist and the doctor you've chosen for your prenatal care. (If you've already conceived, getting that help as soon as possible in your pregnancy is crucial.) For best pregnancy results, close supervision of your condition and possibly frequent adjustment of medication levels will be necessary, as will communication between your doctors.

Most women find that pregnancy does not exacerbate their epilepsy. Half experience no change in their disease, and a smaller percentage find that seizures actually become less frequent and milder. A few discover, however, that their seizures become more frequent and severe.

As for how epilepsy affects pregnancy, expectant moms with epilepsy may be slightly more likely to experience excessive nausea and vomiting (hyperemesis), but they aren't at higher risk for any serious complications.

There seems to be a slight increase in the incidence of certain birth defects in the babies of epileptic mothers, but these appear to be more often caused by the use of certain anticonvulsant medications during pregnancy than by the epilepsy itself.

Discuss with your doctor ahead of time the possibility of being weaned from your medications prior to conception. This may be possible if you've been seizure-free for a period of time. If you have been having seizures, it's important to try to get them under control as soon as possible. You will need medication to do this, but it may be possible to switch to a less risky drug than the one you've been taking. Taking one drug appears to cause fewer problems in pregnancy than multidrug therapy and is the preferred way to go. And it's important not to stop taking a necessary medication for fear of hurting your baby; not taking it—and having frequent seizures—may be more dangerous.

Helping Others with Epilepsy

For more information on epilepsy and pregnancy, check out epilepsyfoundation.org. To help yourself in the future or help other moms with epilepsy, ask your doctor about registering with the Antiepileptic Drug Pregnancy Registry, (888) 233-2334 or aed pregnancyregistry.org. Their goal is to determine which therapies are associated with an increased risk. You will also receive a packet of information about preconception planning and prenatal care.

A detailed structural ultrasound is recommended for anyone on seizure medicine, and certain early pregnancy screening tests may also be ordered. If you've been taking valproic acid (Depakene), the doctor may want to look specifically for neural tube defects, such as spina bifida.

Important for all pregnant women with epilepsy is getting plenty of sleep and the best nutrition, and maintaining adequate fluid levels. Vitamin D supplements may also be recommended, since some epilepsy medications can interfere with metabolism of the vitamin. During the last four weeks of pregnancy, a vitamin K supplement may be prescribed to reduce the risk of hemorrhage, another condition that babies of women taking seizure medications are at slightly greater risk for.

Labor and delivery aren't likely to be more complicated because of your epilepsy, though it is important that anticonvulsant medication continue to be administered during labor to minimize the risk of a seizure during delivery. An epidural anesthesia can be used to manage labor and delivery pain.

Breastfeeding your baby shouldn't be a problem, either. Most epilepsy medications pass into the breast milk in such low doses that they are unlikely to affect a nursing baby.

Making the Most of Your Meds

If you rely on oral medications to control a chronic condition, you may have to do a little adjusting now that you're expecting. For instance, if morning sickness has you down in the first trimester, taking your meds right before going to bed in the evening—so that they can build up in your system before the morning upchucking begins—may keep you from losing most of your medication through vomiting. (Check with your doctor first, because some medications must be taken at certain times of the day.)

Something else that you'll have to keep in mind—and that your team of doctors will have to keep an eye on: Some medications are metabolized differently during pregnancy. So the dosage you're used to isn't necessarily the right dosage now that you're expecting. If you're not sure whether your dosing is correct now that you're pregnant, or if you have a hunch you're not getting enough medication—or you're getting too much—let your doctors know.

Fibromyalgia

"I was diagnosed with fibromyalgia a few years ago. How will this impact my pregnancy?"

The fact that you're aware of your condition actually gives you a head start many women don't have. Fibromyalgia, a condition that affects 8 to 10 million Americans each year and is characterized by pain, burning sensations, and achiness in the muscles and soft tissues of the body, often goes unrecognized in pregnant women, possibly because the fatigue, weakness, and psychological stress it causes are all considered normal signs of pregnancy.

You're probably already used to being frustrated by fibromyalgia and the lack of available information about it and effective treatment for it. Prepare to become even more frustrated because, unfortunately, there's probably even less known about the effect of pregnancy on fibromyalgia and vice versa. From what is known, there is some substantially good news: Babies born to women with fibromyalgia are not affected in any way by the condition. Beyond that, some recent studies and plenty of anecdotal evidence have suggested that pregnancy can be extra tough on a woman with fibromyalgia. You may feel more tired and stiff and experience aches and pains in more parts of your body than an expectant mom without fibromyalgia (though some lucky women do feel better during pregnancy, so you can definitely hope for that). To keep your symptoms to a minimum, try to reduce the amount of stress in your life as much as possible, eat a well-balanced diet, exercise moderately (but never overdo it), and continue doing safe stretches and conditioning exercises (or yoga, water exercises, and so on) that may have helped you before your pregnancy. Women with fibromyalgia do typically gain 25 to 35 pounds during the first year of having the condition, so that during pregnancy, excessive weight gain can be a problem (not to say that you'll balloon up, but you may have trouble staying within the recommended weight gain guidelines). And since the condition is usually treated with antidepressants and pain suppressants, you'll need to make sure your doctor and prenatal practitioner are in contact with each other and only keep you on medications that are safe for use during pregnancy.

Chronic Fatigue Syndrome

Fortunately, having chronic fatigue syndrome (CFS) in no way interferes with having a normal pregnancy and a healthy baby. Unfortunately, that's about all scientists know for sure about the effects of CFS on pregnancy. No studies have been done yet, so the little that is known comes from anecdotal evidence, which tends to suggest that CFS affects different women differently during pregnancy. Some moms-to-be note their symptoms actually improve during pregnancy while others say they get worse. It may be hard to tell, since pregnancy is physically exhausting for all women, even those not dealing with CFS.

If you're pregnant with CFS, it's important that the doctor who has been caring for your condition knows about your pregnancy and the practitioner you've chosen for your prenatal care knows about your CFS. Together, incorporating strategies that have helped you in the past, they will be able to help you cope with your CFS while you're nurturing your baby-to-be.

Hypertension

"I've had hypertension for years. How will my high blood pressure affect my pregnancy?"

With more and more older women conceiving, more and more are also conceiving with chronic hypertension, a condition that becomes more common with age. So you've got lots of company (even if you developed your hypertension earlier on in life).

Your pregnancy is considered high risk, which means you'll be putting in more time at the doctor's office and putting more effort into following doctor's orders. But all for a very good cause.

With well-controlled blood pressure, and carefully monitored self-care and medical care, you're likely to have the best payoff of all—a safe pregnancy and a healthy baby.

All of the following can help increase the odds of a successful pregnancy:

The right medical team. The practitioner who supervises your pregnancy should have plenty of experience caring for mothers-to-be with chronic hypertension and should be joined on your pregnancy care team by the doctor who has been in charge of your hypertension.

Close medical monitoring. Your practitioner will probably schedule more frequent visits for you than for other expectant mothers and may order many more tests—but, again, that's time well spent. Having chronic hypertension increases your risk of developing preeclampsia during pregnancy as well as some other pregnancy complications, so your practitioner will pay particular attention to your well-being during your 40 weeks.

Relaxation. Relaxation exercises are soothing for every expectant soul, but particularly for those with hypertension. Research has shown that these exercises can actually lower blood pressure. Check out—and practice—the one on page 142, or consider using a meditation CD or even taking a class.

Other alternative approaches. Try any CAM techniques recommended by your practitioner, such as biofeedback, acupuncture, or massage.

Plenty of rest. Since both emotional and physical stress can send blood pressure up, don't overdo anything. Take frequent rest breaks during your day, preferably with your feet up. If you work at a high-stress job, rest might not do the trick—you may want to consider a leave of absence or cutting down on hours or responsibilities until after the baby arrives. If you have your hands full at home with other children, get as much help as you can handling the load.

Blood pressure monitoring. You may be asked to keep track of your own blood pressure at home. Take it when you're most rested and relaxed.

Good diet. The Pregnancy Diet is a smart place to start, but modify it with the help of your practitioner to fit your needs. Eating plenty of fruits and vegetables, low-fat or nonfat dairy products, and whole grains may be especially helpful in keeping your blood pressure down.

Adequate fluid. Remember to drink at least eight glasses of fluid a day, which should help relieve any mild swelling of your feet and ankles. In most cases, a diuretic (a drug that draws fluid from the body and is sometimes used in the treatment of hypertension) is not recommended during pregnancy.

Prescribed medication. Whether your medications will be changed or not during pregnancy will depend on what you've been taking. Some medications are considered safe for expectant moms; others are not.

Irritable Bowel Syndrome

"I have irritable bowel syndrome and was wondering if being pregnant will make my symptoms worse."

Since pregnancy seems to affect irritable bowel syndrome (IBS) differently in different women, there's no way to predict how it will affect you. Some women report being entirely symptom free while they're expecting; others find their symptoms get somewhat worse during their nine months.

One reason why it's so hard to pinpoint the effect of pregnancy on IBS—and vice versa—is that bowels are almost always impacted (so to speak) by pregnancy. Expectant women are more prone to constipation (a symptom of IBS, too), though some pregnant women find themselves with looser stools more often (also a symptom of IBS). Same for gas and bloating, which typically worsen when you're expecting, whether or not you have IBS. And since the hormones of pregnancy wreak havoc on all parts of the body, even IBS sufferers are left guessing: A woman who is normally diarrhea-predominant might suddenly find herself dealing with constipation, while a woman who is usually stopped up might find it's become easy—too easy—to move her bowels.

To keep your symptoms manageable, stick to the techniques you're used to using to combat IBS during other times in your life: Eat small, more frequent meals (good advice for any pregnant woman); stay well hydrated (ditto); eat a high-fiber diet to improve digestion (double ditto); avoid spicy foods; avoid excess stress; and steer clear of foods or drinks that make your symptoms worse. You might also want to consider adding some probiotics (in the form of yogurt or yogurt drinks with active cultures, or in powder or capsule form) to your diet. They're surprisingly effective in regulating bowel function and they're safe during pregnancy. Check with your practitioner.

Having IBS does put you at a slightly increased risk for premature delivery (so be sure to be alert to any signs of impending preterm contractions; see page 300). There's also a greater chance you might end up delivering via C-section because of your condition.

Lupus

"My lupus has been pretty quiet lately, but I just became pregnant. Is this likely to bring on a flare-up?"

There are still some unknowns about systemic lupus erythematosus (SLE), particularly when it comes to pregnancy. Studies indicate that pregnancy doesn't affect the long-term course of this autoimmune disorder. During pregnancy itself, some women find that their condition improves; other women find it worsens. More confusing still, what happens in one pregnancy doesn't necessarily predict what will happen in subsequent ones. In the postpartum period, there does appear to be an increased risk of flare-ups.

Whether and how SLE affects pregnancy, however, isn't absolutely clear. It does seem that the women who do best are those who, like you, conceive during a quiet period in their disease. Though the risk of pregnancy loss is slightly increased, in general, their chances of having a healthy baby are excellent. Those with the poorest prognosis are women with SLE who have severe kidney impairment (ideally, kidney function should be stable for at least six months before conception). If you have lupus anticoagulant or related antiphospholipid antibody, daily doses of aspirin and heparin may be prescribed.

Because of your lupus, your pregnancy care will include more, and more frequent, tests, medications (such as corticosteroids), and possibly more limitations. But if you, your obstetrician or maternal-fetal medicine specialist, and the physician who treats your lupus all work together, the odds are very much in favor of a happy outcome that will make all that extra effort completely worthwhile.

Multiple Sclerosis

"I was diagnosed several years ago as having multiple sclerosis. I've only had two episodes of MS, and they were relatively mild. Will the MS affect my pregnancy? Will my pregnancy affect my MS?"

There's good news for both you and your baby. Women with MS can definitely have normal pregnancies and healthy babies. Good prenatal care, beginning early (and better yet, modifying therapies even before conception), coupled with regular visits to your neurologist, will help you achieve that most wonderful of outcomes. And the good news carries over to childbirth, too. Labor and delivery aren't usually affected by MS, and neither are pain relief options. Epidurals and other types of anesthesia appear to be completely safe for delivering moms with MS.

As for pregnancy's effect on MS, some women experience relapses when they're expecting, as well as in the postpartum period, but most women are back to their prepregnancy condition within about three to six months of baby's arrival. Some women with ambulatory problems find that as weight gain increases during pregnancy, walking becomes more difficult, not surprisingly. Avoiding excessive weight gain may help minimize this problem. The happy bottom line: Whether or not you experience relapses, pregnancy doesn't seem to affect the overall lifetime relapse rate or the extent of ultimate disability.

To stay as healthy as possible while you're expecting, try to minimize stress and get enough rest. Also try to avoid raising your body temperature too much (stay out of hot tubs and too-warm baths, and don't exercise too hard or outside in hot weather). Do your best to fight off infections, particularly UTIs, which are more common during pregnancy (see page 498 for preventative measures).

Pregnancy can have some impact on MS treatment. Though low to moderate doses of prednisone are considered safe to use during pregnancy, some other medications used for MS may not be. You'll need to work out a medication regimen with your doctors that's safe for your baby and as effective as possible for you.

After delivery, there's a good chance that you'll be able to breastfeed, at least partially. If breastfeeding isn't an option, either because of the meds you need to take or because it's just too physically stressful, don't worry. Not only do babies thrive on good formula, they always do best when mom's feeling well.

Since going back to work early in the postpartum period may increase both exhaustion and stress—which might exacerbate your symptoms—you may want to consider taking that return slowly, finances permitting. If MS does interfere with your functioning while your child is young, see the next page for tips on baby care for parents with disabilities.

One other note: Many women with MS are concerned about passing the disease on to their children. Though there is a genetic component to the disease, placing these children at increased risk of being affected as adults, the risk is really quite small. Between 95 and 98 percent of children of MS mothers end up MS free.

Phenylketonuria

"I was born with PKU. My doctor let me off my low-phenylalanine diet when I was in my teens, and I was fine. But when I talked about getting pregnant, my OB said I should go back on the diet. Is that really necessary?"

A low-phenylalanine diet, which consists of a phenylalanine-free medical formula and precisely measured amounts of fruits, vegetables, bread, and pasta (and which eliminates all high-protein foods, including meat, poultry, fish, dairy products, eggs, beans, and nuts), definitely isn't tasty or easy to follow. But for pregnant women with phenylketonuria (PKU), it's absolutely necessary. Not sticking to the diet while you're pregnant would put your baby at great risk for a variety of problems, including serious mental deficits. Ideally, the low-phenylalanine regimen should be resumed three months before conception, and blood levels of phenylalanine kept low through delivery. (Even starting the diet early in pregnancy may reduce the seriousness of developmental delay in children of mothers with PKU.) And, of course, all foods sweetened with aspartame (Equal or NutraSweet) are absolutely off-limits.

Without a doubt, it'll be tough to return to the diet after so many years of being off of it—but clearly, the benefits to your developing baby will be well worth the sacrifice. If in spite of this incentive you find yourself slipping off the diet, it might help to get some professional help from a therapist who is familiar with your type of condition. A support group of other mothers with PKU may be even more helpful; the misery of such dietary deprivation definitely benefits from the company of those similarly deprived. For more information, check out pkunetwork.org.

Physical Disability

"I'm a paraplegic because of a spinal cord injury, and I use a wheelchair. My husband and I have wanted a baby for a long while, and I've finally become pregnant. Now what?"

Like every pregnant woman, you'll need to deal with first things first: selecting a practitioner. And as with every pregnant woman who falls into a high-risk category, your practitioner should ideally be an obstetrician or maternal-fetal medicine specialist who has experience dealing with women who face the same challenges as you do. That may be easier to find than you'd think because a growing number of hospitals are developing special programs to provide women with physical disabilities better prenatal and obstetrical care. If such a program or practitioner isn't available in your area, you'll need a doctor who is willing to learn "on the job" and who is able to offer you and your husband all the support you'll need.

Just which additional measures will be necessary to make your pregnancy successful will depend on your physical disabilities. In any case, restricting your weight gain to within the recommended range will help minimize the stress on your body. Eating the best possible diet will improve your general physical well-being and decrease the likelihood of pregnancy complications. And keeping up your exercise regimen will help ensure that you have maximum strength and mobility when the baby arrives; water therapy may be particularly helpful and safe.

It should be reassuring to know that, though pregnancy may be more difficult for you than for other pregnant women, it should not be any more stressful for your baby. And no evidence indicates an increase in fetal abnormalities among babies of women with spinal cord injury (or of those with other physical disabilities not related to hereditary or systemic disease). Women with spinal cord injuries, however, are more susceptible to such pregnancy problems as kidney infections and bladder difficulties, palpitations and sweating, anemia, and muscle spasms. Childbirth, too, may pose special problems, though in most cases a vaginal delivery will be possible. Because uterine contractions may be painless, depending on the kind of damage to your spinal cord, you will have to be instructed to note other signs of impending labor—such as bloody show or rupture of the membranes—or you may be asked to feel your uterus periodically to see if contractions have begun.

Long before your due date, devise a fail-safe plan for getting to the hospital, one that takes into account the fact that you may be home alone when labor strikes (you may want to plan to leave for the hospital early in labor to avoid any problems caused by delays en route). You'll also want to be sure the hospital staff is prepared for your additional needs.

Parenting is always a challenge, particularly in the early weeks, and it's not surprising that it will be even more so for you and your husband (who will have to be your more-than-equal parenting partner). Planning ahead will help you meet this challenge more successfully. Make any necessary modifications to your home to accommodate child care; sign on help (paid or otherwise) to at least get you started. Breastfeeding, which is usually possible, will make life simpler (no rushing off to the kitchen to prepare bottles and no shopping for formula). Getting your diapers and other baby needs delivered will also save effort and time. The changing table should be tailored for you to use from your wheelchair, the crib should have a drop side so you can take baby in and out easily, and—if you'll be doing all or some of the baby bathing—the baby tub should be set up somewhere that's accessible (daily tub baths aren't a must, so you can sponge baby on the changing table or on your lap on alternate days). Wearing your baby in a carrier or sling will probably be the most convenient way to tote him or her, since it'll leave your hands free (putting it on first thing in the morning will allow you to slide baby in and out as needed). Joining a support group of parents with disabilities (or checking out online groups) will provide lots of comfort and empathy and also give you a gold mine of ideas and advice.

For more information, contact Through the Looking Glass at (800) 644-2666 or online at lookingglass.org; or the National Spinal Cord Injury Association at (800) 962-9629 or online at spinalcord.org.

Rheumatoid Arthritis

"I have rheumatoid arthritis. How will this affect my pregnancy?"

Your condition isn't likely to affect your pregnancy very much, but pregnancy is likely to affect your condition—and, happily, for the better. Most women with rheumatoid arthritis (RA) notice a significant decrease in the pain and swelling in their joints during pregnancy, though there is also a somewhat greater risk of temporary symptom flare-up in the postpartum period.

The greatest change you may experience while you're pregnant is in the management of your condition. Because some of the medicines used to treat RA (such as ibuprofen and naproxen) are not safe for use later in pregnancy or at all, your physician will need to switch you over to treatments that are safer, such as steroids.

During labor and delivery, it will be important to choose positions that don't put too much stress or strain on affected joints. Discuss with the physician who manages your arthritis, as well as with your prenatal practitioner, which positions might work best.

Scoliosis

"I was diagnosed with mild scoliosis as a teenager. What effects will the curve of my spine have on my pregnancy?"

Thankfully, not much. Women with scoliosis usually go on to have uneventful pregnancies and deliveries, with healthy babies as the happy outcome. In fact, studies have shown that no significant problems occur during pregnancy that could be specifically attributed to scoliosis.

Women with severe curvature of the spine, or those whose scoliosis involves the hips, pelvis, or shoulders, may experience more discomfort, breathing problems, or weight-bearing difficulties during later pregnancy. If you find your back pain increases during pregnancy, stay off your feet as much as possible, take warm baths, enlist your spouse to give you some back rubs, and try the tips on page 237 for combating back pain. You can also ask your practitioner for the name of an obstetric physiotherapist who may be able to help you with some exercises specific to your scoliosis-related pain. Also discuss which CAM approaches (page 85) might be helpful.

If you think you might want an epidural during labor, talk to your practitioner about finding an anesthesiologist who has experience with moms with scoliosis. Though the condition usually does not interfere with the epidural, it may make it a little more difficult to place. An experienced anesthesiologist, however, should have no problem getting the needle where it needs to go.

Sickle Cell Anemia

"I have sickle cell disease, and I just found out that I'm pregnant. Will my baby be okay?"

Not too many years ago, the answer would not have been reassuring. Today, there's much happier news. Thanks to major medical advances, women with sickle cell disease—even those with such related complications as heart or kidney disease—have a good chance of having a safe pregnancy and delivery and a healthy baby.

Pregnancy for the woman with sickle cell anemia, however, is usually classified as high risk. The added physical stress of pregnancy increases her chances of having a sickle cell crisis, and the added stress of sickle cell disease increases the risks of certain complications, such as miscarriage, preterm delivery, and fetal growth restriction. Preeclampsia is also more common in women with sickle cell anemia.

The prognosis for both you and your baby will be best if you receive state-of-the-art medical care. You'll likely have prenatal checkups more frequently than other pregnant patients—possibly every two to three weeks up to the 32nd week, and every week after that. Your care should take a team approach: Your obstetrician should be familiar with sickle cell disease and work closely with a hematologist who's knowledgeable about sickle cell in pregnancy. Though it's not certain whether it's a beneficial therapy or not, it's possible that you'll be given a blood transfusion at least once (usually in early labor or just prior to delivery) or even periodically throughout pregnancy.

As far as childbirth is concerned, you're as likely as any other mother to have a vaginal delivery. Postpartum, you may be given antibiotics to prevent infection.

If both parents carry a gene for sickle cell anemia, the risk that their baby will inherit a form of the disease is increased. For that reason, your spouse should be tested for the trait early in your pregnancy (if he wasn't before conception). If he turns out to be a carrier, you may want to see a genetic counselor and possibly undergo amniocentesis to see if your baby is affected.

Thyroid Disease

"I was diagnosed as being hypothyroid when I was a teenager and am still taking thyroid pills. Is it safe to keep taking them while I'm pregnant?"

It's not only safe to continue taking your medication, it's vital to both your baby's well-being and your own. One reason is that women with untreated hypothyroidism (a condition in which the thyroid gland does not produce adequate amounts of the hormone thyroxine) are more likely to miscarry. Another reason is that maternal thyroid hormones are necessary for early fetal brain development; babies who don't get enough of these hormones in the first trimester can be born with neurological development problems and, possibly, deafness. (After the first trimester, the fetus makes its own thyroid hormones and is protected even if mom's levels are low.) Low thyroid levels are also linked to maternal depression during pregnancy and post-

partum—another compelling reason to continue your treatment.

Your dose, however, may need to be adjusted, since the body requires more thyroid hormone when it's in baby-making mode. Check with your endocrinologist and your obstetrician to be sure your dose is appropriate now, but keep in mind that your levels will probably be monitored periodically during pregnancy and postpartum to see if your dose needs further adjustment. Be on the lookout, too, for signs that your thyroid level is too low or too high and report these to your practitioner (though many of those probably familiar symptoms of hypothyroidism, such as fatigue, constipation, and dry skin, are so similar to those of pregnancy that it's often tough to tell which have you down, report them anyway).

Iodine deficiency, which is becoming more common among women of childbearing age in the United States because of reduced iodized salt consumption, can interfere with the production of thyroid hormone, so be sure you are getting adequate amounts of this trace mineral. It's most commonly found in iodized salt and seafood.

"I have Graves disease. Is this a problem for my pregnancy?"

Graves disease is the most common form of hyperthyroidism, a condition in which the thyroid gland produces excessive amounts of thyroid hormones. Mild cases of hyperthyroidism sometimes improve during pregnancy because the pregnant body requires more thyroid hormone than usual. But moderate to severe hyperthyroidism is a different story. Left untreated, these conditions could lead to serious complications for both you and your baby, including miscarriage and preterm birth, so appropriate treatment is necessary. Happily, when the disease is treated properly during pregnancy, the outcome is likely to be good for both mother and baby.

During pregnancy, the treatment of choice is the antithyroid medication propylthiouracil (PTU) in the lowest effective dose. If a woman is allergic to PTU, methimazole (Tapazole) may be used. If neither drug can be used, then surgery to remove the thyroid gland may be needed, but it should be performed early in the second trimester to avoid the risk of miscarriage (in the first trimester) or preterm birth (in the late second and third trimester). Radioactive iodine is not safe to use during pregnancy, so it won't be part of your treatment plan.

If you had surgery or radioactive iodine treatment for Graves before you became pregnant, you'll need to continue your thyroid replacement therapy during pregnancy (which is not only safe but essential for your baby's development).

ALL ABOUT

Getting the Support You Need

Though it's true that every expectant woman needs plenty of support, it's also true that moms-to-be with a chronic condition could use even more. Even if you've had your condition for years, you know everything there is to know about it, and you're an old pro at handling it, you'll probably find that pregnancy changes the rules (including the ones you had memorized).

Enter, that extra support. No pregnant woman should ever have to go it alone, but as a pregnant woman with a chronic condition, you may want and need even more company. Among the kinds of support you'll benefit from:

Medical support. Just like every expectant mom, you'll need to find (if you don't already have one) a prenatal practitioner who can consult with you before you conceive (if possible), care for you during your pregnancy, and make that special delivery when the time comes. Unlike with a lot of other expectant moms, that practitioner won't be the only member of your obstetrical team. You'll also need to bring the doctor or doctors who care for your chronic condition on board. Your team of doctors will work together to ensure that you and baby are both well taken care of—that your baby's best interests are represented in the care of your chronic condition, and your best interests are represented in the care of your baby. Communication will be a vital part of that teamwork—so make sure your doctors are all kept in the loop about tests, medications, and other care components.

All your doctors have lots of other patients, so it's best not to assume that communication's always taking place. If your chronic-care specialist prescribes a new medication, ask if it's been okayed by your prenatal practitioner, and vice versa.

Emotional support. Everyone needs somebody to lean on, but you may find you need plenty of somebodies. Somebody to vent to when you're feeling resentful over your special diet (Easter eggs instead of chocolate bunnies?). To complain to about being stuck in a revolving door of medical procedures (six tests in three days?).

To cry to when you're feeling particularly anxious. To confide in, share with, unload on. To give you the emotional support every expectant mom craves—since you might crave a little more.

Your partner is a perfect source of this support, of course, especially because he sees what you're going through and would do anything to help you. Your friends and relatives may lend a sympathetic ear when you need one, too, even if their own pregnancies were more "normal" and they can't always relate. But you'll probably find that no one quite gets it like another mom in the same situation—and that no one else gives you as much comfort, empathy, and satisfying support.

Depending on your chronic condition and where you live, you may be able to find a support group geared to expectant moms or new moms who are in the same or a similar boat as you. Or with a little help from your medical team, you might even be able to start one (even if it's just a group of two—another mom you can have lunch with or chat with on the phone). Or reach out online, either on pregnancy message boards or chat rooms for those who have the same chronic condition. Not only will you find the emotional hand-holding you're in the market for, but you'll find practical support, too—advice, treatment tips, strategies, diet ideas, and other resources to help you cope with your important dual mission: caring for your chronic condition and nurturing your baby-to-be.

Physical support. Again, there isn't an expectant mom who doesn't need it at some point in her pregnancy (probably at many points): someone to do the shopping when she's too tired to move, to scrub the toilet so she doesn't have to breathe in those fumes, to cook dinner when coming face-to-breast with uncooked chicken makes her heave. But for moms who are juggling the physical demands of pregnancy with the physical challenges of a chronic condition, there's no such thing as too much help. Get it wherever you can, and don't be shy about asking for it. Enlist your partner to pick up the slack (and the dry cleaning and groceries) that you don't have the energy to pick up, but also look to friends, relatives, and, if you can afford it, paid household help.

PART 7

The Complicated Pregnancy

CHAPTER 22

Managing a Complicated Pregnancy

I F YOU'VE BEEN DIAGNOSED WITH A complication or suspect that you're having one, you'll find symptoms and treatments in this chapter. If you've had a problem-free pregnancy so far, though, this need-to-know chapter is not for you (you don't need to know any of it). Most women sail through pregnancy and childbirth without any complications. While information is definitely empowering when you need it, reading about all the things that could go wrong when they're not going wrong is only going to stress you out—and for no good reason. Skip it, and save yourself some unneeded worry.

Pregnancy Complications

The following complications, though more common than some pregnancy complications, are still unlikely to be experienced by the average pregnant woman. So read this section only if you've been diagnosed with a complication or you're experiencing symptoms that might indicate a complication. If you are diagnosed with one, use the discussion of the condition in this section as a general overview—so you have an idea of what you're dealing with—but expect to receive more specific (and possibly different) advice from your practitioner.

Early Miscarriage

What is it? A miscarriage—known in medical speak as a spontaneous abortion—is the spontaneous expulsion of an embryo or fetus from the uterus

Types of Miscarriage

If you've experienced an early pregnancy loss, the sadness you'll feel is the same no matter the cause or the official medical name. Still, it's helpful to know about the different types of miscarriage so you're familiar with the terms your practitioner might be using.

Chemical pregnancy. A chemical pregnancy occurs when an egg is fertilized but fails to develop successfully or implant fully in the uterus. A woman may miss her period and suspect she is pregnant; she may even have a positive pregnancy test because her body has produced some low—but detectable—levels of the pregnancy hormone hCG, but in a chemical pregnancy, there will be no gestational sac or placenta on ultrasound examination.

Blighted ovum. A blighted ovum (or anembryonic pregnancy) refers to a fertilized egg that attaches to the wall of the uterus, begins to develop a placenta (which produces hCG), but then fails to develop into an embryo. What is left behind is an empty gestational sac (which can be visualized on an ultrasound).

Missed miscarriage. A missed miscarriage, which is very rare, is when the embryo or fetus dies but continues to stay in the uterus. Often, the only signs of a missed miscarriage are the loss of all pregnancy symptoms, and less commonly, a brownish discharge. Confirmation of the miscarriage occurs when an ultrasound shows no fetal heartbeat.

Incomplete miscarriage. An incomplete miscarriage is when some of the tissue from the placenta stays inside the uterus and some is passed through the vagina via bleeding. With an incomplete miscarriage, a woman continues to cramp and bleed (sometimes heavily), her cervix remains dilated, pregnancy tests still come back positive (or blood hCG levels are still detectable and don't fall as expected), and parts of the pregnancy are still visible on an ultrasound.

Threatened miscarriage. When there is some vaginal bleeding but the cervix remains closed and the fetal heartbeat (as seen on ultrasound) is still detectable, it is considered a threatened miscarriage. Roughly half of those women with a threatened miscarriage go on to have a perfectly healthy pregnancy.

before the fetus is able to live on the outside (in other words, the unplanned end of a pregnancy). Such a loss in the first trimester is referred to as an early miscarriage. Eighty percent of miscarriages occur in the first trimester. (A miscarriage that occurs between the end of the first trimester and week 20 is considered a late miscarriage; see page 540).

Early miscarriage is usually related to a chromosomal or other genetic defect in the embryo, but it can also be caused by hormonal and other factors. Most often, the cause can't be identified.

How common is it? Miscarriage is one of the most common complications of early pregnancy. It's hard to know for sure, but researchers have estimated that over 40 percent of conceptions end in miscarriages. And well over half of those occur so early that pregnancy is not even suspected yet—meaning these miscarriages often go unnoticed, passing for a normal or sometimes heavier period. See the box above for more on the different types of early miscarriage.

Miscarriage can happen to any woman, and in fact, most women who

> ## You'll Want to Know...
>
> In a normal pregnancy, miscarriage is *not* caused by exercise, sex, working hard, lifting heavy objects, a sudden scare, emotional stress, a fall, or a blow to the abdomen. The nausea and vomiting of morning sickness, even when it's severe, will not cause a miscarriage. In fact, morning sickness has been linked with a lower risk of miscarriage. Happily, the vast majority of women who experience miscarriage go on to have a normal pregnancy in the future.

have one have no known risk factors. Still, some factors somewhat increase the risk of miscarriage. One is age; the older eggs of older mothers (and possibly their older partner's sperm) are more likely to contain a genetic defect (a 40-year-old has a 33 percent chance of miscarrying, while a 20-year-old's odds of losing a pregnancy are 15 percent). Other risk factors include vitamin deficiencies (especially of folic acid); being very overweight or underweight; smoking; possibly hormonal insufficiency or imbalance, including an untreated thyroid condition; certain sexually transmitted diseases (STDs); and certain chronic conditions.

What are the signs and symptoms? The symptoms of a miscarriage can include some or all of the following:

- Cramping or pain (sometimes severe) in the center of the lower abdomen or back

- Heavy vaginal bleeding (possibly with clots and/or tissue) similar to a period

- Light staining continuing for more than three days

- A pronounced decrease in or loss of the usual signs of early pregnancy, such as breast tenderness and nausea

What can you and your practitioner do? Not all bleeding or spotting means you're having a miscarriage. In fact, many situations (other than miscarriage) could account for bleeding (see page 139).

If you do notice some bleeding or spotting, call your practitioner. He or she will assess the bleeding and probably perform an ultrasound. If the pregnancy still appears to be viable (in other words, a heartbeat is detected on the ultrasound), your practitioner may put you on some sort of temporary bed rest, your hormone levels will be monitored if you're still very early in your pregnancy (rising hCG levels are a good sign), and the bleeding will most likely stop on its own.

If your practitioner finds that your cervix is dilated and/or no fetal heartbeat is detected on ultrasound (and your dates are correct), it is assumed a miscarriage has occurred or is in progress. In such a case, unfortunately, nothing can be done to prevent the loss.

> ## You'll Want to Know...
>
> Sometimes it's too early to see a fetal heartbeat or visualize the fetal sac on ultrasound, even in a healthy pregnancy. Dates could be off or the ultrasound equipment not sophisticated enough. If your cervix is still closed, you are spotting only lightly, and the ultrasound is ambiguous, a repeat sonogram will be performed in a week or so to let you know what's really going on. Your hCG levels will also be followed.

If You've Had a Miscarriage

Though it is hard for parents to accept it at the time, when an early miscarriage occurs, it's usually because the condition of the embryo or fetus is incompatible with normal life. Early miscarriage is generally a natural selection process in which a defective embryo or fetus (defective because of genetic abnormality; or damaged by environmental factors, such as radiation or drugs; or because of poor implantation in the uterus, maternal infection, random accident, or other, unknown reasons) is lost because it is incapable of survival.

All that said, losing a baby, even this early, is tragic and traumatic. But don't let guilt compound your misery. A miscarriage is not your fault. Do allow yourself to grieve, a necessary step in the healing process. Expect to be sad, even depressed, for a while. Sharing your feelings with your spouse, your practitioner, a relative, or a friend will help. So will joining or forming a support group for couples or singles who have experienced pregnancy loss or reaching out to others online. This sharing with others who truly know how you feel may be especially important if you've experienced more than one pregnancy loss. For more suggestions on coping with your loss, see Chapter 23.

For some women, the best therapy is getting pregnant again as soon as it is safe. But before you do, discuss possible causes of the miscarriage with your doctor. Most often, miscarriage is simply a random one-time occurrence caused by chromosomal abnormality, infection, chemical or other teratogenic (birth defect–causing) exposure, or chance, and it is not likely to recur.

Whatever the cause of your miscarriage, some practitioners suggest waiting two to three months before trying to conceive again, though intercourse can often be resumed as soon as you feel up to it. Other practitioners let nature take over; they tell their patients that their bodies will know when it's time to conceive again. Some studies have shown that women actually have a higher than normal fertility rate in the first three cycles following a first-trimester loss. If your practitioner does recommend a waiting period, however, use reliable contraception, preferably of the barrier type—condom, diaphragm—until the waiting time is up. Take advantage of this waiting period by getting your body into the best baby-making shape possible (see Chapter 1).

Happily, the chances are excellent that next time around you'll have a normal pregnancy and a healthy baby. Most women who have had one miscarriage do not miscarry again. In fact, a miscarriage is an assurance that you're capable of conceiving, and the great majority of women who lose a pregnancy this way go on to complete a normal one.

If you're in a lot of pain from the cramping, your practitioner may recommend or prescribe a pain reliever. Don't hesitate to ask for relief if you need it.

Can it be prevented? Most miscarriages are a result of a defect in the embryo or fetus and can't be prevented. There are steps you can take, however, to reduce the risk of preventable miscarriage:

- Get chronic conditions under control before conception.

- Be sure to take a daily prenatal supplement that includes folic acid and other B vitamins. New research has shown that some women have trouble

Management of a Miscarriage

Most miscarriages are complete, meaning all the contents of the uterus are expelled via the vagina (that's why there is often so much bleeding). But sometimes—especially the later in the first trimester you are—a miscarriage isn't complete, and parts of the pregnancy remain in the uterus (known as an incomplete miscarriage). Or a heartbeat is no longer detected on ultrasound, which means the embryo or fetus has died, but no bleeding has occurred (this is called a missed miscarriage). In both cases, your uterus will eventually be—or need to be—emptied so your normal menstrual cycle can resume (and you can try to get pregnant again, if you choose to). There are a number of ways this can be accomplished:

Expectant management. You may choose to let nature take its course and wait until the pregnancy is naturally expelled. Waiting out a missed or incomplete miscarriage can take any-

where from a few days to, in some cases, three to four weeks.

Medication. Medication—usually a misoprostol pill taken orally, or vaginally as a suppository—can prompt your body to expel the fetal tissue and placenta. Just how long this takes varies from one woman to another, but, typically, it's only a matter of days at the most before the bleeding begins. Side effects of the medication can include nausea, vomiting, cramping, and diarrhea.

Surgery. Another option is to undergo a minor surgical procedure called dilation and curettage (D and C). During this procedure, the doctor dilates your cervix and gently removes (either by suction, scraping, or both) the fetal tissue and placenta from your uterus. Bleeding following the procedure usually lasts no more than a week. Though side effects are rare, there is a slight risk of infection following a D and C.

conceiving and/or sustaining a pregnancy because of a folic acid or vitamin B_{12} deficiency. Once these women begin the appropriate supplementation, they may be able to conceive and carry to term.

- Try to get your weight as close to ideal as possible before conceiving: Being extremely overweight or extremely underweight puts a pregnancy at higher risk.

- Avoid lifestyle practices that increase the risk of miscarriage, such as alcohol use and smoking.

- Use caution when taking medications. Take only those that are okayed by a doctor who knows you are pregnant

and avoid those that are known to be risky during pregnancy.

- Take steps to avoid infections, such as STDs.

If you've had two or more miscarriages, you can have tests to try to determine the possible cause so future pregnancy losses might be prevented (see box, page 542, for more).

Late Miscarriage

What is it? Any spontaneous expulsion of a fetus between the end of the first trimester and the 20th week is termed a late miscarriage. After the 20th week, the loss of the baby in utero is called a stillbirth.

How should you decide which route to take? Some factors you and your practitioner will take into account include:

- How far along the miscarriage is. If bleeding and cramping are already heavy, the miscarriage is probably already well under way. In that case, allowing it to progress naturally may be preferable to a D and C. But if there is no bleeding (as in a missed miscarriage), misoprostol or a D and C might be better alternatives.

- How far along the pregnancy is. The more fetal tissue there is, the more likely a D and C will be necessary to clean the uterus out completely.

- Your emotional and physical state. Waiting for a natural miscarriage to occur after a fetus has died in utero can be psychologically debilitating for a woman, as well as for her spouse. It's likely that you won't be able to begin coming to terms with—and grieving for—your loss while the pregnancy is still inside you. Completing the process faster will also allow you to resume your menstrual cycles soon, and when and if the time is right, to try to conceive again.

- Risks and benefits. Because a D and C is invasive, it carries a slightly higher (though still very low) risk of infection. The benefit of having the miscarriage complete sooner, however, may greatly outweigh that small risk for most women. With a naturally occurring miscarriage, there is also the risk that it won't completely empty the uterus, in which case a D and C may be necessary to finish what nature has started.

- Evaluation of the miscarriage. When a D and C is performed, evaluating the cause of the miscarriage through an examination of the fetal tissue will be easier.

No matter what course is taken, and whether the ordeal is over sooner or later, the loss will likely be difficult for you. See Chapter 23 for help in coping.

The cause of late miscarriage is usually related to the mother's health, the condition of her cervix or uterus, her exposure to certain drugs or other toxic substances, or to problems of the placenta.

How common is it? Late miscarriages occur in about 1 in 1,000 pregnancies.

What are the signs and symptoms? After the first trimester, a pink discharge for several days or a scant brown discharge for several weeks may indicate a threatened late miscarriage. Heavier bleeding, especially when accompanied by cramping, often means a miscarriage is inevitable, especially if the cervix is dilated. (There may be other causes of heavy bleeding, such as placenta previa, page 551; placental abruption, page 553; a tear in the uterine lining; or premature labor, page 556).

What can you and your practitioner do? If you're spotting light pink or brown, call your practitioner. He or she will evaluate the bleeding, possibly do an ultrasound and check your cervix, and probably prescribe bed rest. If the spotting stops, it's likely it wasn't related to miscarriage (sometimes it's triggered by sexual intercourse or an internal exam), which means normal activity can usually be resumed. If your cervix has started to dilate and you have had no bleeding or pain, a diagnosis of incompetent cervix may be made and cerclage (stitching

Repeat Miscarriages

Though having one miscarriage definitely doesn't mean that you're likely to miscarry again, some women do suffer recurring miscarriages (defined as two or three in a row). If you've had several, you may wonder whether you'll ever be able to have a healthy pregnancy. First, know that there's a good chance you will, although you may need to manage future pregnancies differently. The causes of repeated miscarriages are sometimes unknown, but there are tests that may shed light on why the miscarriages took place—even if they each had a different cause.

Trying to determine the cause of a single loss usually isn't worthwhile, but a medical evaluation might be rec-ommended if you have two or more miscarriages in a row. Some factors that might be related to recurrent miscarriage include a thyroid problem, autoimmune problems (in which the mother's immune system attacks the embryo), a vitamin deficiency, or a misshapen uterus. There are now many tests that may pick up risk factors for pregnancy loss and suggest possible ways of preventing it, in some cases very easily. Both parents might also have blood tests to screen for chromosomal problems that can be passed on to a fetus. You may be tested, too, for blood-clotting disorders (some women produce antibodies that attack their own tissues, causing blood clots that can clog the maternal blood vessels

the cervix closed; see page 47) may prevent a late miscarriage.

If you're experiencing the type of heavy bleeding and painful cramping that signal a miscarriage, there's usually nothing, unfortunately, that can be done to stop the inevitable. The further along your pregnancy, the more likely your practitioner might bring you into the hospital. Performing a D and C may be necessary to remove any remnants of the pregnancy.

Can it be prevented? Once a late miscarriage is under way, it isn't preventable. But if the cause of a late miscarriage can be determined, it may be possible to prevent a repeat of the tragedy. If a previously undiagnosed incompetent cervix was responsible, future miscarriages can be prevented by cerclage early in pregnancy, before the cervix begins to dilate. If chronic disease, such as dia-betes, hypertension, or a thyroid condition, is responsible, the condition can be brought under control prior to any future pregnancy. Acute infection can be prevented or treated. And an abnormally shaped uterus or one that is distorted by the growth of fibroids or other benign tumors in some instances can be corrected by surgery. The presence of antibodies that trigger placental inflammation and/or clotting may be treated with low-dose aspirin and heparin injections in a subsequent pregnancy.

Ectopic Pregnancy

What is it? An ectopic pregnancy (also known as a tubal pregnancy) is one that implants outside the uterus, most commonly in a fallopian tube, usually because something (such as scarring in the fallopian tube) obstructs or slows the that feed the placenta). An ultrasound, MRI, or CT scan may be performed on your uterus, your uterine cavity may be assessed with hysteroscopy, and the miscarried fetus itself can be tested for chromosomal abnormalities.

Once you know the cause, or causes, you can talk to your practitioner about treatment options, as well as how best to care for the next pregnancy. Surgery may correct some uterine and cervical issues; thyroid medication can easily treat a thyroid condition, and medically supervised supplementation can just as easily resolve a vitamin deficiency; hormone treatments may also help, as can tests for antibodies and treatment to prevent blood clots (low-dose aspirin and/or heparin). In some instances, patients with a history of early miscarriages who appear to be producing too little progesterone may benefit from taking the hormone, though this treatment is controversial. Or, if excess prolactin is the cause, medication to reduce prolactin levels in the mother's blood may allow a pregnancy to proceed to term.

Even if you've had repeated miscarriages, you still have a good chance of sustaining a successful pregnancy in the future. But that may be hard for you to believe or even to hope for. It will be important to find ways of managing your understandable fear that becoming pregnant again will mean you'll miscarry again. Yoga, visualization techniques, and deep-breathing exercises can help with the anxiety, and support can come from other women who've suffered similar losses. Sharing your feelings openly with your partner may also help. Remember, you're in this together.

movement of the fertilized egg into the uterus. An ectopic pregnancy can also occur in the cervix, on the ovary, or in the abdomen. Unfortunately, there is no way for an ectopic pregnancy to continue normally.

Ultrasound can detect an ectopic pregnancy, often as early as five weeks. But without early diagnosis and treatment of an ectopic pregnancy, the fertilized egg might continue to grow in the fallopian tube, leading to a rupture of the tube. If the tube bursts, its ability in the future to carry a fertilized egg to the uterus is destroyed, and if the rupture is not cared for, it can result in severe, even life-threatening, internal bleeding and shock. Luckily, quick treatment (usually surgery or medication) can help avoid such a rupture and removes most of the risk for the mother while greatly improving the chances of preserving her fertility.

How common is it? About 2 percent of all pregnancies are ectopic. Women at risk of having an ectopic pregnancy include those with a history of endometriosis, pelvic inflammatory disease, a prior ectopic pregnancy, or tubal surgery (conceiving after getting your tubes tied carries a 60 percent chance of an ectopic pregnancy). Also included in the at-risk group are those who became pregnant while using progesterone-only birth control pills; women who became pregnant with an IUD in place (though

You'll Want to Know ...

More than half of the women who are treated for ectopic pregnancies conceive and have a normal pregnancy within a year.

Ectopic Pregnancy

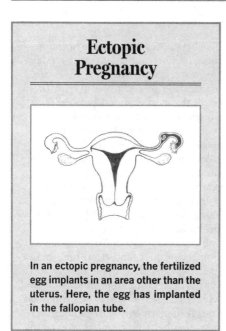

In an ectopic pregnancy, the fertilized egg implants in an area other than the uterus. Here, the egg has implanted in the fallopian tube.

- Dizziness and/or fainting
- Severe sharp abdominal pain
- Rectal pressure
- Shoulder pain (due to blood accumulating under the diaphragm)
- Heavier vaginal bleeding

What can you and your practitioner do? Occasional cramping and even slight spotting early in pregnancy is not cause for alarm, but do let your practitioner know if you experience any type of pain, spotting, or bleeding. Call right away if you experience sharp, crampy pain in the lower abdomen, heavy bleeding, or any of the other symptoms of a ruptured ectopic pregnancy just listed. If it is determined that you have an ectopic pregnancy (usually diagnosed through ultrasound and blood tests), there is, unfortunately, no way to save the pregnancy. You'll most likely have to undergo surgery (laparoscopically) to remove the tubal pregnancy or be given drugs (methotrexate), which will end the abnormally occurring pregnancy. In some cases, it can be determined that the ectopic pregnancy is no longer developing and can be expected to disappear over time on its own, which would also eliminate the need for surgery.

with today's newer IUDs, especially the hormonal kinds, the chance of an ectopic pregnancy is significantly lower); women with STDs; and women who smoke.

What are the signs and symptoms? Early symptoms of an ectopic pregnancy include:

- Sharp, crampy pain with tenderness, usually in the lower abdomen (it often begins as a dull ache that progresses to spasms and cramps); pain may worsen on straining of bowels, coughing, or moving
- Abnormal bleeding (brown spotting or light bleeding that precedes the pain)

If the ectopic pregnancy goes unnoticed and your fallopian tube ruptures, you may experience:

- Nausea and vomiting
- Weakness

You'll Want to Know . . .

Occasional cramping in your lower abdomen early in pregnancy is probably the result of implantation, normally increased blood flow, or ligaments stretching as the uterus grows, not a sign of an ectopic pregnancy.

Because residual material from a pregnancy left in the tube could damage it, a follow-up test of hCG levels is performed to be sure the entire tubal pregnancy was removed or has reabsorbed.

Can it be prevented? Getting treated for sexually transmitted diseases (STDs), and the prevention of STDs (through the practice of safe sex) can help reduce the risk of an ectopic pregnancy, as can quitting smoking.

Subchorionic Bleed

What is it? A subchorionic bleed (also called a subchorionic hematoma) is the accumulation of blood between the uterine lining and the chorion (the outer fetal membrane, next to the uterus) or under the placenta itself, often (but not always) causing noticeable spotting or bleeding.

In the vast majority of cases, women who have a subchorionic bleed go on to have perfectly healthy pregnancies. But because (in rare cases) bleeds or clots that occur under the placenta can cause problems if they get too large, all subchorionic bleeds are monitored.

How common is it? Around 1 percent of all pregnancies have a subchorionic bleed. Of those women who experience first-trimester bleeding, 20 percent of them are diagnosed with a subchorionic bleed as the cause of the spotting.

What are the signs and symptoms? Spotting or bleeding may be a sign, often beginning in the first trimester. But many subchorionic bleeds are detected during a routine ultrasound, without there being any noticeable signs or symptoms.

> ### You'll Want to Know . . .
>
> A subchorionic bleed does not affect the baby, and since you'll be checked with ultrasounds until the hematoma corrects itself, you'll get reassurance each time you see your baby's heartbeat (and that will be more often than most expectant parents get!).

What can you and your practitioner do? If you have spotting or bleeding, call your practitioner; an ultrasound may be ordered to see whether there is indeed a subchorionic bleed, how large it is, and where it's located.

Hyperemesis Gravidarum

What is it? Hyperemesis gravidarum is the medical term for severe pregnancy nausea and vomiting that is continuous and debilitating (not to be confused with typical morning sickness, even a pretty bad case). Hyperemesis usually starts to lift between weeks 12 and 16, but some cases can continue throughout pregnancy.

Hyperemesis gravidarum can lead to weight loss, malnutrition, and dehydration if it's left untreated. Treatment of severe hyperemesis often requires hospitalization—mostly for the administration of IV fluids and antinausea drugs, which can effectively safeguard your well-being and your baby's.

How common is it? Hyperemesis gravidarum occurs in about 1 in 200 pregnancies. This pregnancy complication is more common in first-time mothers, in young mothers, in obese women, in women carrying multiple fetuses, and in women who've had it in a previous pregnancy. Extreme emotional stress can also increase your risk, as can endocrine imbalances and vitamin B deficiencies.

What are the signs and symptoms? The symptoms of hyperemesis gravidarum include:

- Very frequent and severe nausea and vomiting

- The inability to keep any food or even liquid down

- Signs of dehydration, such as infrequent urination or dark yellow urine

- Weight loss of more than 5 percent

- Blood in the vomit

What can you and your practitioner do? If your symptoms are relatively mild, you can first try some of the natural remedies used to fight morning sickness, including ginger, acupuncture, and acupressure wristbands (see page 130). If those don't do the trick, ask your practitioner about medications that can help (a combination of vitamin B_6 and Unisom Sleep Tabs is often prescribed for tough morning sickness cases). But if you're vomiting continually and/or losing significant amounts of weight, your practitioner will assess your need for

intravenous fluids and/or hospitalization, and possibly prescribe some sort of antiemetic (antinausea) drug. Once you're able to keep food down again, it may help to tweak your diet to eliminate fatty and spicy foods, which are more likely to cause nausea, as well as to avoid any smells or tastes that tend to set you off. In addition, try to graze on many small high-carb and high-protein meals throughout the day, and be sure your fluid intake is adequate (keeping an eye on your urinary output is the best way to assess that; dark scant urine is a sign you're not getting, or keeping down, enough fluids).

Gestational Diabetes

What is it? Gestational diabetes (GD)—a form of diabetes that appears only during pregnancy—occurs when the body does not produce adequate amounts of insulin (the hormone that lets the body turn blood sugar into energy) to regulate blood sugar effectively. GD usually begins between weeks 24 and 28 of pregnancy (which explains why a glucose screening test is routine at around 28 weeks). GD almost always goes away after delivery, but if you've had it, you'll be checked postpartum to make sure it's gone.

Diabetes, both the kind that begins in pregnancy and the kind that started before conception, is not harmful to either the fetus or the mother if it is well controlled. But if excessive sugar is allowed to circulate in a mother's blood and thus to enter the fetal circulation through the placenta, the potential problems for both mother and baby are serious. Women who have uncontrolled GD are more likely to have a too-large baby, which can complicate delivery. They are also at risk for developing pre-

You'll Want to Know . . .

As miserable as hyperemesis gravidarum makes you feel, it's unlikely to affect your baby. Most studies show no health or developmental differences between infants of women who experience hyperemesis gravidarum and those who don't.

eclampsia (pregnancy-induced hypertension). Uncontrolled diabetes could also lead to potential problems for the baby after birth, such as jaundice, breathing difficulties, and low blood sugar levels. Later in life, he or she may be at an increased risk for obesity and type 2 diabetes.

How common is it? GD is fairly common, affecting 4 to 7 percent of expectant women. Because it's more common among obese women, rates of GD are rising along with rising obesity rates in the United States. Older moms-to-be are more likely to develop GD, as are women with a family history of diabetes or GD. Native Americans, Latin Americans, and African Americans are also at somewhat greater risk for GD.

What are the signs and symptoms? Most women with GD have no symptoms, though a few may experience:

- Unusual thirst

- Frequent and very copious urination (as distinguished from the also frequent but usually light urination of early pregnancy)

- Fatigue (which may be difficult to differentiate from pregnancy fatigue)

- Sugar in the urine (detected at a routine practitioner visit)

What can you and your practitioner do? Around your 28th week, you'll be given a glucose screening test (see page 297) and, if necessary, a more elaborate three-hour glucose tolerance test. If these tests show you have GD, your practitioner will likely put you on a special diet (similar to the Pregnancy Diet) and suggest exercises to keep your GD under control. You may also need to check your glucose levels at home using a glucose meter or strips.

If diet and exercise alone aren't enough to control your blood sugar level (they usually are), you may need supplementary insulin. The insulin can be given in shots, but the oral drug glyburide is being used more and more often as an alternative treatment for GD. Fortunately, virtually all of the potential risks associated with diabetes in pregnancy can be eliminated through the careful control of blood sugar levels achieved by good self- and medical care. For more on diabetes control, see page 519.

You'll Want to Know...

There's little reason for concern if your GD is well controlled. Your pregnancy will progress normally and your baby shouldn't be affected.

Can it be prevented? Keeping an eye on your weight gain (both before and during pregnancy) can help prevent GD. So, too, can good diet habits (eating plenty of fruits and vegetables, and whole grains, keeping refined sugar intake down, and making sure you're getting enough folic acid) and regular exercise (research shows that obese women who exercise cut their risk of developing GD by half). Continuing these preventive steps after the baby's born also significantly reduces the risk of diabetes occurring later in life.

Keep in mind, too, that having GD during pregnancy puts you at greater risk of developing type 2 diabetes after pregnancy. Keeping your diet healthy, staying at a normal weight, and, even more important, continuing to exercise after the baby is born (and beyond) significantly cuts that risk.

Preeclampsia

What is it? Preeclampsia (also known as pregnancy-induced hypertension or toxemia) is a disorder that generally develops late in pregnancy (after week 20) and is characterized by a sudden onset of high blood pressure, excessive swelling (edema), and protein in the urine.

If preeclampsia goes untreated, it could progress to eclampsia, a much more serious condition involving seizures (see page 562). Unmanaged preeclampsia can also cause a number of other pregnancy complications, such as premature delivery or intrauterine growth restriction.

How common is it? About 8 percent of pregnant women are diagnosed with preeclampsia. Women carrying multiple fetuses, women over 40, and women with high blood pressure or diabetes are at greater risk of developing preeclampsia. If you're diagnosed with preeclampsia in one of your pregnancies, you have a 1 in 3 chance of developing the condition in future pregnancies. That risk is higher if you are diagnosed with preeclampsia in your first pregnancy or if you develop preeclampsia early in any pregnancy.

What are the signs and symptoms? Symptoms of preeclampsia can include any or all of the following:

The Reasons Behind Preeclampsia

No one knows for sure what causes preeclampsia, though there are a number of theories:

- A genetic link. Researchers hypothesize that the genetic makeup of the fetus could be one of the factors that predisposes a pregnancy to preeclampsia. So, if your mother or your spouse's mother had preeclampsia during their pregnancies with either of you, you are somewhat more likely to have preeclampsia during your pregnancies.

- A blood vessel defect. It has been suggested that this defect causes the blood vessels in some women to constrict during pregnancy instead of widen (as usually happens). As a result of this vessel defect, theorize researchers, there is a drop in the blood supply to organs like the kidney and liver, leading to preeclampsia. The fact that women who experience preeclampsia during pregnancy are at an increased risk later in life of having some sort of

cardiovascular condition also seems to indicate that the condition may be the result of a predisposition in some women to high blood pressure.

- Gum disease. Pregnant women with severe gum disease are more than twice as likely to also have preeclampsia compared to women with healthy gums. Experts theorize that the infection causing the periodontal disease may travel to the placenta or produce chemicals that can cause preeclampsia. Still, it is not known if periodontal disease causes preeclampsia or if it is just associated with it.

- An immune response to a foreign intruder: the baby. This theory implies that the woman's body becomes "allergic" to the baby and placenta. This "allergy" causes a reaction in the mother's body that can damage her blood and blood vessels. The more similar the father's and mother's genetic markers, the more likely this immune response will occur.

- Severe swelling of hands and face

- Swelling of the ankles that doesn't go away after 12 hours of rest

- Sudden excessive weight gain unrelated to eating

- Headaches that don't respond to over-the-counter pain relievers

- Pain in the upper abdomen

- Blurred or double vision

- A rise in blood pressure (to 140/90 or more in a woman who has never before had high blood pressure)

- Protein in the urine

- Rapid heartbeat

- Scant urine output

- Abnormal kidney function

- Exaggerated reflex reactions

What can you and your practitioner do? Regular prenatal care is the best way to catch preeclampsia in its early stages (your practitioner might be tipped off by protein in your urine and a rise in your blood pressure, or the symptoms just listed). Being alert to any such symptoms (and alerting your practitioner if you notice them) also helps, particularly if you had a history of hypertension before pregnancy.

If you're diagnosed with preeclampsia, your treatment will probably include bed rest at home and careful blood pressure and fetal monitoring (though more pronounced cases may require hospital bed rest). With severe preeclampsia, the treatment is usually more aggressive and includes delivery within three days of diagnosis. Intravenous magnesium sulfate is begun promptly because it almost always prevents progression to eclampsia.

Though treatments are available to control preeclampsia for short periods of time, there is no cure except for delivery of your baby, which will likely be recommended as soon as the baby is physically mature enough or after medications are given to speed lung maturity. The good news is that 97 percent of women with preeclampsia recover completely, with a speedy return to normal blood pressure, after delivery.

On the research horizon: Scientists are developing simple blood and urine tests that can predict which moms-to-be are likely to develop this complication. They've found that women who eventually develop preeclampsia show high levels of a substance called soluble FH-1 in the blood and urine. Another substance called endoglin may also prove to predict the condition. Ideally, the research will lead to much earlier detection of preeclampsia.

Can it be prevented? Research has suggested that for women at risk for preeclampsia, aspirin or other anticlotting drugs during pregnancy may reduce the risk, though the benefits of this medically induced therapy need to be weighed against its theoretical risks. Some research has suggested that good nutrition, which ensures adequate intakes of antioxidants, magnesium, vitamins, and minerals,

You'll Want to Know...

Fortunately, in women who are receiving regular medical care, preeclampsia is almost invariably caught early on and managed successfully. With appropriate and prompt medical care, a woman with preeclampsia near term has virtually the same excellent chance of having a positive pregnancy outcome as a woman with normal blood pressure.

may reduce the risk of preeclampsia, as may proper dental care.

HELLP Syndrome

What is it? HELLP syndrome is a combination of conditions that can affect a pregnant woman, either by itself or in conjunction with preeclampsia, almost always in the last trimester. The acronym stands for hemolysis (H), in which red blood cells are destroyed too soon, causing a low red-cell count; elevated liver enzymes (EL), which indicates that the liver is functioning poorly and is unable to process toxins in the body efficiently; and low platelet count (LP), which makes it difficult for the blood to form clots.

When HELLP develops, it can threaten both a mother's life and that of her baby. Women who aren't diagnosed and treated quickly run about a 1 in 4 chance of suffering serious complications, primarily in the form of extensive liver damage or stroke.

How common is it? HELLP syndrome occurs in fewer than 1 in 10 preeclamptic or eclamptic pregnancies and fewer than 1 in 500 pregnancies.

Women who develop preeclampsia or eclampsia are at risk, as are women who have had HELLP in a previous pregnancy.

What are the signs and symptoms? The symptoms of HELLP are very vague, consisting of (in the third trimester):

- Nausea

- Vomiting

- Headaches

- General malaise

- Pain and tenderness in the upper right side of the abdomen

- Viral-type illness symptoms

Blood tests reveal a low platelet count, elevated liver enzymes, and hemolysis (the breakdown of red blood cells). Liver function rapidly deteriorates in women with HELLP, so treatment is critical.

What can you and your practitioner do? The only effective treatment for HELLP syndrome is delivery of your baby, so the best thing you can do is be aware of the symptoms of the condition (especially if you already have or are at risk for preeclampsia) and call your practitioner immediately if you develop any. If you have HELLP, you might also be given steroids (to treat the condition and help mature the baby's lungs) and magnesium sulfate (to prevent seizures).

Can it be prevented? Because a woman who has had HELLP in a previous pregnancy is likely to have it again, close monitoring is necessary in any subsequent pregnancy. Unfortunately, nothing can be done to prevent the condition.

Intrauterine Growth Restriction

What is it? Intrauterine growth restriction (IUGR) is a term used for a baby who is smaller than normal during pregnancy. A diagnosis of IUGR is given if your baby's weight is below the 10th percentile for his or her gestational age. IUGR can occur if the health of the placenta or its blood supply is impaired or if the mother's nutrition, health, or lifestyle prevents the healthy growth of her fetus.

How common is it? IUGR occurs in about 10 percent of all pregnancies. It's more common in first pregnancies, in fifth and subsequent ones, in women who are under age 17 or over age 35, in those who had a previous low-birthweight baby, as well as in those who have placental problems or uterine abnormalities. Carrying multiples is also a risk factor, but that's probably due more to the crowded conditions (it's hard to fit more than one 7-pounder in a single womb) than to problems with the placenta. Having been small at birth yourself also puts you at an increased risk of having a small baby, and the risk is also higher if the baby's father was born small.

What are the signs and symptoms? Surprisingly, carrying small is not usually a tip-off to IUGR. In fact, there are rarely any obvious outward signs that the baby isn't growing as he or she should be. Instead, IUGR is usually detected during a routine prenatal exam when the practitioner measures the fundal height—the distance from your pubic bone to the top of your uterus—and finds that it's measuring too small for the baby's gestational age. An ultrasound can also detect a baby whose growth is slower than expected for his or her gestational age.

What can you and your practitioner do? One of the best predictors of a baby's good health is birthweight, so having

IUGR can present some health problems for the newborn, including having difficulty maintaining a normal body temperature or fighting infection. That's why it's so important to diagnose the problem early and try to boost baby's chances of a healthy bottom line at birth. A variety of approaches may be tried, depending on the suspected cause, including bed rest, intravenous feedings if necessary, and medications to improve placental blood flow or to correct a diagnosed problem that may be contributing to the IUGR. If the intrauterine environment is poor and can't be improved, and the fetal lungs are known to be mature, prompt delivery—which allows baby to start living under healthier conditions—is usually the best way to go.

Can it be prevented? Optimum nutrition and the elimination of risk factors can greatly improve the chances for normal fetal growth and a normal birthweight. Controlling certain maternal risk factors (such as chronic high blood pressure, smoking, drinking alcohol, or using recreational drugs) that contribute to poor fetal growth can help prevent IUGR. Good prenatal care can also minimize the risks, as can excellent diet, proper weight gain within recommended guidelines, as well as minimizing physical and excessive psychological stress (including chronic lack of rest). Happily, even when prevention and treatment are unsuccessful and a baby is born smaller than normal, the chances that he or she will do well are increasingly good, thanks to the many advances in neonatal (newborn) care.

Placenta Previa

What is it? The definition of placenta previa is a placenta that partially or completely covers the opening of the cervix. In early pregnancy, a low-lying placenta is fairly common but as pregnancy progresses and the uterus grows, the placenta usually moves upward and away from the cervix. If it doesn't move up and partially covers or touches the cervix, it's called partial previa. If it completely covers the cervix, it's called total or complete previa. Either can physically block your baby's passage into the birth canal, making a vaginal delivery impossible. It can also trigger bleeding late in pregnancy and at delivery. The closer to the cervix the placenta is situated, the greater the possibility of bleeding.

How common is it? Placenta previa occurs in 1 out of every 200 deliveries. It is more likely to occur in women over the age of 30 than in women under the age of 20, and it is also more common in women who have had at least one other pregnancy or any kind of uterine surgery (such as a previous C-section or a D and C following miscarriage). Smoking or carrying multiple fetuses also increases the risks.

What are the signs and symptoms? Placenta previa is most often discovered not on the basis of symptoms but during a routine second-trimester ultrasound (though there isn't even the potential for problems with a previa until the third trimester). Sometimes the condition announces itself in the third trimester (occasionally earlier) with bright-red bleeding. Typically, bleeding is the only symptom. There's usually no pain involved.

What can you and your practitioner do? Nothing needs to be done (and you don't have to give your low-lying placenta a second thought) until the third trimester, by which point most early cases of placenta previa have corrected themselves. Even later on, there is no treatment necessary if you've been diagnosed with previa but aren't experiencing any bleeding (you'll just need to be alert to any bleeding or to signs of premature labor, which is more common with placenta previa). If you're experiencing bleeding related to a diagnosed previa, your practitioner will likely put you on bed rest, pelvic rest (no sex),

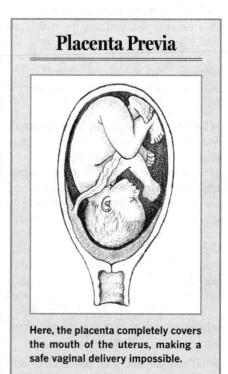

Placenta Previa

Here, the placenta completely covers the mouth of the uterus, making a safe vaginal delivery impossible.

You'll Want to Know...

Placenta previa is considered to be the most common cause of bleeding in the latter part of pregnancy. Most previas are found early and managed well, with the baby delivered successfully by a cesarean (about 75 percent of cases are delivered by C-section before labor starts).

and will monitor you closely. If premature labor seems imminent, you may receive steroid shots to mature your baby's lungs more rapidly. Even if the condition hasn't presented your pregnancy with any problems at all (you haven't had any bleeding and you've carried to term), your baby will still be delivered via C-section.

Placental Abruption

What is it? Placental abruption (also called abruptio placenta) is the early separation of the placenta (the baby's support system) from the uterine wall during pregnancy, rather than after delivery. If the separation is slight, there is usually little danger to the mother or baby as long as treatment is prompt and proper precautions are taken. If the abruption is more severe, however, the risk to the baby is considerably higher. That's because a placenta's complete detachment from the uterine wall means the baby is no longer getting oxygen or nutrition.

How common is it? It occurs in less than 1 percent of pregnancies, almost always in the second half of the pregnancy and most often in the third trimester. Placental abruption can happen to

anyone, but it occurs more commonly in women who are carrying multiples, who have had a previous abruption, who smoke or use cocaine, or who have gestational diabetes, a predisposition to clotting, preeclampsia, or other high blood pressure conditions of pregnancy. A short umbilical cord or trauma due to an accident is occasionally the cause of an abruption.

What are the signs and symptoms? The symptoms of placental abruption depend on the severity of the detachment, but will usually include:

- Bleeding (that could be light to heavy, with or without clots)

- Abdominal cramping or achiness

- Uterine tenderness

- Pain in the back or abdomen

What can you and your practitioner do? Let your practitioner know immediately if you have abdominal pain accompanied by bleeding in the second half of your pregnancy. A diagnosis is usually made using patient history, physical exam, and observation of uterine contractions and the fetal response to them. Ultrasound may be helpful, but only about 25 percent of abruptions can actually be seen on ultrasound. If it's been determined that your placenta has separated slightly from the uterine wall but has not completely detached, and if your baby's vital signs stay regular, you'll probably be put on bed rest. If the bleeding continues, you may require intravenous fluids. Your practitioner may also administer steroids to speed up your baby's lung maturation in case you need to deliver early. If the abruption is significant or if it continues to progress, the only way to treat it is to deliver the baby, most often by C-section.

Chorioamnionitis

What is it? Chorioamnionitis is a bacterial infection of the amniotic membranes and fluid that surround and protect your baby. It's caused by common bacteria such as E. coli or by group B strep (which you'll be tested for around week 36 of your pregnancy). The infection is believed to be a major cause of preterm premature rupture of the membranes (PPROM) as well as of premature delivery.

How common is it? Chorioamnionitis occurs in 1 to 2 percent of pregnancies. Women who experience premature rupture of the membranes are at increased risk for chorioamnionitis because bacteria from the vagina can seep into the amniotic sac after it has ruptured. Women who've had the infection during their first pregnancy are more likely to have it again in a subsequent pregnancy.

What are the signs and symptoms? Diagnosis of chorioamnionitis is complicated by the fact that no simple test can confirm the presence of infection. The symptoms of chorioamnionitis can include:

- Fever

- Tender, painful uterus

- Increased heart rate in both you and your baby

- Leaking, foul-smelling amniotic fluid (if membranes have already ruptured)

- Unpleasant-smelling vaginal discharge (if membranes are intact)

- Increased white blood count (a sign the body is fighting an infection)

What can you and your practitioner do? Be sure to call your practitioner if you

---

You'll Want to Know...

Rapid diagnosis and treatment of chorioamnionitis greatly reduces the risks to both mother and baby.

---

notice any leaking of amniotic fluid, no matter how small, or if you notice a foul-smelling discharge or any other of the symptoms listed above. If you are diagnosed with chorioamnionitis, you will likely be prescribed antibiotics to wipe out the bacteria, and be delivered immediately. You and your baby will also be given antibiotics after delivery to make sure no further infections develop.

Oligohydramnios

What is it? Oligohydramnios is a condition in which there is not enough amniotic fluid surrounding and cushioning the baby. It usually develops in the latter part of the third trimester, though it could show up earlier in pregnancy. Though the majority of women diagnosed with oligohydramnios will have a completely normal pregnancy, there is a slight risk of umbilical cord constriction if there's too little fluid for your baby to float around in. Often, the condition is simply the result of a fluid leak or puncture in the amniotic sac (one you wouldn't necessarily notice). Less commonly, a low level of amniotic fluid can suggest a problem in the baby, such as poor fetal growth or a kidney or urinary tract condition.

How common is it? Four to 8 percent of pregnant women are diagnosed with oligohydramnios during their pregnancy, but among overdue women (those two weeks past their due dates), the number rises to 12 percent. Women with a post-term pregnancy are most likely to have oligohydramnios, as are those who have premature rupture of membranes.

What are the signs and symptoms? There are no symptoms in the mother, but signs that would point to the condition are a uterus that measures smaller than it should and a decreased amount of amniotic fluid, detected via ultrasound. There might also be a noticeable decrease of fetal activity and sudden drops in the fetal heart rate in some cases.

What can you and your practitioner do? If you're diagnosed with oligohydramnios, you'll need to get a lot of rest and drink plenty of water. The amount of amniotic fluid will be closely monitored. If at any point oligohydramnios endangers the well-being of your baby, your practitioner may suggest amnioinfusion (in which fluid levels are augmented with sterile saline) or may opt for an early delivery.

Hydramnios

What is it? Too much amniotic fluid surrounding the fetus causes the condition known as hydramnios (also called polyhydramnios). Most cases of hydramnios are mild and transient, simply the result of a temporary change in the normal balance of the amniotic fluid production, with any extra fluid likely to be reabsorbed without any treatment.

But when fluid accumulation is severe (which is rare), it may signal a problem with the baby, such as a central nervous system or gastrointestinal defect, or an inability to swallow (babies typically swallow amniotic fluid). Too much amniotic fluid can put your pregnancy at risk for premature rupture of membranes, preterm labor, placental abruption, breech presentation, or umbilical cord prolapse.

How common is it? Hydramnios occurs in 3 to 4 percent of all pregnancies. It is more likely to occur when there are multiple fetuses and can be related to untreated diabetes in the mother.

What are the signs and symptoms? More often than not, there are no symptoms at all with hydramnios, though some women may notice:

- Difficulty feeling fetal movements (because there's too much of a cushion)

- Unusually rapid growth of the uterus

- Discomfort in the abdomen

- Indigestion

- Swelling in the legs

- Breathlessness

- Possibly, uterine contractions

Hydramnios is usually detected during a prenatal exam, when your fundal height—the distance from your pubic bone to the top of your uterus—measures larger than normal, or during an ultrasound that measures the amount of fluid in the amniotic sac.

What can you and your practitioner do? Unless the fluid accumulation is fairly severe, there's absolutely nothing you need to do except to keep your appointments with your practitioner, who will continue to monitor your condition. If the accumulation is more severe, your practitioner may suggest you undergo a procedure called therapeutic amniocentesis, during which fluid is withdrawn from the amniotic sac to reduce the amount. Since hydramnios puts you at increased risk for cord prolapse, call your practitioner right away if your water breaks on its own before labor.

Preterm Premature Rupture of the Membranes (PPROM)

What is it? PPROM refers to the rupture of the membranes (or "bag of waters") that cradle the fetus in the uterus, before 37 weeks (in other words, before term, when the baby is still premature). The major risk of PPROM is a premature birth; other risks include infection of the amniotic fluid and prolapse or compression of the umbilical cord. (Premature rupture of the membranes, or PROM, that isn't preterm—that is, it takes place after 37 weeks, but before labor begins—is discussed on page 363.)

How common is it? Preterm premature rupture of membranes occurs in fewer than 3 percent of pregnancies. Women most at risk are those who smoke during pregnancy, have certain STDs, have chronic vaginal bleeding or placental abruption, have had a previous early membrane rupture, have bacterial vaginosis (BV), or who are carrying multiples.

What are the signs and symptoms? The symptoms are leaking or gushing of fluid from the vagina. The way to tell whether you're leaking amniotic fluid and not urine is by taking the sniff test: If it smells like ammonia, it's probably urine. If it has a somewhat sweet smell, it's probably amniotic fluid (unless it's infected; then the fluid will be more foul smelling). If you have any doubts about what you're leaking, call your practitioner to be on the safe side.

What can you and your practitioner do? If your membranes have ruptured after 34 weeks, you'll likely be induced and your baby delivered. If it's too soon for your baby to be delivered safely, chances are you'll be put on in-hospital bed rest

> ## You'll Want to Know . . .
>
> With prompt and appropriate diagnosis and management of PPROM, both mother and baby should be fine, though if the birth is premature, there may be a long stay in the neonatal intensive care unit for baby.

and be given antibiotics to ward off infection, as well as steroids to mature your baby's lungs as quickly as possible for a safer early delivery. If contractions begin and the baby is believed to be too immature for delivery, medication may be given to try to stop them.

Rarely, the break in the membranes heals and the leakage of amniotic fluid stops on its own. If that happens, you'll be allowed to go home and resume your normal routine while remaining on the alert for signs of further leakage.

Can it be prevented? Vaginal infections, particularly BV, can lead to PPROM; therefore, watching out for and treating these infections may be effective in preventing some cases of PPROM.

Preterm or Premature Labor

What is it? Labor that kicks in after week 20 but before the end of week 37 of pregnancy is considered to be preterm labor.

How common is it? Preterm labor is a fairly common problem; about 12 percent of babies are born premature in the United States.

Risk factors leading to premature labor include smoking, alcohol use, drug abuse, too little weight gain, too much weight gain, inadequate nutrition, gum infection, other infections (such as STDs, bacterial vaginosis, urinary tract infections, amniotic fluid infection), incompetent cervix, uterine irritability, chronic maternal illness, placental abruption, and placenta previa. Women who are younger than 17 or older than 35 years old, those who are carrying multiples, and those with a history of premature delivery are also at increased risk. Preterm births are also more common among African American and disadvantaged women. In addition, a fairly large number of premature labors are induced by practitioners in an appropriate response to a medical condition that requires an early birth, such as preeclampsia or PPROM.

Still, much more needs to be learned about what causes labor to begin early; at least half of the women who go into preterm labor have no known risk factors.

What are the signs and symptoms? Signs of premature labor can include all or some of the following:

- Menstrual-like cramps

- Regular contractions that intensify and become more frequent even if you change positions

- Back pressure

- Unusual pressure in your pelvis

- Bloody discharge from your vagina

- Rupture of membranes

- Changes in the cervix (thinning, opening, or shortening) as measured by ultrasound

What can you and your practitioner do? Because each day a baby remains in the womb improves the chances of both survival and good health, holding off labor as long as possible will be the

You'll Want to Know...

A baby born prematurely will likely need to spend time in a neonatal intensive care unit, (NICU) for the first few days, weeks, or, in some cases, months of his or her life. Though prematurity has been linked to slow growth and developmental delays, most babies who arrive too early catch up and have no lasting problems at all. Thanks to advances in medical care, your chances of bringing home a normal, healthy infant after a premature birth are very good.

primary goal. If you're experiencing early contractions, your practitioner may—depending on how far along you are—put you on bed rest at home or admit you to the hospital to administer intravenous fluids (the better hydrated you are, the lower the chances of continued contractions—so if you're at home, keep the fluids flowing, too). Antibiotics may be given, especially if infection is believed to have triggered labor. There are also medications (tocolytic agents such as terbutaline or magnesium sulfate) that you may be given to temporarily halt contractions. Steroids may be administered, too, in order to help your baby's lungs mature more quickly, so that he or she will fare better should a preterm birth become inevitable or necessary. If at any point your practitioner determines that the risk to you or your baby from continuing the pregnancy outweighs the risk of preterm birth, no attempt will be made to postpone delivery.

Can it be prevented? Not all preterm births can be avoided, since not all are due to preventable risk factors.

Predicting Preterm Labor

Even among women who are at high risk for preterm labor, most will carry to term. One way to predict preterm labor is to examine cervical or vaginal secretions for a substance known as fetal fibronectin (fFN). Studies show that some women who test positive for fFN stand a good chance of going into preterm labor within one to two weeks of the test. The test, however, is better at diagnosing women who are *not* at risk for going into preterm labor (by detecting no fFN) than as an accurate predictor of women who are at risk. When fFN is detected, steps should be taken to reduce the chances of preterm labor. The test is now widely available, but is usually reserved for high-risk women only. If you aren't considered high risk for preterm birth, you don't need to be tested for fFN.

Another screening test is one for cervical length. Via ultrasound, the length of your cervix is measured, and if there are any signs that the cervix is shortening or opening, your practitioner may take some steps to prevent early labor—such as putting you on bed rest.

However, all the following measures may reduce the risk of preterm delivery (while boosting your chances of having the healthiest pregnancy possible): taking folic acid before pregnancy; getting early prenatal care; eating well and staying hydrated; getting good dental care; avoiding smoking, cocaine, alcohol, and other drugs not prescribed by your doctor; getting tested for and, if necessary, treated for any infections such as BV and UTIs; and following your practitioner's recommendations as to limitations on strenuous activity, including sexual intercourse and hours spent standing or walking on the job, especially if you have had previous preterm deliveries. Those with previous preterm deliveries or with a short cervix may benefit from supplementary progesterone, given daily or weekly, as a gel or a shot.

Symphysis Pubis Dysfunction (SPD)

What is it? Symphysis pubis dysfunction, or SPD, means the ligaments that normally keep your pelvic bone aligned become too relaxed and stretchy too soon before birth (as delivery nears, things are supposed to start loosening up). This, in turn, can make the pelvic joint—aka the symphysis pubis—unstable, causing mild to severe pain.

How common is it? The incidence of diagnosed SPD is about 1 in 300 pregnancies, though some experts think that more than 2 percent of all pregnant women will experience SPD (but not all will have it diagnosed).

What are the signs and symptoms? The most common symptom is a wrenching pain (as though your pelvis is coming apart) and difficulty when walking. Typically, the pain is focused on the pubic area, but in some women it radiates to the upper thighs and perineum. The pain can worsen when you're walking and doing any weight-bearing activity, particularly one that involves lifting one leg, such as when you're climbing up stairs, getting dressed, getting in and out of a car, even turning over in bed. In very rare cases, the joint may gape apart, a condition called diastasis symphysis pubis or symphyseal separation, which can cause more serious pain in your pelvis, groin, hips, and buttocks.

What can you and your practitioner do? Avoid aggravating the condition by limiting weight-bearing positions and minimizing as best you can any activity that involves lifting or separating your legs—even walking, if it's very uncomfortable. Try stabilizing those floppy ligaments by wearing a pelvic support belt, which "corsets" the bones back into place. Kegels and pelvic tilts can help to strengthen the muscles of the pelvis. If the pain is severe, ask your practitioner about pain relievers or turn to CAM techniques, such as acupuncture or chiropractic.

Very rarely, SPD can make a vaginal delivery impossible and your practitioner may opt for a C-section instead. And in even rarer cases, SPD can worsen after delivery, requiring medical intervention. But for most moms, once your baby is born and production of relaxin (that ligament-relaxing hormone) stops, your ligaments will return to normal.

Cord Knots and Tangles

What is it? Once in a while, the umbilical cord becomes knotted, tangled, or wrapped around a fetus, often at the neck (when it is known as a nuchal cord). Some knots form during delivery; others form during pregnancy when the baby moves around. As long as the knot remains loose, it's not likely to cause any problems at all. But if the knot becomes tight, it could interfere with the circulation of blood from the placenta to the baby and cause oxygen deprivation. Such an event happens only rarely, but when it does, it is most likely to occur during your baby's descent through the birth canal.

How common is it? True umbilical cord knots occur in about 1 in every 100 pregnancies, but only in 1 in 2,000 deliveries will a knot be tight enough to present problems for the baby. The more common nuchal cords occur in as many as a quarter of all pregnancies but very rarely pose risks to the baby. Babies with long cords and those who are large-for-gestational age are at greater risk for developing true knots. Researchers speculate that nutritional deficiencies that affect the structure and protective barrier of the cord, or other risk factors, such as smoking or drug use, carrying multiples, or having hydramnios, may make a woman more prone to having a pregnancy with a cord knot.

What are the signs and symptoms? The most common sign of a cord knot is decreased fetal activity after week 37. If the knot occurs during labor, a fetal monitor will detect an abnormal heart rate.

What can you and your practitioner do? You can keep a general eye on how your baby is doing, especially later in your pregnancy, by doing regular kick counts and calling your practitioner if you notice any change in fetal activity. If a loose knot tightens during delivery, your practitioner will be able to detect the drop in your baby's heart rate, and will make the appropriate decisions to ensure your baby's safe entry into the world. Immediate delivery, usually via C-section, is often the best approach.

Two-Vessel Cord

What is it? In a normal umbilical cord, there are three blood vessels—one vein (which brings nutrients and oxygen to the baby) and two arteries (which transport waste from the baby back to the placenta and the mother's blood). But in some cases, the umbilical cord contains only two blood vessels—one vein and one artery.

How common is it? About 1 percent of singletons and 5 percent of multiple pregnancies will have a two-vessel cord. Those at greater risk include Caucasian women, women over age 40, those carrying a multiple pregnancy, and those with diabetes. Female fetuses are more likely to be affected by a two-vessel cord than males.

What are the signs and symptoms? There are no signs or symptoms with this condition; it's detected on ultrasound examination.

What can you and your practitioner do? In the absence of any other abnormalities, a two-vessel cord in no way harms the pregnancy. The baby is most likely to be born completely healthy. So the first thing you can do is not worry.

If you've been found to have a two-vessel cord, your pregnancy will be monitored more closely, since the condition comes with a small increased risk of poor fetal growth.

Uncommon Pregnancy Complications

The following complications of pregnancy are, for the most part, rare. The average pregnant woman is extremely unlikely to encounter any of them. So, again (and this deserves repeating), read this section *only* if you need to—and even then, read just what applies to you. If you are diagnosed with any of these complications during your pregnancy, use the information here to learn about the condition and its typical treatment (as well as how to prevent it in future pregnancies), but realize that your practitioner's protocol for treating you may be different.

Molar Pregnancy

What is it? In a molar pregnancy, the placenta grows improperly, becoming a mass of cysts (also called a hydatidiform mole), but there is no accompanying fetus. In some cases, identifiable—but not viable—embryonic or fetal tissue

is present; this is called a partial molar pregnancy.

The cause of a molar pregnancy is an abnormality during fertilization, in which two sets of chromosomes from the father become mixed in with either one set of chromosomes from the mother (partial mole)—or none of her chromosomes at all (complete mole). Most molar pregnancies are discovered within weeks of conception. All molar pregnancies end in miscarriage.

You'll Want to Know . . .

Having had one molar pregnancy doesn't put you at much higher risk for having another one. In fact, only 1 to 2 percent of women who have had one molar pregnancy go on to experience a second.

How common is it? Luckily, molar pregnancies are relatively rare, occurring only in 1 out of 1,000 pregnancies. Women under the age of 15 or over the age of 45, as well as women who have had multiple miscarriages are at a slightly increased risk for a molar pregnancy.

What are the signs and symptoms? The symptoms of a molar pregnancy can include:

- A continuous or intermittent brownish discharge

- Severe nausea and vomiting

- Uncomfortable cramping

- High blood pressure

- Larger than expected uterus

- Doughy uterus (rather than firm)

- Absence of embryonic or fetal tissue (as seen on ultrasound)

- Excessive levels of thyroid hormone in the mother's system

What can you and your practitioner do? Call your practitioner if you experience any of the symptoms listed above. Some of these symptoms can be difficult to differentiate from normal early pregnancy signs and symptoms (many completely normal pregnancies include some spotting and cramping, and most include nausea), but trust your instincts. If you think something's wrong, talk to your practitioner—if only to get some much-needed reassurance.

If an ultrasound shows you do have a molar pregnancy, the abnormal tissue must be removed via a dilation and curettage (D and C). Follow-up is crucial to make sure it doesn't progress to choriocarcinoma (see next column), though luckily, the chances of a treated molar pregnancy turning malignant are very low. Your practitioner will probably suggest that you not get pregnant for a year following a molar pregnancy.

Choriocarcinoma

What is it? Choriocarcinoma, an extremely rare form of cancer related to pregnancy, grows from the cells of the placenta. This malignancy most often occurs after a molar pregnancy, miscarriage, abortion, or ectopic pregnancy, when any left-behind placental tissues continue to grow despite the absence of a fetus. Only 15 percent of choriocarcinomas occur after a normal pregnancy.

How common is it? Choriocarcinoma is extremely rare, occurring in only 1 out of every 40,000 pregnancies.

What are the signs and symptoms? The signs of the disease include:

- Intermittent bleeding following a miscarriage, a pregnancy, or the removal of a molar pregnancy

- Abnormal tissue discharge

- Elevated hCG levels that do not return to normal after a pregnancy has ended

- A tumor in the vagina, uterus, or lungs

- Abdominal pain

What can you and your practitioner do? Call your practitioner if you experience any of the above symptoms, but keep in mind that it's extremely

---

You'll Want to Know...

With early diagnosis and treatment of choriocarcinoma, fertility is unaffected, though it's usually recommended that pregnancy be deferred for one year after treatment for choriocarcinoma is complete and there is no evidence of residual disease.

unlikely that they indicate a choriocarcinoma. If you are diagnosed, the news is very reassuring. While any type of cancer carries with it some risk, choriocarcinoma responds extremely well to chemotherapy and radiation treatments and has a cure rate of more than 90 percent. Hysterectomy is almost never necessary because of this type of tumor's excellent response to chemotherapy drugs.

Eclampsia

What is it? Eclampsia is the result of uncontrolled or unresolved preeclampsia (see page 548). Depending on what stage of pregnancy a woman is in when she becomes eclamptic, her baby may be at risk of being born prematurely since immediate delivery is often the only treatment. Although eclampsia is life-threatening for the mother, maternal deaths from it are quite rare in the United States. With optimum treatment and careful follow-up, the majority of women with eclampsia return to normal health after delivery.

How common is it? Eclampsia is much less common than preeclampsia and occurs in only 1 out of every 2,000 to 3,000 pregnancies, typically among women who have not been receiving regular prenatal care.

What are the signs and symptoms? Seizures—usually close to or during delivery—are the most characteristic symptom of eclampsia. Postpartum seizures can also occur, usually within the first 48 hours after delivery.

What can you and your practitioner do? If you already have preeclampsia and start to seize, you'll be given oxygen and drugs to arrest the seizures and your labor will be induced or a C-section performed when you're stable. The major-

ity of women rapidly return to normal after delivery, though careful follow-up is necessary to be certain blood pressure doesn't stay up and seizures don't continue.

Can it be prevented? Regular checkups with your practitioner will allow him or her to pick up on any of the symptoms of preeclampsia. If you are diagnosed with preeclampsia, your practitioner will keep a close eye on you (and your blood pressure) to make sure your condition doesn't progress to eclampsia. Taking steps to try to prevent preeclampsia can also help avoid eclampsia.

You'll Want to Know . . .

Very few women receiving regular prenatal care ever progress from the manageable preeclampsia to the more serious eclampsia.

Cholestasis

What is it? Cholestasis of pregnancy is a condition in which the normal flow of bile in the gallbladder is slowed (as a result of pregnancy hormones), causing the buildup of bile acids in the liver, which in turn can spill into the bloodstream. Cholestasis is most likely to occur in the last trimester, when hormones are at their peak. It usually goes away after delivery.

Cholestasis may increase the risks for fetal distress, preterm birth, or stillbirth, which is why early diagnosis and treatment are crucial.

How common is it? Cholestasis affects 1 to 2 pregnancies in 1,000. It's more common in women carrying multiples, women who have previous liver damage, and in women whose mother or sisters had cholestasis.

What are the signs and symptoms? Most often, the only symptom noticed is severe itching, particularly on the hands and feet, usually late in pregnancy.

What can you and your practitioner do? The goals of treating cholestasis of pregnancy are to relieve the itching and prevent pregnancy complications. Itching can be treated with topical anti-itch medications, lotions, or corticosteroids. Medication is sometimes used to help decrease the concentration of bile acids. If cholestasis is endangering the well-being of the mother or fetus, an early delivery may be necessary.

Deep Venous Thrombosis

What is it? Deep venous thrombosis, or DVT, is the development of a blood clot in a deep vein. These clots show up most commonly in the lower extremities, particularly the thigh. Women are more susceptible to clots during pregnancy and delivery, and particularly in the postpartum period. This happens because nature, wisely worried about too much bleeding at childbirth, tends to increase the blood's clotting ability—occasionally too much. Another factor that can contribute is the enlarged uterus, which makes it difficult for blood in the lower body to return to the heart. If untreated, a DVT can result in the clot moving to the lungs and becoming life threatening.

How common is it? Deep venous thrombosis occurs once in every 1,000 to 2,000 pregnancies (it can also occur postpartum). DVT is more common if you are older, a smoker, have a family or personal history of clots, or have hypertension, diabetes, or a variety of other conditions, including vascular diseases.

What are the signs and symptoms? The most common symptoms of a deep vein thrombosis include:

- A heavy or painful feeling in the leg
- Tenderness in the calf or thigh
- Slight to severe swelling
- Distention of the superficial veins
- Calf pain on flexing the foot (turning the toes up toward the chin)

If the blood clot has moved to the lungs (a pulmonary embolus), there may be:

- Chest pain
- Shortness of breath
- Coughing with frothy, bloodstained sputum
- Rapid heartbeat and breathing rate
- Blueness of lips and fingertips
- Fever

What can you and your practitioner do? If you've been diagnosed with DVT or any kind of blood clot in previous pregnancies, let your practitioner know. In addition, if you notice swelling and pain in just one leg at any time during your pregnancy, call your practitioner right away.

Ultrasound or MRI may be used to diagnose the blood clot. If it turns out that you do have a clot, you might be treated with heparin to thin your blood and prevent further clotting (though the heparin may need to be discontinued as you near labor to prevent you from bleeding excessively during childbirth). Your clotting ability will be monitored along the way.

With a clot that reaches the lungs, clot-dissolving drugs (and, rarely, surgery) may be needed, as well as treatment for any accompanying side effects.

Can it be prevented? You can prevent clots by keeping your blood flowing—getting enough exercise and avoiding long periods of sitting will help you do this. If you're at high risk, you can also wear support hose to prevent clots from developing in your legs.

Placenta Accreta

What is it? Placenta accreta is an abnormally firm attachment of the placenta to the uterine wall. Depending on how deeply the placental cells invade, the condition may be called placenta percreta or placenta increta. Placenta accreta increases the risk of heavy bleeding or hemorrhaging during delivery of the placenta.

How common is it? One out of 2,500 pregnancies will have this attachment abnormality. Placenta accreta is by far the most common of these attachment problems, accounting for 75 percent of cases. In placenta accreta, the placenta digs deeply into the uterine wall, but does not pierce the uterine muscles. In placenta increta, which accounts for 15 percent of cases, the placenta pierces the uterine muscles. In placenta percreta, which accounts for the final 10 percent, the placenta not only burrows into the uterine wall and its muscles, but also pierces the outer part of the wall and may even attach itself to other nearby organs.

Your risk of placenta accreta increases if you have placenta previa and have had one or more cesarean deliveries in the past.

What are the signs and symptoms? There are usually no apparent symptoms. The condition is usually diagnosed via color Doppler ultrasound or may only be noticed during delivery when the placenta doesn't detach (as it normally would) from the uterine wall after the baby is born.

What can you and your practitioner do? Unfortunately, there is little you can do. In most cases, the placenta must be removed surgically after delivery to stop the bleeding. Very rarely, when the bleeding cannot be controlled by tying off the exposed blood vessels, removal of the entire uterus may be necessary.

Vasa Previa

What is it? Vasa previa is a condition in which some of the fetal blood vessels that connect the baby to the mother run outside the umbilical cord and along the membrane over the cervix. When labor begins, the contractions and opening of the cervix can cause the vessels to rupture, possibly causing harm to the baby. If the condition is diagnosed before labor, a C-section will be scheduled and the baby will be born healthy nearly 100 percent of the time.

How common is it? Vasa previa is rare, affecting 1 in 5,200 pregnancies. Women who also have placenta previa, a history of uterine surgery, or a multiple pregnancy are at greater risk.

What are the signs and symptoms? There are usually no signs of this condition, though there may be some bleeding in the second or third trimester.

What can you and your practitioner do? Diagnostic testing, such as with ultrasound or, better yet, a color Doppler ultrasound, can detect vasa previa. Women who are diagnosed with the condition will deliver their babies via C-section, usually before 37 weeks, to make sure labor doesn't begin on its own. Researchers are studying whether vasa previa can be treated using laser therapy to seal off the abnormally positioned vessels.

Childbirth and Postpartum Complications

Many of the following conditions can't be anticipated prior to labor and delivery—and there's no need to read up on them (and start worrying) ahead of time, since they're very unlikely to occur during or after your childbirth. They are included here so that in the unlikely event you experience one, you can learn about it after the fact, or in some cases, learn how you can prevent it from happening in your next labor and delivery.

Fetal Distress

What is it? Fetal distress is a term used to describe what occurs when a baby's oxygen supply is compromised in the uterus, either before or during labor. The distress may be caused by a number of factors, such as preeclampsia, uncontrolled diabetes, placental abruption, too little or too much amniotic fluid, umbilical cord compression or entanglement, intrauterine growth restriction, or simply because the mother is in a position that puts pressure on major blood vessels, depriving the baby of oxygen. Sustained oxygen deprivation and/or decreased heart rate can be serious for the baby and must be corrected as quickly as possible—usually with immediate delivery (most often by C-section, unless a vaginal birth is imminent).

How common is it? The exact incidence of fetal distress is uncertain, but estimates range from 1 in every 25 births to 1 in every 100 births.

What are the signs and symptoms? Babies who are doing well in utero have strong, stable heartbeats and respond to stimuli with appropriate movements. Babies in distress experience a decrease in their heart rate, a change in their pattern of movement (or even no movement altogether), and/or pass their first stool, called meconium, while still in the uterus.

What can you and your practitioner do? If you think your baby might be in distress because you've noticed a change in fetal activity (it seems to have slowed down significantly, stopped, become very jerky and frantic, or otherwise has you concerned), call your practitioner immediately. Once you are in your practitioner's office or in the hospital (or in labor), you'll be put on a fetal monitor to see whether your baby is indeed showing signs of distress. You may be given oxygen and extra fluids via an IV to help better oxygenate your blood and return your baby's heart rate to normal. Turning onto your left side to take pressure off your major blood vessels may also do the trick. If these techniques don't work, the best treatment is a quick delivery.

Cord Prolapse

What is it? A cord prolapse occurs during labor when the umbilical cord slips through the cervix and into the birth canal before the baby does. If the cord becomes compressed during delivery (such as when your baby's head is pushing against a prolapsed cord), the baby's oxygen supply is compromised.

How common is it? Fortunately, cord prolapse is not common, occurring in 1 out of every 300 births. Certain pregnancy complications increase the risk of prolapse. These include hydramnios, breech delivery or any position in which the baby's head does not cover the cervix, and premature delivery. It can also occur during delivery of a second twin. Prolapse is also a potential risk if your water breaks before your baby's head has begun to "engage," or settle into the birth canal.

What are the signs and symptoms? If the cord slips down into the vagina, you may actually be able to feel it or even see it. If the cord is compressed by the baby's head, the baby will show signs of fetal distress on a fetal monitor.

What can you and your practitioner do? There's really no way to know in advance if your baby's cord is going to prolapse. In fact, without fetal monitoring, you may not know until after the fact. If you suspect that your baby's umbilical cord has prolapsed and you are not in the hospital yet, get on your hands and knees with your head down and pelvis up to take pressure off the cord. If you notice the cord protruding from your vagina, gently support it with a clean towel. Call 911 or have someone rush you to the hospital (on the way to the hospital, lie down on the back seat, with your bottom elevated). If you are already in the hospital when the cord prolapses, your practitioner may ask you to move quickly into a different position, one in which it will be easier to disengage the baby's head and take pressure off the umbilical cord. Delivery of your baby will need to be very quick, most likely by C-section.

Shoulder Dystocia

What is it? Shoulder dystocia is a complication of labor and delivery in which one or both of the baby's shoulders become stuck behind the mother's pelvic bone as the baby descends into the birth canal.

How common is it? Size definitely matters when it comes to shoulder dystocia, which occurs most frequently in larger babies. Fewer than 1 percent of babies weighing 6 pounds have shoulder dystocia, but the rate is considerably higher in babies weighing more than 9 pounds. For that reason, mothers who have uncontrolled diabetes or gestational diabetes—and therefore may give birth to very large babies—are more likely to encounter this complication during delivery. The chances also rise if you go past your due date before delivering (since your baby will probably be larger) or if you've previously delivered a baby with shoulder dystocia. Still, many cases of shoulder dystocia occur during labors without any of these risk factors.

What are the signs and symptoms? Delivery stalls after the head emerges and before the shoulders are out. This can occur unexpectedly in a labor that has progressed normally up to that point.

What can you and your practitioner do? A variety of approaches may be used to deliver the baby whose shoulder is lodged in the pelvis, such as changing the mother's position by sharply flexing her legs onto her abdomen or applying pressure on her abdomen, right above the pubic bone.

Can it be prevented? Keeping your weight gain within the recommended range can help ensure that your baby doesn't get too big to maneuver through the birth canal, as can carefully controlling diabetes or gestational diabetes. Picking a labor position that allows your pelvis to open as widely as possible might also help you avoid dystocia.

Serious Perineal Tears

What is it? The pressure of your baby's large head pushing through the delicate tissues of your cervix and vagina can cause tears and lacerations in your perineum, the area between your vagina and your anus.

First-degree tears (when only the skin is torn) and second-degree tears (when skin and vaginal muscle are torn) are common. But severe tears—those that get close to the rectum and involve the vaginal skin, tissues, and perineal muscles (third degree) or those that actually cut into the muscles of the anal sphincter (fourth degree)—cause pain and increase not only your postpartum recovery time, but your risk of incontinence, as well as other pelvic floor problems. Tears can also occur in the cervix.

How common is it? Anyone having a vaginal delivery is at risk for a tear, and as many as half of all women will have at least a small tear after childbirth. Third- and fourth-degree tears are much less common.

What are the signs and symptoms? Bleeding is the immediate symptom; after the tear is repaired, you may also experience pain and tenderness at the site as it heals.

What can you and your practitioner do? Generally, all lacerations that are longer than 2 cm (about 1 inch) or that continue to bleed are stitched. A local anesthetic may be given first, if one wasn't administered during delivery.

If you end up tearing or having an episiotomy, sitz baths, ice packs, witch hazel, anesthetic sprays, and simply exposing the area to air can help it heal more quickly and with less pain (see page 423).

Can it be prevented? Perineal massage and Kegel exercises (see pages 352 and 295), done during the month or so before your due date, may help make the perineal area more supple and better able to stretch over your baby's head as he or she emerges. Warm compresses on the perineum and perineal massage during labor may help avoid tearing.

Uterine Rupture

What is it? A uterine rupture occurs when a weakened spot on your uterine wall—almost always the site of a previous uterine surgery such as a C-section or fibroid removal—tears due to the strain put on it during labor and delivery. A uterine rupture can result in uncontrolled bleeding into your abdomen or, rarely, lead to part of the placenta or baby entering your abdomen.

How common is it? Fortunately, ruptures are rare in women who've never had a previous C-section or uterine surgery. Even women who labor after a previous C-section have only a 1 in 100 chance of rupture (and the risk is far lower when a woman undergoes a repeat C-section without labor). Women at greatest risk of uterine rupture are those who are attempting a vaginal birth after cesarean (VBAC) and have been induced with prostaglandins and/or Pitocin (oxytocin). Abnormalities related to the placenta (such as placental abruption, a placenta that separates prematurely; or placenta accreta, a placenta that is attached deeply in the uterine wall) or to the fetus's position (such as a fetus lying crosswise) can also increase the risk of uterine rupture. Uterine rupture is more common in women who have already had six or more children or have a very distended uterus (because of multiple fetuses or excess amniotic fluid).

What are the signs and symptoms? Searing abdominal pain (a sensation that something is "ripping") followed by diffuse pain and tenderness in the abdomen during labor are the most common signs of uterine rupture. Most typically, the fetal monitor will show a significant drop in the baby's heart rate. The mother may develop signs of low blood volume, such as an increased heart rate, low blood pressure, dizziness, shortness of breath, or loss of consciousness.

What can you and your practitioner do? If you have had a previous C-section or abdominal surgery in which the uterine wall was cut through completely, you'll need to weigh your risks when considering your labor options, especially if you want to attempt a vaginal birth. Discuss with your practitioner the data that show that prostaglandins should not be used to induce labor in a woman who's had previous uterine surgery.

If you do have a uterine rupture, an immediate C-section is necessary, followed by repair of the uterus. You may also be given antibiotics to prevent infection.

Can it be prevented? For women with increased risk factors, fetal monitoring during labor can alert your practitioner to an impending or occurring rupture. Women who are trying for a VBAC delivery should not be induced.

Uterine Inversion

What is it? Uterine inversion is a rare complication of childbirth that occurs when part of the uterine wall collapses and turns inside out (in effect, very much like a sock being pulled inside out), sometimes even protruding through the cervix and into the vagina. The full range of problems that can cause uterine inversion is not fully understood, but in many cases it includes the incomplete separation of the placenta from the uterine wall; the placenta then pulls the uterus with it when it emerges from the birth canal. Uterine inversion, when unnoticed and/or untreated, can result in hemorrhage and shock. But that's a remote possibility; the condition occurs rarely and is unlikely to go unnoticed and untreated.

How common is it? Uterine inversion is very rare; reported rates vary from 1 in 2,000 births to 1 in several hundred thousand. You are at greatest risk for a uterine inversion if you've had an inversion during a previous delivery. Other factors that slightly increase the very remote risk of an inversion include an extended labor (lasting more than 24 hours), several previous vaginal deliveries, or use of drugs like magnesium sulfate or terbutaline (given to halt preterm labor). The uterus also may be more likely to invert if it is overly relaxed or if the cord is pulled too hard in the third stage of childbirth.

What are the signs and symptoms? Symptoms of uterine inversion include:

- Abdominal pain

- Excessive bleeding

- Signs of shock in the mother

- In a complete inversion, the uterus will be visible in the vagina

What can you and your practitioner do? Know your risk factors and inform your practitioner if you've had a uterine inversion in the past. If you do have one, your physician will try to push your uterus back up where it belongs, and then give you drugs like Pitocin (oxytocin) to encourage any floppy muscles to contract. In rare cases, where this does not work, surgery is an option. In either case, you might need a blood transfusion to make up for blood lost during the inversion. Antibiotics may be given to prevent infection.

Can it be prevented? Because a woman who has had one uterine inversion is at an increased risk for another, let your practitioner know if you've had one in the past.

Postpartum Hemorrhage

What is it? Bleeding after delivery, called lochia, is normal. But sometimes the uterus doesn't contract as it should after birth, leading to postpartum hemorrhage—excessive or uncontrolled bleeding from the site where the placenta was attached. Postpartum hemorrhage can also be caused by unrepaired vaginal or cervical lacerations.

Hemorrhage can also occur up to a week or two after delivery when fragments of the placenta are retained in, or adhere to, the uterus. Infection can also cause postpartum hemorrhage, right after delivery or weeks later.

How common is it? Postpartum hemorrhage occurs in somewhere between 2 and 4 percent of deliveries. Excessive bleeding may be more likely to occur if the uterus is too relaxed and doesn't contract due to a long, exhausting labor; a traumatic delivery; a uterus that was overdistended because of multiple births, a large baby, or excess amniotic fluid; an oddly shaped placenta, or one that separated prematurely; fibroids that prevent symmetrical contraction of the uterus; or a generally weakened condition of the mother at the time of delivery (due to, for example, anemia, preeclampsia, or extreme fatigue). Women taking drugs or herbs that interfere with blood clotting (such as aspirin, ibuprofen, ginkgo biloba, or large doses of vitamin E) are also at greater risk for postpartum hemorrhage. Rarely, the cause of the hemorrhage is a previously undiagnosed bleeding disorder in the mother that is genetic.

What are the signs and symptoms? The symptoms of postpartum hemorrhage include:

- Bleeding that soaks through more than one pad an hour for several hours in a row

- Heavy, bright-red bleeding for more than just a few days

- Passing very large clots (lemon size or larger)

- Pain or swelling in the lower abdominal area beyond the first few days after delivery

The loss of large amounts of blood can make a woman feel faint, breathless, dizzy, or cause her heart to speed up.

What can you and your practitioner do? After the placenta is delivered, your practitioner will examine it to make certain that it's complete—that no part of it is remaining in your uterus. He or she will probably give you Pitocin (oxytocin) and may also massage your uterus to encourage it to contract, in order to minimize bleeding. Breastfeeding (if you will be nursing) as soon as possible will also help your uterus to contract.

You should expect bleeding following delivery, but alert your practitioner immediately if you notice abnormally heavy bleeding or any of the other symptoms listed above during the first postpartum week. If the bleeding is severe enough to be categorized as hemorrhage, you may need intravenous fluids or possibly even a blood transfusion.

Can it be prevented? Avoiding any supplement or medication that may interfere with blood clotting (such as the ones listed on the previous page), especially in the last trimester and the immediate postpartum period, will reduce the possibility of abnormal postpartum bleeding.

Postpartum Infection

What is it? The vast majority of women recover from delivery without any problems at all, but childbirth can occasionally leave you open to infection. That's because it can leave you with a variety of open wounds—in your uterus (where the placenta was attached), in your cervix, vagina, or perineum (especially if you tore or had an episiotomy, even if it was repaired), or at the site of a C-section incision. Postpartum infections can also occur in your bladder or kidney if you were catheterized. A fragment of the placenta inadvertently left behind in the uterus can lead to infection, too. But the most common postpartum infection is endometritis, an infection of the lining of the uterus (the endometrium).

While some infections can be dangerous, especially if they go undetected or untreated, most often infections simply make your postpartum recovery slower and more difficult, and they take time and energy away from your most important priority: getting to know your baby. For that reason alone, it's important to get help for any suspected infection as quickly as possible.

How common is it? As many as 8 percent of deliveries result in an infection. Women who had a cesarean delivery or those who had premature rupture of the membranes are at greater risk of infection.

What are the signs and symptoms? Symptoms of postpartum infection vary, depending on where the infection is, but there's almost always:

- Fever

- Pain or tenderness in the infected area

- Foul-smelling discharge (from the vagina in the case of a uterine infection, or from a wound)

- Chills

What can you and your practitioner do? Call your practitioner if you're running a postpartum fever of around 100°F for more than a day; call sooner if the fever is higher or if you notice any of the other symptoms above. If you have an infection, you'll probably receive a prescription for antibiotics, which you should take as prescribed for the entire course, even if you begin to feel better quickly. You should also get plenty of rest (a near impossibility with a newborn in the house, but do the best you can) and drink lots of fluids. If you're breastfeeding, check with your physician and your pharmacist to be sure that any medication you're given is breastfeeding-friendly (most antibiotics are).

Can it be prevented? Meticulous wound care and cleanliness after delivery (wash your hands before touching the perineal area, wipe from front to back after going to the bathroom, and only use maxi pads—not tampons—for postpartum bleeding) can definitely help prevent infections.

If You're Put on Bed Rest

The thought of lying in bed with a stack of magazines and the TV remote may sound pretty appealing—until it's prescribed in the form of bed rest. Bed rest, unfortunately, is no pajama party. Once reality sets in and you realize that you can't even run out for milk or meet some friends for a latte, the appeal of lounging around all day is quickly lost. That's why it's important not to lose sight of the big picture (healthy pregnancy, healthy baby) and to remind yourself that your practitioner probably has good reason for keeping you off your feet.

If you've been put on bed rest, you're in good company. A million pregnancies a year (that's one quarter of pregnancies) are classified as "high-risk" or "at-risk." And 70 percent of these moms will be put on bed rest at some point during their 40 weeks. Even though there is much controversy surrounding the benefits of bed rest, it continues to be prescribed because many practitioners believe, based on their experience with their patients, that it works in preventing preterm labor or slowing the progress of pre-eclampsia and keeps an otherwise high-risk pregnancy from becoming more complicated. Among the rationales suggested for a prescription of bed rest: Staying off your feet takes pressure off the cervix; it reduces the strain on your heart and improves blood flow to your kidneys, which helps eliminate excess fluids; it increases circulation to your uterus, providing additional oxygen and nutrients to your baby; and it minimizes the level of stress hormones in your bloodstream that can trigger contractions.

Certain moms-to-be are more likely to wind up on bed rest, including those who are over 35, who are carrying multiples, who have a history of miscarriage due to incompetent cervix, who have particular pregnancy complications, or who have certain chronic conditions.

Whether bed rest truly helps prevent preterm labor or minimizes the risks of other complications, it is clear that being off your feet for a long period of time comes with its share of drawbacks. Women on prolonged bed rest can suffer hip and muscle pain, headaches, muscle loss (which can make it much harder to bounce back after delivery), skin irritations, and depression, and may be more prone to blood clots. Not being able to get moving may also aggravate many of the normal symptoms of pregnancy, such as heartburn, constipation, leg swelling, and backaches. Finally, bed rest may decrease your appetite, which might be good for your waistline (what waistline?) but not so good for your growing baby (or babies), who counts on those extra calories and nutrients.

The good—and reassuring—news is that many of the side effects of bed rest can be minimized with these tips:

- Keep things circulating. Maximize blood flow to your uterus by lying on your side, not your back. To feel cradled and comfortable, put a pillow under your head, a body pillow under your belly and between your knees (or two pillows), and perhaps a pillow behind you as well, if that helps you balance. Change sides every hour or so to lessen body aches and prevent skin irritations.

Types of Bed Rest

"Bed rest" is the general term used when your practitioner wants you to limit your activities. But it's likely your marching (or in this case, nonmarching) orders came with a list of very specific can-dos and definitely don't-dos. That's because bed rest comes in a variety of packages, from just getting off your feet every couple hours, to resting in bed but being allowed to get up periodically, to staying in bed with bathroom privileges, to staying in bed 24/7 (sometimes in the hospital). What kind of bed rest you're prescribed depends a lot on why you've been put on bed rest to begin with. Here's the lowdown on each type of bed rest:

Scheduled resting. In the hopes of preventing full bed rest later, some practitioners ask moms-to-be with certain risk factors (such as multiples or advanced maternal age) to rest for a prescribed amount of time every day. The recommendation may be to sit with your feet up or lie down (better yet, nap) for two hours at the end of every workday or rest for an hour, lying down on your side, for every four hours that you're awake. Some practitioners may ask you to simply shorten your workday in your third trimester and restrict activities such as exercise, stair-climbing, and walking or standing for extended lengths of time.

Modified bed rest. With modified bed rest, you're generally prohibited from working, driving, and doing household chores (now that's something to celebrate!). Sitting up at your desk to surf the web is okay, as is standing just long enough to make yourself a sandwich or take a shower. You may even be granted one night a week to go out, as long as your outing doesn't involve a long walk or any stairs. Women on modified bed rest may split their day between the couch and the bed, but going up or down stairs should be kept to a minimum.

Strict bed rest. This usually means you need to be horizontal all day except for bathroom trips and a brief shower (a tepid bath is preferred). If there are stairs in your house, you're going to have to pick a floor and stay there. (Some women will be allowed to make a roundtrip once a day; for others it might be once a week.) And your spouse (or your mom or a friend or the person you hire to help you) is going to have to make sure that the chores are getting done and that you have all you need to get by for the day. This may mean keeping a cooler or a mini fridge with breakfast, lunch, dinner, and lots of healthy snacks by the side of your bed.

Hospital bed rest. If you need constant monitoring as well as IV drugs because preterm labor has already begun, you will be admitted to the hospital. And if your labor is successfully stalled, you may need to extend your hospital stay to ensure total bed rest. Your bed may even be positioned at a slight angle (feet higher than head) so that gravity can help keep your babies growing in your womb for as long as possible.

■ Move what you can. Talk to your practitioner about doing arm exercises each day (using light weights) to keep your upper-body muscles from weakening—usually allowed if you're on modified bed rest. If you get the go-ahead, you can perform bicep curls, tricep curls, and overhead presses, all in a sitting position. Follow with stretching and shoulder rolls.

- Stretch what you can, as much as you can. Also check with your practitioner about whether gentle leg stretches— flexing your feet and circling your ankles (without lifting them above hip level)—can be on the bed rest agenda. This can prevent blood clotting in the legs and may keep your muscles a little stronger.

- Watch what you eat, and how much you eat. A significant dip in a mom's appetite can lead to weight loss for her and a lower birthweight for her baby—so if you find yours slacking, fight back by grazing on nutritious, easy-to-digest snacks (high-fiber ones, like dried fruit, will also combat constipation). Of course, if you find yourself eating too much (out of boredom or depression), excessive weight gain might also become an issue—so keep an eye on nonstop nibbling, too, especially high-calorie nibbling.

- Keep the fluids flowing. Staying hydrated is always important when you're expecting, but especially on bed rest (getting enough fluids will minimize swelling and constipation, and possibly prevent contractions). So make sure your bedstand is stocked with water and other beverages.

- Beat heartburn with gravity. More lying can spell more heartburn. Sitting up slightly in bed (if you're allowed), especially after eating, will keep the burn at bay.

- Keep your expectations realistic after delivery. Cut yourself some postpartum slack, factoring in all that your body has been through. You just won't have the same aerobic capacity or muscular strength that you had before you took to bed, even if you were off your feet for just weeks. So give yourself a chance to recover, and plan on building back up to your former fitness level slowly. Walking, postpartum yoga, and swimming are good beginning activities when your practitioner green-lights exercise again.

Bed rest doesn't just impact your physical well-being. It could also affect your sanity. To stay sane while you're staying horizontal:

Reach out. Keep the phone by your side, and let family and friends know they need to be on call for venting (or whining, or worrying, or giggling). Stay connected through e-mail as well (this is one of the many reasons why you'll also want a computer by your side—or a laptop on your lap, or where your lap used to be). And don't forget to visit websites and message boards, where you'll meet other moms-to-be in the exact same shoes (or slippers).

Be prepared. Anticipate what you're going to need each day, and ask your spouse to gather it together for you before he leaves in the morning. Stock a bedside mini fridge or cooler with lots of water, fruit, yogurt, cheese, and sandwiches. Be sure the phone, magazines, books, and TV remote are all within arm's reach.

Structure the day. Try to establish a routine—even if the highlight is a soak in a tepid tub followed by a nap, or a morning on the couch followed by an afternoon in bed. You'll feel a little better if you give the day some sort of structure.

Work from home. If you're on modified bed rest and work in a fully wired field, it may be possible to work from home for all or part of the time you are on

Moms Helping Moms

Every pregnancy comes with some challenges, but a pregnancy that's high risk (or one that's been complicated) can come with a whole lot more. Facing those challenges is always easier when you've got company—other moms who know exactly what you're going through because they're going through it, too (or have already gone through it) themselves. There may be support groups in your area for the specific pregnancy challenge you're facing (ask your practitioner), but you're also likely to find that support online.

bed rest. Between conference calls and e-mails, you can actually be very productive as a gestating telecommuter. Speak to both your practitioner and your boss to be sure everyone is on the same page about what your capabilities and your limits are (and if your job is emotionally stressful, you may not get the go-ahead from the obstetric powers that be).

Get your baby shopping done. Pretty much anything you can do in a store, you can do online. So use this bed-rest time to get baby-ready on the web. Register for your layette, order your crib, or find your future doula, lactation consultant, and babysitter online. And while you're at it, order your groceries, too (you're out of milk again, aren't you?).

Deliver dinner. While you're waiting for your special delivery, tap into your neighborhood network of restaurants that deliver. Keep those menus within arm's reach, or look for them online.

Try some movie magic. Sign up with a DVD-by-mail service and catch all those films you didn't have a chance to see in the theater—and won't have time to see once you have a baby in the house.

Entertain in bed. Get your friends together for a bedroom potluck or pizza and a movie. (Best part of this plan: They'll have to clean up the crumbs, not you.)

Get crafty. Teach yourself to knit, crochet, or quilt. Better yet, have a talented pal come over and teach you. You'll be creating sweet treasures for your little one and getting some much-needed companionship, too. Or take up scrapbooking (you'll soon have more mementos to save than ever before).

Get organized. Put all those old photos into an album (finally), or enter your address book into a computer database. You'll be glad you did when you're able to print out those address labels (for your baby announcements, thank-you notes, party invites, holiday cards . . .) instead of hand-writing them.

Sit pretty. Do the things that make you feel good each day, even when it sometimes seems pointless. Brush your hair, put on makeup, slather your tummy in yummy-smelling lotion (your skin will be itchy and dry anyway). If you can afford it, consider having a hairstylist or manicurist make a house call. (Drop the hint to your friends that this would make a great shower gift.) Don't fall into that "nobody's going to see me anyway" trap—looking good makes you feel good, whether anyone else sees you or not.

Freshen up. Charge your spouse with changing the sheets on your well-used bed once a week. Keep baby wipes and hand sanitizers nearby to keep yourself clean and relatively fresh between showers and baths.

Start a journal. Think of the bright side: Now's the perfect time to begin recording your thoughts or feelings about pregnancy or bed rest, or writing a few letters to your baby that you can share with him or her in years to come. Check out *The What to Expect Pregnancy Journal and Organizer,* which can help you preserve pregnancy moments. Writing your feelings down is also a great way to vent.

Keep your eyes on the prize. Frame one of your ultrasound pictures, and keep it by your side—so when the going gets tough, you can remind yourself that you have the best reason in the world not to go anywhere at all.

Coping with Pregnancy Loss

PREGNANCY IS SUPPOSED TO BE a joyous time, filled with excitement, anticipation, and pink-and-blue daydreams about life with your baby-to-be (mixed in with a little normal trepidation and anxiety). And usually, it is all of those things, but it isn't always. If you've experienced the loss of a pregnancy or a newborn, you know firsthand that the depth of your pain can be beyond words. This chapter is dedicated to helping you handle that pain and cope with one of life's most difficult losses.

Miscarriage

Just because it often takes place very early in pregnancy doesn't mean that miscarriage isn't painful for expectant parents. The grief that can come with a miscarriage is real, no matter how early in pregnancy you lost your baby. Even though you never saw your baby, except perhaps on ultrasound, you knew that he or she was growing inside of you, and you may have already formed a bond, however abstract. From the moment you found out you were pregnant, you may have daydreamed about your baby and imagined yourself a mother. And then, all the excitement of months (and years, and decades) to come abruptly came to a stop. Understandably, you may feel a range of emotions: sad and disheartened over the loss; angry and resentful that it happened to you; possibly withdrawn from friends and family (especially those who are pregnant or just had babies). You may have trouble sleeping and eating at first and accepting the finality of it all. You may cry a lot, or you may not cry at all. These are among the many natural, healthy responses to a pregnancy loss. (Remember that your reaction is what's normal for you.)

In fact, for some couples, coping with early pregnancy loss may be, at least in certain ways, just as difficult as coping with a loss later on. Why? First of all, because so many couples hold off on spreading the word about their pregnancy until the third month has passed, even close friends and family may not have been told yet, which can mean that support may be hard to come by. Even those who knew about the pregnancy and/or are told about the miscarriage may offer less support than they would have if the pregnancy had been further along. They may try to minimize the significance of the loss with a "Don't worry, you can try again," not realizing that the loss of a baby, no matter how early in pregnancy it occurs, can be devastating. Second, the fact that there is no possibility of holding the baby, taking a photo, having a funeral and burial—rituals of grieving that can all help offer some closure for parents of stillborn infants—may complicate the recovery process.

Still, if you've suffered a miscarriage (or an ectopic or molar pregnancy), it's important to remember that you have the right to grieve as much—or as little—as you need to. Do this in any way that helps you heal and eventually move on.

Perhaps you'll find closure in a private ceremony with close family members or just you and your spouse. Or by sharing your feelings—individually, through a support group, or online—with others who experienced early miscarriage. Since so many women suffer a miscarriage at least once during their

A Personal Process

When it comes to dealing with a miscarriage or other pregnancy loss, no one emotional formula must be followed. Different couples confront, cope with, and process their feelings in completely different ways. You may find yourself deeply saddened, even devastated by the loss—and discover that healing comes surprisingly slowly. Or you may handle the loss more matter-of-factly, seeing it as a bump in the road to having a baby. You may find that after some momentary sadness, you're able to put the experience behind you more quickly than you might have expected—instead of lingering over the loss, you may choose to look ahead to trying again. Just remember: The normal reaction to a pregnancy loss is the reaction that's normal for you. Feel whatever you need to feel in order to heal and move ahead.

reproductive years, you may be surprised to find how many others you know have had the same experience as you but never talked about it with you, or maybe even talked about it at all. (If you don't feel like sharing your feelings—or don't feel you need to—don't. Do only what's right for you.) Some of the tips for those who have later pregnancy losses may be helpful for you, too. You may also want to read about the Stages of Grief (see box on page 585), which may or may not apply to you.

Accept that you may always have a place in your heart for the pregnancy you lost, and you may feel sad or down on the anniversary of the due date of your lost baby or on the anniversary of the miscarriage itself, even years later. If you

Coping with Repeat Miscarriages

Suffering one pregnancy loss can be hard enough to cope with. But if you've suffered more than one, you may find it infinitely harder—with each loss hitting you a little harder than the last. You may be discouraged, depressed, angry, irritable, unable to focus on the rest of your life (or on anything beyond your losses). The healing of your psyche may not only take a lot longer than the healing of your body, but the sadness can be literally debilitating. What's more, the emotional pain may lead to physical symptoms, including headaches, appetite loss or overeating, insomnia, and overwhelming fatigue. (Some couples handle even repeat losses more matter-of-factly, and that's completely normal, too.)

Time may not heal all, but it will definitely help eventually. In the meantime, patience, knowledge, and support may be your best remedies. Pregnancy loss support groups may be available in your area, so ask your practitioner, or find a support group online, if you think that might help you (some couples prefer to turn to each other for support). Sharing with others who have suffered through pregnancy losses, especially multiple losses, can help you feel less alone, as well as more hopeful. Most of all, don't let guilt add to your burden. Miscarriage is not your fault. Instead, try to focus on how strong you've been (even if you haven't always felt that strong) and how determined you are to have a baby.

find it helps, plan on doing something special at that time—at least for the first year or so—that will be cheering yet allows you to remember: planting some new flowers or a tree, having a quiet picnic in the park, sharing a commemorative dinner with your spouse.

While it's normal to mourn your loss—and important to come to terms with it your way—you should also start to feel gradually better as time passes. If you don't, or if you have continued trouble coping with everyday life—you're not eating or sleeping, you're not able to focus at work, you're becoming isolated from family and friends—or if you continue to feel very anxious (anxiety is an even more common sympton following miscarriage than depression is), professional counseling can help you recover.

Try to remind yourself that you can—and most likely will—become pregnant again and give birth to a healthy baby. For the vast majority of women,

a miscarriage is a onetime event—and actually, an indication of future fertility.

Loss in the Uterus

When you don't hear from (or feel) your baby for several hours or more, it's natural to fear the worst. And the worst is that your unborn baby has died.

You are likely to be in a fog of disbelief and grief after being told your baby's heartbeat can't be located and that he or she has died in your uterus. It may be difficult or even impossible for you to carry on with any semblance of your usual life while carrying around a fetus that is no longer living, and studies show that a woman is much more likely to suffer severe depression after the delivery of a stillborn if the delivery is delayed more than three days after the death is diagnosed. For this reason, your emotional state will be taken into account while your practitioner decides what to do next. If labor is imminent, or has already started, your stillborn baby will probably be delivered. If labor isn't clearly about to start, the decision of whether or not to induce labor immediately, or to allow you to return home until it begins spontaneously, will depend on how far you are from your due date, on your physical condition, and on how you're doing emotionally.

The grieving process you will go through if your fetus has died in utero will probably be very similar to that of parents whose baby has died during or after birth. The same steps will help you begin the long healing process, including, when possible and practical, holding your baby in your arms and having a funeral or memorial service. See below for more.

Loss During or After Birth

Sometimes the loss of a baby occurs during labor or delivery, sometimes just after delivery. Either way, your world comes crashing down. You've waited for this baby for months—and now you're going home empty-handed.

There's probably no greater pain than that inflicted by the loss of a child. And though nothing can completely heal the hurt you're feeling, there are steps you can take now to lessen the inevitable sadness that follows such a tragedy:

- See your baby, hold your baby, name your baby. Grieving is a vital step in accepting and recovering from your loss, and it's difficult to grieve for a nameless child you've never seen. Even if your child has malformations, experts advise that it is better to see him or her than not to because what is imagined is usually worse than the

reality. Holding and naming your baby will make the death more real to you and ultimately easier to recover from. So will arranging for a funeral and burial or a memorial service, which will give you another opportunity to say good-bye. If there is a burial, the grave will provide a permanent site where you can visit your baby in future years.

- Save a photo or other mementos (a lock of hair, a footprint), so you'll have some tangible reminders to cherish when you think about your lost baby in the future. Try to focus on the details you'll want to remember later—big

Postpartum Depression and Pregnancy Loss

Every parent who loses a baby has reason to feel sad. But for some, the sadness can be deepened by postpartum depression and/or anxiety. Untreated, postpartum depression can prevent you from experiencing the stages of grief that are essential to healing. Though it might be hard to distinguish postpartum depression from the depression brought on by the tragic loss of a baby, any kind of depression requires help. If you're exhibiting signs of depression (loss of interest in everyday activities, inability to sleep, loss of appetite, extreme sadness that interferes with your ability to function), don't hesitate to get the help you need. Speak to your prenatal practitioner or your regular doctor, and ask to be referred to a mental health professional. Therapy—and, if necessary, medication—can help you feel better.

Lactation Suppression When a Baby Dies

If you've suffered the devastating loss of your baby, the last thing you need is another reminder of what would have been. Sadly, nature can deliver that reminder when the end of pregnancy (even when it has ended tragically) automatically signals the beginning of lactation, and your breasts fill with the milk that was intended to feed your baby. This can be incredibly painful to cope with, both physically and emotionally—as can handling milk production that has already been fully initiated (because your baby died after you started nursing or pumping in the NICU).

If your baby died in utero or at birth, and you never had a chance to nurse, you'll have to deal with breast engorgement. Ice packs, mild pain relievers, and a supportive bra can help minimize the physical discomfort you'll feel. Avoiding hot showers, nipple stimulation, and expressing milk from your breasts will help avoid further milk production. The engorgement will pass within a few days.

If your baby died after you already began nursing or pumping (as might happen with a baby in the NICU), ask the nurses in the hospital or a lactation consultant for help. You'll likely be advised to remove enough milk (using a pump, or manually if you prefer) to reduce the pressure in your breasts but not enough to empty them and encourage more production. The frequency and duration of pumping varies from one woman to another, depending on the amount of milk you've been producing, the frequency of feedings, and the length of time since the birth of your baby, but, in general, you should gradually go longer between expressions and pump for a shorter period of time. Be aware that it's normal for drops of milk to be present in your breasts for weeks or even months after breastfeeding and/or pumping is discontinued.

If you have a large amount of milk, either in storage or in production (if you're producing a lot of milk or if you were pumping for twins, for instance), you might want to consider donating your breast milk to a milk bank. Donation of the milk may help you find some meaning in the death of your baby. But, as always, do what helps you most.

---

eyes and long lashes, beautiful hands and delicate fingers, a headful of hair.

- Discuss autopsy findings and other medical reports with your practitioner to help you accept the reality of what happened and to help you in the grieving process. You may have been given a lot of details in the delivery room, but medications, your hormonal status, and the shock you were feeling probably prevented you from fully understanding them.

- Ask friends or relatives to leave the preparations you made for baby at home. Coming home to a house that looks as though a baby was never expected will only make it more difficult to accept what has happened.

- Keep in mind that the grieving process usually has many steps, including denial and isolation, anger, depression, and acceptance. Don't be surprised if you feel these emotions, though not necessarily in this order. And don't be surprised if you don't feel all of them or if you experience other emotions instead or in addition. Everyone is different and everyone reacts differently, even in a similar situation—especially such a personal one.

■ Expect a difficult time. For a while, you may be depressed, very anxious, or just deeply sad and have trouble sleeping, eating, or focusing at work. You may be short-tempered with your spouse and with your other children, if you have any. You may feel lonely—even if you're surrounded with people who love you—and empty, and you may even imagine you hear your baby crying in the middle of the night. You will probably feel the need to be a child yourself, to be loved, coddled, and cared for. All this is normal.

■ Cry—for as long and as often as you feel you need to.

■ Recognize that fathers grieve, too. His grief may seem less intense or more short-lived—partly because, unlike you, he didn't carry the baby inside him for so many months. But that doesn't make the pain he's feeling any less real or the process of mourning any less vital to healing. Sometimes, fathers may have a harder time expressing their grief, or they may bottle up their emotions in an effort to be strong for their partners. If you sense that's the case with your spouse, you may both find comforting release in talking the pain out. Encourage him to share with you, with a counselor, or with another father who's been through such a loss.

■ Take care of each other. Grief can be very self-absorbing. You and your spouse may find yourselves so consumed by your own pain that you don't have the emotional reserves left to comfort each other. Unfortunately, relationship problems can sometimes result when partners shut each other out that way, making recovering even more difficult. Although there will almost certainly be times when you'll want to be alone with your thoughts, also make time for sharing them with your spouse. Consider seeking grief counseling together, too, or joining a couples support group. It may not only help you both find comfort but also help preserve—and even deepen—your relationship.

■ Don't face the world alone. If you're dreading the friendly faces asking, "So, did you have your baby?" take a friend who can field the questions for you on the first several trips to the supermarket, dry cleaners, and so on. Be sure that those at work, at your place of worship, at other organizations in which you're active, are informed before you return, so you don't have to do any more difficult explaining than is absolutely necessary.

■ Realize that some friends and family may not know what to do or say. Some may be so uncomfortable that they withdraw during the mourning period. Others may say things that hurt more than help: "I know just how you feel," or "Oh, you can have another baby," or "It's a good thing the baby died before you became attached to it." Though they certainly mean well, they may not understand that no one who hasn't lost a baby can know how it feels, that another baby can never take the place of the one you lost, or that parents can become attached to a baby long before birth. If you're hearing such comments frequently, ask a close friend or relative to explain your feelings and to let others know that you would rather they just say they are sorry about your loss.

■ Look for support from those who've been there. Like many other parents, you may derive strength from joining a support group for parents who have lost infants. There are support groups online, too, that may offer some solace. (Try compassionatefriends.org or missingangel.org.) But try not to let such a group become a way of holding on to—rather than letting go of—your grief. If after a year you're still having problems coming to terms with your loss (sooner, if you're having trouble functioning), seek individual therapy.

- Take care of yourself. In the face of so much emotional pain, your physical needs may be the last thing on your mind. They shouldn't be. Eating right, getting enough sleep, and exercising are vital not just in maintaining your health but also in aiding your recovery. Make a conscious effort to sit down for meals, even if you're not feeling very much like eating. Take a warm bath or do some relaxation exercises to help you unwind before bed, so you'll sleep better at night. Try to build some physical activity into your day, even if it's just a walk before dinner. And let yourself take a break from grieving once in a while. See a movie, accept an invitation to visit friends, take a weekend in the country—and enjoy yourself without feeling guilty. For life to go on, after all, you need to go on living.

- Remember your baby as privately or publicly as you need to. When it comes to a memorial service, do whatever feels right to you. That might be a completely private ceremony—which allows you and your spouse to share your feelings alone—or one that surrounds you with the love and support of family, friends, and community.

- Honor your child's memory in a way that has meaning to you, if that helps. Buy books for a child care center that serves kids in need, or donate to an organization that helps disadvantaged

expectant and new moms; plant a tree or a new flower bed in your backyard or in a local park.

- Turn to religion, if you find it comforting. For some grieving parents, faith is a great solace.

- Do become pregnant again, if that's what you want—but not in an effort to feel better or to replace the child you've lost. It's best to wait until the period of deepest sorrow has passed before contemplating conceiving again. See page 586 for more.

- Expect your pain to lessen over time. At first, there will be only bad days, then a few good days mixed in; eventually, there will be more good days than bad. But be prepared for the possibility that remnants of the pain may last a lot longer. The grieving process, which may include nightmares and fleeting but painful flashbacks, is often not fully completed for as long as two years, but the worst is usually over three to six months after the loss. If after six to nine months your grief remains the center of your life, if you're having trouble functioning or focusing, or have little interest in anything else, seek help. Also seek help if, from the beginning, you haven't been able to grieve at all. And remember that postpartum depression can cloud the healing process, too; see page 579.

- Recognize that guilt can unnecessarily compound grief and make adjusting to a loss more difficult. If you feel that the loss of your baby was your punishment for having been ambivalent about your pregnancy, or for lacking the nurturing or other qualities necessary for motherhood, or for any other reason, seek professional support to help you understand that you are in no way responsible for your loss.

Seek help, too, if you've suffered self-doubts in the past and now believe your doubts have been confirmed (you couldn't produce a live baby). If you feel guilty even thinking about getting your life back to normal because you sense it would be disloyal to the child you've lost, it may help to ask your baby, in spirit, for forgiveness or for permission to enjoy life again. You might try doing it in a "letter," in which you express all your feelings, hopes, and dreams.

- Sometimes, organ donation may be possible when a baby is born alive and with some functioning organs but has a hopeless prognosis. The possibility of helping another baby live may bring some comfort in that case.

Loss of One Twin

The parent who loses one twin (or more babies, in the case of triplets or quads) faces celebrating a birth (or births) and mourning a death (or deaths) at the same time. If this happens, you may feel too conflicted to either mourn your lost child or enjoy your living one—both vitally important processes. Understanding why you feel the way you do may help you better cope with your feelings, which may include all or just some of these:

- You may feel heartbroken. You've lost a baby, and the fact that you have another doesn't minimize your loss. Realize that you're entitled to mourn the baby you've lost, even as you're celebrating your other baby's birth. In fact, mourning that loss is an important part of the healing process. Taking the steps for grieving parents described in the previous section can help you more easily accept your baby's death as a reality.

Why?

The painful question "Why?" may never be answered. But it may be helpful to attach some reality to the tragedy by learning about the physical causes of the death of a fetus or newborn. Often, the baby looks perfectly normal, and the only way to uncover the cause of death is to carefully examine the history of the pregnancy and do a complete examination of the fetus or baby. If the fetus died in utero or was stillborn, pathological examination of the placenta by an expert pathologist is also important. Knowing what happened (and this isn't always possible to determine) doesn't really tell you why it happened to you and your baby, but it helps bring closure to the event, and it will help you prepare for a future pregnancy.

- You may be happy, too, but ambivalent about showing it. It may seem somehow inappropriate to be excited about the arrival of your surviving baby or even disloyal to the one who didn't live. That's a natural feeling but one you'll need to try to let go of. Loving and nurturing the sibling is a wonderful way of honoring your lost baby—besides, it's essential to your living baby's well-being.

- You may want to celebrate, but don't know if it's okay to. A new baby is always something to celebrate, even when the happy news comes with sadness. If you're uncomfortable holding a baby-welcoming event without acknowledging your loss, consider first holding a memorial ceremony or farewell for the baby who has passed away.

Pregnancy Reduction

Sometimes an ultrasound reveals that one (or more) of the fetuses in a multiple pregnancy can't survive or is so severely malformed that the chances of survival outside the womb are minimal—and worse yet, that the ailing fetus may be endangering your other healthy one(s). Or there are so many fetuses that there is a significant risk to the mother and all her babies. In such cases, your practitioner may recommend a pregnancy reduction. Contemplating this procedure can be agonizing—it may seem like sacrificing one child to protect another—and may leave you plagued with guilt, confusion, and conflicted feelings. You may come to your decision of whether to proceed (or not proceed) easily, or it may be an excruciating decision-making process.

There may be no easy answers, and there are definitely no perfect options, but you'll want to do whatever you can to make peace with the decision you end up making. Review the situation with your practitioner, and seek a second opinion, or third, or fourth, until you're as confident as you can be about your choice. You can also ask your practitioner to put you in touch with someone from the bioethics staff of the hospital (if that's available). You may want to share your feelings with close friends, or you may want to keep this personal decision private. If religion plays an important role in your life, you'll probably want to look to spiritual guidance. Once you make your decision, try not to second-guess: Accept that it's the best decision you can make under the difficult circumstances. Also try not to burden yourself with guilt, no matter what you choose. Because none of this is your fault, there's no reason to feel guilty about it.

If you end up undergoing pregnancy reduction, you may expect to experience the same grief as any parent who has lost one or more babies.

- You may view your baby's death as punishment, perhaps because you really weren't sure you wanted or could handle being the parent of multiples or because you wanted a girl more than you wanted a boy (or vice versa). Though this kind of guilt is common among parents who experience a pregnancy loss of any kind, it's completely unwarranted. Nothing you did—or thought or imagined or wished for—could have caused the loss.

- You may feel disappointed that you won't be a parent of multiples. It's normal to be sad over the loss of this excitement, especially if you've been imagining and planning for the arrival of multiples for months. You may even feel twinges of regret when seeing sets of multiples. Don't feel guilty about feeling that way; it's completely understandable.

- You may be afraid that explaining your situation to family and friends will be awkward and difficult, especially if they've been eagerly awaiting the twins. To make facing the world a little easier, enlist a friend or close relative to spread the word so you won't have to. In the first few weeks, try to take someone with you when you go out with your baby, so they can anticipate and answer the inevitable—and possibly painful—questions.

- You may have trouble handling the reactions and comments of family and friends. In trying to help, friends and family may overdo the excitement when welcoming your living child, without acknowledging the one you've lost. Or they may urge you to forget your lost baby and appreciate your living one. As well intentioned as their actions and words may be, they can hurt and upset you. So don't hesitate to tell people—especially the ones who are closest to you—how you feel. Let them know that you need to grieve for what you have lost as well as celebrate the new arrival.

- You may feel too depressed over your loss to care for your new baby—or, if you're still pregnant, to care for your baby by taking the best possible care of yourself. Don't beat yourself up over your unhappy or conflicted feelings. They're normal, and completely understandable. But do make sure that you get the help you need so you can start meeting your baby's needs—both physical and emotional. Support groups may help, and so can counseling.

- You may feel that you're alone in your pain. Getting support from others who know what you're going through can help more than you can imagine. Find that support in a local support group or online. You can contact Centers for Loss in Multiple Births (CLIMB), at climb-support.org.

Stages of Grief

Whether the loss of a baby comes early in pregnancy, near term, or at delivery, you'll likely experience many feelings and reactions. Though you can't wish them away, understanding them will eventually help you come to terms with your loss. Many people who suffer a loss go through a number of steps on their road to emotional healing. These steps are common, though the order in which the first three occur may vary; so, too, may the feelings you experience.

- Shock and denial. There may be numbness and disbelief, the feeling that "this couldn't have happened to me." This is a mental mechanism designed to protect your psyche from the trauma of the loss.

- Guilt and anger. Desperate to pin the blame for such a senseless tragedy on something, you may blame it on yourself ("I must have done something wrong to cause the miscarriage" or "If I'd been happier about the pregnancy, the baby would still be alive"). Or you may blame others—God, for letting this happen, or your practitioner (even if there is no reason to). You may feel resentful and envious of those around you who are pregnant or who are parents, and even have fleeting feelings of hatred for them.

- Depression and despair. You may find yourself feeling sad most or all of the time, crying constantly, unable to eat, sleep, be interested in anything, or otherwise function. You may also wonder if you'll never be able to have a healthy baby.

- Acceptance. Finally, you'll come to terms with the loss. Keep in mind that this doesn't mean you'll forget the loss—just that you'll be able to accept it and get back to the business of life.

No matter what you're feeling—and given your situation, your feelings may be all over the emotional map—give yourself time. Chances are that you'll feel progressively better—and better about feeling better.

Trying Again

Making the decision to try again for a new pregnancy—and a new baby—after a loss isn't always easy, and definitely is not as easy as those around you might think. It's an intensely personal decision, and it can also be a painful one. Here are some things that you might want to consider when deciding when—and if—you try again:

- Trying again for another baby after losing one (or more) takes courage. Give yourself the credit you deserve—and the pat on the back you need—as you embark on this process.

- The right time is the time that's right for you. It may take just a short time for you to feel emotionally ready to try for another baby—or it may take a much longer time. Don't push yourself (or let others push you) into trying too soon. And don't second-guess yourself (or paralyze yourself) into waiting longer than you have to. Listen to your heart, and you'll know when you're emotionally healed and when you're ready to contemplate a new pregnancy.

- You'll need to be physically ready, too. Check with your practitioner to see whether a waiting period will be necessary in your case. Often, you can try as soon as you feel up to it (and as soon as your cycle begins cooperating). If there's a reason why you have to wait longer than you want to (as may be the case after a molar pregnancy), use the time to get yourself into the best physical condition possible for conception (see Chapter 1), if you're not already.

- A new pregnancy may be less innocent. Now you know that not all pregnancies end happily, which means you probably won't take anything about your new pregnancy for granted. You may feel more nervous than you did the first time, especially until you've passed the anniversary of the week you lost your last pregnancy (and if you lost your baby at or just before or after birth, you may worry more the entire time). You may try to keep your excitement in check, and you may find that your joy is tempered by trepidation—so much so that you may even hesitate to attach yourself to your new baby until that fear of loving and losing again has dissipated. You may be extra-attuned to every pregnancy symptom: the ones that give you hope (swollen breasts, morning sickness, those frequent runs to the bathroom) and those that trigger anxiety (those pelvic twinges, those crampy feelings). All of this is completely understandable and completely normal, as you'll find out if you reach out to others who've carried a new pregnancy to term after experiencing a loss. Just make sure that if these kinds of feelings keep you from nurturing and nourishing your new pregnancy, you quickly get some help working them out.

Looking forward to the ultimate reward—that baby you're so anxious to cuddle—instead of looking back on your loss will help you stay positive. Remember, the vast majority of women who have experienced a pregnancy loss or the loss of a baby go on to have completely normal pregnancies and completely healthy babies.

Index

More from *What to Expect*®

What to Expect® the First Year

The reassuring and comprehensive month-by-month guide to child care in the first year.

"It delivers on its promise. . . .
Better than any current book on infant care."
—MARK D. WIDOME, MD, MPH, PROFESSOR OF PEDIATRICS,
THE PENN STATE CHILDREN'S HOSPITAL

♦ ♦ ♦

What to Expect® the Toddler Years

An all-inclusive guide for the parent of toddlers.

"This wonderful guide . . .
is essential in every parent's library."
—MARIAN WRIGHT EDELMAN, PRESIDENT AND FOUNDER OF
THE CHILDREN'S DEFENSE FUND

♦ ♦ ♦

What to Expect® Eating Well When You're Expecting

Everything you need to know to nourish a healthy pregnancy, including 175 delicious recipes.

"The recipes are delicious—
and just right for today's mother-to-be."
—SHEILA LUKINS, FOOD EDITOR, *PARADE;*
CO-AUTHOR, *THE NEW BASICS* AND *SILVER PALATE* COOKBOOKS

♦ ♦ ♦

What to Expect® Pregnancy Journal & Organizer

The all-in-one planner that helps an expectant mother keep track of every detail of pregnancy, from diet to checkups to shopping for baby's layette.

What to Expect® Pregnancy Planner

An indispensable "dateless" pregnancy planner, appointment calendar, and record-keeper in a handy wall-calendar format.

◆ ◆ ◆

What to Expect® Baby-Sitter's Handbook

Everything a baby-sitter needs to know about caring for a child, from newborn to preschooler.

◆ ◆ ◆

Available at your local retailer or visit www.workman.com. For more information, please contact:

WORKMAN PUBLISHING COMPANY, INC.
225 Varick Street
New York, NY 10014-4381